Arthritis Sourcebook

Basic Consumer Health Information about Specific Forms of Arthritis and Related Disorders, Including Rheumatoid Arthritis, Osteoarthritis, Gout, Polymyalgia Rheumatica, Psoriatic Arthritis, Spondyloarthropathies, Juvenile Rheumatoid Arthritis, and Juvenile Ankylosing Spondylitis; Along with Information about Medical, Surgical, and Alternative Treatment Options, and Including Strategies for Coping with Pain, Fatigue, and Stress

Edited by Allan R. Cook. 575 pages. 1998. 0-7808-0201-2. $78.

Back & Neck Disorders Sourcebook

Basic Information about Disorders and Injuries of the Spinal Cord and Vertebrae, Including Facts on Chiropractic Treatment, Surgical Interventions, Paralysis, and Rehabilitation, Along with Advice for Preventing Back Trouble

Edited by Karen Bellenir. 548 pages. 1997. 0-7808-0202-0. $78.

"The strength of this work is its basic, easy-to-read format. Recommended."
— *Reference and User Services Quarterly, Winter '97*

Blood & Circulatory Disorders Sourcebook

Basic Information about Blood and Its Components, Anemias, Leukemias, Bleeding Disorders, and Circulatory Disorders, Including Aplastic Anemia, Thalassemia, Sickle-Cell Disease, Hemochromatosis, Hemophilia, Von Willebrand Disease, and Vascular Diseases; Along with a Special Section on Blood Transfusions and Blood Supply Safety, a Glossary, and Source Listings for Further Help and Information

Edited by Karen Bellenir and Linda M. Shin. 575 pages. 1998. 0-7808-0203-9. $78.

Brain Disorders Sourcebook

Basic Consumer Health Information about Strokes, Epilepsy, Amyotrophic Lateral Sclerosis (ALS/Lou Gehrig's Disease), Parkinson's Disease, Brain Tumors, Cerebral Palsy, Headache, Tourette Syndrome, and More; Along with Statistical Data, Treatment and Rehabilitation Options, Coping Strategies, Reports on Current Research Initiatives, a Glossary, and Resource Listings for Additional Help and Information

Edited by Karen Bellenir. 600 pages. 1999. 0-7808-0229-2. $78.

Burns Sourcebook

Basic Information about Various Types of Burns and Scalds, Including Flame, Heat, Electrical, Chemical, and Sun; Along with Short- and Long-Term Treatments, Tissue Reconstruction, Plastic Surgery, Prevention Suggestions, and First Aid

Edited by Allan R. Cook. 600 pages. 1999. 0-7808-0204-7. $78.

Cancer Sourcebook, 1st Edition

Basic Information on Cancer Types, Symptoms, Diagnostic Methods, and Treatments, Including Statistics on Cancer Occurrences Worldwide and the Risks Associated with Known Carcinogens and Activities

Edited by Frank E. Bair. 932 pages. 1990. 1-55888-888-8. $78.

"Written in nontechnical language. Useful for patients, their families, medical professionals, and librarians."
— *Guide to Reference Books, '96*

"Designed with the non-medical professional in mind. Libraries and medical facilities interested in patient education should certainly consider adding the *Cancer Sourcebook* to their holdings. This compact collection of reliable information . . . is an invaluable tool for helping patients and patients' families and friends to take the first steps in coping with the many difficulties of cancer."
— *Medical Reference Services Quarterly, Winter '91*

"Specifically created for the nontechnical reader . . . an important resource for the general reader trying to understand the complexities of cancer."
— *American Reference Books Annual, '91*

"This publication's nontechnical nature and very comprehensive format make it useful for both the general public and undergraduate students." — *Choice, Oct '90*

New Cancer Sourcebook, 2nd Edition

Basic Information about Major Forms and Stages of Cancer, Featuring Facts about Primary and Secondary Tumors of the Respiratory, Nervous, Lymphatic, Circulatory, Skeletal, and Gastrointestinal Systems, and Specific Organs; Statistical and Demographic Data; Treatment Options; and Strategies for Coping

Edited by Allan R. Cook. 1,313 pages. 1996. 0-7808-0041-9. $78.

"This book is an excellent resource for patients with newly diagnosed cancer and their families. The dialogue is simple, direct, and comprehensive. Highly recommended for patients and families to aid in their understanding of cancer and its treatment."
— *Booklist Health Sciences Supplement, Oct '97*

"The amount of factual and useful information is extensive. The writing is very clear, geared to general readers. Recommended for all levels." — *Choice, Jan '97*

Continues next page

Cancer Sourcebook, 3rd Edition

Basic Information about Major Forms and Stages of Cancer, Featuring Facts about Primary and Secondary Tumors of the Respiratory, Nervous, Lymphatic, Circulatory, Skeletal, and Gastrointestinal Systems, and Specific Organs, Statistical and Demographic Data, Treatment Options, and Strategies for Coping

Edited by Edward J. Prucha. 800 pages. 1999. 0-7808-0227-6. $78.

Cancer Sourcebook for Women

Basic Information about Specific Forms of Cancer That Affect Women, Featuring Facts about Breast Cancer, Cervical Cancer, Ovarian Cancer, Cancer of the Uterus and Uterine Sarcoma, Cancer of the Vagina, and Cancer of the Vulva; Statistical and Demographic Data; Treatments, Self-Help Management Suggestions, and Current Research Initiatives

Edited by Allan R. Cook and Peter D. Dresser. 524 pages. 1996. 0-7808-0076-1. $78.

". . . written in easily understandable, non-technical language. Recommended for public libraries or hospital and academic libraries that collect patient education or consumer health materials."
— *Medical Reference Services Quarterly, Spring '97*

"Would be of value in a consumer health library. . . . written with the health care consumer in mind. Medical jargon is at a minimum, and medical terms are explained in clear, understandable sentences."
— *Bulletin of the MLA, Oct '96*

"The availability under one cover of all these pertinent publications, grouped under cohesive headings, makes this certainly a most useful sourcebook."
— *Choice, Jun '96*

"Presents a comprehensive knowledge base for general readers. Men and women both benefit from the gold mine of information nestled between the two covers of this book. Recommended."
— *Academic Library Book Review, Summer '96*

"This timely book is highly recommended for consumer health and patient education collections in all libraries."
— *Library Journal, Apr '96*

Cancer Sourcebook for Women, 2nd Edition

Basic Information about Specific Forms of Cancer That Affect Women, Featuring Facts about Breast Cancer, Cervical Cancer, Ovarian Cancer, Cancer of the Uterus and Uterine Sarcoma, Cancer of the Vagina, and Cancer of the Vulva, Statistical and Demographic Data, Treatments, Self-Help Management Suggestions, and Current Research Initiatives

Edited by Edward J. Prucha. 600 pages. 1999. 0-7808-0226-8. $78.

Cardiovascular Diseases & Disorders Sourcebook

Basic Information about Cardiovascular Diseases and Disorders, Featuring Facts about the Cardiovascular System, Demographic and Statistical Data, Descriptions of Pharmacological and Surgical Interventions, Lifestyle Modifications, and a Special Section Focusing on Heart Disorders in Children

Edited by Karen Bellenir and Peter D. Dresser. 683 pages. 1995. 0-7808-0032-X. $78.

". . . comprehensive format provides an extensive overview on this subject."
— *Choice, Jun '96*

". . . an easily understood, complete, up-to-date resource. This well executed public health tool will make valuable information available to those that need it most, patients and their families. The typeface, sturdy non-reflective paper, and library binding add a feel of quality found wanting in other publications. Highly recommended for academic and general libraries. "
— *Academic Library Book Review, Summer '96*

Communication Disorders Sourcebook

Basic Information about Deafness and Hearing Loss, Speech and Language Disorders, Voice Disorders, Balance and Vestibular Disorders, and Disorders of Smell, Taste, and Touch

Edited by Linda M. Ross. 533 pages. 1996. 0-7808-0077-X. $78.

"This is skillfully edited and is a welcome resource for the layperson. It should be found in every public and medical library."
— *Booklist Health Sciences Supplement, Oct '97*

Congenital Disorders Sourcebook

Basic Information about Disorders Acquired during Gestation, Including Spina Bifida, Hydrocephalus, Cerebral Palsy, Heart Defects, Craniofacial Abnormalities, Fetal Alcohol Syndrome, and More, Along with Current Treatment Options and Statistical Data

Edited by Karen Bellenir. 607 pages. 1997. 0-7808-0205-5. $78.

"Recommended reference source." — *Booklist, Oct '97*

Consumer Issues in Health Care Sourcebook

Basic Information about Health Care Fundamentals and Related Consumer Issues, Including Exams and Screening Tests, Physician Specialties, Choosing a Doctor, Using Prescription and Over-the-Counter Medications Safely, Avoiding Health Scams, Managing Common Health Risks in the Home, Care Options for Chronically or Terminally Ill Patients, and a List of Resources for Obtaining Help and Further Information

Edited by Karen Bellenir. 592 pages. 1998. 0-7808-0221-7. $78.

Continues in back end sheets

AIDS

SOURCEBOOK

Second Edition

Health Reference Series

AIDS Sourcebook, 1st Edition

AIDS Sourcebook, 2nd Edition

Allergies Sourcebook

Alternative Medicine Sourcebook

Alzheimer's, Stroke & 29 Other
Neurological Disorders Sourcebook

Alzheimer's Disease Sourcebook,
2nd Edition

Arthritis Sourcebook

Back & Neck Disorders Sourcebook

Blood & Circulatory Disorders Sourcebook

Brain Disorders Sourcebook

Burns Sourcebook

Cancer Sourcebook, 1st Edition

New Cancer Sourcebook, 2nd Edition

Cancer Sourcebook, 3rd Edition

Cancer Sourcebook for Women

Cancer Sourcebook for Women,
2nd Edition

Cardiovascular Diseases & Disorders
Sourcebook

Communication Disorders Sourcebook

Congenital Disorders Sourcebook

Consumer Issues in Health Care
Sourcebook

Contagious & Non-Contagious Infectious
Diseases Sourcebook

Death & Dying Sourcebook

Diabetes Sourcebook, 1st Edition

Diabetes Sourcebook, 2nd Edition

Diet & Nutrition Sourcebook, 1st Edition

Diet & Nutrition Sourcebook, 2nd Edition

Domestic Violence Sourcebook

Ear, Nose & Throat Disorders Sourcebook

Endocrine & Metabolic Disorders
Sourcebook

Environmentally Induced Disorders
Sourcebook

Ethical Issues in Medicine Sourcebook

Fitness & Exercise Sourcebook

Food & Animal Borne Diseases
Sourcebook

Forensic Medicine Sourcebook

Gastrointestinal Diseases & Disorders
Sourcebook

Genetic Disorders Sourcebook

Head Trauma Sourcebook

Health Insurance Sourcebook

Healthy Aging Sourcebook

Immune System Disorders Sourcebook

Kidney & Urinary Tract Diseases &
Disorders Sourcebook

Learning Disabilities Sourcebook

Medical Tests Sourcebook

Men's Health Concerns Sourcebook

Mental Health Disorders Sourcebook

Ophthalmic Disorders Sourcebook

Oral Health Sourcebook

Pain Sourcebook

Physical & Mental Issues in Aging
Sourcebook

Pregnancy & Birth Sourcebook

Public Health Sourcebook

Rehabilitation Sourcebook

Respiratory Diseases & Disorders
Sourcebook

Sexually Transmitted Diseases Sourcebook

Skin Disorders Sourcebook

Sleep Disorders Sourcebook

Sports Injuries Sourcebook

Substance Abuse Sourcebook

Women's Health Concerns Sourcebook

Workplace Health & Safety Sourcebook

Health Reference Series

Second Edition

AIDS
SOURCEBOOK

*Basic Consumer Health Information about
Acquired Immune Deficiency Syndrome (AIDS)
and Human Immunodeficiency Virus (HIV)
Infection, Featuring Updated Statistical Data,
Reports on Recent Research and Prevention
Initiatives, and Other Special Topics of Interest
for Persons Living with AIDS, Including New
Antiretroviral Treatment Options, Strategies for
Combating Opportunistic Infections, Information
about Clinical Trials, and More; Along with a
Glossary of Important Terms and Resource
Listings for Further Help and Information*

Edited by
Karen Bellenir

Omnigraphics, Inc.

Penobscot Building / Detroit, MI 48226

Bibliographic Note

Because this page cannot legibly accommodate all the copyright notices, the Bibliographic Note portion of the Preface constitutes an extension of the copyright notice.

Beginning with books published in 1999, each volume of the *Health Reference Series* on a new topic will be individually titled and called a "First Edition." Subsequent updates will carry sequential edition numbers. To help avoid confusion and to provide maximum flexibility in our ability to respond to informational needs, the practice of consecutively numbering each volume will be discontinued.

Edited by Karen Bellenir

Health Reference Series

Karen Bellenir, *Series Editor*
Peter D. Dresser, *Managing Editor*
Joan Margeson, *Research Associate*
Dawn Matthews, *Verification Assistant*
Margaret Mary Missar, *Research Coordinator*
Jenifer Swanson, *Research Associate*

Omnigraphics, Inc.

Tamekia Nichole Ashford, *Production Associate*
Matthew P. Barbour, *Manager, Production and Fulfillment*
Laurie Lanzen Harris, *Vice President, Editorial Director*
Peter E. Ruffner, *Vice President, Administration*
James A. Sellgren, *Vice President, Operations and Finance*
Jane J. Steele, *Marketing Consultant*

Robert R. Tyler, Executive Vice President and Associate Publisher
Frederick G. Ruffner, Jr., Publisher

©1999, Omnigraphics, Inc.
Library of Congress Cataloging-in-Publication Data

AIDS sourcebook : basic consumer health information about acquired immune deficiency syndrome (AIDS) and human immunodeficiency virus (HIV) infection, featuring updated statistical data, reorts on recent research and prevention initiatives, and other special topics of interest for persons living with AIDS, including new antiretroviral treatment options, strategies for combating opportunistic infections, information about clinical trials, and more ; along with a glosary of important terms and resource listings for further help and information / edited by Karen Bellenir.— 2nd ed.
    p. cm. — (Health reference series ; v. 48)
    Includes bibliographical references and index.
    ISBN 0-7808-0225-X (lib. bdg. : alk. paper)
    1. AIDS (Disease) I. Bellenir, Karen. II. Series.
RC607.A26A3573 1998   98-53294
362.1'969792 — dc21   CIP

∞

This book is printed on acid-free paper meeting the ANSI Z39.48 Standard. The infinity symbol that appears above indicates that the paper in this book meets that standard.

Printed in the United States

Table of Contents

v

Part III: Information for People Living with HIV/AIDS

Part IV: HIV/AIDS Prevention

Part V: HIV/AIDS Research and Clinical Trials

Part VI: Additional Help and Information

Preface

About This Book

The battle against acquired immune deficiency syndrome (AIDS) has made significant progress since the publication of the first edition of *AIDS Sourcebook* in 1995. In recent years, researchers have developed new methods of combating human immunodeficiency virus (HIV) infection and its associated opportunistic infections. In addition, a new class of drugs, called protease inhibitors, has been approved to treat HIV infection.

Although the war against HIV/AIDS is far from over, the encouraging new therapies can help:

- slow the spread of HIV in the body

- interrupt virus replication

- delay the onset of opportunistic infections, such as tuberculosis, *Pneumocystis carinii* pneumonia (PCP), toxoplasmosis, and *Mycobacterium avium* complex (MAC),

- protect the health of fetuses with HIV-infected mothers

This *Second Edition* of Omnigraphics' acclaimed *AIDS Sourcebook* provides updated information for AIDS patients, their families and caregivers, and the general public. It offers statistical data, reports on research and prevention initiatives, and outlines new treatment strategies. All the documents included are either updated or new to this edition. A comprehensive glossary is provided, and extensive resource listings will guide readers to organizations able to provide further help. Readers seeking for information on pediatric AIDS will find this topic addressed in greater depth in *Pediatric AIDS Sourcebook*, a forthcoming volume of the *Health Reference Series*.

How to Use This Book

This book is divided into parts and chapters. Parts focus on broad areas of interest. Chapters are devoted to single topics within a part.

Part I: General Information about Acquired Immune Deficiency Syndrome (AIDS) and the Human Immunodeficiency Virus (HIV) describes HIV infection, transmission, and the process by which it leads to AIDS. Information about HIV Type 2, typical risk behaviors, and the unique characteristics of HIV/AIDS at various ages is also presented.

Part II: HIV/AIDS Statistics and Trends provides demographic information about HIV and AIDS in various U.S. sub-populations, such as men, women, minorities, children, inmates, and health care workers. A report on the global HIV/AIDS epidemic is also included.

Part III: Information for People Living with HIV/AIDS offers patients and caregivers updated information on coping with the day-to-day issues surrounding HIV/AIDS. Topics include HIV testing, viral load, new antiretroviral therapies, home care, and management of opportunistic infections.

Part IV: HIV/AIDS Prevention reports on current progress and related issues in stopping the spread of AIDS through the prevention of HIV transmission.

Part V: HIV/AIDS Research and Clinical Trials describes the process by which new drugs are developed and tested, reports on current research initiatives, and offers an update on the quest for an AIDS vaccine.

Part VI: Additional Help and Information includes an extensive glossary of HIV/AIDS-related terms, a chapter devoted HIV/AIDS information on the internet, and other chapters with full contact information for organizations able to provide specific help to people with HIV/AIDS.

Bibliographic Note

This volume contains documents and excerpts from publications issued by the following U.S. government agencies: AIDS Clinical Trial Information Service (ACTIS); AIDS Treatment Information Service (ATIS); CDC National AIDS Clearinghouse (CDC NAC); Center for Mental Health Services (CMHS); Centers for Disease Control and Prevention (CDC); Federal Trade Commission (FTC); National Cancer Institute (NCI); National Center for HIV, STD and TB Prevention (NCHSTP); National Institute of Allergy and Infectious Diseases (NIAID); National Institute on Aging (NIA); NIH (National Institutes of Health) Consensus Program; Office of National AIDS Policy (ONAP); Social Security Administration (SSA); U.S. Department of Health and Human Services (DHHS); U.S. Department of Justice (DoJ); and the U.S. Food and Drug Administration (FDA).

In addition, this volume contains copyrighted documents from the following organizations: American Dietetic Association (ADA); American Red Cross (ARC); Joint United Nations Programme on HIV/AIDS (UNAIDS); and the National Association of People with AIDS (NAPWA). Full citation information is provided on the first page of each chapter. Every effort has been made to secure all necessary rights to reprint the copyrighted material. If any omissions have been made, please contact Omnigraphics to make corrections for future editions.

Acknowledgements

In addition to the many organizations listed above that provided the material presented in this volume, special thanks are due to researchers Margaret Mary Missar and Jenifer Swanson, permissions specialist Maria Franklin, verification assistant Dawn Matthews, indexer Edward J. Prucha, and document engineer Bruce Bellenir.

Note from the Editor

This book is part of Omnigraphics' *Health Reference Series*. The series provides basic consumer health information about a broad range of medical concerns. It is not intended to serve as a tool for diagnosing illness, in prescribing treatments, or as a substitute for the physician/patient relationship. All persons concerned about medical symptoms or the possibility of disease are encouraged to seek professional care from an appropriate health care provider.

Our Advisory Board

The *Health Reference Series* is reviewed by an Advisory Board comprised of librarians from public, academic, and medical libraries. We would like to thank the following board members for providing guidance to the development of this series:

Health Reference Series *Update Policy*

The inaugural book in the *Health Reference Series* was the first edition of *Cancer Sourcebook* published in 1992. Since then, the *Series* has been enthusiastically received by librarians and in the medical community. In order to maintain the standard of providing high-quality health information for the lay person, the editorial staff at Omnigraphics felt it was necessary to implement a policy of updating volumes when warranted.

Medical researchers have been making tremendous strides, and the challenge to stay current with the most recent advances is one our editors take seriously. Each decision to update a volume will be made on an individual basis. Some of the considerations will include how much new information is available and the feedback we receive from people who use the books. If there's a topic you would like to see added to the update list, or an area of medical concern you feel has not been adequately addressed, please write to:

Editor
Health Reference Series
Omnigraphics, Inc.
2500 Penobscot Bldg.
Detroit, MI 48226

The commitment to providing on-going coverage of important medical developments has also led to some technical changes in the *Health Reference Series*. Beginning with books published in 1999, each volume on a new topic will be individually titled and called a "First Edition." Subsequent updates will carry sequential edition numbers. To help avoid confusion and to provide maximum flexibility in our ability to respond to informational needs, the practice of consecutively numbering each volume will be discontinued.

Part One

General Information about Acquired Immune Deficiency Syndrome (AIDS) and the Human Immunodeficiency Virus (HIV)

Chapter 1

HIV Infection and AIDS

AIDS—acquired immune deficiency syndrome—was first reported in the United States in 1981 and has since become a major worldwide epidemic. AIDS is caused by the human immunodeficiency virus (HIV). By killing or impairing cells of the immune system, HIV progressively destroys the body's ability to fight infections and certain cancers. Individuals diagnosed with AIDS are susceptible to life-threatening diseases called opportunistic infections, which are caused by microbes that usually do not cause illness in healthy people.

More than 500,000 cases of AIDS have been reported in the United States since 1981, and as many as 900,000 Americans may be infected with HIV. The epidemic is growing most rapidly among minority populations and is a leading killer of African-American males. According to the U.S. Centers for Disease Control and Prevention (CDC), the prevalence of AIDS is six times higher in African-Americans and three times higher among Hispanics than among whites.

Transmission

HIV is spread most commonly by sexual contact with an infected partner. The virus can enter the body through the lining of the vagina, vulva, penis, rectum or mouth during sex.

HIV also is spread through contact with infected blood. Prior to the screening of blood for evidence of HIV infection and before the introduction in 1985 of heat-treating techniques to destroy HIV in

National Institute of Allergy and Infectious Diseases (NIAID), May 1997.

3

blood products, HIV was transmitted through transfusions of contaminated blood or blood components. Today, the risk of acquiring HIV from such transfusions is extremely small.

HIV frequently is spread among injection drug users by the sharing of needles or syringes contaminated with minute quantities of blood of someone infected with the virus. However, transmission from patient to health-care worker or vice-versa via accidental sticks with contaminated needles or other medical instruments is rare.

Women can transmit HIV to their fetuses during pregnancy or birth. Approximately one-quarter to one-third of all untreated pregnant women infected with HIV will pass the infection to their babies. HIV also can be spread to babies through the breast milk of mothers infected with the virus. If the drug AZT is taken during pregnancy, the chance of transmitting HIV to the baby is reduced significantly.

Although researchers have detected HIV in the saliva of infected individuals, no evidence exists that the virus is spread by contact with saliva. Laboratory studies reveal that saliva has natural compounds that inhibit the infectiousness of HIV. Studies of people infected with HIV have found no evidence that the virus is spread to others through saliva such as by kissing. However, the risk of infection from so-called "deep" kissing, involving the exchange of large amounts of saliva, is unknown. Scientists also have found no evidence that HIV is spread through sweat, tears, urine or feces.

Studies of families of HIV-infected people have shown clearly that HIV is not spread through casual contact such as the sharing of food utensils, towels and bedding, swimming pools, telephones or toilet seats. HIV is not spread by biting insects such as mosquitoes or bedbugs.

HIV can infect anyone who practices risky behaviors such as:

- sharing drug needles or syringes;
- having unprotected sexual contact with an infected person or with someone whose HIV status is unknown.

Having another sexually transmitted disease such as syphilis, herpes, chlamydia or gonorrhea appears to make someone more susceptible to acquiring HIV infection during sex with an infected partner.

Early Symptoms

Many people do not develop any symptoms when they first become infected with HIV. Some people, however, have a flu-like illness within a month or two after exposure to the virus. They may have fever, headache, malaise and enlarged lymph nodes (organs of the immune system easily felt in the neck and groin). These symptoms usually disappear within a week to a month and are often mistaken for those of another viral infection.

AIDS

The term AIDS applies to the most advanced stages of HIV infection. Official criteria for the definition of AIDS are developed by the U.S. Centers for Disease Control and Prevention (CDC) in Atlanta, Ga., which is responsible for tracking the spread of AIDS in the United States.

In 1993, CDC revised its definition of AIDS to include all HIV-infected people who have fewer than 200 CD4+ T cells. (Healthy adults usually have CD4+ T-cell counts of 1,000 or more.) In addition, the definition includes 26 clinical conditions that affect people with advanced HIV disease. Most AIDS-defining conditions are opportunistic infections, which rarely cause harm in healthy individuals. In people with AIDS, however, these infections are often severe and sometimes fatal because the immune system is so ravaged by HIV that the body cannot fight off certain bacteria, viruses and other microbes.

Opportunistic infections common in people with AIDS cause such symptoms as coughing, shortness of breath, seizures, dementia, severe and persistent diarrhea, fever, vision loss, severe headaches, wasting, extreme fatigue, nausea, vomiting, lack of coordination, coma, abdominal cramps, or difficult or painful swallowing.

Although children with AIDS are susceptible to the same opportunistic infections as adults with the disease, they also experience severe forms of the bacterial infections to which children are especially prone, such as conjunctivitis (pink eye), ear infections and tonsillitis.

People with AIDS are particularly prone to developing various cancers such as Kaposi's sarcoma or cancers of the immune system known as lymphomas. These cancers are usually more aggressive and difficult to treat in people with AIDS. Hallmarks of Kaposi's sarcoma in light-skinned people are round brown, reddish or purple spots that develop in the skin or in the mouth. In dark-skinned people, the spots are more pigmented.

During the course of HIV infection, most people experience a gradual decline in the number of CD4+ T cells, although some individuals may have abrupt and dramatic drops in their CD4+ T-cell counts. A person with CD4+ T cells above 200 may experience some of the early symptoms of HIV disease. Others may have no symptoms even though their CD4+ T-cell count is below 200.

Many people are so debilitated by the symptoms of AIDS that they are unable to hold steady employment or do household chores. Other people with AIDS may experience phases of intense life-threatening illness followed by phases of normal functioning.

A small number of people initially infected with HIV 10 or more years ago have not developed symptoms of AIDS. Scientists are trying to determine what factors may account for their lack of progression to AIDS, such as particular characteristics of their immune systems or whether they were infected with a less aggressive strain of the virus or if their genetic make-up may protect them from the effects of HIV.

Diagnosis

Because early HIV infection often causes no symptoms, it is primarily detected by testing a person's blood for the presence of antibodies (disease-fighting proteins) to HIV. HIV antibodies generally do not reach detectable levels until one to three months following infection and may take as long as six months to be generated in quantities large enough to show up in standard blood tests.

People exposed to HIV should be tested for HIV infection as soon as they are likely to develop antibodies to the virus. Such early testing will enable them to receive appropriate treatment at a time when they are most able to combat HIV and prevent the emergence of certain opportunistic infections (see "Treatment" below). Early testing also alerts HIV-infected people to avoid high-risk behaviors that could spread HIV to others.

HIV testing is done in most doctors' offices or health clinics and should be accompanied by counseling. Individuals can be tested anonymously at many sites if they have particular concerns about confidentiality.

Two different types of antibody tests, ELISA and Western Blot, are used to diagnose HIV infection. If a person is highly likely to be infected with HIV and yet both tests are negative, a doctor may test for the presence of HIV itself in the blood. The person also may be told to repeat antibody testing at a later date, when antibodies to HIV are more likely to have developed.

Babies born to mothers infected with HIV may or may not be infected with the virus, but all carry their mothers' antibodies to HIV for several months. If these babies lack symptoms, a definitive diagnosis of

HIV infection using standard antibody tests cannot be made until after 15 months of age. By then, babies are unlikely to still carry their mothers' antibodies and will have produced their own, if they are infected. New technologies to detect HIV itself are being used to more accurately determine HIV infection in infants between ages 3 months and 15 months. A number of blood tests are being evaluated to determine if they can diagnose HIV infection in babies younger than 3 months.

Treatment

When AIDS first surfaced in the United States, no drugs were available to combat the underlying immune deficiency and few treatments existed for the opportunistic diseases that resulted. Over the past 10 years, however, therapies have been developed to fight both HIV infection and its associated infections and cancers.

The Food and Drug Administration has approved a number of drugs for the treatment of HIV infection. The first group of drugs used to treat HIV infection, called reverse transcriptase (RT) inhibitors, interrupt an early stage of virus replication. Included in this class of drugs are AZT (also known as zidovudine), ddC (zalcitabine), ddI (dideoxyinosine), d4T (stavudine), and 3TC (lamivudine). These drugs may slow the spread of HIV in the body and delay the onset of opportunistic infections. Importantly, they do not prevent transmission of HIV to other individuals.

Non-nucleoside reverse transcriptase inhibitors (NNRTIs) such as delavirdine (Rescriptor) and nevirapine (Viramune) are also available for use in combination with other antiretroviral drugs.

More recently, a second class of drugs has been approved for treating HIV infection. These drugs, called protease inhibitors, interrupt virus replication at a later step in its life cycle. They include ritonavir (Norvir), saquinivir (Invirase), indinavir (Crixivan), and nelfinavir (Viracept). Because HIV can become resistant to both classes of drugs, combination treatment using both is necessary to effectively suppress the virus.

Currently available antiretroviral drugs do not cure people of HIV infection or AIDS, however, and they all have side effects that can be severe. AZT may cause a depletion of red or white blood cells, especially when taken in the later stages of the disease. If the loss of blood cells is severe, treatment with AZT must be stopped. DdI can cause an inflammation of the pancreas and painful nerve damage.

The most common side effects associated with protease inhibitors include nausea, diarrhea and other gastrointestinal symptoms. In addition, protease inhibitors can interact with other drugs resulting in serious side effects.

A number of drugs are available to help treat opportunistic infections to which people with HIV are especially prone. These drugs include foscarnet and ganciclovir, used to treat cytomegalovirus eye infections, fluconazole to treat yeast and other fungal infections, and TMP/SMX or pentamidine to treat *Pneumocystis carinii* pneumonia (PCP).

In addition to antiretroviral therapy, adults with HIV whose CD4+ T-cell counts drop below 200 are given treatment to prevent the occurrence of PCP, which is one of the most common and deadly opportunistic infections associated with HIV. Children are given PCP preventive therapy when their CD4+ T-cell counts drop to levels considered below normal for their age group. Regardless of their CD4+ T-cell counts, HIV-infected children and adults who have survived an episode of PCP are given drugs for the rest of their lives to prevent a recurrence of the pneumonia.

HIV-infected individuals who develop Kaposi's sarcoma or other cancers are treated with radiation, chemotherapy or injections of alpha interferon, a genetically engineered naturally occurring protein.

Prevention

Since no vaccine for HIV is available, the only way to prevent infection by the virus is to avoid behaviors that put a person at risk of infection, such as sharing needles and having unprotected sex.

Because many people infected with HIV have no symptoms, there is no way of knowing with certainty whether a sexual partner is infected unless he or she has been repeatedly tested for the virus or has not engaged in any risky behavior. The Public Health Service recommends that people either abstain from sex or protect themselves by using latex condoms whenever having oral, anal or vaginal sex with someone they aren't certain is free of HIV or other sexually transmitted diseases. Only condoms made of latex should be used, and water-based lubricants should be used with latex condoms.

Although some laboratory evidence shows that spermicides can kill HIV organisms, scientists are still evaluating the usefulness of spermicides in preventing HIV infection.

The risk of HIV transmission from a pregnant woman to her fetus is significantly reduced if she takes AZT during pregnancy, labor and delivery, and her baby takes it for the first six weeks of life.

Research

NIAID-supported investigators are conducting an abundance of research on HIV infection, including the development and testing of HIV vaccines and new therapies for the disease and some of i+ associated conditions. More than a dozen HIV vaccines are being tested in people, and many drugs for HIV infection or AIDS-associated opportunistic infections are either in development or being tested. Researchers also are investigating exactly how HIV damages the immune system. This research is suggesting new and more effective targets for drugs and vaccines. NIAID-supported investigators also continue to document how the disease progresses in different people.

For information about studies of new HIV therapies, call the AIDS Clinical Trials Information Service:

1-800-TRIALS-A 1-800-243-7012 (TDD/Deaf Access)

For federally approved treatment guidelines on HIV/AIDS, call the HIV/AIDS Treatment Information Service:

1-800-HIV-0440 1-800-243-7012 (TDD/Deaf Access)

NIAID, a component of the National Institutes of Health, supports research on AIDS, tuberculosis and other infectious diseases, as well as allergies and immunology. NIH is an agency of the U.S. Department of Health and Human Services. NIAID press releases, fact sheets and other materials are available on the Internet via the NIAID home page at http://www.niaid.nih.gov.

Chapter 2

Facts about HIV and Its Transmission

Research has revealed a great deal of valuable medical, scientific, and public health information about the human immunodeficiency virus (HIV) and acquired immunodeficiency syndrome (AIDS). The ways in which HIV can be transmitted have been clearly identified. Unfortunately, some materials that conflict with the scientific findings have been widely dispersed. The Centers for Disease Control and Prevention (CDC) provides the following information to correct a few misperceptions about HIV.

Transmission

HIV is spread by sexual contact with an infected person, by sharing needles and/or syringes (primarily for drug injection) with someone who is infected, or, less commonly (and now very rarely in countries where blood is screened for HIV antibodies), through transfusions of infected blood or blood clotting factors. Babies born to HIV-infected women may become infected before or during birth, or through breast-feeding after birth.

In the health-care setting, workers have been infected with HIV after being stuck with needles containing HIV-infected blood or, less frequently, after infected blood contacts the worker's open cut or splashes into a mucous membrane (e.g., eyes or inside of the nose). There has been only one demonstrated instance of patients being infected by a health-care worker; this involved HIV transmission from

HIV/AIDS Prevention, Centers for Disease Control and Prevention, July 1997.

11

an infected dentist to six patients. Investigations have been completed involving more than 22,000 patients of 63 HIV-infected physicians, surgeons, and dentists, and no other cases of this type of transmission have been identified.

Some people fear that HIV might be transmitted in other ways; however, no scientific evidence to support any of these fears has been found. If HIV were being transmitted through other routes (for example, through air, food, water, animals, or insects), the pattern of reported AIDS cases would be much different from what has been observed, and cases would be occurring much more frequently in persons who report no identified risk for infection. All reported cases suggesting new or potentially unknown routes of transmission are thoroughly investigated by state and local health departments with the assistance, guidance, and laboratory support from CDC; no additional routes of transmission have been recorded, despite a national sentinel system designed to detect just such an occurrence.

The following paragraphs specifically address some of the more common misperceptions about HIV transmission.

HIV in the Environment

Scientists and medical authorities agree that HIV does not survive well in the environment, making the possibility of environmental transmission remote. HIV is found in varying concentrations or amounts in blood, semen, vaginal fluid, breast milk, saliva, and tears. To obtain data on the survival of HIV, laboratory studies have required the use of artificially high concentrations of laboratory-grown virus. Although these unnatural concentrations of HIV can be kept alive for days or even weeks under precisely controlled and limited laboratory conditions, CDC studies have shown that drying of even these high concentrations of HIV reduces the amount of infectious virus by 90 to 99 percent within several hours. Since the HIV concentrations used in laboratory studies are much higher than those actually found in blood or other specimens, drying of HIV-infected human blood or other body fluids reduces the theoretical risk of environmental transmission to that which has been observed—essentially zero. Incorrect interpretation of conclusions drawn from laboratory studies have unnecessarily alarmed some people.

Results from laboratory studies should not be used to assess specific personal risk of infection because 1) the amount of virus studied is not found in human specimens or elsewhere in nature, and 2) no one has been identified as infected with HIV due to contact with an environmental surface. Additionally, HIV is unable to reproduce outside its living host (unlike many bacteria or fungi, which may do so under suitable conditions), except under laboratory conditions, therefore, it does not spread or maintain infectiousness outside its host.

Households and Other Settings

Although HIV has been transmitted between family members in a household setting, this type of transmission is very rare. These transmissions are believed to have resulted from contact between skin or mucous membranes and infected blood. To prevent even such rare occurrences, precautions, as described in previously published guidelines, should be taken in all settings—including the home—to prevent exposures to the blood of persons who are HIV infected, at risk for HIV infection, or whose infection and risk status are unknown. For example, gloves should be worn during contact with blood or other body fluids that could possibly contain visible blood, such as urine, feces, or vomit. Cuts, sores, or breaks on both the care giver's and patient's exposed skin should be covered with bandages. Hands and other parts of the body should be washed immediately after contact with blood or other body fluids, and surfaces soiled with blood should be disinfected appropriately. Practices that increase the likelihood of blood contact, such as sharing of razors and toothbrushes, should be avoided. Needles and other sharp instruments should be used only when medically necessary and handled according to recommendations for health-care settings. (Do not put caps back on needles by hand or remove needles from syringes. Dispose of needles in puncture-proof containers out of the reach of children and visitors.)

There is no known risk of HIV transmission to co-workers, clients, or consumers from contact in industries such as food-service establishments (see information on survival of HIV in the environment). Food-service workers known to be infected with HIV need not be restricted from work unless they have other infections or illnesses (such as diarrhea or hepatitis A) for which any food-service worker, regardless of HIV infection status, should be restricted. The Public Health Service recommends that all food-service workers follow recommended standards and practices of good personal hygiene and food sanitation.

In 1985, CDC issued routine precautions that all personal-service workers (e.g., hairdressers, barbers, cosmetologists, massage therapists) should follow, even though there is no evidence of transmission from a personal-service worker to a client or vice versa. Instruments that are intended to penetrate the skin (e.g., tattooing and acupuncture needles, ear piercing devices) should be used once and disposed of or thoroughly cleaned and sterilized. Instruments not intended to penetrate the skin but which may become contaminated with blood (e.g., razors) should be used for only one client and disposed of or thoroughly cleaned and disinfected after each use. Personal-service workers can use the same cleaning procedures that are recommended for health-care institutions.

Kissing

Casual contact through closed-mouth or "social" kissing is not a risk for transmission of HIV. Because of the potential for contact with blood during "French" or open-mouth kissing, CDC recommends against engaging in this activity with a person known to be infected. However, the risk of acquiring HIV during open-mouth kissing is believed to be very low. CDC has investigated only one case of HIV infection that may be attributed to contact with blood during open-mouth kissing.

Biting

Recently, a state health department conducted an investigation of an incident that suggested blood-to-blood transmission of HIV by a human bite. There have been other reports in the medical literature in which HIV appeared to have been transmitted by a bite. Severe trauma with extensive tissue tearing and damage and presence of blood were reported in each of these instances. Biting is not a common way of transmitting HIV. In fact, there are numerous reports of bites that did not result in HIV infection.

Saliva, Tears, and Sweat

HIV has been found in saliva and tears in very low quantities from some AIDS patients. It is important to understand that finding a small amount of HIV in a body fluid does not necessarily mean that HIV can be transmitted by that body fluid. HIV has not been recovered from the sweat of HIV-infected persons. Contact with saliva, tears, or sweat has never been shown to result in transmission of HIV.

Insects

From the onset of the HIV epidemic, there has been concern about transmission of the virus by biting and bloodsucking insects. However, studies conducted by researchers at CDC and elsewhere have shown no evidence of HIV transmission through insects—even in areas where there are many cases of AIDS and large populations of insects such as mosquitoes. Lack of such outbreaks, despite intense efforts to detect them, supports the conclusion that HIV is not transmitted by insects.

The results of experiments and observations of insect biting behavior indicate that when an insect bites a person, it does not inject its own or a previously bitten person's or animal's blood into the next person bitten. Rather, it injects saliva, which acts as a lubricant or anticoagulant so the insect can feed efficiently. Such diseases as yellow fever and malaria are transmitted through the saliva of specific species of mosquitoes. However, HIV lives for only a short time inside an insect and, unlike organisms that are transmitted via insect bites, HIV does not reproduce (and, does not survive) in insects. Thus, even if the virus enters a mosquito or another sucking or biting insect, the insect does not become infected and cannot transmit HIV to the next human it feeds on or bites. HIV is not found in insect feces.

There is also no reason to fear that a biting or bloodsucking insect, such as a mosquito, could transmit HIV from one person to another through HIV-infected blood left on its mouth parts. Two factors serve to explain why this is so—first, infected people do not have constant, high levels of HIV in their bloodstreams and, second, insect mouth parts do not retain large amounts of blood on their surfaces. Further, scientists who study insects have determined that biting insects normally do not travel from one person to the next immediately after ingesting blood. Rather, they fly to a resting place to digest this blood meal.

Effectiveness of Condoms

The proper and consistent use of latex condoms when engaging in sexual intercourse—vaginal, anal, or oral—can greatly reduce a person's risk of acquiring or transmitting sexually transmitted diseases, including HIV infection.

Under laboratory conditions, viruses occasionally have been shown to pass through natural membrane ("skin" or lambskin) condoms, which may contain natural pores and are therefore not recommended for disease prevention (they are documented to be effective for contraception). On the other hand, laboratory studies have consistently demonstrated that latex condoms provide a highly effective mechanical barrier to HIV.

In order for condoms to provide maximum protection, they must be used consistently(every time) and correctly. Incorrect use contributes to the possibility that the condom could leak or break.

When condoms are used reliably, they have been shown to prevent pregnancy up to 98 percent of the time among couples using them as their only method of contraception. Similarly, numerous studies among sexually active people have demonstrated that a properly used latex condom provides a high degree of protection against a variety of sexually transmitted diseases, including HIV infection.

Condoms are classified as medical devices and are regulated by the Food and Drug Administration. Condom manufacturers in the United States test each latex condom for defects, including holes, before it is packaged. Several studies of correct and consistent condom use clearly show that condom breakage rates in this country are less than 2 percent. Even when condoms do break, one study showed that more than half of such breaks occurred prior to ejaculation.

Latex condoms are highly effective in preventing pregnancy and most sexually transmitted diseases, including HIV infection, but only if they are used consistently and correctly.

Chapter 3

How HIV Causes AIDS

An important focus of the National Institute of Allergy and Infectious Diseases (NIAID) is research devoted to the pathogenesis of human immunodeficiency virus (HIV) disease—the complex mechanisms that result in the destruction of the immune system of an HIV-infected person. A detailed understanding of HIV and how it establishes infection and causes the acquired immunodeficiency syndrome (AIDS) is crucial to identifying and developing effective drugs and vaccines to fight HIV and AIDS. This chapter summarizes what scientists are learning about this process.

Overview

HIV disease is characterized by a gradual deterioration of immune function. Most notably, crucial immune cells called CD4+ T cells are disabled and killed during the typical course of infection. These cells, sometimes called "T-helper cells," play a central role in the immune response, signaling other cells in the immune system to perform their special functions.

A healthy, uninfected person usually has 800 to 1,200 CD4+ T cells per cubic millimeter (mm^3) of blood. During HIV infection, the number of these cells in a person's blood progressively declines. When a person's CD4+ T cell count falls below $200/MM^3$, he or she becomes particularly vulnerable to the opportunistic infections and cancers

National Institute of Allergy and Infectious Diseases (NIAID), February 1998.

that typify AIDS, the end stage of HIV disease. People with AIDS often suffer infections of the intestinal tract, lungs, brain, eyes and other organs, as well as debilitating weight loss, diarrhea, neurologic conditions and cancers such as Kaposi's sarcoma and lymphomas.

Most scientists think that HIV causes AIDS by directly killing CD4+ T cells or interfering with their normal function, and by triggering other events that weaken a person's immune function. For example, the network of signaling molecules that normally regulates a person's immune response is disrupted during HIV disease, impairing a person's ability to fight other infections. The HIV-mediated destruction of the lymph nodes and related immunologic organs also plays a major role in causing the immunosuppression seen in people with AIDS.

Scope of the HIV Epidemic

Although HIV was first identified in 1983, studies of previously stored blood samples indicate that the virus entered the U.S. population sometime in the late 1970s. In the United States, 612,078 cases of AIDS, and 379,258 deaths among people with AIDS had been reported to the Centers for Disease Control and Prevention (CDC) as of June 30, 1997. AIDS is now the second leading killer of people aged 25 to 44 in this country. Despite an overall stabilization in the number of new AIDS cases in this country, the epidemic continues to accelerate in certain segments of the population, notably among women and injection drug users.

Worldwide, an estimated 30.6 million people were living with HIV/AIDS as of December 1997, a figure that is projected to reach 40 million by the year 2000. More than 75 percent of all adult HIV infections have resulted from heterosexual intercourse. Through 1997, cumulative HIV/AIDS-associated deaths worldwide numbered approximately 11.7 million—9 million adults and 2.7 million children.

HIV Is a Retrovirus

HIV belongs to a class of viruses called retroviruses, which have genes composed of ribonucleic acid (RNA) molecules. The genes of humans and most other organisms are made of a related molecule, deoxyribonucleic acid (DNA).

Like all viruses, HIV can replicate only inside cells, commandeering the cell's machinery to reproduce. However, only HIV and other retroviruses, once inside a cell, use an enzyme called reverse transcriptase to convert their RNA into DNA, which can be incorporated into the host cell's genes.

Slow Viruses

HIV belongs to a subgroup of retroviruses known as lentiviruses, or "slow" viruses. The course of infection with these viruses is characterized by a long interval between initial infection and the onset of serious symptoms.

Other lentiviruses infect nonhuman species. For example, the feline immunodeficiency virus (FIV) infects cats and the simian immunodeficiency virus (SIV) infects monkeys and other nonhuman primates. Like HIV in humans, these animal viruses primarily infect immune system cells, often causing immunodeficiency and AIDS-like symptoms. These viruses and their hosts have provided researchers with useful, albeit imperfect, models of the HIV disease process in people.

Structure of HIV

The Viral Envelope

HIV has a diameter of 1/10,000 of a millimeter and is spherical in shape. The outer coat of the virus, known as the viral envelope, is composed of two layers of fatty molecules called lipids, taken from the membrane of a human cell when a newly formed virus particle buds from the cell.

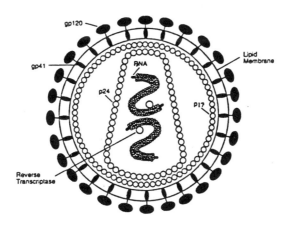

Figure 3.1. *Organization of the HIV-1 Virion*

19

Embedded in the viral envelope are proteins from the host cell, as well as 72 copies (on average) of a complex HIV protein that protrudes from the envelope surface. This protein, known as Env, consists of a cap made of three or four molecules called glycoprotein (gp)120, and a stem consisting of three or four gp41 molecules that anchor the structure in the viral envelope. Much of the research to develop a vaccine against HIV has focused on these envelope proteins.

The Viral Core

Within the envelope of a mature HIV particle is a bullet-shaped core or capsid, made of 2000 copies of another viral protein, p24. The capsid surrounds two single strands of HIV RNA, each of which has a copy of the virus's nine genes. Three of these, *gag*, *pol* and *env*, contain information needed to make structural proteins for new virus particles. The *env* gene, for example, codes for a protein called gp160 that is broken down by a viral enzyme to form gp120 and gp41, the components of Env.

Three regulatory genes, *tat*, *rev*, and *nef*, and three auxiliary genes, *vif*, *vpr* and *vpu*, contain information necessary for the production of proteins that control the ability of HIV to infect a cell, produce new copies of virus or cause disease. The protein encoded by *nef*, for instance, appears necessary for the virus to replicate efficiently, and the *vpu*-encoded protein influences the release of new virus particles from infected cells.

The ends of each strand of HIV RNA contain an RNA sequence called the long terminal repeat (LTR). Regions in the LTR act as switches to control production of new viruses and can be triggered by proteins from either HIV or the host cell.

The core of HIV also includes a protein called p7, the HIV nucleocapsid protein; and three enzymes that carry out later steps in the virus's life cycle: reverse transcriptase, integrase and protease. Another HIV protein called p17, or the HIV matrix protein, lies between the viral core and the viral envelope.

Replication Cycle of HIV

Entry of HIV into Cells

Infection typically begins when an HIV particle, which contains two copies of the HIV RNA, encounters a cell with a surface molecule called cluster designation 4 (CD4). Cells with this molecule are known as CD4 positive (CD4+) cells.

One or more of the virus's gp120 molecules binds tightly to CD4 molecule(s) on the cell's surface. The membranes of the virus and the cell fuse, a process that probably involves the envelope of HIV and a second "coreceptor" molecule on the cell surface. Following fusion, the virus's RNA, proteins and enzymes are released into the cell.

Recent studies by NIAID intramural and extramural researchers have identified multiple coreceptors for different types of HIV strains; these coreceptors are promising targets for new anti-HIV drugs. In the early stage of HIV disease, most people harbor viruses that use, in addition to CD4, a receptor called CCR5 to enter their target cells. With disease progression, the spectrum of coreceptor usage expands to include others, notably a molecule called CXCR4.

Steps in Viral Replication

1) Attachment/Entry

2) Reverse Transcription and DNA Synthesis

3) Transport to Nucleus

4) Integration

5) Viral Transcription

6) Viral Protein Synthesis

7) Assembly of Virus

8) Release of Virus

9) Maturation

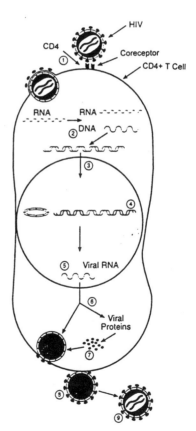

Figure 3.2. Life Cycle of HIV

Although CD4+ T cells appear to be HIV's main target, other immune system cells with CD4 molecules on their surfaces are infected as well. Among these are long-lived cells called monocytes and macrophages, which apparently can harbor large quantities of the virus without being killed, thus acting as reservoirs of HIV. CD4+ T cells also serve as important reservoirs of HIV: a small proportion of these cells harbor HIV in a stable, inactive form. Normal immune processes may activate these cells, resulting in the production of new HIV virions.

Cell-to-cell spread of HIV also can occur through the CD4-mediated fusion of an infected cell with an uninfected cell.

Reverse Transcription

In the cytoplasm of the cell, HIV reverse transcriptase converts viral RNA into DNA, the nucleic acid form in which the cell carries its genes. Seven of the 11 antiviral drugs approved in the United States for the treatment of people with HIV infection—AZT, ddC, ddI, d4T, 3TC, nevirapine, and delavirdine—work by interfering with this stage of the viral life cycle.

Integration

The newly made HIV DNA moves to the cell's nucleus, where it is spliced into the host's DNA with the help of HIV integrase. Once incorporated into the cell's genes, HIV DNA is called a "provirus." Integrase is an important target for the development of new drugs.

Transcription

For a provirus to produce new viruses, RNA copies must be made that can be read by the host cell's protein-making machinery. These copies are called messenger RNA (mRNA), and production of mRNA is called transcription, a process that involves the host cell's own enzymes. Viral genes in concert with the cellular machinery control this process: the *tat* gene, for example, encodes a protein that accelerates transcription.

Cytokines, proteins involved in the normal regulation of the immune response, also may regulate transcription. Molecules such as tumor necrosis factor (TNF)-alpha and interleukin (IL)-6, secreted in elevated levels by the cells of HIV-infected people, may help to activate HIV proviruses. Other infections, by organisms such as *Mycobacterium tuberculosis*, may also enhance transcription.

Translation

After HIV mRNA is processed in the cell's nucleus, it is transported to the cytoplasm. HIV proteins are critical to this process: for example, a protein encoded by the rev gene allows mRNA encoding HIV structural proteins to be transferred from the nucleus to the cytoplasm. Without the *rev* protein, structural proteins are not made.

In the cytoplasm, the virus co-opts the cell's protein-making machinery—including structures called ribosomes—to make long chains of viral proteins and enzymes, using HIV mRNA as a template. This process is called translation.

Assembly and Budding

Newly made HIV core proteins, enzymes and RNA gather just inside the cell's membrane, while the viral envelope proteins aggregate within the membrane. An immature viral particle forms and pinches off from the cell, acquiring an envelope that includes both cellular and HIV proteins from the cell membrane. During this part of the viral life cycle, the core of the virus is immature and the virus is not yet infectious. The long chains of proteins and enzymes that make up the immature viral core are now cleaved into smaller pieces by a viral enzyme called protease. This step results in infectious viral particles.

Drugs called protease inhibitors interfere with this step of the viral life cycle. Four such drugs—saquinavir, ritonavir, indinavir and nelfinavir—have been approved for marketing in the United States.

Transmission of HIV

Among adults, HIV is spread most commonly during sexual intercourse with an infected partner. During sex, the virus can enter the body through the mucosal linings of the vagina, vulva, penis, rectum or, rarely, via the mouth. The likelihood of transmission is increased by factors that may damage these linings, especially other sexually transmitted diseases that cause ulcers or inflammation.

Research suggests that immune system cells called dendritic cells, which reside in the mucosa, may begin the infection process after sexual exposure by binding to and carrying the virus from the site of infection to the lymph nodes where other immune system cells become infected.

HIV also can be transmitted by contact with infected blood, most often by the sharing of drug needles or syringes contaminated with minute quantities of blood containing the virus. The risk of acquiring

HIV from blood transfusions is now extremely small in the United States, as all blood products in this country are screened routinely for evidence of the virus.

Almost all HIV-infected children acquire the virus from their mothers before or during birth. In the United States, approximately 25 percent of pregnant HIV-infected women not receiving antiretroviral therapy have passed on the virus to their babies. NIAID-sponsored researchers have shown that a specific regimen of the drug zidovudine (AZT) can reduce the risk of transmission of HIV from mother to baby by two-thirds. Research using combinations of approved anti-HIV drugs is underway to determine if the transmission rate can be further reduced.

The virus also may be transmitted from a nursing HIV-infected mother to her infant.

Early Events in HIV Infection

Once it enters the body, HIV infects a large number of CD4+ cells and replicates rapidly. During this acute or primary phase of infection, the blood contains many viral particles that spread throughout the body, seeding various organs, particularly the lymphoid organs. Lymphoid organs include the lymph nodes, spleen, tonsils and adenoids.

During the acute phase of infection, the number of CD4+ T cells in the bloodstream decreases by 20 to 40 percent. Scientists do not yet know whether these cells are killed by HIV or if they leave the blood and go to the lymphoid organs in preparation to mount an immune response.

Two to four weeks after exposure to the virus, up to 70 percent of HIV-infected persons suffer flu-like symptoms related to the acute infection. The patient's immune system fights back with killer T cells (CD8+ T cells) and B-cell-produced antibodies, which dramatically reduce HIV levels. A patient's CD4+ T cell count may rebound to 80 to 90 percent of its original level. A person then may remain free of HIV-related symptoms for years despite continuous replication of HIV in the lymphoid organs seeded during the acute phase of infection.

One reason HIV is unique is that despite the body's aggressive immune responses, which are sufficient to clear most viral infections, some HIV invariably escapes. This is due in large part to the high rate of mutations that occur during the process of HIV replication. Even when the virus does not avoid the immune system by mutating, the body's best soldiers in the fight against HIV—certain subsets of killer T cells—may multiply so rapidly following initial infection that they become exhausted and disappear, allowing HIV to escape and continue replication.

In addition, early in the course of HIV infection, patients may lose HIV-specific CD4+ T cell responses that normally slow the replication of viruses. Such responses include the secretion of interferons and other antiviral factors, and the orchestration of CD8+ T cells.

Course of HIV Infection

Among patients enrolled in large epidemiologic studies in western countries, the median time from infection with HIV to the development of AIDS-related symptoms has been approximately 10 to 12 years. However, researchers have observed a wide variation in disease progression. Approximately 10 percent of HIV-infected people in these studies have progressed to AIDS within the first two to three years following infection, while up to 5 percent of individuals in the studies have stable CD4+ T cell counts and no symptoms even after 12 or more years.

Factors such as age or genetic differences among individuals, the level of virulence of an individual strain of virus, and co-infection with other microbes may influence the rate and severity of disease progression. Drugs that fight the infections associated with AIDS have improved and prolonged the lives of HIV-infected people by preventing or treating conditions such as *Pneumocystis carinii* pneumonia.

HIV Co-Receptors and Disease Progression

Recent research has shown that most infecting strains of HIV use a co-receptor molecule called CCR5, in addition to the CD4 molecule, to enter certain of its target cells. HIV-infected people with a specific mutation in one of their two copies of the gene for this receptor generally have a slower disease course than people with two normal copies of the gene. Rare individuals with two mutant copies of the CCR5 gene appear—in most cases—to be completely protected from HIV infection. Mutations in the gene for other HIV coreceptors also may influence the rate of disease progression.

Viral Burden Predicts Disease Progression

Numerous studies show that people with high levels of HIV in their bloodstream are more likely to develop new AIDS-related symptoms or die than individuals with lower levels of virus. For instance, in the

Multicenter AIDS Cohort Study (MACS), NIAID-supported investigators demonstrated that the level of HIV in an individual's plasma soon after infection—the so-called viral "set point"—is highly predictive of the rate of disease progression; that is, patients with high levels of virus are much more likely to get sicker, faster, than those with low levels of virus. The MACS and other studies have provided the rationale for providing aggressive antiretroviral therapy to HIV-infected people, as well as for routinely using newly available blood tests to measure viral load when initiating, monitoring and modifying anti-HIV therapy.

New anti-HIV drug combinations—which generally include a protease inhibitor taken with two reverse transcriptase inhibitors—can reduce a person's "viral burden" to very low levels and in many cases delay the progression of HIV disease for prolonged periods. However, antiretroviral regimens have yet to completely and permanently suppress the virus in HIV-infected people. Recent studies have shown that HIV persists in a replication-competent form in resting CD4+ T cells even in patients receiving aggressive antiretroviral therapy who have no easily detectable HIV in their blood. Investigators around the world are working to develop the next generation of anti-HIV drugs.

HIV Is Active in the Lymph Nodes

Although HIV-infected individuals often exhibit an extended period of clinical latency with little evidence of disease, the virus is never truly latent. NIAID researchers have shown that even early in disease, HIV actively replicates within the lymph nodes and related organs, where large amounts of virus become trapped in networks of specialized cells with long, tentacle-like extensions. These cells are called follicular dendritic cells (FDCs).

FDCs are located in hot spots of immune activity called germinal centers. They act like flypaper, trapping invading pathogens (including HIV) and holding them until B cells come along to initiate an immune response.

Close on the heels of B cells are CD4+ T cells, which rush into the germinal centers to help B cells fight the invaders. CD4+ T cells, the primary targets of HIV, may become infected as they encounter HIV trapped on FDCs. Research suggests that HIV trapped on FDCs remains infectious, even when coated with antibodies. Thus, FDCs are an important reservoir of HIV, and the large quantity of infectious HIV trapped on FDCs may explain in part how the momentum of HIV infection is maintained.

Once infected, CD4+ T cells may leave the germinal center and infect other CD4+ cells that congregate in the region of the lymph node surrounding the germinal center.

Over a period of years, even when little virus is readily detectable in the blood, significant amounts of virus accumulate in the germinal centers, both within infected cells and bound to FDCs. In and around the germinal centers, numerous CD4+ T cells are probably activated by the increased production of cytokines such as TNF-alpha and IL-6, possibly secreted by B cells. Activation allows uninfected cells to be more easily infected and increases replication of HIV in already infected cells.

While greater quantities of certain cytokines such as TNF-alpha and IL-6 are secreted during HIV infection, others with key roles in the regulation of normal immune function may be secreted in **decreased** amounts. For example, CD4+ T cells may lose their capacity to produce interleukin 2 (IL-2), a cytokine that enhances the growth of other T cells and helps to stimulate other cells' response to invaders. Infected cells also have low levels of receptors for IL-2, which may reduce their ability to respond to signals from other cells.

Breakdown of FDC Networks

Ultimately, accumulated HIV overwhelms the FDC networks. As these networks break down, their trapping capacity is impaired, and large quantities of virus enter the bloodstream.

Although it remains unclear why FDCs die and the FDC networks dissolve, some scientists think that this process may be as important in HIV pathogenesis as the loss of CD4+ T cells. The destruction of the lymph node structure seen late in HIV disease may preclude a successful immune response against not only HIV but other pathogens as well. This devastation heralds the onset of the opportunistic infections and cancers that characterize AIDS.

Role of CD8+ T Cells

CD8+ T cells are important in the immune response to HIV during the acute infection and the clinically latent stage of disease. These cells attack and kill infected cells that are producing virus.

CD8+ T cells also appear to secrete soluble factors that suppress HIV replication. Several molecules, including RANTES, MIP-1 alpha, MIP-1 beta, and MDC appear to block HIV replication by occupying the co-receptors necessary for the entry of many strains of HIV into their target cells. There may be many other immune system molecules—yet undiscovered—that can suppress HIV replication to some degree.

Rapid Replication and Mutation of HIV

HIV replicates rapidly; several billion new virus particles may be produced every day. In addition, the HIV reverse transcriptase enzyme makes many mistakes while making DNA copies from HIV RNA. As a consequence, many variants of HIV develop in an individual, some of which may escape destruction by antibodies or killer T cells. Additionally, HIV can recombine with itself to produce a wide range of variants or strains.

During the course of HIV disease, viral strains emerge in an infected individual that differ widely in their ability to infect and kill different cell types, as well as in their rate of replication. Scientists are investigating why strains of HIV from patients with advanced disease appear to be more virulent and infect more cell types than strains obtained earlier from the same individual.

Theories of Immune System Cell Loss in HIV Infection

Researchers around the world are studying how HIV destroys or disables CD4+ T cells, and many think that a number of mechanisms may occur simultaneously in an HIV-infected individual. Recent data suggest that billions of CD4+ T cells may be destroyed every day, eventually overwhelming the immune system's regenerative capacity.

Direct Cell Killing

Infected CD4+ T cells may be killed directly when large amounts of virus are produced and bud off from the cell surface, disrupting the cell membrane, or when viral proteins and nucleic acids collect inside the cell, interfering with cellular machinery.

Syncytia Formation

Infected cells also may fuse with nearby uninfected cells, forming balloon-like giant cells called syncytia. In test-tube experiments at NIAID and elsewhere, these giant cells have been associated with the death of uninfected cells. The presence of so-called syncytia-inducing variants of HIV has been correlated with rapid disease progression in HIV-infected individuals.

Apoptosis

Infected CD4+ T cells may be killed when cellular regulation is distorted by HIV proteins, probably leading to their suicide by a process known as programmed cell death or apoptosis. Recent reports indicate that apoptosis occurs to a greater extent in HIV-infected individuals, both in the bloodstream and lymph nodes.

Uninfected cells also may undergo apoptosis. Investigators have shown in cell cultures that the HIV envelope alone or bound to antibodies sends an inappropriate signal to CD4+ T cells causing them to undergo apoptosis even if not infected by HIV.

Innocent Bystanders

Uninfected cells may die in an innocent bystander scenario: HIV particles may bind to the cell surface, giving them the appearance of an infected cell and marking them for destruction by killer T cells.

Killer T cells also may mistakenly destroy uninfected cells that have consumed HIV particles and that display HIV fragments on their surfaces. Alternatively, because HIV envelope proteins bear some resemblance to certain molecules that may appear on CD4+ T cells, the body's immune responses may mistakenly damage such cells as well.

Anergy

Researchers have shown in cell cultures that CD4+ T cells can be turned off by a signal from HIV that leaves them unable to respond to further immune stimulation. This inactivated state is known as anergy.

Superantigens

Other investigators have proposed that a molecule known as a superantigen, either made by HIV or an unrelated agent, may stimulate massive quantities of CD4+ T cells at once, rendering them highly susceptible to HIV infection and subsequent cell death.

Damage to Precursor Cells

Studies suggest that HIV also destroys precursor cells that mature to have special immune functions, as well as the parts of the bone marrow and the thymus needed for the development of such cells. These organs probably lose the ability to regenerate, further compounding the suppression of the immune system.

Central Nervous System Damage

Although monocytes and macrophages can be infected by HIV, they appear to be relatively resistant to killing. However, these cells travel throughout the body and carry HIV to various organs, especially the lungs and brain. People infected with HIV often experience abnormalities in the central nervous system. Neurologic manifestations of HIV disease, seen in 40 to 50 percent of HIV-infected people, are the subject of many research projects. Investigators have hypothesized that an accumulation of HIV in brain and nerve cells, or the inappropriate release of cytokines or toxic byproducts by these cells, may be to blame.

Role of Immune Activation in HIV Disease

During a normal immune response, many components of the immune system are mobilized to fight an invader. CD4+ T cells, for instance, may quickly proliferate and increase their cytokine secretion, thereby signaling other cells to perform their special functions. Scavenger cells called macrophages may double in size and develop numerous organelles, including lysosomes that contain digestive enzymes used to process ingested pathogens. Once the immune system clears the foreign antigen, it returns to a relative state of quiescence.

Paradoxically, although it ultimately causes immune deficiency, HIV disease for most of its course is characterized by immune system hyperactivation, which has negative consequences. As noted above, HIV replication and spread are much more efficient in activated CD4+ cells. Chronic immune system activation during HIV disease may also result in a massive stimulation of a person's B cells, impairing the ability of these cells to make antibodies against other pathogens.

Chronic immune activation also can result in apoptosis, and an increased production of cytokines that may not only increase HIV replication but also have other deleterious effects. Increased levels of TNF-alpha, for example, may be at least partly responsible for the severe weight loss or wasting syndrome seen in many HIV-infected individuals.

The persistence of HIV and HIV replication probably plays an important role in the chronic state of immune activation seen in HIV-infected people. In addition, researchers have shown that infections with other organisms activate immune system cells and increase production of the virus in HIV-infected people. Chronic immune activation due to persistent infections, or the cumulative effects of multiple episodes of immune activation and bursts of virus production, likely contribute to the progression of HIV disease.

NIAID Research on the Pathogenesis of AIDS

NIAID-supported scientists conduct HIV pathogenesis research in laboratories on the campus of the National Institutes of Health (NIH) in Bethesda, Md., at the Institute's Rocky Mountain Laboratories in Hamilton, Mont., and at universities and medical centers in the United States and abroad.

An NIAID-supported collaborative center of the World Health Organization, known as the NIH AIDS Research and Reference Reagent Program, provides AIDS-related research materials free to qualified researchers around the world.

In addition, the Institute convenes groups of investigators and advisory committees to exchange scientific information, clarify research priorities and bring research needs and opportunities to the attention of the scientific community.

The NIAID HIV/AIDS Research Agenda and fact sheets on NIAID HIV/AIDS vaccine research, clinical trials for AIDS therapies and vaccines, and AIDS-related opportunistic infections are available from the NIAID Office of Communications. To receive free copies, call (301) 496-5717, Monday through Friday, 8:30 a.m. to 5:00 p.m. Eastern Time. These materials also are available via the NIAID home page on the Internet at http://www.niaid.nih.gov.

NIAID, a component of the National Institutes of Health, supports research on AIDS, tuberculosis, malaria and other infectious diseases, as well as allergies and immunology. NIH is an agency of the U.S. Department of Health and Human Services. Press releases, fact sheets and other NIAID-related materials are available on the Internet via the NIAID home page at http://www.niaid.nih.gov.

Chapter 4

Human Immunodeficiency Virus Type 2

In 1984, 3 years after the first reports of a disease that was to become known as AIDS, researchers discovered the primary causative viral agent, the human immunodeficiency virus type 1 (HIV-1). In 1986, a second type of HIV, called HIV-2, was isolated from AIDS patients in West Africa, where it may have been present decades earlier. Studies of the natural history of HIV-2 are limited, but to date comparisons with HIV-1 show some similarities while suggesting differences. Both HIV-1 and HIV-2 have the same modes of transmission and are associated with similar opportunistic infections and AIDS. In persons infected with HIV-2, immunodeficiency seems to develop more slowly and to be milder. Compared with persons infected with HIV-1, those with HIV-2 are less infectious early in the course of infection. As the disease advances, HIV-2 infectiousness seems to increase; however, compared with HIV-1, the duration of this increased infectiousness is shorter. HIV-1 and HIV-2 also differ in geographic patterns of infection; the United States has few reported cases.

Which Countries Have a High Prevalence of HIV-2 Infection?

HIV-2 infections are predominantly found in Africa. West African nations with a prevalence of HIV-2 of more than 1% in the general population are Cape Verde, Côte d'Ivoire (Ivory Coast), Gambia, Guinea-Bissau, Mali, Mauritania, Nigeria, and Sierra Leone. Other

CDC Facts, National Center for HIV, STD, and TB Prevention, April 1998.

West African countries reporting HIV-2 are Benin, Burkina Faso, Ghana, Guinea, Liberia, Niger, São Tomé, Senegal, and Togo. Angola and Mozambique are other African nations where the prevalence of HIV-2 is more than 1%.

Prevalence is the proportion of cases present in a population at a given point in time.

What Is Known about HIV-2 in the United States?

The first case of HIV-2 infection in the United States was diagnosed in 1987. Since then, the Centers for Disease Control and Prevention (CDC) has worked with state and local health departments to collect demographic, clinical, and laboratory data on persons with HIV-2 infection.

Of the 77 infected persons, 65 are black and 50 are male. Fifty-two were born in West Africa, 7 in the United States, 2 in India, and 2 in Europe. The region of origin was not known for 14 of the persons, although 4 of them had a malaria-antibody profile consistent with

State of Report	No.	State of Report	No.
California	2	Mississippi	1
Colorado	1	New Jersey	4
Connecticut	1	New York	26
Delaware	1	North Carolina	1
District of Columbia	2	Ohio	1
Florida	1	Pennsylvania	1
Georgia	4	Rhode Island	3
Illinois	1	Texas	1
Maryland	9	Washington	1
Massachusetts	10	West Virginia	1
Michigan	2	Wisconsin	3
		Total	77

Figure 4.1. HIV-2 cases by state, reported through December 31, 1997

residence in West Africa. AIDS-defining conditions have developed in 15, and 8 have died. These case counts represent minimal estimates because completeness of reporting has not been assessed. Although AIDS is reported uniformly nationwide, the reporting of HIV infection, including HIV-2 infection, differs from state to state according to state policy.

Who Should Be Tested for HIV-2?

Because epidemiologic data indicate that the prevalence of HIV-2 in the United States is very low, CDC does not recommend routine HIV-2 testing at U.S. HIV counseling and test sites or in settings other than blood centers. However, when HIV testing is to be performed, tests for antibodies to both HIV-1 and HIV-2 should be obtained if demographic or behavioral information suggests that HIV-2 infection might be present.

Persons at Risk for HIV-2 Infection Include

- Sex partners of a person from a country where HIV-2 is endemic (refer to countries listed earlier)
- Sex partners of a person known to be infected with HIV-2
- People who received a blood transfusion or a nonsterile injection in a country where HIV-2 is endemic
- People who shared needles with a person from a country where HIV-2 is endemic or with a person known to be infected with HIV-2
- Children of women who have risk factors for HIV-2 infection or are known to be infected with HIV-2

HIV-2 Testing Also Is Indicated for

- People with an illness that suggests HIV infection (such as an HIV-associated opportunistic infection) but whose HIV-1 test result is not positive
- People for whom HIV-1 Western blot exhibits the unusual indeterminate test band pattern of gag (p55, p24, or p17) plus pol (p66, p51, or p32) in the absence of env (gpl60, gpl20, or gp41)

Among all HIV-infected people, the prevalence of HIV-2 is very low compared with HIV-1. However, the potential risk for HIV-2 infection in some populations (such as those listed) may justify routine IIIV-2 testing for all people for whom HIV-1 testing is warranted. The decision to implement routine HIV-2 testing requires consideration of the number of HIV-2-infected persons whose infection would remain undiagnosed without routine HIV-2 testing compared with the problems and costs associated with the implementation of HIV-2 testing.

The development of antibodies is similar in HIV-1 and HIV-2. Antibodies generally become detectable within 3 months of infection. Testing for HIV-2 antibodies is available through private physicians or state and local health departments.

Are Blood Donors Tested for HIV-2?

Since 1992, all U.S. blood donations have been tested with a combination HIV-1/HIV-2 enzyme immunoassay test kit that is sensitive to antibodies to both viruses. This testing has demonstrated that HIV-2 infection in blood donors is extremely rare. All donations detected with either HIV-1 or HIV-2 are excluded from any clinical use, and donors are deferred from further donations.

Is the Clinical Treatment of HIV-2 Different from That of HIV-1?

Little is known about the best approach to the clinical treatment and care of patients infected with HIV-2. Given the slower development of immunodeficiency and the limited clinical experience with HIV-2, it is unclear whether antiretroviral therapy significantly slows progression. Not all of the drugs used to treat HIV-1 infection are as effective against HIV-2. *In vitro* (laboratory) studies suggest that nucleoside analogs are active against HIV-2, though not as active as against HIV-1. Protease inhibitors should be active against HIV-2. However, non-nucleoside reverse transcriptase inhibitors (NNRTIs) are not active against HIV-2. Whether any potential benefits would outweigh the possible adverse effects of treatment is unknown.

Monitoring the treatment response of patients infected with HIV-2 is more difficult than monitoring people infected with HIV-1. No FDA-licensed HIV-2 viral load assay is available yet. Viral load assays used for HIV-1 are not reliable for monitoring HIV-2. Response to treatment for HIV-2 infection may be monitored by following CD4$^+$ T-cell counts and other indicators of immune system deterioration, such as weight loss, oral candidiasis, unexplained fever, and the appearance of a new AIDS-defining illness. More research and clinical experience is needed to determine the most effective treatment for HIV-2.

The optimal timing for antiretroviral therapy (i.e., soon after infection, when symptoms appear, or when CD4+ T-cell counts fall below a certain level) remains under review by clinical experts. *Guidelines for the Use of Antiretroviral Agents in HIV-Infected Adults and Adolescents*, by the Department of Health and Human Services Panel on Clinical Practices for Treatment of HIV Infection, may be helpful to the clinician who is caring for a patient infected with HIV-2; however, the recommendations on viral load monitoring and the use of NNRTIs would not apply to patients with HIV-2 infection. Copies of the guidelines are available from the CDC National Prevention Information Network (1-800-458-5231) and from their Web site (www.cdcnac.org). The guidelines also are available from the HIV/AIDS Treatment Information Service (1-800-448-0440; Fax 301-519-6616; TTY 1-800-243-7012) and on the ATIS Web site (www.hivatis.org).

What Is Known about HIV-2 Infection in Children?

HIV-2 infection in children is rare. Compared with HIV-1, HIV-2 seems to be less transmissible from an infected mother to her child. However, cases of transmission from an infected woman to her fetus or newborn have been reported among women who had primary HIV-2 infection during their pregnancy. Zidovudine therapy has been demonstrated to reduce the risk for perinatal HIV-1 transmission and also might prove effective for reducing perinatal HIV-2 transmission. Zidovudine therapy should be considered for HIV-2-infected expectant mothers and their newborns, especially for women who become infected during pregnancy.

How Should Physicians and Patients Decide Whether to Start Treatment for HIV-2?

Physicians caring for patients with HIV-2 infection should decide whether to initiate antiretroviral therapy after discussing with their patients what is known, what is not known, and the possible adverse effects of treatment.

What Can Be Done to Control the Spread of HIV-2?

Continued surveillance is needed to monitor HIV-2 in the U.S. population because the possibility for further spread of HIV-2 exists, especially among injecting drug users and people with multiple sex partners. Programs aimed at preventing the transmission of HIV-1 also can help to prevent and control the spread of HIV-2.

Suggested Reading

CDC. Testing for antibodies to human immunodeficiency virus type 2 in the United States. *MMWR* 1992;41(No. RR-12).

CDC. Update: HIV-2 infection among blood and plasma donors— United States, June 1992–June 1995. *MMWR* 1995;44:603-06.

De Cock KM, Adjorlolo G, Ekpini E, et al. Epidemiology and transmission of HIV-2: why there is no HIV-2 pandemic. *JAMA* 1993;270: 2083-86.

Faye A, Burgard M, Crosnier H, Retbi J, Blanche S. Human immunodeficiency virus type 2 infection in children. *J Pediatr* 1997;130:994-97.

Markovitz DM. Infection with the human immunodeficiency virus type 2. *Ann Intern Med* 1993; 118:211-18.

O'Brien TR, George JR, Holmberg SD. Human immunodeficiency virus type 2 infection in the United States. *JAMA* 1992;267:2775-79.

Chapter 5

HIV and AIDS: Are You at Risk?

While it's almost certain that you've heard quite a bit about AIDS in the past few years, the term HIV might be new to you.

HIV and AIDS are closely related, and if you understand HIV infection, you can better understand AIDS.

What Is AIDS?

AIDS stands for acquired immunodeficiency syndrome, a disease in which the body's immune system breaks down. Normally, the immune system fights off infections and certain other diseases. When the system fails, a person with AIDS can develop a variety of life-threatening illnesses.

AIDS Is Caused by HIV

AIDS is caused by a virus called the human immunodeficiency virus, or HIV. A virus is one of the smallest "germs" that can cause disease.

If you have unprotected sex (sexual intercourse without consistent and correct condom use) or share needles or syringes with an infected person, you may become infected with HIV. Specific blood tests can show evidence of HIV infection. You can be infected with HIV and have no symptoms at all. You might feel perfectly healthy, but if you're infected, you can pass the virus to anyone with whom you have unprotected sex or share needles or syringes.

Centers for Disease Control and Prevention, September 1994.

Will You Get AIDS If You Are Infected with HIV?

About half of the people infected with HIV develop AIDS within 10 years, but the time between infection with HIV and the onset of AIDS can vary greatly. The severity of the HIV-related illness or illnesses will differ from person to person, according to many factors, including the overall health of the individual.

Today there are promising medical treatments that can postpone many of the illnesses associated with AIDS. This is a step in the right direction, and scientists are becoming optimistic that HIV infection will someday be controllable. In the meantime, people who get medical care to monitor and treat their HIV infection can carry on with their lives, including their jobs, for longer than ever before.

How Can You Become Infected with HIV?

You can become infected with HIV in two main ways:

• Having unprotected sexual intercourse—anal, vaginal, or oral—with an infected person.

• Sharing drug needles or syringes with an infected person.

Also, women infected with HIV can pass the virus to their babies during pregnancy or during birth. They can also pass it on when breast-feeding. Some people have become infected by receiving blood transfusions. Since 1985, however, when careful screening and laboratory testing of all blood donations began, this possibility has been greatly reduced.

You cannot be infected by giving blood at a blood bank.

You Can Get HIV from Sexual Intercourse

HIV can be spread through sexual intercourse, from male to male, male to female, female to male, and from female to female.

HIV is sexually transmitted, and HIV is not the only infection that is passed through intimate sexual contact. Other sexually transmitted diseases (STDs), such as gonorrhea, syphilis, herpes, and chlamydia, can also be contracted through anal, vaginal, and oral intercourse. If you have one of these STDs and engage in sexual behaviors that can transmit HIV, you are at greater risk of getting infected with HIV.

HIV may be in an infected person's blood, semen, or vaginal secretions. HIV can enter the body through cuts or sores in the skin.

HIV can also enter the body through the moist lining of the vagina, penis, rectum, or even the mouth, in which case cuts and sores in these areas greatly increase the risk of infection. Some of these cuts or sores are so small you may not even know they're there. Anal intercourse with an infected person is one of the ways HIV has been most frequently transmitted. Other forms of sexual intercourse, including oral sex, can spread it as well. During oral sex, a person who takes semen, blood, or vaginal secretions into their mouth is at risk of becoming infected.

Many infected people have no symptoms and have not been tested. If you have unprotected sex with one of them, you put yourself in danger. Also, the more sex partners you have, the greater your chances of encountering one or more who are infected and of becoming infected yourself. The only sure way to avoid infection through sex is to abstain from sexual intercourse or engage in sexual intercourse only with someone who is not infected and only has sex with you. Latex condoms have been shown to prevent HIV infection and other sexually transmitted diseases. But you have to use condoms correctly every time you have sex—vaginal, anal, or oral. Condoms made of plastics such as polyurethane should also be highly effective. Condoms made of lambskin, however, do not offer good protection.

You Can Get HIV from Sharing Needles

Sharing needles or syringes with an infected person, even once, is very risky. Many people have become infected with HIV and other germs this way. HIV from an infected person can remain in a needle or syringe and then be injected directly into the body of the next person who uses it. Sharing needles to inject drugs is the most dangerous form of needle sharing.

Sharing needles for other purposes may also transmit HIV and other germs. These types of needles include those used to inject steroids or vitamins and those used for tattooing or ear-piercing.

If you plan to have your ears pierced or get a tattoo, make sure you go to a qualified person who uses brand-new or sterile equipment. Don't be shy about asking questions. Responsible technicians will explain the safety measures they follow.

HIV and Babies

A woman infected with HIV can pass the virus on to her baby during pregnancy, while giving birth, or when breast-feeding. If a woman is infected before or during pregnancy, without medical treatment her child has about one chance in four of being born with HIV infection. Medical treatment with AZT during pregnancy and labor may reduce the risk of infecting the baby to about 1 in 12. There must be no breast-feeding by the infected mother and the baby must be given AZT for the first several weeks of life. Even then, the risk of infecting the child cannot be totally eliminated.

Any woman who is considering having a baby and who thinks she might have done something that could have caused her to become infected with HIV—even if this occurred years ago—should seek counseling and testing for HIV infection to help her make an informed choice about becoming pregnant. To find out where to go in your area for counseling and testing, call your local health department or the CDC National AIDS Hotline (1-800-342-AIDS).

Blood Transfusions and HIV

In the past some people became infected with HIV from receiving blood transfusions. This risk has been practically eliminated. Since a 1983 Public Health Service recommendation, potential blood donors at risk of HIV infection have been asked not to donate blood. Since 1985 all donated blood has been tested for evidence of HIV. All blood found to contain evidence of HIV infection is discarded. Currently in the United States, there is only a very small chance of infection with HIV through a blood transfusion.

You cannot get HIV from giving blood at a blood bank or other blood collection center. The needles used for blood donations are sterile. They are used once, then destroyed.

How You Cannot Get HIV

HIV infection doesn't "just happen." You can't "catch" it like a cold or flu. Unlike cold or flu viruses, HIV is not spread by coughs or sneezes. Again, you get HIV by coming in contact with infected blood, semen, or vaginal fluids from another person.

- You won't get HIV through everyday contact with infected people at school, work, home, or anywhere else.

- You won't get HIV from clothes, drinking fountains, phones, or toilet seats. It isn't passed on by things like forks, cups, or other objects that someone who is infected with the virus has used.

- You won't get HIV from eating food prepared by an infected person.

- You won't get HIV from a mosquito bite. HIV does not live in a mosquito, and it is not transmitted through a mosquito's bite like other germs, such as the ones that cause malaria. You won't get it from bedbugs, lice, flies, or other insects, either.

- You won't get HIV from contact with sweat, saliva, or tears.

- You won't get HIV from a simple kiss. Most scientists agree that although transmission of HIV through deep or prolonged kissing may be possible because of potential blood contact, it would be unlikely.

Who Is Really at Risk for HIV Infection?

There is evidence that HIV, the virus that causes AIDS, has been in the United States at least since 1978. The following are known risk factors for HIV. You may be at increased risk of infection if any of the following have applied to you since 1978.

- Have you shared needles or syringes to inject drugs or steroids?

- If you are a male, have you had unprotected sex with other males?

- Have you had unprotected sex with someone who you believe may have been infected with HIV?

- Have you had a sexually transmitted disease (STD)?

- Have you received blood transfusions or blood clotting factor between 1978 and 1985?

- Have you had unprotected sex with someone who would answer yes to any of the above questions?

If you answered yes to any of the above questions, you should discuss your need for testing with a trained counselor. If you are a woman in any of the above categories and you plan to become pregnant, counseling and testing are even more important.

If you have had unprotected sex with someone and you didn't know their risk behavior, or you have had many sex partners in the last ten years, then you have increased the chances that you might be HIV-infected.

What about the HIV Test?

The only way to tell if you have been infected with HIV is by taking an HIV-antibody blood test. This test should be done through a testing site, doctor's office, or clinic familiar with the test. It is important that you discuss what the test may mean with a qualified health professional, both before and after the test is done.

Do You Need More Information about HIV or HIV Counseling and Testing?

You can receive free publications from the Centers for Disease Control and Prevention. To receive brochures, or to ask any questions about HIV infection or AIDS, call the CDC National AIDS Hotline at 1-800-342-AIDS (Spanish: 1-800-344-7432; deaf access: 1-800-243-7889 [TTY]). The Hotline is staffed with information specialists who can offer a wide variety of written materials or answer your questions about HIV infection and AIDS in a prompt, confidential manner. There are also local groups that can help you find the information you need. Contact your State or local health department, AIDS service organization, or other community-based organization dealing with HIV and AIDS. The CDC National AIDS Hotline can tell you how to contact all of these.

Chapter 6

Pediatric AIDS

Overview

The National Institute of Allergy and Infectious Diseases (NIAID) has a lead role in research devoted to children infected with the human immunodeficiency virus (HIV), the virus that causes the acquired immunodeficiency syndrome (AIDS).

NIAID-supported researchers are developing and refining treatments to prolong the survival and improve the quality of life of HIV-infected infants, children and adolescents. Many promising therapies are being tested in the Pediatric AIDS Clinical Trials Group (ACTG), a nationwide clinical trials network jointly sponsored by NIAID and the National Institute of Child Health and Human Development (NICHD). Scientists also are improving tests for diagnosing HIV infection in infants soon after birth so that therapy can begin as soon as possible.

Epidemiologic studies are examining risk factors for transmission as well as the course of HIV disease in pregnant women and their babies in an era of antiretroviral therapy. Researchers have helped illuminate the mechanisms of HIV transmission as well as the distinct features of pediatric HIV infection and how the course of disease and the usefulness of therapies can differ in children and adults.

Researchers also are studying ways to prevent transmission of HIV from mother to infant. Notably, Pediatric ACTG investigators have demonstrated that a specific regimen of zidovudine (AZT) treatment,

National Institute of Allergy and Infectious Diseases (NIAID), April 1997.

given to an HIV-infected woman during pregnancy and to her baby after birth, can reduce maternal transmission of HIV by two-thirds. Many consider this finding to be one of the most significant research advances to date in the fight against HIV and AIDS.

The Scope of the Problem

The Joint United Nations Programme on HIV/AIDS (UNAIDS) and the World Health Organization (WHO) estimate that by late 1996, 2.6 million children worldwide had been infected with HIV and 1.3 million had died as a result. By 2000, the WHO projects that 5 to 10 million children will have been infected with HIV, with another 5 to 10 million children orphaned by the HIV/AIDS pandemic.

In the United States, through December 1996, 7,629 cases of AIDS in children younger than 13 and 2,754 cases in those aged 13 through 19 had been reported to the Centers for Disease Control and Prevention (CDC). Many other children are currently infected with HIV but have not yet developed AIDS.

HIV infection ranks seventh among the leading causes of death for U.S. children 1 to 14 years of age. In many cities in the northeastern United States, HIV disease is the leading cause of death among children ages 2 to 5.

Transmission

Almost all HIV-infected children acquire the virus from their mothers before or during birth, a process called perinatal transmission. In the United States, approximately 25 percent of pregnant HIV-infected women not receiving AZT therapy have passed on the virus to their babies.

Most perinatal transmission, causing an estimated 50 to 80 percent of infections in children, probably occurs late in pregnancy or during birth. Although the precise mechanisms are unknown, scientists think HIV may be transmitted when maternal blood enters the fetal circulation, or by mucosal exposure to virus during labor and delivery. The role of the placenta in maternal-fetal transmission is unclear and the focus of ongoing research.

The risk of perinatal transmission is significantly increased if the mother has advanced HIV disease, increased levels of HIV in her bloodstream, or fewer numbers of the immune system cells—CD4+ T cells—that are the main targets of HIV.

Other factors that may increase the risk of perinatal transmission are maternal drug use, severe inflammation of fetal membranes, or a prolonged period between membrane rupture and delivery. A recent study sponsored by NIAID and others found that HIV-infected women who gave birth more than four hours after the rupture of the fetal membranes were nearly twice as likely to transmit HIV to their infants, as compared to women who delivered within four hours of membrane rupture.

HIV also may be transmitted from a nursing mother to her infant. Recent studies suggest that breast-feeding introduces an additional risk of HIV transmission of approximately 14 percent among women with chronic HIV infection. The WHO recommends that all HIV-infected women be advised as to both the risks and benefits of breast-feeding of their infants so that they can make informed decisions. In countries where safe alternatives to breast-feeding are readily available and economically feasible, this alternative should be encouraged. In general, in developing countries where safe alternatives to breast-feeding are not readily available, the benefits of breast-feeding in terms of decreased illness and death due to other infectious diseases greatly outweigh the potential risk of HIV transmission.

Prior to 1985 when screening of the nation's blood supply for HIV began, some children were infected through transfusions with blood or blood products contaminated with HIV. A small number of children also have been infected through sexual or physical abuse by HIV-infected adults.

Preventing Perinatal HIV Transmission

In 1994, a landmark study conducted by the Pediatric ACTG demonstrated that AZT, given to HIV-infected women who had very little or no prior antiretroviral therapy and CD4+ T cell counts above 200/ mm^3 reduced the risk of maternal-infant transmission by two-thirds, from 25 percent to 8 percent.

In the study, known as ACTG 076, AZT therapy was initiated in the second or third trimester and continued during labor, and infants were treated for six weeks following birth. AZT produced no serious side effects in mothers or infants; long-term follow-up of the infants and mothers is ongoing.

Researchers have subsequently shown that this AZT regimen has reduced perinatal transmission in other populations in which it has been used. Several recent observational studies in the United States and Europe indicate that similar reductions in perinatal HIV transmission can be achieved by using this regimen in regular clinical care settings.

Following up on the success of ACTG 076, the Pediatric ACTG has begun new perinatal HIV prevention trials that build on the AZT regimen. These trials include additional antiretrovirals in an attempt to reduce perinatal HIV transmission even more than that achieved by AZT alone.

The AZT regimen used in ACTG 076 is not always available because of cost and logistical demands. Therefore, NIAID is pursuing a global strategy that assesses whether simpler and less costly regimens for preventing mother-to-infant HIV transmission can be effective in various settings.

Because a significant amount of perinatal HIV transmission occurs around the time of birth, and the risk of maternal-fetal transmission depends, in part, on the amount of HIV in the mother's blood, it may be possible to reduce transmission using drug therapy only around the time of birth.

NIAID has planned other studies that will assess the effectiveness of this approach as well as the role of new antiretrovirals, microbicides and other innovative strategies in reducing the risk of perinatal transmission.

Diagnosis

HIV infection is often difficult to diagnose in very young children. Infected babies, especially in the first few months of life, often appear normal and may exhibit no telltale signs that would allow a definitive diagnosis of HIV infection. Moreover, all children born to infected mothers have antibodies to HIV, made by the mother's immune system, that cross the placenta to the baby's bloodstream before birth and persist for up to 18 months. Because these maternal antibodies reflect the mother's but not the infant's infection status, the test is not useful in newborns or young infants.

In the past few years, investigators have demonstrated the utility of highly accurate blood tests in diagnosing HIV infection in children 6 months of age and younger. One laboratory technique called polymerase chain reaction (PCR) can detect minute quantities of the virus in an infant's blood. Another procedure allows physicians to culture a sample of an infant's blood and test it for the presence of HIV.

Currently, PCR assays or HIV culture techniques can identify at birth about one-third of infants who are truly HIV-infected. With these techniques, approximately 90 percent of HIV-infected infants are identifiable by 2 months of age, and 95 percent by 3 months of age. One innovative new approach to both RNA and DNA PCR testing uses dried blood spot specimens, which should make it much simpler to gather and store specimens in field settings.

Progression of HIV Disease in Children

Researchers have observed two general patterns of illness in HIV-infected children. About 20 percent of children develop serious disease in the first year of life; most of these children die by age 4 years.

The remaining 80 percent of infected children have a slower rate of disease progression, many not developing the most serious symptoms of AIDS until school entry or even adolescence.

A recent report from a large European registry of HIV-infected children indicated that half of the children with perinatally acquired HIV disease were alive at age 9. Another study, of 42 perinatally HIV-infected children who survived beyond 9 years of age, found about one-quarter of the children to be asymptomatic with relatively intact immune systems.

The factors responsible for the wide variation observed in the rate of disease progression in HIV-infected children are a major focus of the NIAID pediatric AIDS research effort. The Women and Infants Transmission Study, a multisite perinatal HIV study funded by NIH, has found that maternal factors including Vitamin A level and CD4 counts during pregnancy, as well as infant viral load and CD4 counts in the first several months of life, can help identify those infants at risk for rapid disease progression who may benefit from early aggressive therapy.

Signs and Symptoms of Pediatric HIV Disease

Many children with HIV infection do not gain weight or grow normally. HIV-infected children frequently are slow to reach important milestones in motor skills and mental development such as crawling, walking and speaking. As the disease progresses, many children develop neurologic problems such as difficulty walking, poor school performance, seizures, mental retardation and cerebral palsy.

Like adults with HIV infection, children with HIV develop life-threatening opportunistic infections (OIs), although the incidence of various OIs differs in adults and children. For example, toxoplasmosis is seen less frequently in HIV-infected children than in HIV-infected adults, while serious bacterial infections occur more commonly in children than in adults. Also, as children with HIV become sicker, they may suffer from chronic diarrhea due to opportunistic pathogens.

Pneumocystis carinii pneumonia (PCP) is the leading cause of death in HIV-infected children with AIDS. PCP, as well as cytomegalovirus (CMV) disease, usually are new infections in children, whereas in adults these diseases result from the reactivation of latent infections.

A lung disease called lymphocytic interstitial pneumonitis (LIP), rarely seen in adults, also occurs frequently in HIV-infected children. This condition, like PCP, can make breathing progressively more difficult and often results in hospitalization.

Children with HIV suffer the usual childhood bacterial infections—only more frequently and more severely than uninfected children. These bacterial infections can cause seizures, fever, pneumonia, recurrent colds, diarrhea, dehydration and other problems that often result in extended hospital stays and nutritional problems.

HIV-infected children frequently have severe candidiasis, a yeast infection that can cause unrelenting diaper rash and infections in the mouth and throat that make eating difficult.

Treatment of HIV-Infected Children

Anti-HIV Therapies

NIAID investigators are defining the best treatments for pediatric patients. Largely due to studies in the Pediatric ACTG, four anti-HIV agents are currently approved for use in children. In addition, two protease inhibitors are now approved for children with HIV disease. Most doctors consider giving anti-HIV therapy to children who have HIV-related symptoms or who have laboratory evidence of immunosuppression.

NIAID-supported researchers have demonstrated that two treatment regimens—ddI alone or in combination with AZT—are each superior to AZT alone in children who have had little or no previous antiretroviral therapy. Many other promising new antiretroviral regimens are being assessed for use in children in the Pediatric ACTG, including various combinations of nevirapine, d4T, lamivudine (3TC), and 1592U89. The Institute also is undertaking clinical trials of new protease inhibitors in pediatric patients, as well as novel treatment approaches such as gene therapy. The overall trend in both adult and pediatric HIV disease management is for early and aggressive use of combination antiretroviral therapy to keep HIV virus replication at as low a level as possible.

Opportunistic Infections

Many medications used to treat adults with opportunistic infections are effective in children when given in appropriate doses. For example, 85 percent of HIV-infected children are able to tolerate trimethoprim-sulfamethoxazole (TMP/SMX) for PCP. This drug is extremely effective in preventing new or recurrent PCP in children and is the first choice for pediatric patients, as it is in adult patients. NIAID studies are assessing alternative treatments to prevent PCP in children who do not benefit from or cannot tolerate TMP/SMX.

NIAID investigators are developing pediatric formulations of other agents commonly used against OIs, and to understand how children absorb and metabolize these drugs.

Immune Product Studies

Clinical trials sponsored by NIAID and NICHD have demonstrated that intravenous immunoglobulin (IVIG), a preparation containing many types of antibodies, can reduce bacterial infections frequent in children with AIDS. However, the NIAID study suggested that the benefits of IVIG are confined to those patients who had not received TMP/SMX as preventive therapy for PCP. Studies are now underway to assess whether specially made immune globulin products with extra antibodies to HIV can further improve the health status of children with HIV.

AIDS in Adolescents

Adolescents account for a rapidly growing percentage of the reported AIDS cases in the United States. Although less than 1 percent of AIDS patients in the United States are between 13 and 19 years of age, this figure underestimates the significance of HIV transmission during adolescence. Since the average period of time from HIV infection to the development of AIDS is 10 years, the majority of people in their twenties with AIDS were likely infected as adolescents. Approximately 20 percent of all reported cases of AIDS in the United States have occurred in young adults between the ages of 20 and 29.

Several recent studies have found that increasing numbers of teenagers are becoming infected with HIV, especially in poor, urban areas as well as in rural areas of the South. Surveys of military recruits and Job Corps participants as well as blinded seroprevalance studies indicate that as many as one in 20 individuals aged 15 to 20 years from certain populations in the northeastern and southern United States are HIV-infected.

Psychosocial Issues

A disproportionate number of children with AIDS belong to minority groups: 84 percent of children reported with AIDS in 1996 in the United States were black or Hispanic. Most live in inner cities, where poverty, illicit drug use, poor housing and limited access to and use of medical care and social services add to the challenges of HIV disease. A mother and child with HIV usually are not the only family members with the disease. Often, the mother's sexual partner is infected, and other children in the family may be infected as well. Frequently, a mother with AIDS does not survive to care for her HIV-infected child.

Management of the complex medical and social problems of families affected by HIV requires a multidisciplinary case management team, integrating medical, social, mental health and educational services. NIAID provides special funding to many of its clinical research sites to provide for services, such as transportation, day care, and the expertise of social workers, crucial to families devastated by HIV.

Chapter 7

Youth and HIV/AIDS: A Generation at Risk

Today's youth are tomorrow's future. Yet, every year in the United States half of all new HIV infections occur among people under the age of 25 and one-quarter of new infections occurs among people between the ages of 13 and 21. Based on current trends, that means that an average of two young people are infected with HIV every hour of every day.

While the number of cases of AIDS among teenagers is relatively low, it has grown rapidly from one case in 1981 to 417 cases in 1994. The rate of HIV infection among teenagers becomes more apparent when you examine the number of AIDS cases among people in their 20s. According to the Centers for Disease Control and Prevention (CDC), one in five AIDS cases in the U.S. is diagnosed in the 20-29 year age group. Looking at AIDS cases alone obscures the extent of the epidemic among young people. Since a majority of AIDS cases are likely to have resulted from HIV infections acquired 10 years before, most of these individuals are likely to have been infected as teenagers.

Among adolescents (13-19 years of age), HIV infection is more prevalent among those in their late teens, males, and racial and ethnic minorities. But recent trends also point to a rise in infection and diagnosis among adolescent females—increasing from 14 percent of diagnosed cases of AIDS among adolescents in 1987 to 43 percent in 1994.

Excerpted from *Youth and HIV/AIDS: An American Agenda*, A Report to the President, prepared by the Office of National AIDS Policy, March 1996.

What is also clear is that American adolescents are engaging in behaviors that put them at risk for acquiring HIV infection as well as other sexually transmitted diseases, unintended pregnancy, and infections associated with drug injection. According to the CDC, approximately three-quarters of high school students have had sexual intercourse by the time they complete the twelfth grade. About 50 percent of sexually-active high school seniors report consistent use of latex condoms and surveys indicate that condom use declines with age. In a recent survey, one in 62 high school students reported having injected an illegal drug. Recent reports indicate an increase in the use of non-injectable drugs, including marijuana, cocaine, and alcohol. The use of alcohol and other drugs impairs judgment and can lead to risky sexual behaviors and practices, particularly for young people in the stage of experimentation.

Also according to the CDC, about 12 million cases of sexually transmitted diseases (STDs) are reported in the U.S. each year. Roughly two-thirds of those cases are reported in individuals under the age of 25 and one-quarter are among teenagers. About 3 million teens contract an STD each year, and many of these young people will suffer long-term health consequences as a result.

Without forceful and focused action, these already troubling trends may worsen. This is a particularly complex challenge. Adolescents are neither large children nor small adults, yet they often are treated as one or the other and their unique characteristics and needs are often overlooked. Adolescents are in a developmental stage that can make them particularly vulnerable—both physiologically and emotionally—to activities that put them at risk of becoming infected with HIV.

Young people are at greatest risk of HIV infection if they have unprotected sex outside of a mutually monogamous relationship between two HIV-negative individuals, use injection drugs, or use alcohol or other drugs that impair their decision-making abilities. Adolescents often do not have the maturity, experience, or range of options that adults usually bring to their decision-making processes. Adolescents are engaged in a developmental process that includes development of decision-making skills, sexual maturation and experimentation, emotional and cognitive changes, and the molding of identity and self-worth.

Adolescents live in a world in which their families, cultural institutions, religious institutions, media, and peers compete to instill values, dictate actions, and impart positive and negative messages to them. The mass media often glamorizes youth and sex at the same time that parents and schools are encouraging abstinence. Attempts to turn young people into sex symbols are particularly troublesome because of the message that sends to both young people and adults.

Adolescents, particularly those in their early teens, tend to be short-term thinkers. To many, the present is all important and the future often is perceived in very vague terms. Some adolescents, then, feel invulnerable to harm and often make decisions based on immediate desires rather than after consideration of the long-term consequences of their decisions.

Many young people have an enhanced sense of invincibility and may be unprepared to respond to situations that place them at risk. They may not perceive a need to avoid the risk or be aware that certain behaviors can place them at risk for contracting HIV. At the same time, many young people experience stigmatization and discrimination because of their race, ethnicity, gender, sexual orientation, HIV status, or economic status. Such discrimination hampers their ability to navigate successfully the many challenges and complex situations that they confront.

Set against this backdrop is the fact that young Americans are beginning the physiological and emotional process of puberty earlier in their lives than did previous generations. Yet they are also postponing many traditional adult responsibilities including full-time employment, marriage, or a committed monogamous relationship.

All young people need thoughtful guidance and loving care. The role of parents has never been more important in the successful development of adolescents. But it is a job that has also become much tougher. Parents, too, need assistance in learning how to best communicate with their children about the often difficult subjects of sex, drug use, and death. Many adolescents do not have adults in their lives who can effectively provide the nurturing and guidance that they need.

Some young people are at particular risk of HIV infection due to circumstances that are often beyond their control. Adolescents who are victims of sexual abuse are at risk for direct transmission from their sexual partners and may also suffer emotional problems that lead them to later engage in high-risk behavior that can lead to HIV infection.

There are also those youth who have left or been kicked out of their homes or who have fled abusive family relationships. They are highly susceptible to risky behavior just to survive. Their sense of self-worth is usually low or non-existent. They may trade sex for food, housing, drugs, and affection. Adolescents challenged with homelessness rarely view reducing their risk factors for HIV as a high priority in comparison with their daily struggle for survival.

Gay, lesbian, and bisexual youth often are isolated from positive adult role models and peers. Personal, institutional, and societal homophobia can often deny them access to opportunities to address their developing sexuality and contribute to a feeling of worthlessness.

Adolescents need the tools to successfully navigate an increasingly dangerous world. Young people need to hear from parents and other adults that they are loved, valued, and have worth as individuals so they will internalize those feelings and believe they are worth protecting. They must be shown the dangers they may encounter and taught negotiation and decision-making skills. They need to be engaged in activities that will allow them and their peers to practice those skills. And they need to exert personal responsibility to protect both themselves and others from infection.

Adolescent HIV prevention is a job too big for any one segment of society. All parents, adults, leaders, policymakers, young people, and institutions must become constructively engaged in the important work of preventing HIV infection among our nation's most precious resource.

Prevention

Until a vaccine is found, the only way to prevent new HIV infections is through education. Adolescents can protect themselves if they are given comprehensive information and the tools, skills, and reasons to use them. It is incumbent on all adolescents to demonstrate personal responsibility by protecting themselves and others. Communities promoting the close cooperation of parents, teachers, coaches, clergy, physicians, and other adults interacting with youth can ensure that every young person has access to this information. Every adult who touches a young person's life should be equipped to impart this knowledge in a clear, accurate, sensitive manner.

Parents can be the best teachers for their children and HIV prevention approaches for adolescents should ideally start with parents. Parents should be key participants in HIV prevention efforts. If parents aren't convinced of the risk to their children, they may fail to recognize their child's risk-taking behavior. More must be done to educate the parents of adolescents about the risks their children face and about the means that are available to protect their children from this disease.

Efforts to encourage sexual abstinence should continue to be supported. Teens who are thinking about becoming sexually active should be encouraged to consider the implications of their decision and to examine whether they are prepared to deal responsibly with these behaviors (including taking personal responsibility for the consequences of these behaviors and protecting themselves and their partners against disease and unintended pregnancy). It is important that young people make healthy and safe choices about sex. To help them make those decisions, families and communities should help their young citizens to grow and develop to their full potential and provide them with a safe environment to accomplish that growth through schools, role models, and other opportunities. Without community support and reinforcement, even the best HIV prevention approaches will falter or fail.

Effective HIV prevention is neither a single program nor a single event; it must take place over the course of many years and be developmentally appropriate. Therefore, it is inadvisable to separate HIV prevention from sexually transmitted disease prevention, pregnancy prevention, substance abuse prevention, sexuality education, self-esteem activities, and human development education.

National Institutes of Health (NIH) programs on adolescent risk behavior and HIV infection include programs to identify and develop potential intervention strategies for decreasing the high-risk behaviors of young people. Model programs are being developed to increase adolescent STD/HIV prevention knowledge, improve attitudes, and develop skills to delay adolescent sexual activity. Many of these programs are developing and testing culturally sensitive and gender appropriate interventions that target the reduction of AIDS risk behaviors among diverse groups of adolescents. Some of these interventions have already produced positive behavior change among homeless and runaway youth.

Successful prevention efforts concentrate on providing access to accurate information, personalizing this information to motivate change, providing training in behavioral skills for implementing decisions, and reinforcing and rehearsing skills to build competence, communication, and self-esteem. Reality-based approaches recognize that people sometimes use faulty judgment and incorporate efforts to emphasize the ability of individuals to recommit to their long-term goals.

Schools are a highly effective and appropriate place to teach young people HIV prevention information and skills before they begin the behaviors that put them at risk for HIV infection. An estimated 98 percent of young people between the ages of 5 and 17 are enrolled in schools. The Centers for Disease Control and Prevention (CDC) has implemented a multi-faceted program to help schools and other agencies that serve youth across the nation provide effective health education to prevent the spread of HIV. This program is based on the principle that the specific scope and content of HIV education in schools should be consistent with parental and community values. CDC provides funding and technical assistance to the departments of education in every state, six territories, and 18 large cities. CDC also has developed "Guidelines for Effective School Health Education to Prevent the Spread of AIDS."

Beginning at the earliest appropriate age, young people should receive sexuality and HIV/AIDS education as part of a comprehensive curriculum of health education. Such a curriculum should include accurate information about HIV and modes of transmission, the opportunity to assess personal risk of infection, and skills training. HIV prevention information should be age-, language-, and culturally-relevant and designed to accommodate the context of the lives of young people and their families.

There is a compelling need for comprehensive school-based HIV prevention education, yet those school-based efforts are just one step in a long journey to effectively protecting adolescents from HIV. School-based programs do not reach all youths at risk. Those adolescents not in school—because they have graduated or dropped out— will need to be reached with the same kind of basic information that schools provide to all others.

Misconceptions and misunderstandings about HIV transmission and high-risk behaviors often arise when relevant information is omitted. Sexuality education, when done properly, reflects the needs of the community and acknowledges the value of both abstinence and safer sex as tools to prevent HIV infection. Yet in some school districts, education policies preclude discussion of subjects such as intercourse, homosexuality and bisexuality, and condom use. Discussion of the facts concerning such matters is not inconsistent with also encouraging abstinence or delayed sexual activity.

The job of HIV prevention is too important to be left to health educators alone. As mentioned before, all adults who work with young people should be armed to impart HIV prevention information effectively and sensitively to adolescents in their charge. This requires approaches that work—those designed to work well in a given community—and that can be employed to meet a variety of prevention needs.

Yet, teaching young people something and ensuring that they will follow through with what they've been taught are two separate things.

To be successful, HIV prevention efforts must be targeted and they must be sustained. Lessons learned from efforts to prevent smoking, substance abuse, and teenage pregnancy demonstrate that such efforts can positively affect adolescents' behavior.

In 1994, the Centers for Disease Control and Prevention (CDC) launched the Prevention Marketing Initiative (PMI), a comprehensive HIV/AIDS education and prevention program involving partnerships between Federal, state, and local government and national and community-based organizations throughout the U.S. The PMI specifically targets young adults between the ages of 18 and 25. In 1994 and again in 1995, CDC prepared and distributed public service announcements aimed at young adults that communicate two central messages. First, sexual abstinence or delaying sexual activity is the most effective way to prevent sexual transmission of HIV. Second, for those who are sexually active outside of a mutually monogamous relationship, the correct and consistent use of latex condoms is an effective method of preventing HIV transmission.

Successful HIV prevention efforts also have recognized that behavior isn't changed with knowledge alone. An analysis of approaches that are successful in reducing high risk behavior among young people found that schools often were at the focal point of these efforts and that community-wide, multi-agency efforts were needed both in terms of funding and reinforcement of messages. Successful prevention efforts also have been designed to meet the specific needs of target audiences and offer their services outside the traditional school-based setting.

Community-based organizations are also a valuable and credible source of prevention messages. They can supplement, support, and reinforce messages from within families and schools.

Peer counselors—young people trained in providing HIV/AIDS-specific information—have been shown in NIH-sponsored studies to be particularly successful messengers. Peer educators have repeatedly demonstrated that they can present material in a way that addresses the relevance of HIV and HIV prevention to young people's lives. Adolescents often find prevention messages more believable when they are delivered by their peers.

Peer-led prevention efforts are currently being conducted at a variety of sites around the country but many more such efforts are needed. The challenge lies in supporting the development and application of programs that are innovative and address the needs of adolescents.

59

Testing, Treatment and Care

Advances in science and medical care have enabled individuals living with HIV to live longer, healthier lives. Drugs and treatments now are available to arrest or even prevent opportunistic infections that previously led to death. New classes of drugs now in development may hold promise for dramatic improvements in life expectancy and quality of life. However, in order to access such care, individuals must know their HIV status and be connected to a continuum of care.

Millions of young people who have engaged in high-risk behaviors do not know their HIV status. Adolescents should be strongly encouraged to learn their HIV status. A negative test provides the best opportunity to reinforce the importance and efficacy of risk-reduction behaviors. A positive test provides an immediate opportunity to link those who are HIV-positive to treatment, often at an early stage of disease progression. Such early intervention has been shown to be highly effective at prolonging and improving quality of life.

In 1994, the Centers for Disease Control and Prevention (CDC) supported HIV counseling and testing services in approximately 9,600 sites throughout the U.S. Those sites accommodated approximately 400,000 visits by persons 19 years of age or younger. Many of those services are provided at little or no cost to youth with parental permission. In addition, the CDC supports the National AIDS Hotline and the National AIDS Clearinghouse, which provide referral and information services through toll-free telephone services. Both are private, free, and confidential and are well publicized.

HIV testing should always include appropriate pre- and post-test counseling to ensure that both HIV-negative and HIV-positive young people understand their status and their responsibilities to themselves and others as a result of that status. Pre- and post-test counseling is particularly important for adolescents. Counseling should be appropriate for the adolescents' social and emotional development, language, culture, and sexual orientation. Effective counselors are sensitive to the great anxiety adolescents feel about HIV testing because of fear of the disease as well as the stigma attached to the disease. As with prevention efforts, the use of peer educators in pre- and post-test counseling has been shown to be effective in communicating critical information to adolescents at what is often a highly emotional point.

The process of testing for HIV allows adolescents to evaluate their own behavior and think of the consequences of that behavior. As a result, there are numerous emotional needs that must be dealt with by both adolescent and counselor if the effort is to be a success. The involvement of parents and other family members is critical to an HIV-positive youth's ability to cope with this diagnosis and enter into a continuum of care.

Whether the results are positive or negative, post-test counseling is equally important. For adolescents who test negative, post-test counseling provides an opportunity for further risk reduction. For some, this may be the only opportunity for meaningful prevention education. Positive results require immediate intervention. It is essential that adolescents have an opportunity to talk to knowledgeable persons who can help them understand what their HIV status means and help them deal with issues that may seem overwhelming. HIV-negative youth should have that behavior reinforced.

Adolescents' access to HIV counseling and voluntary testing often is severely limited by a variety of factors. First, many adolescents don't know how to arrange for HIV testing and where to go for such services. Second, adolescents do not have the money or means of transportation necessary to access some forms of counseling and testing. Third, school hours often coincide with the hours of counseling and testing facilities. Finally, parental consent requirements for counseling and voluntary testing also may pose a barrier for many young people—especially those who know or feel they cannot communicate openly with their parents about this subject.

Taken singly, these barriers can make it difficult for an adolescent to get counseled and tested. Combined, they present a formidable barrier that only a truly determined adolescent can surmount.

To address some of these concerns, HIV counseling and voluntary testing sites need to be designed to be accessible to adolescents. Business hours should complement rather than compete with school schedules and facilities should offer their services at low or no cost to adolescents. This would accommodate adolescents who don't own a car and must use public transportation, are in school and involved in extra-curricular activities, and have little money or independent health insurance.

A particularly challenging impediment to counseling and testing is the legal requirement in many states for parental consent. Consent is usually necessary for medical care of individuals under the age of 18. The conditions under which minors may consent to HIV testing vary across states. Ideally, parents, young people, and health care providers should all possess the skills and knowledge necessary to maximize a youth's access to services and support. However, consideration should be given to creating alternative access to counseling and testing where obtaining parental consent is not possible.

Linking HIV-positive adolescents to a system of HIV primary care immediately after a positive diagnosis is vital in order to prevent or delay the onset of HIV-related opportunistic infections, such as *Pneumocystis carinii* pneumonia (PCP), and to prolong the healthy lives of HIV-positive individuals. An integrated care system, in which medical services are connected to mental health, substance abuse, education, juvenile justice, and social support is necessary to meet the needs of these adolescents. For runaway or homeless youth, housing and nutrition services are also critical. Currently, there are few programs that meet the full range of health care needs for HIV-positive youth. Efforts are plagued by insufficient numbers of primary care physicians and other health care providers specifically trained to work with adolescents, lack of insurance and other financial assistance, a fragmented health care system, and geographically remote facilities. NIH is supporting programs to identify better ways of facilitating access, utilization, and adherence to medical, mental health, and substance abuse treatment by adolescents.

Large numbers of young people are uninsured or underinsured, and the sources for funds to pay for necessary services are limited. If an adolescent is HIV-positive access to insurance often is blocked by insurance policies that exclude individuals with pre-existing medical conditions.

Federal grants for program development such as the Health Resources and Services Administration's Ryan White CARE Act, including Special Programs of National Significance (SPNS), have encouraged care models that consider the special needs of the adolescent population and provide communities with the tools they need to conduct effective outreach programs. Title IV of the Ryan White CARE Act provides support for the development of innovative models that link systems of comprehensive primary/community-based research, medical, and social services for children, adolescents, and families.

Besides responding to an HIV-positive adolescent's physical and mental health needs, linkage with important social services is also an important element to care. Social service providers should be trained to offer referrals for legal assistance, other treatment programs, information about housing, job-training assistance, and help in obtaining health insurance. They also are more able to offer outreach services for adolescents who are homeless, pregnant, or trading sex for food and shelter.

Medicaid provides coverage for a comprehensive set of benefits that includes counseling and testing, prescription drugs, physician visits, inpatient hospital care, substance abuse treatment, home care, and hospice care. Medicaid coverage of children and adolescents has been improved in recent years but many low-income families may not be aware of their eligibility for such benefits. The Federal government and states should examine opportunities to ensure that all Medicaid-eligible HIV-positive youth have access to appropriate treatment and care. Medicaid is the largest single payer of direct medical services for people living with AIDS, serving nearly 50 percent of all persons living with AIDS and more than 90 percent of children with AIDS.

Research

HIV/AIDS research has made great strides on many fronts. Physicians have a growing array of medications to treat and even prevent a variety of HIV-related opportunistic infections. As a result, HIV-positive people who have access to care usually are not getting sick as often, their illnesses aren't as severe, and they are spending less time in the hospital than they did 10 years ago. But adolescents have not received the full benefit of recent research discoveries, and there is significant unmet need for adolescent-specific treatment and behavioral research. We clearly do not know enough about adolescents in general, about how HIV affects them physiologically or behaviorally, and about the progress of HIV disease in young people.

HIV/AIDS research efforts have primarily focused on two specific populations: infants and adults. Funding for adolescent-related AIDS research has traditionally come from those pursuing pediatric research. But adolescents are biologically more like adults than infants yet they still are not at the same developmental stage as most adults.

Adolescents are not considered central to the pediatric mission, and researchers who focus on adults usually are not funded to include adolescents in their research programs. The result has been that adolescents appear only peripherally on the radar screens of most AIDS researchers, and when they do, it's only to the extent that they share adults' physical or behavioral traits.

Additionally, a variety of developmental and behavioral factors challenge efforts to draw adolescents into the few adolescent-specific protocols that have been developed for their benefit. Adolescents can sometimes be particularly challenging subjects for research. Researchers have reported difficulty enrolling adolescents in protocols, keeping them enrolled, and ensuring that they are following the guidelines for protocol conduct.

Basic research sponsored by NIH has provided and will continue to provide a better understanding of the pathogenic mechanisms and course of the disease in adolescents.

In recognition of the fact that adolescent development is different from that of both adults and children, NIH is supporting studies on adolescents.

While NIH has opened pediatric clinical trials to adolescents up to age 18 and adults trials to those who are as young as 13, adolescents continue to face barriers to their participation in clinical trials. This lack of participation has left significant gaps in the knowledge base about adolescents. Scientists are quick to acknowledge that a great deal of catching up remains to be done. Basic research on adolescent reproductive and immune system development is lacking. Data are just beginning to be gathered on how the adolescent's immune system differ from that of adults, an important consideration in defining the response of an adolescent's body to HIV. Further studies are needed on the effect HIV has on adolescent growth and puberty.

Additional studies are needed to understand the natural history of HIV in adolescents as well as expanded study of youth and their behaviors. The NIH currently sponsors natural history studies designed to track the shifting demographics and the changing manifestations of HIV/AIDS. But there are things we need to know about HIV-positive adolescents that we don't know, such as how they become infected, how they effectively resist infection, how long they live, and how quickly they die. We don't know enough about the factors that influence the behavior of young people, including why some choose to be sexually active and others do not; why some use drugs or alcohol and others do not; and why certain sexual behaviors are chosen over others.

Surveillance of HIV infection among adolescents in the United States has not been comprehensive enough to accurately estimate the scope of the problem. The family of HIV seroprevalence surveys should be expanded to target and teach us more about the epidemic as it affects young people. Accurate data help to target HIV prevention efforts and to forecast the kinds of services needed. Such studies would help to indicate which communities are experiencing high infection rates, how HIV is being transmitted, how long HIV-infected adolescents are ill, and the general scope of the epidemic among this age group.

The inclusion of adolescents in clinical trials permits the identification of appropriate regimens of treatment for this age group. The development of clinical practice guidelines with correct dosages and times to start treatment can only be developed from such studies. Similarly, the rapid dissemination of information concerning clinical practice guidelines, results of clinical trials, and options for trials, as well as eligibility criteria for trial participation, must be a high priority for the NIH.

There still is not enough information about the optimum time to begin anti-retroviral treatment, which treatments to use, and the correct dosages for adolescents. The lack of a significant base of adolescents enrolled in trials has resulted in little dissemination of information. At this early period in the study of adolescent-related HIV issues, even anecdotal information is important to clinicians and researchers if they are to begin building a response to the epidemic among young people.

The NIH has recognized that current research efforts aimed at young people are few in number and much further behind than those for adults and children. The Adolescent HIV/AIDS Research Network, a collaborative effort between the NIH and the Health Resources and Services Administration (HRSA), has been launched to plan and conduct research on the medical, biobehavioral, and psychosocial aspects of HIV and AIDS in young people. This network, combined with other youth-focused efforts at NIH and CDC, can reduce the barriers to young people participating in research and narrow the information gap. Working together the Federal government and its partners should achieve the goal of providing better treatments and health care to HIV-positive adolescents and crafting Federal responses that best meet their often changing needs.

Chapter 8

HIV, AIDS, and Older Adults

Everyone talks about AIDS (acquired immunodeficiency syndrome), but few talk about how AIDS affects older people. No wonder so many older adults think they are not at risk.

Like many other widespread disease outbreaks of the past, the HIV/AIDS epidemic is having a multigenerational impact on U.S. society. Many persons age 50 or older may have thought that HIV/AIDS would never affect them, but as HIV continues to spread, its impact on older Americans is becoming apparent in a number of ways:

- Approximately 10 percent of all persons diagnosed with AIDS were diagnosed at age 50 or older. According to Centers for Disease Control and Prevention (CDC) statistics, that numbered doubled between 1992 and 1995, rising from 26,053 cases to 52,097.

- Adults in this age group tend to use condoms less frequently than do younger adults practicing the same risky behaviors, according to a study conducted by Ron Stall and Joseph Catania of the Center for AIDS Prevention Studies at the University of California, San Francisco. The study, published in *Archives of Internal Medicine* in 1994, found that older, at-risk heterosexual individuals are one sixth as likely to use condoms during sex and one fifth as likely to have been tested for HIV.

This chapter combines excerpts from "HIV, AIDS, and Older Adults," a fact sheet produced by the National Institute on Aging, 1994, and excerpts from "Locating Basic Resources on HIV/AIDS and Older Americans," CDC National AIDS Clearinghouse, March 1997.

- An estimated one-third of young adults living with HIV/AIDS depend on an older parent—or parents—for financial, physical, and/or emotional support. These parents, in turn, must cope with the fact that they may outlive their children.

- The rate of HIV infection among women of childbearing age is climbing rapidly, especially among certain subpopulations. Their children, in turn, are becoming orphans at a young age; many of these children are left in the care of an aging grandparent.

What Is AIDS?

AIDS is a disease caused by a virus called HIV (short for human immunodeficiency virus). HIV attacks the body's immune system. When the immune system is hurt, it can no longer fight diseases the way it used to.

People with HIV seem to be healthy at first. But after several years, they begin to get sick. Often they get serious infections or cancers. When this happens, they are diagnosed with AIDS. The most common cause of death in people with AIDS is a type of pneumonia called *pneumocystis carinii* pneumonia or PCP.

How Do People Get AIDS?

HIV is spread when body fluids, such as semen and blood, pass from a person who has the infection to another person. For the most part, the virus is spread by sexual contact or by sharing drug needles and syringes.

In older people, sexual activity is the most common cause of HIV infection. Second is blood transfusions received before 1985. Since 1985, blood banks have been testing all blood for HIV, so there is now little danger of getting HIV from transfusions.

Otherwise, HIV is not easy to catch. It is not spread by mosquito bites, using a public telephone or restroom, being coughed or sneezed on by an infected person, or touching someone with the disease.

Is AIDS Different in Older People?

The immune system normally gets weaker with age, but this decline is faster in older AIDS patients. They usually become sick and die sooner than younger patients.

It may be harder to recognize AIDS in older people. Early symptoms of AIDS—feeling tired, confused, having a loss of appetite, and swollen glands—are like other illnesses common in older people. Health professionals may assume these are signs of minor problems.

Prevention

Stopping HIV depends on each person's actions. You can prevent AIDS by thinking about the risk of infection before sexual contact. Use condoms if sexually involved with someone other than a mutually faithful, uninfected partner.

Help and Resources

Older AIDS patients often may not have anyone to take care of them. Help is available from local groups in some cases and from the Social Security Administration (1-800-SSA-1213).

In most cities, health agencies or centers offer HIV testing, counseling, and other services. In addition, the following national organizations offer information:

National AIDS Hotline
1-800-342-AIDS
1-800-344-SIDA for Spanish
1-800-AIDS-889 (TTY)

The hotline operates 24 hours a day, 7 days a week. It offers general information and local referrals.

Senior Action in a Gay Environment (SAGE)
305 7th Avenue
New York, NY 10001
(212) 741-2247
(212) 366-1947 fax
E-mail: sageusa@aol.com

SAGE provides crisis intervention counseling, group and individual counseling, bereavement counseling, safer sex counseling, a buddy program, educational presentations, and professional training for social workers. It also offers support groups for men who are 50 and older with HIV infection, a bereavement support group, and a caregivers support group.

Social Security Administration (SSA)
500 N. Calvert Street
Baltimore, MD 21202
410) 962-0746
Contact local office or call: 1-800-SSA-1213

SSA evaluates disability claims involving HIV/AIDS under two programs: Social Security Disability Insurance (SSDI) and Supplemental Security Income (SSI). To file a claim, an individual may phone his or her local or national Social Security Office.

American Association of Retired Persons (AARP)
Social Outreach and Support (SOS)
Grandparent Information Center
601 E Street, NW
Washington, DC 20049
(202) 434-2260
Website: www.aarp.org

The AARP/SOS program has information on HIV and AIDS and their impact on midlife and older adults. The Grandparent Information Center is maintained for all grandparents who are raising their grandchildren, including those who are caring for their grandchildren due to HIV/AIDS. The Center offers information, referrals, and support groups, and publishes a newsletter titled *Parenting Grandchildren: A Voice for Grandparents*.

Part Two

HIV/AIDS Statistics and Trends

Chapter 9

HIV/AIDS Surveillance Report

Commentary

Through December 1997, 641,086 persons with AIDS have been reported to CDC. From 1995 to 1996, for the first time in the epidemic, the occurrence of AIDS-defining opportunistic illnesses (AIDS-OIs) among infected persons and deaths among persons reported with AIDS decreased 7 percent and 25 percent, respectively. These declines were largely due to the increasing use of combination antiretroviral therapy including protease inhibitors. Perinatally-acquired AIDS incidence continued a pattern of marked decline, principally reflecting successful strategies to promote voluntary prenatal HIV testing and reduce transmission rates through the administration of zidovudine perinatally. These treatment advances have altered the natural history of HIV infection, contributed to an increase in the number of persons living with AIDS, and changed the shape of the epidemic curves. As therapy has improved the health and prospects for AIDS-free survival among HIV-infected persons who receive these new treatment regimens, the ability of AIDS surveillance data to represent the characteristics of affected populations and project the need for resources for prevention and treatment has been diminished. This edition of the *HIV/AIDS Surveillance Report* marks a transition in how CDC will present HIV infection and AIDS data depicting the epidemic.

HIV/AIDS Surveillance Report, Year-end edition, Vol. 9, No.2, Centers for Disease Control and Prevention (CDC), December 1997.

AIDS surveillance data will no longer be adjusted to reflect the incidence of AIDS-OIs. The incidence of AIDS-OIs can no longer be estimated reliably because data are not currently available to model the increasing effects of therapy on the rate of disease progression. The procedure was developed to take into account the 1993 expansion of the AIDS case definition which had a temporary distorting effect on the AIDS incidence curve. In future editions, CDC will publish estimates of AIDS incidence based on the incidence of all AIDS-defining conditions included in the 1993 AIDS surveillance case definition. AIDS data will remain useful as a measure of severe HIV-related morbidity in the population and to represent populations in which treatments have failed or those which were not tested or treated prior to a diagnosis of AIDS.

The proportion of AIDS and HIV infection cases initially reported without risk information has increased in recent years. Several factors have contributed to this increase, including the greater volume of cases after the change in the AIDS case definition in 1993, decreases in surveillance staff in some areas, and increases in heterosexual transmission to persons (especially women) without recognizable high-risk behaviors. In the past, areas that conducted both HIV infection

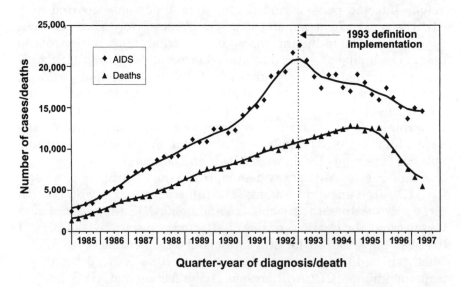

Figure 9.1. Estimated incidence of AIDS and deaths of persons with AIDS, adjusted for delays in reporting, by quarter-year of diagnosis/death, United States, January 1985 through June 1997

74

and AIDS case reporting prioritized the completion of risk information for AIDS rather than HIV infection cases. The high percentage of recent cases that have no reported risk poses difficulties in interpreting the meaning of the proportionate distribution of cases by risk groups. No longer is it possible to compare differences in proportions by risk group for the current year to the previous year without estimating how the cases without risk information will eventually be reclassified. Therefore, in future editions of the *HIV/AIDS Surveillance Report*, tables that present risk data for HIV infection and AIDS cases will be revised to include adjustments for unreported risk in order to enable readers of the report to infer recent trends by risk group.

The trend data for AIDS-OI incidence, deaths, and prevalence are adjusted for delays in reporting of cases and deaths. These adjustments have been routinely applied when presenting trends in AIDS surveillance data for many years, but not for HIV infection surveillance data. HIV infection case surveillance data are currently reported from most, but not all states and the HIV infection and AIDS case reporting systems in these areas were only fully integrated in late 1993. Based on several years experience with delays in reporting of HIV infection cases, delay adjustments for these data have been developed recently. In future editions of the *HIV/AIDS Surveillance Report*, trends in the number of new diagnoses of HIV infection will be presented using these adjustment procedures to enable readers of the report to interpret more recent trends in the epidemic than are reflected in AIDS surveillance data.

Most states and metropolitan statistical areas reported a decrease in the number of AIDS cases reported in 1997 compared to the number reported in 1996. Whereas HIV infection and AIDS incidence are unaffected by surveillance practices, the reporting of HIV infection and AIDS cases to state and territorial health departments can be affected by changes in staffing patterns, evaluation studies which may states that conduct HIV infection case reporting. To interpret unusual patterns in the number of cases reported in some geographic areas, readers of the *HIV/AIDS Surveillance Report* should consult the surveillance staff of the appropriate state or territorial health department.

Since the beginning of the epidemic, CDC has published data on the number and characteristics of AIDS cases reported to CDC by state and territorial health departments. Initially, data were published weekly to help track this previously unrecognized and rapidly burgeoning health threat. Epidemiologic data quickly identified the ways in which the epidemic was spreading and the populations that were at greatest risk of HIV infection. With an increasing number of cases, detecting changes in geographic, demographic, and risk/exposure trends required longer periods of time, and the AIDS data publication schedule was revised to monthly, then quarterly, then semiannually. The ability of AIDS surveillance data to accurately depict the distribution and characteristics of affected populations led to a reliance on these data to describe the epidemic, identify populations in need of HIV prevention programs, and target and allocate resources for medical and other services for infected persons. However, because treatments have affected AIDS incidence rates among infected persons, CDC has stated that all states should implement HIV infection case surveillance as an extension of their AIDS surveillance programs. HIV diagnoses are not affected by treatment. Although all infected persons in the population may not seek or be offered HIV testing, the number of persons diagnosed with HIV infection together with AIDS diagnoses provides a reliable minimum estimate of the number and characteristics of persons who have accessed testing or care. CDC estimates that the majority of infected persons in the U.S. have been tested. The proportion tested among infected persons in the population is expected to increase. Accordingly, integrated HIV infection and AIDS case surveillance data will be useful in planning and evaluating prevention and treatment program needs and outcomes.

While the number and characteristics of reported cases of HIV infection and AIDS in this chapter remain useful as a minimum estimate of the characteristics of persons in need of services and treatment, the HIV/AIDS surveillance system must evolve to meet public health needs for data in a changing epidemic. CDC and state and territorial health departments are currently revising HIV infection and AIDS case finding and reporting methods, changing how surveillance data will be analyzed and presented, and shifting the focus of surveillance program activities from AIDS to HIV infection including AIDS in order to be consistent with current public health recommendations for early voluntary testing, diagnosis, and treatment of HIV-infected persons.

Technical Notes

Surveillance of AIDS

All 50 states, the District of Columbia, U.S. dependencies and possessions, and independent nations in free association with the United

States report AIDS cases to CDC using a uniform surveillance case definition and case report form. The original definition was modified in 1985 (*MMWR* 1985;34:373-75) and 1987 (*MMWR* 1987;36[suppl no. 1S]:1S-15S). The case definition for adults and adolescents was modified again in 1993 (*MMWR* 1992;41 [no. RR-17]:1-19; see also *MMWR* 1995;44:64-67). The revisions incorporated a broader range of AIDS-indicator diseases and conditions and used HIV diagnostic tests to improve the sensitivity and specificity of the definition. The laboratory and diagnostic criteria for the 1987 pediatric case definition (*MMWR* 1987;36:225-30, 235) were updated in 1994 (*MMWR* 1994;43[no. RR-12]:1-19).

For persons with laboratory-confirmed HIV infection, the 1987 revision incorporated HIV encephalopathy, wasting syndrome, and other indicator diseases that are diagnosed presumptively (i.e., without confirmatory laboratory evidence of the opportunistic disease). In addition to the 23 clinical conditions in the 1987 definition, the 1993 case definition for adults and adolescents includes HIV-infected persons with $CD4^+$ T-lymphocyte counts of less than 200 cells/μL or a $CD4^+$ percentage of less than 14, and persons diagnosed with pulmonary tuberculosis, recurrent pneumonia, and invasive cervical cancer. All conditions added to the 1993 definition require laboratory confirmation of HIV infection. Persons who meet the criteria for more than one definition category are classified hierarchically in the following order: pre-1987, 1987, and 1993. Persons in the 1993 definition category meet only the 1993 definition.

The pediatric case definition incorporates the revised 1994 pediatric classification system for evidence of HIV infection. Children with their first positive results on Western blot or HIV detection tests before October 1994 were categorized based on the 1987 classification system. Those tested during or after October 1994 are categorized under the revised 1994 pediatric classification system. For children of any age with an AIDS-defining condition that requires evidence of HIV infection, a single positive HIV-detection test (i.e., HIV culture, HIV PCR, or HIV antigen [p24]) is sufficient for a reportable AIDS diagnosis if the diagnosis is confirmed by a physician.

Although completeness of reporting of diagnosed AIDS cases to state and local health departments varies by geographic region and patient population, studies conducted by state and local health departments indicate that reporting of AIDS cases in most areas of the United States is more than 85 percent complete (*J Acquir Immune Def Syndr*, 1992;5:257-64 and *Am J Public Health* 1992;82:1495-99). In addition, multiple routes of exposure, opportunistic diseases diagnosed after the initial AIDS case report was submitted to CDC, and vital status may not be determined or reported for all cases. However, among persons reported with AIDS, reporting of deaths is estimated to be more than 90 percent complete (*JAMA* 1996;276:126-31).

Included in this report are persons known to be infected with human immunodeficiency virus type 2 (HIV-2). See *MMWR* 1995;44:603-06.

Surveillance of HIV Infection

Through December 31, 1997, 27 states had laws or regulations requiring confidential reporting by name of all persons with confirmed HIV infection, in addition to reporting of persons with AIDS. Two other states, Connecticut and Texas, required reporting by name of HIV infection only for children less than 13 years of age; and Oregon required reporting for children less than 6 years of age. These states initiated reporting at various times after the development of serum HIV-antibody tests in 1985. Before 1991, surveillance of HIV infection was not standardized and reporting of HIV infections was based primarily on passive surveillance. Consequently, many cases reported before 1991 do not have complete information. Since then, CDC has assisted states in conducting active surveillance of HIV infection using standardized report forms and software. However, collection of demographic and risk information still varies among states.

Estimates of the prevalence of HIV infection in the United States in 1992 were between 650,000 and 900,000 (*JAMA* 1996;276:126-31). However, HIV surveillance reports may not be representative of all persons estimated to be infected with HIV since not all infected persons have been tested; HIV infection data should be interpreted with caution. Because many HIV-reporting states also offer anonymous HIV testing in publicly funded sites and through home collection HIV test kits, confidential HIV infection reports may not be representative of all persons being tested in these areas. Furthermore, many factors may influence testing patterns, including the extent that testing is targeted or routinely offered to specific groups and the availability and access to medical care and testing services. These data provide a minimum estimate of the number of persons known to be HIV infected in states with confidential HIV infection reporting.

For this report, persons greater than 18 months of age were considered HIV infected if they had at least one positive Western blot or positive detection test (culture, antigen, or other detection test) or had a diagnosis of HIV infection documented by a physician. Before October 1994, children less than 15 months of age were considered HIV infected if they met the definition stated in the 1987 pediatric classification system for HIV infection (*MMWR* 1987;36:225-30, 235). Beginning October 1994, children less than 18 months of age are considered HIV infected if they meet the definition stated in the 1994 pediatric classification system for HIV infection (*MMWR* 1994;43[no. RR-12]:1-10). This report also includes children who were diagnosed by a physician as HIV infected. Although many states monitor reports of children born to infected mothers, only those with documented diagnosis of HIV infection are included in this report.

Because states initiated reporting on different dates, the length of time reporting has been in place will influence the number of HIV infection cases reported. For example, data presented for a given annual period may include cases reported during only a portion of the year. Prior to statewide HIV reporting, some states collected reports of HIV infection in selected populations. Therefore, these states have reports prior to initiation of statewide confidential reporting. A state with confidential HIV infection reporting also may report persons testing positive in that state who are residents of other states. Therefore, when HIV data are presented by state of residence, persons reported prior to the date a state initiated reporting may have been reported from other states with confidential HIV infection reporting.

Over time, persons with HIV infection will be diagnosed and reported with AIDS. HIV infection cases later reported with AIDS are deleted from the HIV infection tables and added to the AIDS tables. Persons with HIV infection may be tested at any point in the clinical spectrum of disease; therefore, the time between diagnosis of HIV infection and AIDS will vary. In addition, because surveillance practices differ, reporting and updating of clinical and vital status of cases vary among states.

Included in this report are persons known to be infected with human immunodeficiency virus type 2 (HIV-2). See *MMWR* 1995;44:603-06.

Tabulation and Presentation of Data

Data in this report are provisional. Each issue of this report includes information received by CDC through the last day of the reporting period. AIDS data are tabulated by date of report to CDC unless otherwise noted. Data for U.S. dependencies and possessions and for associated independent nations are included in the totals.

Age group tabulations are based on the person's age at first documented positive HIV-antibody test result for HIV infection cases, and age at diagnosis of AIDS for AIDS cases. Adult/adolescent cases include persons 13 years of age and older; pediatric cases include children under 13 years of age.

Tabulations of persons living with HIV infection and AIDS include persons whose vital status was "alive" as of the last update; persons whose vital status is missing or unknown are not included. Tabulations of deaths in persons with AIDS include persons whose vital status was "dead" as of the last update; persons whose vital status is missing or unknown are not included. Caution should be used in interpreting these data because states vary in the frequency with which they review the vital status of persons reported with HIV infection and AIDS. In addition, some cases may be lost to follow-up.

AIDS-indicator conditions data are known to underreport AIDS-indicator conditions and should be interpreted with caution. Reported conditions overrepresent initial AIDS-indicator illness because follow-up for subsequent indicator diseases is resource intensive and has not been systematic or standardized in most health departments. The 1993 AIDS surveillance case definition for adults and adolescents added reporting of HIV-infected persons with severe HIV-related immunosuppression ($CD4^+$ T-lymphocyte count of less than $200/\mu L$ or less than 14 percent). Since implementation of the 1993 definition, reporting of AIDS cases based on AIDS-defining opportunistic infections has decreased (*AIDS* 1994; 8:1489-93).

Estimates of AIDS deaths and estimated persons living with AIDS are not counts of actual numbers of persons reported to the surveillance system. The estimates are adjusted for delays in reporting of cases and deaths and are based on a number of assumptions. While these tables use the best estimates currently available, there is inherent uncertainty in these estimates. Therefore, the estimates in this report are rounded. Other analyses suggest that the uncertainty in these estimates is at least one percent (*J Acquir Immune Def Syndr*, 1997;16:116-21). Therefore, the rounding is to one percent of the upper limit within arbitrarily chosen ranges. State and local surveillance staff are encouraged to adopt similar rounding conventions when presenting estimates. As is standard computational practice, changes in the estimates of the AIDS-OI incidence, estimates of deaths, and estimates of persons living with AIDS should be computed from unrounded numbers, rather than from rounded numbers. That is, an estimate, such as the percent change in annual incidence, should not be computed from the rounded estimates of AIDS-OI incidence. An estimate of change computed from rounded numbers is especially unreliable if the annual estimates are relatively small.

Exposure Categories

For surveillance purposes, HIV infection cases and AIDS cases are counted only once in a hierarchy of exposure categories. Persons with more than one reported mode of exposure to HIV are classified in the exposure category listed first in the hierarchy, except for men with both a history of sexual contact with other men and injecting drug use. They make up a separate exposure category.

"Men who have sex with men" cases include men who report sexual contact with other men (i.e., homosexual contact) and men who report sexual contact with both men and women (i.e., bisexual contact). "Heterosexual contact" cases are in persons who report specific heterosexual contact with a person with, or at increased risk for, HIV infection (e.g., an injecting drug user).

Adults/adolescents born, or who had sex with someone born, in a country where heterosexual transmission was believed to be the predominant mode of HIV transmission (formerly classified as Pattern-II countries by the World Health Organization) are no longer classified as having heterosexually acquired AIDS. Similar to case reports for other persons who are reported without behavioral or transfusion risks for HIV, these reports are now classified (in the absence of other risk information which would classify them into another exposure category) as "no risk reported or identified" (*MMWR* 1994;43:155-60). Children whose mother was born, or whose mother had sex with someone born, in a Pattern-II country are now classified (in the absence of other risk information which would classify them into another exposure category) as "Mother with/at risk for HIV infection: has HIV infection, risk not specified."

"No risk reported or identified" cases are in persons with no reported history of exposure to HIV through any of the routes listed in the hierarchy of exposure categories. "Risk not reported or identified" cases include persons who are currently under investigation by local health department officials; persons whose exposure history is incomplete because they died, declined to be interviewed, or were lost to follow-up; and persons who were interviewed or for whom other follow-up information was available and no exposure mode was identified. Persons who have an exposure mode identified at the time of follow-up are reclassified into the appropriate exposure category. Historically, investigations and follow up for modes of exposure by state health departments were conducted routinely for persons reported with AIDS and as resources allowed for those reported with HIV infection. Therefore, the percentage of HIV infected persons with risk not reported or identified is substantially higher than for those reported with AIDS.

Reporting Delays

Reporting delays (time between diagnosis of HIV infection or AIDS and report to CDC) may vary among exposure, geographic, racial/ethnic, age and sex categories, and have been as long as several years for some AIDS cases. About 50 percent of all AIDS cases were reported to CDC within 3 months of diagnosis and about 80 percent were reported within 1 year. Among persons with AIDS, estimates in delay of reporting of deaths show that approximately 90 percent of deaths are reported within 1 year. For HIV infection cases diagnosed since implementation of uniform reporting through the HIV/AIDS Reporting System on January 1, 1994, about 70 percent of all HIV infection cases were reported to CDC within 3 months of diagnosis and about 95 percent were reported within 1 year. See *MMWR* 1998; 47:309-14.

Reporting delay adjustments to some tables were estimated by a maximum likelihood statistical procedure, taking into account differences in reporting delays among exposure, geographic, racial/ethnic, age, sex, and vital status at diagnosis categories, but assuming that reporting delays within these groups have not changed over time (*Statist Med* 1998; 17:143-54 and *Lecture Notes in Biomathematics* 1989;83:58-88).

Rates

Rates are calculated for 12-month period per 100,000 population for AIDS cases only. Rates are not calculated for HIV infection reports because case counts for HIV infection are believed to be less complete than AIDS case counts. Population denominators for computing AIDS rates for the 50 states and the District of Columbia are based on official postcensus estimates from the U.S. Bureau of Census. Denominators for U.S. dependencies and possessions and associated independent nations are linear extrapolations of official 1980 and 1990 census counts. Each 12-month rate is the number of cases reported during the 12-month period, divided by the 1996 or 1997 population, multiplied by 100,000. The denominators for computing race-specific rates are based on 1997 census estimates published in U.S. Bureau of Census publication PPL-91, "U.S. Population Estimates by Age, Sex, Race, and Hispanic Origin: 1990 to 1997." Race-specific rates are the number of cases reported for a particular racial/ethnic group during the preceding 12-month period divided by the projected population for that race/ ethnicity, multiplied by 100,000.

Case-fatality rates are calculated for each half-year by date of diagnosis of AIDS. Each 6-month case-fatality rate is the number of deaths ever reported among cases diagnosed in that period (regardless of the year of death), divided by the number of total cases diagnosed in that period, multiplied by 100. Reported deaths are not necessarily caused by HIV-related disease. Caution should be used in interpreting case-fatality rates because reporting of deaths is incomplete (*Am J Public Health* 1992;82:1500-05 and *Am J Public Health* 1990;80:1080-86).

Suggested Reading

CDC. Diagnosis and reporting of HIV and AIDS in states with integrated HIV and AIDS surveillance—United States, January 1994-June 1997. *MMWR* 1998;47:309-14.

CDC. HIV/AIDS among American Indians and Alaskan Natives—United States, 1981-1997. *MMWR* 1998;47:154-60.

CDC. AIDS among persons aged 50 years and older—United States, 1991-1996. *MMWR* 1998;47:21-27.

CDC. Update: perinatally acquired HIV/AIDS—United States, 1997. *MMWR* 1997;46:1086-92.

CDC. AIDS rates. *MMWR* 1997;46:903-04.

CDC. Update: trends in AIDS incidence—United States, 1996. *MMWR* 1997;46:861-67.

CDC. Update: trends in AIDS incidence, deaths, and prevalence—United States, 1996. *MMWR* 1997;46:165-73.

CDC. *HIV/AIDS Surveillance Report*, 1997;9(No.1):1-37.

Tables

Selected statistical tables related to HIV/AIDS surveillance begin on page 84.

Table 9.2. AIDS cases and annual rates per 100,000 population, by state, reported in 1996 and 1997; and cumulative totals, by state and age group, through December 1997, United States

State of residence	1996 No.	1996 Rate	1997 No.	1997 Rate	Cumulative totals Adults/ adolescents	Cumulative totals Children < 13 years old	Total
Alabama	607	14.2	570	13.2	4,774	63	4,837
Alaska	36	6.0	52	8.5	407	5	412
Arizona	589	13.3	448	9.8	5,447	21	5,468
Arkansas	267	10.7	242	9.6	2,356	35	2,391
California	9,508	29.8	7,029	21.8	104,201	555	104,756
Colorado	518	13.6	380	9.8	6,103	27	6,130
Connecticut	1,110	34.0	1,222	37.4	9,566	172	9,738
Delaware	285	39.4	231	31.6	1,995	15	2,010
District of Columbia	1,258	233.3	998	188.7	10,255	154	10,409
Florida	7,293	50.6	6,098	41.6	63,617	1,289	64,906
Georgia	2,420	33.0	1,722	23.0	18,555	179	18,734
Hawaii	199	16.8	94	7.9	2,074	14	2,088
Idaho	38	3.2	52	4.3	415	2	417
Illinois	2,193	18.5	1,842	15.5	20,165	233	20,398
Indiana	590	10.1	523	8.9	4,904	34	4,938
Iowa	110	3.9	101	3.5	1,066	9	1,075
Kansas	230	8.9	159	6.1	1,978	10	1,988
Kentucky	401	10.3	361	9.2	2,562	21	2,583
Louisiana	1,463	33.7	1,094	25.1	10,096	112	10,208
Maine	50	4.0	51	4.1	797	9	806
Maryland	2,245	44.4	1,875	36.8	16,864	274	17,138
Massachusetts	1,303	21.4	863	14.1	12,714	198	12,912
Michigan	961	9.9	882	9.0	9,164	94	9,258
Minnesota	304	6.5	214	4.6	3,187	21	3,208
Mississippi	450	16.6	347	12.7	3,160	47	3,207
Missouri	853	15.9	577	10.7	7,773	54	7,827
Montana	34	3.9	41	4.7	265	3	268
Nebraska	99	6.0	91	5.5	870	9	879
Nevada	426	26.6	592	35.3	3,632	25	3,657
New Hampshire	93	8.0	55	4.7	759	8	767
New Jersey	3,580	44.7	3,226	40.1	35,417	693	36,110
New Mexico	206	12.0	169	9.8	1,607	5	1,612
New York	12,364	68.2	13,189	72.7	118,042	2,061	120,103
North Carolina	898	12.3	850	11.4	8,057	109	8,166
North Dakota	12	1.9	13	2.0	90	—	90
Ohio	1,156	10.4	848	7.6	9,453	112	9,565
Oklahoma	272	8.3	283	8.5	2,987	26	3,013
Oregon	460	14.4	305	9.4	4,147	16	4,163
Pennsylvania	2,340	19.4	1,912	15.9	19,058	265	19,323
Rhode Island	177	17.9	152	15.4	1,722	18	1,740
South Carolina	853	23.0	779	20.7	6,956	71	7,027
South Dakota	14	1.9	11	1.5	125	4	129
Tennessee	821	15.5	784	14.6	6,265	46	6,311
Texas	4,799	25.1	4,718	24.3	44,164	337	44,501
Utah	194	9.6	152	7.4	1,513	21	1,534
Vermont	25	4.3	29	4.9	325	3	328
Virginia	1,195	17.9	1,175	17.4	10,116	155	10,271
Washington	799	14.5	641	11.4	8,194	32	8,226
West Virginia	121	6.6	130	7.2	866	8	874
Wisconsin	271	5.3	255	4.9	3,009	25	3,034
Wyoming	7	1.5	16	3.3	155	2	157
Subtotal	**66,497**	**25.1**	**58,443**	**21.8**	**611,989**	**7,701**	**619,690**
U.S. dependencies, possessions, and associated nations							
Guam	4	2.8	2	1.4	19	—	19
Pacific Islands, U.S.	1	0.3	1	0.3	4	—	4
Puerto Rico	2,241	59.2	2,040	53.3	20,241	370	20,611
Virgin Islands, U.S.	18	17.2	99	93.9	363	14	377
Total[1]	**68,808**	**25.5**	**60,634**	**22.3**	**633,000**	**8,086**	**641,086**

[1]U.S. totals presented in this report include data from the United States (50 states and the District of Columbia), and from U.S. dependencies, possessions, and independent nations in free association with the United States. See Technical Notes. Totals include 385 persons whose state of residence is unknown.

Table 9.3. AIDS cases by age group, exposure category, and sex, reported in 1996 and 1997; and cumulative totals, by age group and exposure category, through December 1997, United States

	Males 1996		Males 1997		Females 1996		Females 1997		Totals 1996		Totals 1997		Cumulative total[1]	
	No.	(%)	No.	(%)	No.	(%)	No.	(%)	No.	(%)	No.	(%)	No.	(%)
Adult/adolescent exposure category														
Men who have sex with men	27,861	(51)	21,260	(45)	–	–	–	–	27,861	(41)	21,260	(35)	309,247	(49)
Injecting drug use	12,654	(23)	10,486	(22)	4,895	(36)	4,212	(32)	17,549	(26)	14,698	(24)	161,872	(26)
Men who have sex with men and inject drugs	3,269	(6)	2,374	(5)	–	–	–	–	3,269	(5)	2,374	(4)	40,534	(6)
Hemophilia/coagulation disorder	308	(1)	184	(0)	22	(0)	17	(0)	330	(0)	201	(0)	4,689	(1)
Heterosexual contact:	3,496	(6)	3,105	(7)	6,030	(44)	5,007	(38)	9,526	(14)	8,112	(13)	58,884	(9)
Sex with injecting drug user	913		749		2,047		1,475		2,960		2,224		24,128	
Sex with bisexual male	–		–		338		266		338		266		2,887	
Sex with person with hemophilia	7		4		37		24		44		28		401	
Sex with transfusion recipient with HIV infection	37		28		65		29		102		57		893	
Sex with HIV-infected person, risk not specified	2,539		2,324		3,543		3,213		6,082		5,537		30,575	
Receipt of blood transfusion, blood components, or tissue[2]	278	(1)	224	(0)	273	(2)	185	(1)	551	(1)	409	(1)	8,214	(1)
Other/risk not reported or identified[3]	6,504	(12)	9,423	(20)	2,547	(19)	3,684	(28)	9,051	(13)	13,107	(22)	49,560	(8)
Adult/adolescent subtotal	54,370	(100)	47,056	(100)	13,767	(100)	13,105	(100)	68,137	(100)	60,161	(100)	633,000	(100)
Pediatric (<13 years old) exposure category														
Hemophilia/coagulation disorder	4	(1)	1	(0)	1	(0)	–	–	5	(1)	1	(0)	233	(3)
Mother with/at risk for HIV infection[3]	311	(91)	235	(92)	310	(94)	197	(91)	621	(93)	432	(91)	7,335	(91)
Injecting drug use	84		65		77		42		161		107		2,936	
Sex with an injecting drug user	43		31		44		29		87		60		1,340	
Sex with a bisexual male	4		6		9		1		13		7		159	
Sex with person with hemophilia	1		2		–		–		1		2		28	
Sex with transfusion recipient with HIV infection	–		–		–		–		–		–		24	
Sex with HIV-infected person, risk not specified	57		53		59		49		116		102		1,033	
Receipt of blood transfusion, blood components, or tissue	4		4		5		3		9		7		154	
Has HIV infection, risk not specified	118		74		116		73		234		147		1,661	
Receipt of blood transfusion, blood components, or tissue[2]	5	(1)	1	(0)	3	(1)	1	(0)	8	(1)	2	(0)	374	(5)
Risk not reported or identified[3]	21	(6)	19	(7)	16	(5)	19	(9)	37	(6)	38	(8)	144	(2)
Pediatric subtotal	341	(100)	256	(100)	330	(100)	217	(100)	671	(100)	473	(100)	8,086	(100)
Total	**54,711**		**47,312**		**14,097**		**13,322**		**68,808**		**60,634**		**641,086**	

[1]Includes 12 persons known to be infected with human immunodeficiency virus type 2 (HIV-2). See *MMWR* 1995;44:603-06.
[2]Thirty-seven adults/adolescents and 2 children developed AIDS after receiving blood screened negative for HIV antibody. Thirteen additional adults developed AIDS after receiving tissue, organs, or artificial insemination from HIV-infected donors. Four of the 13 received tissue, organs, or artificial insemination from a donor who was negative for HIV antibody at the time of donation. See *N Engl J Med* 1992;326:726-32.
[3]See table 16 and figure 7 for a discussion of the "other" exposure category. "Other" also includes 82 persons who acquired HIV infection perinatally but were diagnosed with AIDS after age 13. These 82 persons are tabulated under the adult/adolescent, not pediatric, exposure category.

Table 9.4. AIDS cases and annual rates per 100,000 population, by race/ethnicity, age group and sex, reported in 1997, United States

	Adults/adolescents						Children <13 years		Total	
	Males		Females		Total					
Race/ethnicity	No.	Rate	No.	Rate	No.	Rate	No.	Rate	No.	Rate
White, not Hispanic	17,649	22.5	2,485	3.0	20,134	12.4	63	0.2	20,197	10.4
Black, not Hispanic	18,903	163.4	7,880	58.8	26,783	107.2	292	4.0	27,075	83.7
Hispanic	9,778	78.5	2,578	21.5	12,356	50.6	110	1.3	12,466	37.7
Asian/Pacific Islander	381	10.2	64	1.5	445	5.6	3	0.1	448	4.5
American Indian/Alaska Native	168	23.0	36	4.7	204	13.6	2	0.4	206	10.4
Total[1]	47,056	44.0	13,105	11.5	60,161	27.3	473	0.9	60,634	22.3

[1]Totals include 242 persons whose race/ethnicity is unknown.

Table 9.5. AIDS cases by year of diagnosis and definition category, diagnosed through December 1997, United States

	Period of diagnosis											
	Before 1994		1994		1995		1996		1997		Cumulative total	
Definition category	No.	(%)	No.	(%)	No.	(%)	No.	(%)	No.	(%)	No.	(%)
Pre-1987 definition	251,159	(60)	23,542	(33)	18,511	(28)	13,002	(24)	6,358	(20)	312,572	(49)
1987 definition	96,600	(23)	12,550	(18)	10,228	(15)	7,543	(14)	3,752	(12)	130,673	(20)
1993 definition[1]	70,076	(17)	35,117	(49)	37,494	(57)	34,111	(62)	21,043	(68)	197,841	(31)
Pulmonary tuberculosis	5,725		1,607		1,282		955		456		10,025	
Recurrent pneumonia	2,301		980		912		668		345		5,206	
Invasive cervical cancer	307		141		89		56		26		619	
Severe HIV-related immunosuppression[2]	61,880		32,441		35,239		32,454		20,224		182,238	
Total	417,835	(100)	71,209	(100)	66,233	(100)	54,656	(100)	31,153	(100)	641,086	(100)

[1]The sum of diagnoses listed for the four conditions under the 1993 definition do not equal the 1993 definition total because some persons have more than one diagnosis from the added conditions of pulmonary tuberculosis, recurrent pneumonia, and invasive cervical cancer.
[2]Defined as CD4$^+$ T-lymphocyte count of less than 200 cells/μL or a CD4$^+$ percentage less than 14 in persons with laboratory confirmation of HIV infection.

Table 9.6. AIDS-indicator conditions reported in 1997, by age group, United States

AIDS-indicator conditions	Adults/adolescents No.	(%)	Children <13 years old No.	(%)
AIDS-defining opportunistic illness1	23,527	(39)	473	(100)
Bacterial infections, multiple or recurrent	NA[2]		84	(18)
Candidiasis of bronchi, trachea, or lungs	534	(2)	11	(2)
Candidiasis of esophagus				
Definitive diagnosis	2,057	(9)	30	(6)
Presumptive diagnosis	1,255	(5)	20	(4)
Carcinoma, invasive cervical	144	(1)	NA[3]	
Coccidioidomycosis, disseminated or extrapulmonary	74	(0)	1	(0)
Cryptococcosis, extrapulmonary	1,168	(5)	5	(1)
Cryptosporidiosis, chronic intestinal	314	(1)	10	(2)
Cytomegalovirus disease other than retinitis	827	(4)	30	(6)
Cytomegalovirus retinitis				
Definitive diagnosis	551	(2)	4	(1)
Presumptive diagnosis	260	(1)	5	(1)
Herpes simplex, with esophagitis, pneumonitis, or chronic mucocutaneous ulcers	1,250	(5)	15	(3)
Histoplasmosis, disseminated or extrapulmonary	208	(1)	1	(0)
HIV encephalopathy (dementia)	1,196	(5)	108	(23)
HIV wasting syndrome	4,212	(18)	73	(15)
Isosporiasis, chronic intestinal	22	(0)	1	(0)
Kaposi's sarcoma				
Definitive diagnosis	1,088	(5)	—	—
Presumptive diagnosis	412	(2)	—	—
Lymphoid interstitial pneumonia and/or pulmonary lymphoid hyperplasia				
Definitive diagnosis	NA[2]		23	(5)
Presumptive diagnosis	NA[2]		57	(12)
Lymphoma, Burkitt's (or equivalent term)	162	(1)	2	(0)
Lymphoma, immunoblastic (or equivalent term)	518	(2)	3	(1)
Lymphoma, primary in brain	170	(1)	1	(0)
Mycobacterium avium or M. kansasii, disseminated or extrapulmonary				
Definitive diagnosis	941	(4)	22	(5)
Presumptive diagnosis	183	(1)	10	(2)
M. tuberculosis, disseminated or extrapulmonary				
Definitive diagnosis	426	(2)	1	(0)
Presumptive diagnosis	65	(0)	1	(0)
M. tuberculosis, pulmonary				
Definitive diagnosis	1,426	(6)	NA[3]	
Presumptive diagnosis	195	(1)	NA[3]	
Mycobacterial disease, other, disseminated or extrapulmonary				
Definitive diagnosis	221	(1)	4	(1)
Presumptive diagnosis	80	(0)	—	—
Pneumocystis carinii pneumonia				
Definitive diagnosis	5,763	(24)	77	(16)
Presumptive diagnosis	3,382	(14)	41	(9)
Pneumonia, recurrent				
Definitive diagnosis	1,044	(4)	NA[3]	
Presumptive diagnosis	303	(1)	NA[3]	
Progressive multifocal leukoencephalopathy	213	(1)	1	(0)
Salmonella septicemia, recurrent	68	(0)	NA[4]	
Toxoplasmosis of brain				
Definitive diagnosis	576	(2)	1	(0)
Presumptive diagnosis	497	(2)	2	(0)
Immunosuppression, severe HIV-related5	36,634	(61)	NA[3]	
Total	**60,161**	**(100)**	**473**	**(100)**

[1]Percentages for individual AIDS-defining opportunistic illnesses are based upon 23,527 adults/adolescents and 473 children reported to CDC in 1997, with at least one of the illnesses listed above. The sum of percentages is greater than 100 because some patients are reported with more than one illness. Of persons reported with AIDS-defining opportunistic illnesses, 65 percent also were reported with severe HIV-related immunosuppression.
[2]Not applicable as indicator of AIDS in adults/adolescents.
[3]Not applicable as indicator of AIDS in children.
[4]Tabulated above in "bacterial infections, multiple or recurrent."
[5]Defined as a CD4+ T-lymphocyte count of less than 200 cells/μL or a CD4+ percentage less than 14 in adults/adolescents who meet the AIDS surveillance case definition. In 1997, 51,991 adults/adolescents were reported with severe HIV-related immunosuppression. The 36,634 adults/adolescents presented on this table are those persons reported with immunosuppression as their only AIDS-indicator condition. These persons may also have other AIDS-indicator conditions that are unreported.

Table 9.7. Adult/adolescent AIDS cases by single and multiple exposure categories, reported through December 1997, United States

	AIDS cases	
Exposure category	No.	(%)
Single mode of exposure		
Men who have sex with men	296,483	(47)
Injecting drug use	129,990	(21)
Hemophilia/coagulation disorder	3,784	(1)
Heterosexual contact	57,360	(9)
Receipt of transfusion[1]	8,201	(1)
Receipt of transplant of tissues, organs, or artificial insemination[2]	13	(0)
Other[3]	114	(0)
Single mode of exposure subtotal	**495,945**	**(78)**
Multiple modes of exposure		
Men who have sex with men; injecting drug use	34,845	(6)
Men who have sex with men; hemophilia/coagulation disorder	155	(0)
Men who have sex with men; heterosexual contact	8,966	(1)
Men who have sex with men; receipt of transfusion/transplant	3,315	(1)
Injecting drug use; hemophilia/coagulation disorder	183	(0)
Injecting drug use; heterosexual contact	29,051	(5)
Injecting drug use; receipt of transfusion/transplant	1,581	(0)
Hemophilia/coagulation disorder; heterosexual contact	86	(0)
Hemophilia/coagulation disorder; receipt of transfusion/transplant	785	(0)
Heterosexual contact; receipt of transfusion/transplant	1,524	(0)
Men who have sex with men; injecting drug use; hemophilia/coagulation disorder	44	(0)
Men who have sex with men; injecting drug use; heterosexual contact	4,868	(1)
Men who have sex with men; injecting drug use; receipt of transfusion/transplant	587	(0)
Men who have sex with men; hemophilia/coagulation disorder; heterosexual contact	22	(0)
Men who have sex with men; hemophilia/coagulation disorder; receipt of transfusion/transplant	35	(0)
Men who have sex with men; heterosexual contact; receipt of transfusion/transplant	266	(0)
Injecting drug use; hemophilia/coagulation disorder; heterosexual contact	68	(0)
Injecting drug use; hemophilia/coagulation disorder; receipt of transfusion/transplant	38	(0)
Injecting drug use; heterosexual contact; receipt of transfusion/transplant	938	(0)
Hemophilia/coagulation disorder; heterosexual contact; receipt of transfusion/transplant	34	(0)
Men who have sex with men; injecting drug use; hemophilia/coagulation disorder; heterosexual contact	11	(0)
Men who have sex with men; injecting drug use; hemophilia/coagulation disorder; receipt of transfusion/transplant	14	(0)
Men who have sex with men; injecting drug use; heterosexual contact; receipt of transfusion/transplant	160	(0)
Men who have sex with men; hemophilia/coagulation disorder; heterosexual contact; receipt of transfusion/transplant	5	(0)
Injecting drug use; hemophilia/coagulation disorder; heterosexual contact; receipt of transfusion/transplant	23	(0)
Men who have sex with men; injecting drug use; hemophilia/coagulation disorder; heterosexual contact; receipt of transfusion/transplant	5	(0)
Multiple modes of exposure subtotal	**87,609**	**(14)**
Risk not reported or identified[4]	**49,446**	**(8)**
Total	633,000	(100)

[1]Includes 37 adult/adolescents who developed AIDS after receiving blood screened negative for HIV antibody.
[2]Thirteen adults developed AIDS after receiving tissue, organs, or artificial insemination from HIV-infected donors. Four of the 13 received tissue or organs from a single donor who was negative for HIV antibody at the time of donation. See *N Engl J Med* 1992;326:726-32.
[3]See table 16 and figure 7 for a discussion of the "other" exposure category. "Other" also includes 82 persons who acquired HIV infection perinatally, but were diagnosed with AIDS after age 13.
[4]See figure 7.

Table 9.8. Estimated deaths of persons with AIDS, by race/ethnicity and year of death, 1991 through 1996, United States[1]

Race/ethnicity	Year of death					
	1991	1992	1993	1994	1995	1996
White, not Hispanic	19,000	20,500	21,500	22,000	21,500	14,500
Black, not Hispanic	11,000	13,500	15,500	17,500	19,000	16,000
Hispanic	6,300	7,100	7,700	8,800	9,000	6,900
Asian/Pacific Islander	250	270	300	400	350	280
American Indian/ Alaska Native	90	80	130	140	180	100
Total[2]	36,500	41,000	45,000	49,500	50,000	37,500

[1]Estimates are adjusted for delays in the reporting of deaths, but not for incomplete reporting of deaths. Estimates of less than 1,000, 1,000 to 2,499, 2,500 to 4,999, 5,000 to 9,999, and 10,000 or more are rounded to the nearest 10, 25, 50, 100, and 500, respectively. Annual estimates are through the most recent year for which reliable estimates are available. Because there is uncertainty in the estimates of deaths of persons with AIDS, changes over time in the estimates of deaths of persons with AIDS should not be computed from these rounded estimates. See Technical Notes.
[2]Totals include estimates of persons whose race/ethnicity is unknown.

Table 9.9. Estimated deaths of persons with AIDS, by age group, sex, exposure category, and year of death, 1991 through 1996, United States[1]

Male adult/adolescent exposure category	Year of death					
	1991	1992	1993	1994	1995	1996
Men who have sex with men	21,000	23,000	23,500	25,000	24,500	16,500
Injecting drug use	6,900	8,100	9,200	10,500	10,500	8,500
Men who have sex with men and inject drugs	2,450	2,700	3,000	3,300	3,250	2,425
Hemophilia/coagulation disorder	280	320	350	340	320	220
Heterosexual contact	830	1,175	1,550	1,925	2,300	2,050
Reciept of blood transfusion, blood components, or tissue	370	330	320	300	270	230
Risk not reported or identified	210	240	200	160	120	70
Male sutotal	32,000	35,500	38,500	41,500	41,500	30,000
Female adult/adolescent exposure category						
Injecting drug use	2,250	2,700	3,100	3,650	3,750	3,250
Hemophilia/coagulation disorder	10	20	20	20	30	20
Heterosexual contact	1,625	1,975	2,600	3,450	3,900	3,450
Reciept of blood transfusion, blood components, or tissue	250	250	240	240	240	180
Risk not reported or identified	80	110	90	70	60	40
Female subtotal	4,250	5,100	6,000	7,400	8,000	7,000
Pediatric (<13 years old) exposure category	400	420	530	560	530	420
Total[2]	36,500	41,000	45,000	49,500	50,000	37,500

[1]Estimates are adjusted for delays in the reporting of deaths, but not for incomplete reporting of deaths. Estimates of less than 1,000, 1,000 to 2,499, 2,500 to 4,999, 5,000 to 9,999, and 10,000 or more are rounded to the nearest 10, 25, 50, 100, and 500, respectively. Annual estimates are through the most recent year for which reliable estimates are available. Because there is uncertainty in the estimates of deaths of persons with AIDS, changes over time in the estimates of deaths of persons with AIDS should not be computed from these rounded estimates. See Technical Notes.
[2]The sum of the exposure category estimates may not equal the total annual estimates because of rounding.

Table 9.10. Persons reported to be living with HIV infection[1] and with AIDS, by state and age group, reported through December 1997[2]

U.S. state of residence (Date HIV reporting initiated)	Living with HIV infection[3]			Living with AIDS[4]			Cumulative totals		
	Adults/ adolescents	Children <13 years old	Total	Adults/ adolescents	Children <13 years old	Total	Adults/ adolescents	Children <13 years old	Total
Alabama (Jan. 1988)	4,221	35	4,256	2,211	21	2,232	6,432	56	6,488
Alaska	—	—	—	202	2	204	202	2	204
Arizona (Jan. 1987)	3,260	35	3,295	1,941	6	1,947	5,201	41	5,242
Arkansas (July 1989)	1,556	18	1,574	1,173	20	1,193	2,729	38	2,767
California	—	—	—	36,483	200	36,683	36,483	200	36,683
Colorado (Nov. 1985)	5,016	26	5,042	2,441	7	2,448	7,457	33	7,490
Connecticut (July 1992)[5]	—	88	88	4,754	80	4,834	4,754	168	4,922
Delaware	—	—	—	904	8	912	904	8	912
District of Columbia	—	—	—	4,375	86	4,461	4,375	86	4,461
Florida (July 1997)	2,049	19	2,068	26,939	573	27,512	28,988	592	29,580
Georgia	—	—	—	8,067	77	8,144	8,067	77	8,144
Hawaii	—	—	—	716	4	720	716	4	720
Idaho (June 1986)	243	2	245	175	—	175	418	2	420
Illinois	—	—	—	7,217	111	7,328	7,217	111	7,328
Indiana (July 1988)	2,934	27	2,961	2,107	14	2,121	5,041	41	5,082
Iowa	—	—	—	457	4	461	457	4	461
Kansas	—	—	—	746	3	749	746	3	749
Kentucky	—	—	—	1,082	11	1,093	1,082	11	1,093
Louisiana (Feb. 1993)	5,218	90	5,308	4,173	53	4,226	9,391	143	9,534
Maine	—	—	—	348	8	356	348	8	356
Maryland	—	—	—	7,086	148	7,234	7,086	148	7,234
Massachussets	—	—	—	4,288	78	4,366	4,288	78	4,366
Michigan (April 1992)	3,520	83	3,603	3,558	31	3,589	7,078	114	7,192
Minnesota (Oct. 1985)	2,116	22	2,138	1,277	11	1,288	3,393	33	3,426
Mississippi (Aug. 1988)	3,524	39	3,563	1,321	23	1,344	4,845	62	4,907
Missouri (Oct. 1987)	3,587	39	3,626	3,406	18	3,424	6,993	57	7,050
Montana	—	—	—	131	—	131	131	—	131
Nebraska (Sept. 1995)	330	5	335	348	4	352	678	9	687
Nevada (Feb. 1992)	2,197	20	2,217	1,791	13	1,804	3,988	33	4,021
New Hampshire	—	—	—	412	3	415	412	3	415
New Jersey (Jan. 1992)	10,765	340	11,105	12,161	249	12,410	22,926	589	23,515
New Mexico	—	—	—	656	3	659	656	3	659
New York	—	—	—	41,346	754	42,100	41,346	754	42,100
North Carolina (Feb. 1990)	7,172	93	7,265	3,097	51	3,148	10,269	144	10,413
North Dakota (Jan. 1988)	55	—	55	36	—	36	91	—	91
Ohio (June 1990)	3,411	53	3,464	3,296	38	3,334	6,707	91	6,798
Oklahoma (June 1988)	1,773	13	1,786	1,296	10	1,306	3,069	23	3,092
Oregon (Sept. 1988)[5]	—	11	11	1,664	7	1,671	1,664	18	1,682
Pennsylvania	—	—	—	7,676	138	7,814	7,676	138	7,814
Rhode Island	—	—	—	734	4	738	734	4	738
South Carolina (Feb. 1986)	5,885	104	5,989	3,203	26	3,229	9,088	130	9,218
South Dakota (Jan. 1988)	158	5	163	46	1	47	204	6	210
Tennessee (Jan. 1992)	4,292	43	4,335	3,001	18	3,019	7,293	61	7,354
Texas (Feb. 1994)[5]	—	213	213	18,345	134	18,479	18,345	347	18,692
Utah (April 1989)	767	4	771	668	7	675	1,435	11	1,446
Vermont	—	—	—	144	1	145	144	1	145
Virginia (July 1989)	6,404	73	6,477	4,048	82	4,130	10,452	155	10,607
Washington	—	—	—	3,294	14	3,308	3,294	14	3,308
West Virginia (Jan. 1989)	420	1	421	389	3	392	809	4	813
Wisconsin (Nov. 1985)	1,955	29	1,984	1,297	10	1,307	3,252	39	3,291
Wyoming (June 1989)	56	—	56	60	2	62	116	2	118
Subtotal	**82,884**	**1,530**	**84,414**	**236,586**	**3,169**	**239,755**	**319,470**	**4,699**	**324,169**
U.S. dependencies, possessions, and associated nations									
Guam	—	—	—	7	—	7	7	—	7
Pacific Islands, U.S.	—	—	—	2	—	2	2	—	2
Puerto Rico	—	—	—	7,228	169	7,397	7,228	169	7,397
Virgin Islands, U.S.	—	—	—	180	8	188	180	8	188
Total	**82,884**	**1,530**	**84,414**	**244,224**	**3,347**	**247,571**	**327,108**	**4,877**	**331,985**

[1]Includes only persons reported with HIV infection who have not developed AIDS.
[2]Persons reported with vital status "alive" as of the last update. Excludes persons whose vital status is unknown.
[3]Includes only persons reported from states with confidential HIV reporting. Excludes 1,719 adults/adolescents and 47 children reported from states with confidential HIV infection reporting whose state of residence is unknown or are residents of other states.
[4]Includes 221 adults/adolescents and 1 child whose state of residence is unknown.
[5]Connecticut and Texas have confidential HIV infection reporting for pediatric cases only; Oregon has confidential infection reporting for children less than 6 years old.

Chapter 10

Trends in AIDS Incidence

Provisional surveillance data about acquired immunodeficiency syndrome (AIDS) for the first 6 months of 1996 indicated a decrease in deaths among persons with AIDS, attributed primarily to the effect of antiretroviral therapies on the survival of persons infected with human immunodeficiency virus (HIV)[1]. This report describes a decline in AIDS incidence during 1996 compared with 1995 and the continued decline in AIDS deaths; the findings indicate that HIV therapies are having a widespread beneficial impact on the rate of HIV disease progression in the United States.

Cumulative AIDS cases among persons aged 13 years and older reported to CDC through June 1997 from the 50 states, the District of Columbia, and the U.S. territories were analyzed by sex, age, race/ethnicity, and mode of risk/exposure (categories included persons aged 20-64 years of white, black, or Hispanic race/ethnicity but excluded persons infected through receipt of contaminated blood/blood products and persons with other or no risks reported).[2] Estimates of AIDS incidence and deaths were adjusted for delays in reporting. For analyses by risk/exposure, estimates were adjusted for the anticipated reclassification of cases initially reported without an HIV risk/exposure.[2] To adjust for the 1993 expansion of the AIDS reporting criteria (conditions in HIV-infected persons that were added to the AIDS case definition in 1993 included laboratory measures of severe immunosuppression—i.e., CD4+ T-lymphocyte

Morbidity and Mortality Weekly Report (MMWR), Centers for Disease Control and Prevention (CDC), Vol. 46, No. 37, September 19, 1997.

count <200 cells/μL or percentage of total lymphocytes <14—and three clinical conditions: pulmonary tuberculosis, recurrent pneumonia, and invasive cervical cancer), estimates of the incidence of AIDS-opportunistic illnesses (AIDS-OIs) were calculated from the sum of cases reported with an AIDS-OI and cases with estimated dates of diagnosis of an AIDS-OI that were reported based only on immunologic criteria.[2] AIDS-OI incidence was estimated quarterly through December 1996 (the most recent period for which reliable estimates were available). Deaths among persons with AIDS were identified by review of medical records and death certificates and represent both deaths from HIV-related and other causes. AIDS prevalence was estimated as the cumulative incidence of AIDS based on the 1993 expanded AIDS case criteria minus cumulative deaths. Populations with <500 estimated cases were excluded because the estimates of annual percentage change from 1995 to 1996 in AIDS-OI incidence, deaths, and prevalence are not reliable.

AIDS-OI Incidence

During 1996, AIDS-OIs were diagnosed in an estimated 56,730 persons, a decline of 6% compared with 1995 (Figure 10.1). This represents the first calendar year during which AIDS-OI incidence overall did not increase in the United States.

From 1995 to 1996, AIDS-OI incidence declined in all four geographic regions of the United States (West, 12%; Midwest, 10%; Northeast, 8%; and South, 1%. Northeast = Connecticut, Maine, Massachusetts, New Hampshire, New Jersey, New York, Pennsylvania, Rhode Island, and Vermont; Midwest = Illinois, Indiana, Iowa, Kansas, Michigan, Minnesota, Missouri, Nebraska, North Dakota, Ohio, South Dakota, and Wisconsin; South = Alabama, Arkansas, Delaware, District of Columbia, Florida, Georgia, Kentucky, Louisiana, Maryland, Mississippi, North Carolina, Oklahoma, South Carolina, Tennessee, Texas, Virginia, and West Virginia; and West = Alaska, Arizona, California, Colorado, Hawaii, Idaho, Montana, Nevada, New Mexico, Oregon, Utah, Washington, and Wyoming). AIDS-OI incidence decreased in all 5-year age groups; men; non-Hispanic whites and Hispanics; men who have sex with men (MSM); injecting-drug users (IDUs); and men who reported both of these exposures (MSM-IDUs) (Table 10.2). The largest proportionate declines occurred among non-Hispanic white MSM (Figure 10.3) and non-Hispanic white and black MSM-IDUs (Table 10.4). AIDS-OI incidence leveled among non-Hispanic blacks. The greatest proportionate increases in AIDS-OI incidence occurred among non-Hispanic black men (19%), Hispanic men (13%), and non-Hispanic black women (12%) who had heterosexual risk/exposures (Table 10.4).

From 1995 to 1996, annual AIDS incidence changed abruptly compared with the magnitude and direction of the average annual changes in AIDS-OI incidence during 1992-1995. During these years, AIDS-OI incidence increased but was characterized by a slowing in the growth of the epidemic overall (average annual change from 1992 to 1995 was 2%).[1,2] The magnitude and/or the direction of the average annual change in AIDS-OI incidence from 1992 to 1995 was substantially different from the change from 1995 to 1996 among men (1% versus -8%) and women (10% versus 2%); whites (-2% versus -13%), non-Hispanic blacks (7% versus 0), and Hispanics (4% versus -5%); MSM (-1% versus -11%), men and women IDUs (3% versus

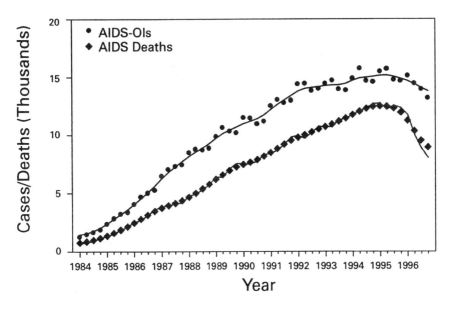

Figure 10.1. Estimated incidence of AIDS-opportunistic illnesses (AIDS-OIs) and estimated number of deaths among persons aged ≥13 years with AIDS (AIDS deaths), adjusted for delays in reporting, by quarter year of diagnosis/death—United States, 1984-1996. Points represent quarterly incidence; lines represent "smoothed" incidence. Estimates are not adjusted for incomplete reporting of AIDS cases.

-6% and 5% versus -4%, respectively), and MSM-IDUs (-3% versus - 15%).

Deaths among Persons Reported with AIDS

Deaths among persons reported with AIDS declined 23% in 1996 compared with 1995, with the largest declines occurring during the last three quarters of 1996 (Figure 10.1). From 1995 to 1996, deaths declined in all four geographic regions (West, 33%; Midwest, 25%; Northeast, 22%; an South, 19%); among men and women; among all racial/ethnic groups; and in all risk/exposure categories (Table 10.2).

Table 10.2. Estimated incidence* of AIDS-opportunistic illnesses (AIDS-OIs) and estimated number of deaths among persons aged 13 years and older reported with AIDS, by sex, race/ethnicity†, exposure category, and percentage change in AIDS-OIs and deaths from 1995 to 1996—United States.

	AIDS-OIs			Deaths		
Characteristic	1995 No.	1996 No.	% Change from 1995 to 1996	1995 No.	1996 No.	% Change from 1995 to 1996
Sex						
Men	49,360	45,240	− 8	42,000	31,440	−25
Women	11,260	11,490	2	8,140	7,340	−10
Race/Ethnicity						
White, non-Hispanic	24,370	21,130	−13	21,700	14,670	−32
Black, non-Hispanic	24,090	24,030	0	18,840	16,460	−13
Hispanic	11,410	10,800	− 5	9,010	7,220	−20
Exposure category						
MSM§	28,640	25,530	−11	24,880	17,310	−30
MSM-IDU¶	3,580	3,030	−15	3,310	2,490	−25
Male-IDU	12,880	12,140	− 6	10,790	8,970	−17
Female-IDU	4,950	4,750	− 4	3,830	3,440	−10
Heterosexual contact						
Male	3,420	3,790	11	2,300	2,120	− 8
Female	5,900	6,320	7	3,980	3,640	− 8
Total**	**60,620**	**56,730**	**− 6**	**50,140**	**38,780**	**−23**

*Estimates are presented rounded to the nearest 10 because they do not represent exact counts of persons with AIDS-OIs but are estimates that are approximately ±3% of the true value.
†Numbers for races other than black and white were too small for meaningful analysis. Persons of Hispanic origin may be of any race.
§Men who have sex with men.
¶Injecting-drug user.
**Includes persons aged ≥13 years with hemophilia/coagulation disorders, transfusion recipients, or with other or no risks reported.

AIDS Prevalence

Approximately 235,470 persons in whom AIDS has been diagnosed are still living, and from 1995 to 1996, the prevalence of AIDS increased 11% (Table 10.5). MSM accounted for the largest proportion (48%) of persons with AIDS, and the largest proportionate increases in prevalence occurred among men and women who acquired AIDS through heterosexual contact (28% and 23%, respectively), the only risk/exposure category that experienced increases in AIDS-OI incidence.

Reported by: State and local health depts. Div of HIV/AIDS Prevention-Surveillance and Epidemiology, National Center for HIV, STD, and TB Prevention, CDC

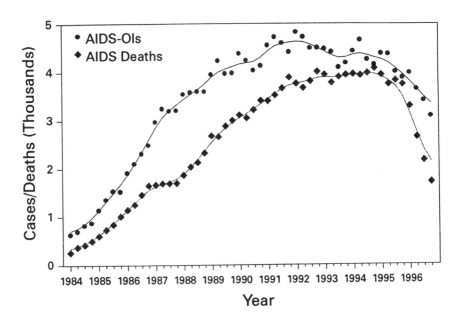

Figure 10.3. *Estimated incidence of AIDS-opportunistic illnesses (AIDS-OIs) and estimated number of deaths among non-Hispanic white men who have sex with men aged 13 years and older with AIDS (AIDS deaths), adjusted for delays in reporting, by quarter year of diagnosis/death—United States, 1984-1996. Points represent quarterly incidence; lines represent "smoothed" incidence. Estimates are not adjusted for incomplete reporting of AIDS cases.*

Editorial Note [in the original document]: The findings in this report document the first overall decline in the annual incidence of AIDS-OIs in the United States. Concurrently, annual deaths among persons aged 13 years and older reported with AIDS also have decreased. Temporal trends in AIDS cases and deaths are the result of changes in the rate of new HIV infections, AIDS diagnoses resulting from progression of HIV disease to AIDS, and deaths of HIV-infected persons. The declines in AIDS-OI incidence and deaths reflect the impact of both HIV prevention efforts and the use of antiretroviral therapies and AIDS-OI prophylaxis.

During 1996, AIDS-OI incidence declined for almost all populations and in all regions of the country, and deaths declined substantially (23%) compared with 1995. The actual decline in AIDS-OI incidence is probably greater than the estimates in this report because there are insufficient longitudinal clinical data to model the impact of the newly available antiretroviral therapies on AIDS-OI incidence. However, the 1996 AIDS surveillance data are consistent with reports that recent improvements in HIV care are preventing or delaying the onset of AIDS-OI and deaths among many populations of HIV-infected

Table 10.4. Estimated incidence* of AIDS-opportunistic illnesses (AIDS-OIs) among persons aged 13 years and older, by race/ethnicity†, sex and exposure category, and percentage change from 1995 to 1996—United States.

Exposure category	White, non-Hispanic			Black, non-Hispanic			Hispanic		
	1995	1996	% Change from 1995 to 1996	1995	1996	% Change from 1995 to 1996	1995	1996	% Change from 1995 to 1996
Men									
MSM§	16,600	14,060	−15	7,330	7,110	− 3	4,250	3,900	− 8
IDU¶	2,470	2,280	− 8	6,840	6,540	− 4	3,470	3,240	− 7
MSM-IDU	1,690	1,410	−17	1,290	1,120	−13	**	**	**
Heterosexual	640	620	− 2††	1,970	2,340	19	780	880	13
Women									
IDU	1,090	1,030	− 5††	2,920	2,860	− 2	900	820	− 9
Heterosexual	1,270	1,220	− 4	3,300	3,700	12	1,270	1,330	5

*Estimates are presented rounded to the nearest 10 because they do not represent exact counts of persons with AIDS-OIs but are estimates that are approximately ±3% of the true value.
†Numbers for races other than black and white were too small for meaningful analysis. Persons of Hispanic origin may be of any race.
§Men who have sex with men.
¶Injecting-drug user.
**Excluded because estimates were <500.
††The annual percentage changes were calculated from modeled point estimates before rounding.

persons.[3] Recent declines in AIDS incidence also have been reported in several western European countries and have been attributed to widespread use of combination antiretroviral therapies.[4]

Data from CDCs Adult/Adolescent Spectrum of Disease (ASD)[5] project indicate that an increasing proportion of HIV-infected persons are receiving combination antiretroviral therapy. Among HIV-infected persons observed in clinical care in ASD during 1995-1996, the prescribed use of combination antiretroviral therapy increased from 24% of 5027 persons in the second half of 1995 to 65% of 2973 persons in the second half of 1996 (CDC, unpublished data, 1997). Use of these therapies is expected to increase because revised HIV treatment guidelines recommend earlier initiation of combination antiretroviral therapy in HIV-infected persons without AIDS-defining conditions.[6]

Ensuring timely access to HIV-care services for HIV-infected persons remains important because in many persons HIV infection is not diagnosed until AIDS is diagnosed.[7] To enable HIV-infected persons to benefit from treatment advances, HIV counseling and testing programs in screening and health-care settings must better facilitate early diagnosis of HIV infection and ensure that HIV-infected persons have access to care and treatment services.

Table 10.5. Estimated prevalence* of AIDS among persons aged 13 years and older, by sex and exposure category, and percentage change from 1995 to 1996—United States.

Exposure category	1995 No.	1995 (%)	1996 No.	1996 (%)	% Change from 1995 to 1996
Men					
MSM[†]	101,970	(48)	111,860	(48)	10
IDU[§]	43,800	(21)	48,000	(20)	10
MSM-IDU	14,170	(7)	14,660	(6)	3
Heterosexual	9,620	(5)	12,300	(5)	28
Total	**173,560**	**(82)**	**191,040**	**(81)**	**10**
Women					
IDU	17,840	(8)	19,700	(8)	10
Heterosexual	18,610	(9)	22,860	(10)	23
Total	**38,080**	**(18)**	**44,440**	**(19)**	**17**
Total[¶]	**211,650**	**(100)**	**235,470**	**(100)**	**11**

*Estimates are presented rounded to the nearest 10 because they do not represent exact counts of persons with AIDS-OIs but are estimates that are approximately ±3% of the true value.
[†]Men who have sex with men.
[§]Injecting-drug users.
[¶]Includes persons aged ≥13 years with hemophilia/coagulation disorders, transfusion recipients, or with other or no risks reported. The sum of the estimates for men and women may not equal total annual estimates because of rounding.

Despite the decreases in AIDS-OI incidence and deaths in 1996, AIDS-OI incidence remained high, and HIV infection remained a leading cause of death among persons aged 25-44 years.[8] AIDS-OI incidence continued to increase among persons who were infected through heterosexual contact. Until effective vaccines are developed, continued emphasis on behavioral risk-reduction and other prevention strategies targeted to these populations is the most effective way to reduce HIV infections.

The 1996 AIDS surveillance trends illustrate how surveillance data are now affected by both patterns of HIV incidence and HIV treatment advances. In comparison, surveillance based on a diagnosis of HIV infection is not affected by changes in the progression of HIV disease. CDC supports both HIV and AIDS surveillance in 30 states. Among these states, the number of prevalent HIV and AIDS cases combined is approximately 2.5 times greater than the number of prevalent AIDS cases alone.[1,2] HIV/AIDS surveillance programs in these states provide a more timely measure of emerging patterns of HIV transmission, a more complete estimate of the number of persons with HIV infection and disease, and a better mechanism to evaluate access to HIV testing and medical and prevention services than AIDS surveillance alone.[9]

Although AIDS surveillance continues to be essential for understanding reasons for the lack of timely access to HIV testing and care and the failure of treatment regimens to delay HIV disease progression, HIV surveillance is becoming increasingly important as more infected persons receive effective antiretroviral therapy. In June 1997, the Council of State and Territorial Epidemiologists (CSTE) recommended that all states implement HIV case reporting by name from health-care providers and laboratories.[10] The Association of State and Territorial Health Officers has provisionally endorsed the CSTE recommendation pending a vote of its full membership. CDC recently provided additional resources to state and local surveillance programs that plan to or are conducting HIV case surveillance in addition to AIDS surveillance.

All states and territories should conduct HIV case surveillance as an extension of their AIDS Surveillance programs, and CDC is developing HIV surveillance policy and technical guidance to assist all states and territories to conduct HIV/AIDS case surveillance. CDC and CSTE recently convened a consultation to discuss the objectives and methods of conducting HIV/AIDS case surveillance. (The Consultation on the Future of HIV/AIDS Surveillance was held in Atlanta on May 21-22, 1997, sponsored by CSTE and CDC; documents presented at the meeting and a meeting transcript can be obtained from the CDC National AIDS Clearinghouse.) CDC will continue to foster a collaborative approach among public health authorities, health-care providers, and the community to meet their information needs and to ensure the confidentiality of HIV/AIDS surveillance data.

References

1. CDC. Update: trends in AIDS incidence, deaths, and prevalence-United States, 1996. *MMWR* 1997;46:165-73.

2. CDC. *HIV / AIDS surveillance report.* Atlanta: US Department of Health and Human Services, Public Health Service, 1996; (vol 8, no. 2).

3. Hammer SM, Squires KE, Hughes MD, et al, A controlled trial of two nucleoside analogues plus indinavir in persons with human immunodeficiency virus infection and CD4 cell counts of 200 per cubic millimeter or less. *N Engl J Med* 1997;337:725-33.

4. Hamers F, Downs A, Alix J, Brunet JB. AIDS trends in Europe: decrease in the west, increase in the east. *Eurosurveillance* 1997;2:36-7.

5. Farizo KM, Buehler JW, Chamberland ME, et al. Spectrum of disease in persons with human immunodeficiency virus infection in the United States. *JAMA* 1992;267:1798-805.

6. Carpenter CC, Fischl MA, Hammer SM, et al. Antiretroviral therapy for HIV infection in 1997: updated recommendations of the International AIDS Society-USA panel. *JAMA* 1997;277:1962-9.

7. Wortley PM, Chu SY, Diaz T, et al. HIV testing patterns: where, why, and when were persons with AIDS tested for HIV? *AIDS* 1995;9:487-92.

8. Ventura SJ, Peters KD, Martin JA, Maurer JD. *Births and deaths: United States, 1996.* Hyattsville, Maryland: US Department of Health and Human Services, Public Health Service, CDC, National Center for Health Statistics, 1997. (Monthly vital statistics report; vol 45, no. 12, suppl).

9. CDC. Public health uses of HIV infection reports—South Carolina, 1986-1991. *MMWR* 1992;41:245-9.

10. Council of State and Territorial Epidemiologists. CSTE: position statement ID-4. National HIV surveillance: addition to the National Public Health Surveillance System. Atlanta: Council of State and Territorial Epidemiologists, 1997.

Chapter 11

HIV/AIDS: Epidemic Shifts Further Toward Young Women and Minorities

In the United States, HIV-related death has the greatest impact on young and middle-aged adults, particularly racial and ethnic minorities. HIV is the second leading cause of death for Americans between the ages of 25 and 44. It is the leading cause of death for African-American men and women in this age group. Many of these young adults likely were infected as teenagers. It is estimated that half of all new HIV infections in the United States are among people under 25, and the majority of young people are infected sexually.

Among 13- to 24-year-olds, 52% of all AIDS cases reported among males in 1997 were among young men who have sex with men (MSM); 10% were among injection drug users (IDUs); and 7% were among young men infected heterosexually. In 1997, among young women the same age, 49% were infected heterosexually and 13% were IDUs.

Because of the long and variable time between HIV infection and AIDS, surveillance of HIV infection provides a much clearer picture of the impact of the epidemic in young people than surveillance of AIDS cases. CDC recently announced results from a study that analyzed data from 25 states (Alabama, Arizona, Arkansas, Colorado, Idaho, Indiana, Louisiana, Michigan, Minnesota, Mississippi, Missouri, Nevada, New Jersey, North Carolina, North Dakota, Ohio, Oklahoma, South Carolina, South Dakota, Tennessee, Utah, Virginia, West Virginia, Wisconsin, Wyoming) that had integrated HIV and AIDS reporting systems for the period between January 1994 and

CDC Update, National Center for HIV, STD, and TB Prevention, June 1998.

101

June 1997. In these states, young people (aged 13 to 24) accounted for a much greater proportion of HIV than AIDS cases (14% versus 3%). Nearly half (44%) of the HIV infections in that age group were reported among young females, and well over half (63%) were among African Americans. The study also showed that even though AIDS incidence (the number of new cases diagnosed during a given time period, usually a year) is declining, there has not been a comparable decline in the number of newly diagnosed HIV cases among young people.

How Can We Improve Prevention Programs for Young People?

CDC's role is to provide communities with the best available science to guide comprehensive HIV prevention programs. As part of this process, CDC conducts an ongoing research synthesis process that seeks to identify the most recent and relevant scientific findings from around the world, both published and unpublished, and make them available to prevention program planners. CDC constantly combs the scientific literature, reviews domestic and international scientific databases, and speaks with colleagues around the world to identify effective interventions for all populations at risk, including youth.

Young people's prevention needs are as diverse as young people themselves. To reduce the toll AIDS takes on young Americans, a wide range of activities must be implemented.

Comprehensive, ongoing prevention efforts are needed for each group entering adolescence and young adulthood. All groups that exert influence over young people—families, schools, peer groups and social systems, youth-serving agencies, religious organizations—must be involved.

- **School-based programs.** Because risk behaviors do not exist independently—for example, a young person's ability to resist peer pressure and social influences to smoke are integrally related to the ability to say no to risky sexual activity—topics such as HIV, STDs, unintended pregnancy, tobacco, nutrition, and physical activity should be integrated and ongoing for all students in kindergarten through high school. The specific scope and content of school health programs, especially those related to HIV and STD prevention, should be locally determined and consistent with parental and community values. For communities and schools that seek assistance, CDC and other

102

organizations have identified elements of successful HIV education programs, and this information is widely available from
CDC and other youth-serving agencies. Research has clearly
shown that the most effective programs are comprehensive ones
that include a focus on delaying sexual behavior and provide information on how sexually active young people can protect
themselves.

- **Community-based programs.** Addressing the needs of adolescents who are most vulnerable to HIV infection, such as homeless or runaway youth, juvenile offenders, or school drop-outs, is
  critically important. For example, a 1993 serosurveillance survey of females in four juvenile detention centers found that between 1% and 5% were HIV infected (median 2.8%). Increased
  HIV seroprevalence rates may be associated with higher rates
  of drug injection or high-risk sexual practices in these populations of adolescents. Community outreach programs play an important role in reaching these young people.

- **Sustaining prevention efforts for young gay and bisexual
  men.** Targeted, sustained prevention efforts are urgently
  needed for young MSM as they come of age and initiate high-
  risk sexual behavior. Ongoing studies show that both HIV
  prevalence and risk behaviors remain high among young MSM.
  In a sample of young MSM ages 15-22 in 6 urban counties, researchers found that, overall, between 5% and 8% were infected
  with HIV. HIV prevalence was higher among young African
  Americans (13%) and Hispanics (5%) compared with young
  white MSM (4%).

- **Need to address sexual and drug-related risk.** Many students report using alcohol or drugs when they have sex, and 1
  in 50 high school students reports having injected an illegal
  drug. Surveillance data from the 25 states with integrated HIV
  and AIDS reporting systems between January 1994 and June
  1997 showed that drug injection led to 6% of HIV diagnoses reported among those aged 13-24 during that time period, with an
  additional 57% attributed to sexual transmission (26% heterosexual, 31% from male-to-male sex).

- **Role of STD treatment in comprehensive HIV prevention
  programs for young people.** An estimated 12 million cases of
  STDs other than HIV are diagnosed annually in the United

States, and about two-thirds (roughly 8 million) of those are among people under the age of 25. A large body of research has shown that biological factors make people who are infected with an STD more likely to become infected with HIV if exposed sexually; and HIV-infected people with STDs also are more likely to transmit HIV to their sex partners. Expanding STD treatment services is critical to reducing the consequences of these diseases and also helping reduce risks of transmitting HIV among youth.

- **Ongoing evaluation of factors influencing risk behavior.** To better understand adolescent behaviors and the impact of selected family, social, and cultural factors on risk behaviors, CDC conducts broad-based surveys of the extent of risk behaviors among young people, as well as focused studies of the factors contributing to risk and behavioral intent among specific groups of adolescents.

  Eight-year trends from the Youth Risk Behavior Survey (YRBS) show both a leveling of sexual risk behavior rates and increased condom use among sexually active young people. Still, more than one-quarter of adolescents report initiating intercourse by age 15. From 1990 through 1997 the percentages of high school students who reported ever having had sex, having four or more partners, or having intercourse in the 3 months prior to the survey all remained steady. In contrast, overall condom use at last intercourse was up significantly, from 46% in 1990 to 57% in 1997. Female and African-American students posted the largest increases in condom use. While increased condom use is encouraging, YRBS findings indicate that more must be done, and done earlier, to help young people delay initiation of sexual activity and reduce risky sexual behaviors.

For young people, it is critical to prevent patterns of risky behaviors before they start. HIV prevention efforts must be sustained and designed to reach each new generation of Americans.

Chapter 12

HIV/AIDS among Hispanics in the United States

Hispanics in the United States include a diverse mixture of ethnic groups and cultures. With more than 25 million Hispanics, the United States has the fifth largest Hispanic population in the world, following Mexico, Spain, Argentina, and Colombia. Although Hispanics represent an estimated 10% of the total U.S. population, they account for 18% of the 641,086 AIDS cases reported in the United States through December 1997.

In 1997, 60,634 new AIDS cases were reported to CDC. Of these, 12,466 (21%) occurred among Hispanics. The AIDS incidence rate (the number of new cases of a disease that occurs during a specific time period) among Hispanics was 37.7 per 100,000 population in 1997, almost 4 times the rate for whites (10.4 per 100,000) and almost half the rate of African Americans (83.7 per 100,000 population).

A recent CDC study examined data from the 25 states (Alabama, Arizona, Arkansas, Colorado, Idaho, Indiana, Louisiana, Michigan, Minnesota, Mississippi, Missouri, Nevada, New Jersey, North Carolina, North Dakota, Ohio, Oklahoma, South Carolina, South Dakota, Tennessee, Utah, Virginia, West Virginia, Wisconsin, Wyoming) that had integrated HIV and AIDS surveillance from January 1994 through June 1997. This study showed that HIV diagnoses increased 10% among Hispanics between 1995 and 1996 (the most recent year for which overall trends can be examined). However, the number of cases reported among Hispanics was relatively small, since many

CDC Update, National Center for HIV, STD, and TB Prevention, June 1998.

states with large Hispanic populations have not implemented integrated HIV and AIDS reporting and were not included in the study. At the same time, HIV diagnoses declined slightly among African Americans (-3%) and among whites (-2%) in these states. Of the 7,200 young people ages 13-24 years who were diagnosed with HIV from January 1994 to June 1997, 5% were Hispanic.

Historical Trends in HIV and AIDS Cases

Most HIV and AIDS cases reported to date among Hispanics have been among men, although the proportion of cases among women is rising. Among Hispanic men, the majority of reported cases have been among gay and bisexual men and injection drug users. Among Hispanic women, most cases have been the result of heterosexual exposures, although drug use also plays a major role in the spread of infection to women. A large proportion of Hispanic women were infected through injection drug use or by having sex with an injection drug user. To reduce the toll of the epidemic among Hispanic men, women, and children, prevention programs must address the intersection of sexual and drug-related risks.

CDC's HIV Prevention Efforts Targeting Hispanic Populations

Since early in the HIV/AIDS epidemic, CDC recognized that Hispanic populations were being disproportionately affected and took a number of steps to better target HIV prevention efforts in these communities. The following is a brief overview of some of those activities.

- CDC currently provides $253 million in funding to state and local health departments for HIV prevention programs. Since December 1993, CDC has funded a process designed to put more of the decisions about how these prevention funds are directed in the hands of the communities affected. Under this process, HIV Prevention Community Planning, health departments are required to establish priorities in conjunction with a planning group that brings together health department staff, representatives of affected populations, epidemiologists, behavioral scientists, service providers, and other community members to identify prevention needs and interventions to meet these needs. This process helps ensure that HIV prevention efforts are locally relevant and address the unique epidemic and prevention needs of each community.

CDC has conducted several recent assessments to determine what proportion of these funds are used to reach minority populations. While not all programs are targeted by race (some, for example, target high-risk communities such as injection drug users or people being treated in STD clinics, which include individuals from multiple races), it is clear that a significant proportion of funding for major programs, such as counseling and testing and risk-reduction programs, are targeted to Hispanics. Of programs identified as specifically targeting a racial/ethnic group (representing $143 million), 22% of funds ($31.4 million) target Hispanics.

- CDC also directly funds minority and other community-based organizations to design and implement HIV prevention programs that are highly targeted to high-risk individuals within racial and ethnic minority populations. Many serve gay and bisexual men of color or injection drug users as their primary focus. CDC currently provides $18 million to fund 94 community-based organizations through this program. Sixty-four of these organizations direct their programs to Hispanics. CDC recently announced the availability of an additional $4 million in fiscal year 1998 for community-based organizations for HIV prevention activities directed to African-American and Hispanic populations.

- CDC funds a $9.5 million program to assist National and Regional Minority Organizations in building capacity to deliver HIV prevention programs and services within minority communities. Of these 22 organizations, 8 exclusively serve Latino/Latina populations and 3 others serve several minority populations including Latino/Latinas.

- Additionally, CDC conducts a number of behavioral research projects aimed at reducing HIV infection in the Hispanic community.

  - The *People of Color Initiative*, designed to reduce the disproportionate spread of HIV/AIDS among minority populations, will develop, strengthen, support, and, as needed, redesign HIV prevention strategies targeting racial and ethnic minority communities.

107

— The *Women and Infants Demonstration Project* is a community-level behavioral intervention research project targeting young women ages 15 to 34, most of whom are members of racial/ethnic minority populations. This project is designed to improve understanding of factors influencing women's behavior changes regarding condom and contraceptive use and to improve the development and delivery of interventions.

—The *Prevention of HIV Infection in Youth at Risk* project focuses primarily on young men of color. This program is developing and evaluating approaches to encourage young African-American and Hispanic men who have sex with men to reduce behaviors that put them at risk for HIV.

Building Better Prevention Programs for Hispanics

While race and ethnicity alone are not risk factors for HIV infection, underlying social and economic conditions (such as language or cultural diversity, higher rates of poverty and substance abuse, or limited access to health care) may increase the risk for infection in some Hispanic-American communities.

In addition to addressing these underlying conditions, improved prevention efforts for Hispanics will require focusing on several key challenges. To reduce the infection risk for Hispanic women, efforts to prevent drug use and HIV must be better integrated. And to adequately address the prevention needs of Hispanic gay and bisexual men, homophobia must be confronted on a national, societal, and community level. Finally, we must apply lessons learned in designing culturally appropriate prevention efforts to developing effective programs for communities not yet effectively reached. Despite successes to date, this epidemic is far from over. As long as we continue to see preventable infections occur each year, we can and must do better.

Chapter 13

AIDS among Children

As of September 30,1996, a total of 566,002 acquired immunodeficiency syndrome (AIDS) cases, including 7472 cases among children aged <13 years (1%), had been reported to CDC by state and territorial health departments. Most children reported with AIDS, acquired human immunodeficiency virus (HIV) infection perinatally from their mothers[1]. During 1988-1993, an estimated 6000-7000 children were born each year to HIV-infected women; an estimated 1000-2000 of these children were infected annually[2]. In 1994, results of clinical trials demonstrating effective therapy for reducing perinatal HIV transmission indicated a two-thirds decrease in such transmission associated with zidovudine (ZDV) therapy for HIV-infected pregnant women and their newborns. The Public Health Service (PHS) issued recommendations in 1994 for ZDV treatment to reduce perinatal HIV transmission, and in 1995 for routine HIV counseling and voluntary testing for all pregnant women in the United States.[3,4] This report summarizes the epidemiology of AIDS in children in the United States reported cumulatively from 1982 through September 1996, presents rates for 1995 (the most recent year for which census estimates are available), and describes a recent decrease in the rate of perinatally acquired AIDS.

AIDS among Children

Of the 7472 children reported with AIDS, 58% were non-Hispanic black, 23% were Hispanic, 18% were non-Hispanic white, and 1% were

Morbidity and Mortality Weekly Report (MMWR), Centers for Disease Control and Prevention, November 22, 1996, Vol. 45, No. 46, pp. 1005-1010.

of other racial/ethnic groups. During 1995, the rates of reported AIDS cases per 100,000 children were 6.4 for non-Hispanic blacks, 2.3 for Hispanics, 0.4 for non-Hispanic whites, 0.4 for American Indians/Alaskan Natives, and 0.3 for Asians/Pacific Islanders. Among all U.S. children with AIDS, 6750 (90%) acquired HIV perinatally, 370 (5%) through receipt of contaminated blood transfusions, and 231 (3%) through receipt of contaminated blood products for coagulation disorders; 121 (2%) had no reported risk factor. Among children with perinatally acquired AIDS, the median age at diagnosis was 18 months. Approximately 80% of all children with AIDS had AIDS diagnosed before age 5 years. The highest numbers of cases were reported from New York (1901), Florida (1199), New Jersey (661), California (524), Puerto Rico (347), and Texas (296); combined, these cases accounted for 66% of all AIDS cases reported among children.

Risk exposures for HIV infection among the mothers of the 6750 children with perinatally acquired AIDS included injecting-drug use (IDU) (41%), sexual contact with a partner with or at risk for HIV/AIDS (34%), and receipt of contaminated blood or blood products (2%); for 13%, no risk was specified.

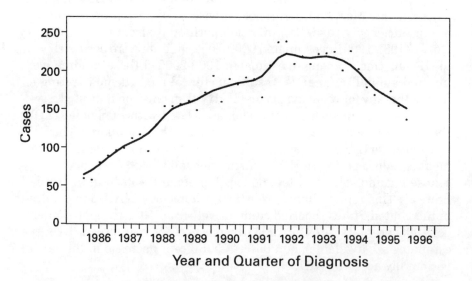

Figure 13.1. Number of perinatally acquired AIDS cases among children aged <13 years, by quarter of diagnosis—United States, 1986–March 1996. Estimates were based on cases reported through September 1996, adjusted for reporting delays and unreported risk but not for incomplete reporting of diagnosed AIDS cases. Points represent estimated quarterly incidence, and the line represents "smoothed" incidence.

Trends in Perinatally Acquired AIDS

To examine trends in the incidence of AIDS among children born to HIV-infected mothers, the number of perinatally acquired AIDS cases diagnosed each quarter from 1986 through March 1996 was estimated using standard statistical adjustments that account for delays in reporting cases to CDC and estimates of behavioral risk among persons reported without a risk[1]. The estimated number of children with perinatally acquired AIDS peaked at 905 during 1992, followed by a decline in incidence (Figure 13.1).

From 1992 through 1995, the estimated annual number of perinatally acquired AIDS cases declined 27%, from 905 to 663. During this time, the estimated annual number of cases declined 39% among non-Hispanic white, 26% among non-Hispanic black, and 25% among Hispanic children. The proportionate decrease in the number of children with perinatally acquired AIDS from the six areas reporting the highest number of cases was greater than the decrease for all remaining areas and for all areas combined.

HIV Infection among Children

To enhance the usefulness of surveillance systems to characterize affected populations and to improve the targeting of resources for prevention and care, 28 states require confidential reporting of children with HIV infection without a diagnosis of AIDS as well as those with AIDS[1]. Through September 1996, these states reported 29% (2155) of all children with AIDS and 1447 children with HIV infection. During 1995, these states reported 228 AIDS cases among children and 302 children with documented HIV infection who had not developed AIDS (Table 13.2). During 1995, these states received 1464 additional reports of children who were born to HIV-infected mothers but who require follow-up with providers to determine their HIV-infection status.

Among the six reporting areas with the highest cumulative number of children with AIDS, only New Jersey and Texas require reports of HIV infection among children.

Reported by state, territorial, and local health departments. Div of HIV/AIDS Prevention, National Center for HIV, STD, and TB Prevention, CDC.

Editorial Note [in original document]: The findings in this report document a decline in the incidence of perinatally acquired AIDS before and after the release of Public Health Service (PHS) recommendations for HIV counseling and voluntary testing for pregnant women and for ZDV therapy to prevent perinatal transmission.[3,4] The recommendations were issued to promote the adoption of these HIV-prevention strategies as standard medical practice in the United States. Because the number of HIV-infected women who gave birth each year was stable during 1989-1994[5], this decline suggests that the decrease in perinatal HIV transmission rates probably reflected the effect of perinatal ZDV therapy. Increasing proportions of women may be accepting voluntary prenatal HIV testing and using ZDV to prevent perinatal transmission.[6,7]

Because the incidence of perinatally acquired AIDS declined slightly before the PHS recommendations on ZDV therapy were issued in 1994, other factors may have contributed to the decrease in

Table 13.2. Number of children aged <l3 years reported with HIV infection* and AIDS—United States and territories, 1995†

Area	HIV	AIDS	Area	HIV	AIDS
Alabama	8	4	Nebraska	2	1
Alaska	—	0	Nevada	1	4
Arizona	6	1	New Hampshire	—	0
Arkansas	8	3	New Jersey	48	61
California	—	89	New Mexico	—	0
Colorado	4	1	New York	—	166
Connecticut	12	18	North Carolina	25	12
Delaware	—	1	North Dakota	0	0
District of Columbia	—	13	Ohio	14	14
Florida	—	111	Oklahoma	3	0
Georgia	—	28	Oregon	—	2
Hawaii	—	0	Pennsylvania	—	19
Idaho	0	0	Puerto Rico	—	46
Illinois	—	26	Rhode Island	—	0
Indiana	4	3	South Carolina	24	7
Iowa	—	0	South Dakota	1	0
Kansas	—	2	Tennessee	12	10
Kentucky	—	1	Texas	51	31
Louisiana	23	12	Utah	0	0
Maine	—	1	Vermont	—	0
Maryland	—	37	Virginia	10	19
Massachusetts	—	19	Virgin Islands	—	5
Michigan	19	9	Washington	—	3
Minnesota	3	3	West Virginia	0	2
Mississippi	7	8	Wisconsin	7	0
Missouri	10	5	Wyoming	0	0
Montana	—	0	**Total**	**302**	**797**

*Twenty-eight states reported children with HIV infection without a diagnosis of AIDS in addition to children with AIDS.
†Data reported to CDC through September 1996.

112

perinatally acquired AIDS cases during this period. For example, the proportion of HIV-infected childbearing women who received ZDV therapy before and during pregnancy for treatment of their HIV disease was increasing.[8] Among children, increased use of prophylaxis to prevent AIDS opportunistic infections may have delayed the development of these conditions. However, the incidence of *Pneumocystis carinii* pneumonia, the most common AIDS-defining condition among children, has not decreased substantially among young children.[9,10]

AIDS surveillance conducted in all reporting areas provides a standardized means to monitor AIDS incidence in children as a measure of the effectiveness of perinatal prevention efforts. To further characterize implementation of counseling, testing, and treatment for HIV-infected mothers and their children, CDC and other federal agencies are initiating facility-based program evaluations in selected high-incidence areas. These studies also will examine factors that may contribute to a change in perinatal HIV transmission rates (e.g., changing obstetrical practices and womens' attitudes toward and adherence to ZDV and other preventive therapy). In states that conduct confidential HIV reporting for children, timely assessment of HIV-prevention measures in mother-infant pairs (e.g., prenatal care and prenatal and neonatal ZDV therapy) will measure changes in perinatal HIV transmission rates statewide and permit refinement and redirection of prevention efforts. The Council of State and Territorial Epidemiologists has recommended that all states implement HIV infection reporting for children and consider reporting of all children of indeterminate HIV status who were born to infected mothers.

In the United States, HIV and AIDS disproportionately affect non-Hispanic black and Hispanic women and their children. This disparity probably reflects socioeconomic factors, access to and use of medical services, or differences in behaviors associated with HIV transmission risks among women. Health-care providers in the public and private sectors should implement comprehensive integrated-service delivery programs to ensure that all women have access to HIV counseling and voluntary testing and to services for related health needs (e.g., antiretroviral therapy, substance-abuse treatment, and social and support services).

The ZDV regimen recommended in the United States is not an affordable prevention strategy in many countries where HIV prevalence rates among women are highest. Worldwide, an estimated 8.8 million women and 800,000 children have HIV/AIDS; most of these persons reside in sub-Saharan Africa where resources for health services infrastructure are limited (World Health Organization, unpublished

113

data, 1996). CDC and other organizations are collaborating with ministries of health in Africa and Asia to evaluate the effectiveness of shorter and simplified ZDV regimens, other antiretroviral medications, and other interventions for reducing perinatal HIV transmission. However, because ZDV treatment or other potential interventions are not universally effective in preventing perinatal transmission, primary prevention of HIV infection among children will continue to require preventing new HIV infections among women in the United States and other countries.

References

1. CDC. *HIV/AIDS surveillance report*. Atlanta: US Department of Health and Human Services, Public Health Service, 1996:3-4, 30-3. (Vol 8, no. 1).

2. Davis SF, Byers RH, Jr, Lindegren ML, Caldwell MB, Karon JM, Gwinn M. Prevalence and incidence of vertically acquired HIV infection in the United States. *JAMA* 1995;274:952-5.

3. CDC. Recommendations of the U.S. Public Health Service Task Force on the use of zidovudine to reduce perinatal transmission of human immunodeficiency virus. *MMWR* 1994;43(no. RR-11).

4. CDC. U.S. Public Health Service recommendations for human immunodeficiency virus counseling and voluntary testing for pregnant women. *MMWR* 1995;44(no. RR-7).

5. Davis SF, Steinberg S, Jean-Simon M, Rosen D, Gwinn M. HIV prevalence among U.S. childbearing women, 1989-1994 [Abstract]. Vancouver, British Columbia: XI International Conference on AIDS, 1996.

6. Lindsay MK, Peterson HB, Feng TI, Slade BA, Willis S, Klein L. Routine antepartum human immunodeficiency virus infection screening in an inner-city population. *Obstet Gynecol* 1989; 74:289-94.

7. Thomas P, Singh T, Lindegren ML, Saletan S, Brooks A, Forlenza S. Patterns of zidovudine (ZDV) use in pregnant HIV-infected women in New York City (NYC) [Abstract].

Vancouver, British Columbia: XI International Conference on AIDS, 1996.

8. Simonds RJ, Nesheim S, Matheson P, et al. Declining mother-to-child HIV transmission following perinatal zidovudine recommendations, United States [Abstract]. Vancouver, British Columbia: XI International Conference on AIDS, 1996.

9. Lindegren ML, Byers R, Fleming P, et al. A decline in the incidence of perinatally acquired (PA) AIDS in the United States [Abstract]. Vancouver, British Columbia: XI International Conference on AIDS, 1996.

10. CDC. 1995 Revised guidelines for prophylaxis against *Pneumocystis carinii* pneumonia for children infected with or perinatally exposed to human immunodeficiency virus. *MMWR* 1995; 44(no. RR-4).

Chapter 14

HIV/AIDS in Women

The proportion of total AIDS cases attributable to women is increasing. From 1985 through 1996, the proportion of adolescent/adult women reported to the Centers for Disease Control and Prevention (CDC) with AIDS increased steadily each year, from 7% to 20% of reported cases. Of the total cases reported among women, the proportion attributed to heterosexual contact is also increasing. In 1994, AIDS cases in women attributable to transmission via heterosexual contact surpassed the number attributable to transmission via injecting drug use; however, sexual contact with a man who injects drugs accounts for the majority of heterosexually acquired AIDS cases. HIV infection is the third leading cause of death among women ages 25-44; the leading cause of death among Black women in this same age group. This chapter presents data from the 1996 year-end edition of the CDC *HIV/AIDS Surveillance Report*. The figure and Tabular data are from the 1997 year-end edition.

Magnitude of the Problem

From June 1982 through December 1996, CDC had received reports of 581,429 cases of AIDS among persons of all ages and racial/ethnic groups in the United States, including 85,500 cases (15%) among women.

Centers for Disease Control and Prevention (CDC), National Center for HIV, STD and TB Prevention, Update, July 1997; Tables and Figure from *HIV/AIDS Surveillance Report: U.S. HIV and AIDS cases reported through December 1997*, CDC, 1998.

Table 14.1. Female adult/adolescent AIDS cases by exposure category and race/ethnicity, reported in 1997, and cumulative totals, through December 1997, United States.

Exposure category	White, not Hispanic 1997 No.	(%)	White, not Hispanic Cumulative total No.	(%)	Black, not Hispanic 1997 No.	(%)	Black, not Hispanic Cumulative total No.	(%)	Hispanic 1997 No.	(%)	Hispanic Cumulative total No.	(%)
Injecting drug use	907	(36)	9,614	(43)	2,511	(32)	24,981	(45)	750	(29)	8,359	(42)
Hemophilia/coagulation disorder	2	(0)	91	(0)	10	(0)	74	(0)	3	(0)	36	(0)
Heterosexual contact:	991	(40)	8,838	(39)	2,790	(35)	19,981	(36)	1,174	(46)	9,193	(46)
Sex with injecting drug user	316		3,734		779		8,402		368		4,531	
Sex with bisexual male	102		1,277		1144		1,091		42		440	
Sex with person with hemophilia	16		257		7		65		1		30	
Sex with transfusion recipient with HIV infection	10		279		13		147		5		93	
Sex with HIV-infected person, risk not specified	547		3,291		1,877		10,276		758		4,099	
Receipt of blood transfusion, blood components, or tissue	39	(2)	1,739	(8)	112	(1)	1,146	(2)	28	(1)	517	(3)
Risk not reported or identified	546	(22)	2,181	(10)	2,457	(31)	9,009	(16)	623	(24)	1,789	(9)
Total	**2,485**	**(100)**	**22,463**	**(100)**	**7,880**	**(100)**	**55,191**	**(100)**	**2,578**	**(100)**	**19,894**	**(100)**

Exposure category	Asian/Pacific Islander 1997 No.	(%)	Asian/Pacific Islander Cumulative total No.	(%)	American Indian/Alaska Native 1997 No.	(%)	American Indian/Alaska Native Cumulative total No.	(%)	Cumulative totals[1] 1997 No.	(%)	Cumulative totals[1] Cumulative total No.	(%)
Injecting drug use	11	(17)	87	(17)	14	(39)	128	(46)	4,212	(32)	43,214	(44)
Hemophilia/coagulation disorder	1	(2)	4	(1)	1	(3)	1	(0)	17	(0)	206	(0)
Heterosexual contact:	30	(47)	239	(47)	13	(36)	105	(38)	5,007	(38)	38,391	(39)
Sex with injecting drug user	7		69		4		54		1,475		16,800	
Sex with bisexual male	5		58		2		15		266		2,887	
Sex with person with hemophilia	–		4		–		2		24		358	
Sex with transfusion recipient with HIV infection	1		17		–		–		29		537	
Sex with HIV-infected person, risk not specified	17		91		7		34		3,213		17,809	
Receipt of blood transfusion, blood components, or tissue	4	(6)	91	(18)	1	(3)	13	(5)	185	(1)	3,509	(4)
Risk not reported or identified	18	(28)	87	(17)	7	(19)	32	(11)	3,684	(28)	13,148	(13)
Total	**64**	**(100)**	**508**	**(100)**	**36**	**(100)**	**279**	**(100)**	**13,105**	**(100)**	**98,468**	**(100)**

[1] *Includes 133 women whose race/ethnicity is unknown.*

In 1996, 69,151 AIDS cases were reported to CDC and of these cases, 13,820 (20%) were reported among women. Over 80% of these cases were reported from Metropolitan Statistical Areas with populations greater than 500,000. Black and Hispanic women have been disproportionately affected, accounting for 59% and 19% of women reported in 1996. AIDS rates for Black and Hispanic women are 17 and 6 times higher than for white women (61.7 and 22.7 and 3.5 per 100,000, respectively). Women under 30 accounted for 22% of reported cases in 1996. Because the time from initial infection with HIV to the development of AIDS can be long and variable, many of these young women acquired their infections in their teens and early twenties. The states with the highest AIDS rates in 1996 were New York, New Jersey, Florida, Maryland, and Delaware. The states with the highest number reported were New York (3249), Florida (1825), New Jersey (1050), California (940), and Texas (722).

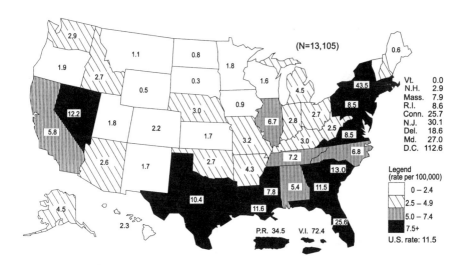

Figure 14.2. Female adult/adolescent AIDS annual rates per 100,000 population, for cases reported in 1997, United States.

119

Table 14.3. Female adult/adolescent HIV infection cases[1] by exposure category and race/ethnicity, reported in 1997, and cumulative totals, through December 1997, from states with confidential HIV infection reporting.

Exposure category	White, not Hispanic 1997 No.	(%)	White Cumulative total No.	(%)	Black, not Hispanic 1997 No.	(%)	Black Cumulative total No.	(%)	Hispanic 1997 No.	(%)	Hispanic Cumulative total No.	(%)
Injecting drug use	204	(21)	1,629	(29)	386	(13)	3,370	(22)	57	(19)	368	(26)
Hemophilia/coagulation disorder	1	(0)	10	(0)	2	(0)	10	(0)	—	—	—	—
Heterosexual contact:	375	(39)	2,310	(41)	992	(33)	5,767	(37)	112	(37)	573	(41)
Sex with an injecting drug user	104		838		229		1,722		35		240	
Sex with a bisexual male	36		271		75		434		4		22	
Sex with person with hemophilia	5		58		3		29		1		7	
Sex with transfusion recipient with HIV infection	3		28		7		42		2		5	
Sex with HIV-infected person, risk not specified	227		1,115		678		3,540		70		299	
Receipt of blood tranfusion, blood components, or tissue	12	(1)	119	(2)	21	(1)	218	(1)	2	(1)	20	(1)
Risk not reported or identified[2]	362	(38)	1,620	(28)	1,615	(54)	6,122	(40)	134	(44)	438	(31)
Total	**954**	**(100)**	**5,688**	**(100)**	**3,016**	**(100)**	**15,487**	**(100)**	**305**	**(100)**	**1,399**	**(100)**

Exposure category	Asian/Pacific Islander 1997 No.	(%)	A/PI Cumulative total No.	(%)	American Indian/Alaska Native 1997 No.	(%)	AI/AN Cumulative total No.	(%)	Cumulative totals[3] 1997 No.	(%)	Cumulative total No.	(%)
Injecting drug use	1	(7)	7	(10)	9	(43)	54	(38)	663	(15)	5,455	(24)
Hemophilia/coagulation disorder	—	—	—	—	—	—	—	—	3	(0)	20	(0)
Heterosexual contact:	4	(29)	26	(36)	5	(24)	54	(38)	1,491	(34)	8,764	(38)
Sex with an injecting drug user	—		6		4		32		373		2,846	
Sex with a bisexual male	—		1		—		7		115		739	
Sex with person with hemophilia	—		—		—		—		9		94	
Sex with transfusion recipient with HIV infection	—		—		—		—		12		75	
Sex with HIV-infected person, risk not specified	4		19		1		15		982		5,010	
Receipt of blood tranfusion, blood components, or tissue	—	—	1	(1)	—	—	1	(1)	35	(1)	361	(2)
Risk not reported or identified	9	(64)	38	(53)	7	(33)	34	(24)	2,170	(50)	8,458	(37)
Total	**14**	**(100)**	**72**	**(100)**	**21**	**(100)**	**143**	**(100)**	**4,362**	**(100)**	**23,058**	**(100)**

[1]Includes only persons reported with HIV infection who have not developed AIDS.

[2]For HIV infection cases, "risk not reported or identified" refers primarily to persons whose mode of exposure was not reported and who have not been followed up to determine their mode of exposure, and to a smaller number of persons who are not reported with one of the exposures listed above after follow-up.

[3]Includes 269 women whose race/ethnicity is unknown.

Suggested Reading

CDC. "Update: Trends in AIDS Incidence, Deaths, and Prevalence—United States, 1996." *MMWR* 1997;46:165-73.

CDC. "AIDS Associated with Injecting-Drug Use—United States, 1995." *MMWR* 1996;45:392-8.

CDC. "Update: AIDS Among Women—United States, 1994." *MMWR* 1995;44:81-4. Erratum: *MMWR* 1995:44-135.

Kennedy MB, Scarlett MI, Duerr AC, Chu SY. "Assessing HIV Risk among Women Who Have Sex with Women: Scientific and Communication Issues." *JAMWA* 1995;50:103-7.

Ellerbrock TV, Bush TJ, Chamberland ME, *et al.* "Epidemiology of Women with AIDS in the United States, 1981 through 1990: A Comparison with Heterosexual Men with AIDS." *JAMA* 1991;265:2971-5.

Selik RM, Chu SY, Buehler JW. "HIV Infection as Leading Cause of Death Among Young Adults in U.S. Cities and States." *JAMA* 1993;269:2991-4.

Additional Information

For further analysis of surveillance and trends in HIV/AIDS, consult the *HIV/AIDS Surveillance Report*. The most recent issue of the report, as well as many other resources, can be obtained by contacting:

CDC National AIDS Clearinghouse
P.O. Box 6003
Rockville, MD 20849-6003
(800) 458-5231
e-mail: aidsinfo@cdcnac.org
website: http://www.cdcnac.org

Chapter 15

HIV/AIDS among Women Who Have Sex with Women

The biologic risk of transmission through female-to-female sex is unknown, but case reports of female-to-female transmission of HIV and the well documented risk of female-to-male transmission of HIV indicate that vaginal secretions and menstrual blood are potentially infectious and that mucous membrane (e.g. oral, vaginal) exposure to these secretions can potentially lead to HIV infection. Information from HIV/AIDS surveillance, however, suggests that female-to-female transmission of HIV is a rare occurrence.

What Do Surveillance Tools Tell Us about Transmission between Women?

Through December 1996, 85,500 women were reported with AIDS. Of these, 1,648 were reported to have had sex with women; however, the vast majority had other risks (such as injection drug use, sex with high-risk men, or receipt of blood or blood products). Of the 333 (out of 1,648) who were reported to have had sex *only* with women, 97% of these women also had another risk—injection drug use in most cases.

Note: Information on whether a woman had sex with women is missing in half of the 85,500 case reports, possibly because the physician did not elicit the information or the woman did not volunteer it.

CDC Facts, Centers for Disease Control and Prevention, July 1997.

What Do Investigations of Female-to-Female Transmission Show?

Women with AIDS whose only reported risk initially is sex with women are prioritized for follow up investigation. As of December 1996, none of these investigations had resulted in a confirmed AIDS case report of female-to-female transmission, either because other risks were subsequently identified or because, in a few cases, women declined to be interviewed. A separate study of over 1 million female blood donors found no HIV-infected women whose only risk was sex with women. These findings suggest that female-to-female transmission of HIV is uncommon. However, they do not negate the possibility because it could be masked by other behaviors.

What Are the Behaviors that May Place Women Who Have Sex with Women (WSW) at Risk?

Surveys of risk behaviors have been conducted in groups of WSW. These surveys have generally been surveys of convenient samples of WSW that differ in sampling, location, and definition of WSW. As a result, their findings are not generalizable to all populations of WSW. These surveys suggest that some groups of WSW have relatively high rates of high-risk behaviors, such as injection drug use and unprotected vaginal sex with gay/bisexual men and injection drug users.

What Can WSW Do to Reduce Their Risk of Contracting HIV?

Although female-to-female transmission of HIV is apparently rare, female sexual contact should be considered a possible means of transmission among WSW. These women need to know:

- that exposure of a mucous membrane, like the mouth, (especially non-intact) to vaginal secretions and menstrual blood is potentially infectious, particularly during early and late-stage HIV infection when the amount of virus in the blood is expected to be highest.

- that condoms should be used consistently and correctly each and every time for sexual contact with men or when using sex toys. Sex toys should not be shared. No barrier methods for use during oral sex have been evaluated as effective barriers or been approved by the FDA. However, women can use dental dams, cut open condoms, or plastic wrap to help protect themselves from contact with body fluids during oral sex.

• their own and their partner's HIV status. This knowledge can help uninfected women begin and maintain behavioral changes that reduce their risk of becoming infected and can assist infected women in getting early treatment and avoiding infecting others.

Health professionals also need to remember:

• that sexual identity does not necessarily predict behavior, and that women who identify as lesbian may be at risk for HIV through unprotected sex with men.

• that prevention interventions targeting WSW must address behaviors that put WSW at risk for HIV infection, specifically injection drug use and unprotected vaginal-penile intercourse.

References

Chu SY, Buehler JW, Fleming PL, Berkelman RL. Epidemiology of reported cases of AIDS in lesbians: United States, 1980-89. *Am J Pub Health* 1990,80:1380-81.

Chu SY, Hammett TA, Buehler JW. Update: epidemiology of reported cases of AIDS in women who report only sex with other women, United States, 1980-91. *AIDS* 1992;6:518-19.

Kennedy, MB, Scarlett MI, Duerr AC, Chu SY. Assessing HIV risk among women who have sex with women: Scientific and Communication issues. *J Am Med Wom Assoc* 1995;50:103-107.

Lemp GF, Jones M, Kellog TA, et al. HIV seroprevalence and risk behaviors among lesbians and bisexual women in San Francisco and Berkeley, California. *Am J Pub Health* 1995;85:1549-52.

Petersen LR, Doll L, White C, Chu S, and the blood donor study group. *J Acquir Immun Defic Synd* 1992;5:853-855.

Chapter 16

HIV/AIDS Trends among Men Who Have Sex with Men

The AIDS rate for men who have sex with men (MSM—The term MSM is meant to identify men whose primary risk category for HIV infection is unprotected sex with other men. The MSM term is not intended to imply that all sex between men is inherently risky, but that unprotected sex between men of discordant or unknown serostatus may pose a risk for HIV transmission. Also, the term MSM includes all men who have had unprotected sex with men, whether they identify themselves as gay, bisexual, heterosexual, or other.) continues to rise, but more slowly than earlier in the epidemic. Due to behavior changes that began in the 1980s, there has been a slowing in the overall rate or new AIDS cases among MSM, and declines in new HIV infections have occurred in many areas. Although the overall numbers of AIDS cases among MSM have leveled, cases have steadily risen in some populations of MSM. Racial/ethnic minority MSM have had large increases in AIDS rates, whereas AIDS rates have decreased slightly for white MSM. AIDS rates also have continued to rise among MSM in small cities and rural areas.

The statistics and trends analyzed in this chapter pertain to men whose primary risk factor for acquiring HIV infection was sex with other men. Therefore, this analysis does not include MSM who inject drugs.

Centers for Disease Control and Prevention (CDC), CDC Facts, November 1997; tabular data and figure from *HIV/AIDS Surveillance Report: U.S. HIV and AIDS cases reported through December 1997*, CDC, 1998.

This chapter is presented in a question-and-answer format that includes current statistics and trends and addresses the changing face of HIV/AIDS among MSM.

Magnitude of the Problem

How many reported AIDS cases in the United States have been among MSM?

From June 1982 through December 1996, the Centers for Disease Control and Prevention (CDC) received reports of 581,429 cases of AIDS in the United States. Of these cases 287,576, or 49%, were among MSM. The same 287,576 cases accounted for 59% of all reported AIDS cases among adolescent/adult men.

Through December 1996, the breakdown of AIDS cases reported among MSM by race/ethnicity shows:

- 65% of cases were among white MSM;
- 20% were among African-American MSM;
- 13% were among Hispanic MSM;
- 1% were among Asian/Pacific Islander MSM; and
- less than 1% were among American Indian/Alaska native MSM.

What was the reported number of new AIDS cases among MSM in 1996?

In 1996, there were 27,316 new cases of AIDS reported among MSM. This represented 40% of all reported AIDS cases in 1996. The same 27,316 represented 50% of reported AIDS cases among adolescent/adult males in 1996.

How has the racial/ethnic distribution of AIDS cases among MSM changed between 1990 and 1996?

The proportion of African-American and Hispanic MSM among new AIDS cases has increased. In 1990, African-American and Hispanic MSM accounted for 19% and 11%, respectively, of new AIDS cases among MSM. In 1996, the percentages increased to 24% and 15%, respectively. In contrast, the proportion for MSM with AIDS who were Asian/Pacific Islander or American Indian/Alaska Native did not differ substantially between 1990 and 1996, and the proportion who were white decreased from 69% to 59%.

Table 16.1. Male adult/adolescent AIDS cases by exposure category and race/ethnicity, reported in 1997, and cumulative totals, through December 1997, United States.

Exposure category	White, not Hispanic 1997 No.	(%)	Cumulative total No.	(%)	Black, not Hispanic 1997 No.	(%)	Cumulative total No.	(%)	Hispanic 1997 No.	(%)	Cumulative total No.	(%)
Men who have sex with men	11,787	(67)	199,776	(75)	5,749	(30)	64,879	(38)	3,355	(34)	40,399	(43)
Injecting drug use	2,008	(11)	23,905	(9)	5,494	(29)	60,118	(35)	2,895	(30)	34,063	(36)
Men who have sex with men and inject drugs	1,078	(6)	21,066	(8)	897	(5)	12,842	(8)	367	(4)	6,230	(7)
Hemophilia/coagulation disorder	137	(1)	3,509	(1)	26	(0)	490	(0)	17	(0)	390	(0)
Heterosexual contact:	545	(3)	4,178	(2)	1,740	(9)	11,464	(7)	776	(8)	4,674	(5)
Sex with an injecting drug user	*155*		*1,599*		*416*		*4,252*		*171*		*1,430*	
Sex with person with hemophilia	*–*		*23*		*2*		*12*		*2*		*8*	
Sex with transfusion recipient with HIV infection	*10*		*142*		*15*		*130*		*3*		*75*	
Sex with HIV-infected person, risk not specified	*380*		*2,414*		*1,307*		*7,070*		*600*		*3,161*	
Receipt of blood tranfusion, blood components, or tissue	108	(1)	3,059	(1)	72	(0)	989	(1)	38	(0)	539	(1)
Risk not reported or identified	1,986	(11)	9,159	(3)	4,925	(26)	19,359	(11)	2,330	(24)	7,289	(8)
Total	17,649	(100)	264,652	(100)	18,903	(100)	170,141	(100)	9,778	(100)	93,584	(100)

Exposure category	Asian/Pacific Islander 1997 No.	(%)	Cumulative total No.	(%)	American Indian/Alaska Native 1997 No.	(%)	Cumulative total No.	(%)	Cumulative totals[1] 1997 No.	(%)	Cumulative total No.	(%)
Men who have sex with men	229	(60)	3,020	(75)	79	(47)	868	(59)	21,260	(45)	309,247	(58)
Injecting drug use	25	(7)	214	(5)	33	(20)	224	(15)	10,486	(22)	118,658	(22)
Men who have sex with men and inject drugs	12	(3)	138	(3)	19	(11)	242	(16)	2,374	(5)	40,534	(8)
Hemophilia/coagulation disorder	3	(1)	62	(2)	1	(1)	26	(2)	184	(0)	4,483	(1)
Heterosexual contact:	24	(6)	119	(3)	12	(7)	37	(3)	3,105	(7)	20,493	(4)
Sex with an injecting drug user	*5*		*31*		*1*		*13*		*749*		*7,328*	
Sex with person with hemophilia	*–*		*–*		*–*		*–*		*4*		*43*	
Sex with transfusion recipient with HIV infection	*–*		*7*		*–*		*1*		*28*		*356*	
Sex with HIV-infected person, risk not specified	*19*		*81*		*11*		*23*		*2,324*		*12,766*	
Receipt of blood tranfusion, blood components, or tissue	4	(1)	101	(3)	2	(1)	8	(1)	224	(0)	4,705	(1)
Risk not reported or identified	84	(22)	383	(9)	22	(13)	72	(5)	9,423	(20)	36,412	(7)
Total	381	(100)	4,037	(100)	168	(100)	1,477	(100)	47,056	(100)	534,532	(100)

[1]*Includes 641 men whose race/ethnicity is unknown.*

What is the AIDS prevalence among MSM?

Prevalence refers to the number of people living with a particular disease. In June of 1996, MSM accounted for the largest number of persons living with AIDS (approximately 98,000), and from July 1995 to June 1996, MSM accounted for the largest absolute increase (5,100) in the number of persons living with AIDS.

Current Trends

Because of changes in the AIDS case reporting system over time and to adjust for reporting delays, CDC uses a statistical technique to estimate AIDS incidence and analyze trends in the epidemic. (To more accurately analyze trends, CDC uses estimates based on when people will develop opportunistic infections—OIs. Most HIV-infected people become severely immunosuppressed *before* the onset of one of the numerous illnesses indicative of AIDS. The estimates of when these AIDS-related opportunistic illnesses—AIDS-OIs—will occur are used to determine the annual AIDS incidence—or the number of people diagnosed each year with AIDS. The use of this technique adjusts for reporting delays and changes in the reporting system over time.) Some of the trends among MSM described in this section were analyzed using this technique.

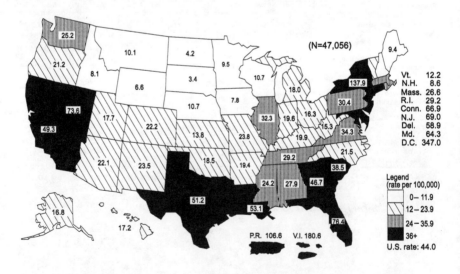

Figure 16.2. Male adult/adolescent AIDS annual rates per 100,000 population, for cases reported in 1997, United States.

130

Table 16.3. Male adult/adolescent HIV infection cases[1] by exposure category and race/ethnicity, reported in 1997, and cumulative totals through December 1997, from states with confidential HIV infection reporting.

	White, not Hispanic				Black, not Hispanic				Hispanic			
	1997		Cumulative total		1997		Cumulative total		1997		Cumulative total	
Exposure category	No.	(%)	No.	(%)	No.	(%)	No.	(%)	No.	(%)	No.	(%)
Men who have sex with men	2,286	(59)	18,296	(61)	1,342	(27)	10,002	(32)	274	(35)	1,489	(35)
Injecting drug use	351	(9)	2,710	(9)	740	(15)	6,470	(21)	132	(17)	1,113	(26)
Men who have sex with men and inject drugs	242	(6)	2,480	(8)	146	(3)	1,581	(5)	18	(2)	246	(6)
Hemophilia/coagulation disorder	19	(0)	319	(1)	9	(0)	77	(0)	1	(0)	9	(0)
Heterosexual contact:	126	(3)	771	(3)	492	(10)	2,875	(9)	55	(7)	253	(6)
Sex with an injecting drug user	*26*		*207*		*98*		*704*		*16*		*83*	
Sex with person with hemophilia	*—*		*3*		*1*		*8*		*—*		*—*	
Sex with transfusion recipient with HIV infection	*2*		*17*		*7*		*46*		*—*		*2*	
Sex with HIV-infected person, risk not specified	*98*		*544*		*386*		*2,117*		*39*		*168*	
Receipt of blood tranfusion, blood components, or tissue	10	(0)	170	(1)	12	(0)	152	(0)	3	(0)	25	(1)
Risk not reported or identified[2]	845	(22)	5,207	(17)	2,201	(45)	10,331	(33)	309	(39)	1,076	(26)
Total	3,879	(100)	29,953	(100)	4,942	(100)	31,488	(100)	792	(100)	4,211	(100)

	Asian/Pacific Islander				American Indian/Alaska Native				Cumulative totals[3]			
	1997		Cumulative total		1997		Cumulative total		1997		Cumulative total	
Exposure category	No.	(%)	No.	(%)	No.	(%)	No.	(%)	No.	(%)	No.	(%)
Men who have sex with men	16	(42)	95	(48)	29	(47)	189	(48)	3,985	(40)	30,315	(45)
Injecting drug use	1		16	(8)	8	(13)	58	(15)	1,242	(13)	10,432	(15)
Men who have sex with men and inject drugs	—		3	(2)	7	(11)	58	(15)	419	(4)	4,393	(7)
Hemophilia/coagulation disorder	1		2	(1)	—	—	2	(1)	30	(0)	413	(1)
Heterosexual contact:	3		11	(6)	1	(2)	19	(5)	680	(7)	3,945	(6)
Sex with an injecting drug user	*1*		*5*		*1*		*8*		*142*		*1,010*	
Sex with person with hemophilia	*—*		*—*		*—*		*—*		*1*		*11*	
Sex with transfusion recipient with HIV infection	*—*		*—*		*—*		*—*		*10*		*66*	
Sex with HIV-infected person, risk not specified	*2*		*6*		*—*		*11*		*527*		*2,858*	
Receipt of blood tranfusion, blood components, or tissue	—		1	(1)	—	—	2	(1)	25	(0)	355	(1)
Risk not reported or identified	17	(45)	70	(35)	17	(27)	62	(16)	3,513	(36)	17,519	(26)
Total	38	(100)	198	(100)	62	(100)	390	(100)	9,894	(100)	67,372	(100)

[1]Includes only persons reported with HIV infection who have not developed AIDS.

[2]For HIV infection cases, "risk not reported or identified" refers primarily to persons whose mode of exposure was not reported and who have not been followed up to determine their mode of exposure, and to a smaller number of persons who are not reported with one of the exposures listed above after follow-up.

[3]Includes 1,132 men whose race/ethnicity is unknown.

131

What were the trends in AIDS incidence among MSM in the 1990s?

Among All MSM

From 1990 through 1992, the AIDS incidence among MSM increased 17%. Annual increases in incidence then began to slow, and from 1994 through 1995, estimated cases among MSM remained relatively constant at about 29,500 each year.

Among Young MSM

Betwen 1990 and 1995, AIDS incidence among MSM aged 13 to 25 years declined 29%. However, trends in incidence varied greatly by race/ethnicity. While AIDS incidence decreased 50% among young white MSM during this period, incidence fell just 2% among young black MSM and rose 5% among young Hispanic MSM.

What were the trends in AIDS incidence rates among MSM from 1990 through 1995?

For regional analysis in this section, only data from the 50 states and the District of Columbia were used. National analysis also included Puerto Rico and other U.S. dependencies, possessions, and associated nations.

By Age

AIDS rates over the 5-year period increased for men age 30 and older, but decreased for men ages 13 to 29. The largest increase was for men over 59 years old (32%); however, the rates in this age group were low.

By Geographic Region

AIDS incidence rates in the West decreased slightly (-2%), but rates increased in all other regions. Although racial/ethnic rate differences were fairly consistent within regions, the highest race/region-specific increase in AIDS rates occurred among African-American MSM in the South (59%) and the Midwest (59%). The only race/region-specific decrease was among white MSM in the West (-8%); in all other regions, rates among white MSM were stable.

By Metropolitan Area

Larger increases in AIDS incidence rates occurred in rural areas and areas with 50,000 to 249,000 residents; however, these smaller metropolitan areas had lower rates than large metropolitan areas in 1990. The largest race/metropolitan area-specific increases in rates occurred among African-Americans (132%) and Hispanic (100%) MSM in rural areas, African-American (83%) MSM in metropolitan areas between 50,000 and 249,000 residents, and African-Americans (100%) and American Indian/Alaska Native (100%) MSM in metropolitan areas of 250,000 to 999,999 residents. The only decrease in rates occurred among white MSM (-9%) in metropolitan areas of more than 2.5 million residents.

In the 10 metropolitan areas with the largest cumulative numbers of estimated AIDS cases among MSM, the AIDS incidence rates and changes in the rates have differed. Rates for African-American MSM increased in all 10 areas, and rates for Hispanic MSM increased in 6 of the 8 metropolitan areas with enough data for analysis. In contrast, rates for white MSM decreased in 7 of the 10 metropolitan areas. The largest decrease in AIDS incidence rates occurred in Houston (-21%), and the largest increase occurred in Miami (34%) and was associated with a large increase among African-American MSM (110%).

What are the trends in AIDS mortality among MSM?

The estimated number of deaths among MSM reported with AIDS rose steadily in the 1980s and early 1990s, and then leveled at approximately 25,000 deaths in 1994 and 1995. In 1996, overall AIDS deaths declined for the first time. Compared with the first half of 1995, AIDS among MSM fell 19% in the first half of 1996. While AIDS deaths among MSM have shown a decline, AIDS remains the leading cause of death among all men ages 25-44.

References

Centers for Disease Control and Prevention (CDC). *HIV/AIDS Surveillance Report* 1996;8(2)1-39.

CDC Update: Trends in AIDS incidence, deaths, and prevalence—United States, 1996. *MMWR* 1997;46(8):165-172.

Denning PH, Jones JL, Ward JW. Recent trends in the HIV epidemic among adolescent and young adult gay and bisexual men. *J Acquir Immune Defic Syndr*. In press.

Sullivan PS, Chu SY, Fleming PL, Ward JW. Changes in AIDS incidence for men who have sex with men, United States, 1990 through 1995. *AIDS*. In press.

For further analysis of surveillance and trends in HIV/AIDS, consult the *HIV/AIDS Surveillance Report*. The most recent issue of the report, as well as many other resources, can be obtained from:

CDC National AIDS Clearinghouse
P.O. Box 6003
Rockville, MD 20849-6003
(800) 458-5231
e-mail: aidsinfo@cdcnac.org
website: http://www.cdcnac.org

Chapter 17

HIV/AIDS among Inmate Populations

Introduction

Because of their comparatively high rates of drug abuse, jail and prison inmates are at greater risk of contracting AIDS. In 1991 an estimated 1 in 4 State prisoners had been using cocaine or crack in the month before their imprisonment offense, and about 1 in 10 reported use of heroin or other opiates. During their lives, nearly 1 in 4 State prisoners had used a needle to inject illegal drugs.

This report provides the most recent information from BJS statistical programs covering State prisons and the largest jails nationwide on AIDS testing and the prevalence of AIDS and HIV seropositivity. It also provides information from State prisoners reporting on their personal characteristics and how these relate to HIV test results.

Lawrence A. Greenfeld, Acting Director

Summary of Findings

In 1991, 2.2% of Federal and State prison inmates—17,479 of 792,176 inmates held in U.S. prisons—were infected with the human immunodeficiency virus (HIV) that causes AIDS. Of the total prison population 0.6% exhibited symptoms of HIV infection, including 0.2% with confirmed AIDS.

Excerpted from "HIV in U.S. Prisons and Jails," *Bureau of Justice Statistics: Special Report*, U. S. Department of Justice, September 1993.

This report uses data from three Bureau of Justice Statistics (BJS) data series. Some information on prisoners with HIV comes from the annual reports made by State and Federal correctional authorities (National Prisoner Statistics or NPS). Other data on prisoner characteristics and drug use resulted from interviews with inmates (1991 Survey of Inmates in State Correctional Facilities). Jail data were provided by the Nation's 503 largest jail jurisdictions (1992 Annual Survey of Jails).

Additional findings about HIV in U.S. prisons and jails include the following:

- State prisons reported 2.3% of inmates were HIV positive, and Federal prisons reported 1.0%.

- Of HIV-positive inmates in State or Federal prisons, 9.6% had confirmed AIDS. In State prisons in the West, 21.1 % of HIV-positive inmates had AIDS.

- All prison jurisdictions tested at least some inmates for HIV; 17 tested all prisoners.

- In 1991, 28% of all deaths in State prisons were attributable to AIDS. Between July 1, 1991, and June 30,1992, 24% of deaths in jails were AIDS related.

- In 1991, about 51 % of State prison inmates reported having been tested for HIV and knowing the results.

- In 1991, among those prison inmates tested, an estimated 3.3% of women, 3.7% of Hispanics, and 3.7% of those between age 35 and 44 tested positive to HIV.

- In 1991, an estimated 0.8% of tested prison inmates who said they never used drugs were HIV positive, as were 2.5% who ever used drugs, 4.9% who used needles to inject drugs, and 7.1 % who shared needles.

Data Sources

The NPS-1 program includes midyear and yearend numbers and movements of prison inmates, provided to BJS by the departments of corrections in the 50 States and the District of Columbia and by the U.S. Bureau of Prisons. In 1991 questions were added to the yearend report to determine the numbers of HIV-positive prisoners and the department policies on testing for the virus.

136

The 1991 Survey of Inmates in State Correctional Facilities questioned a nationally representative sample of almost 14,000 State prisoners about current offenses, prior drug use and treatment, personal characteristics, and other aspects of their life. Questions on whether prisoners had ever been tested for HIV and the results of the test were included in the interviews.

The Annual Survey of Jails obtains data on populations and movements of jail inmates. The sample includes all jail jurisdictions with 100 or more inmates and a sample of smaller jurisdictions. The 503 large jail jurisdictions provide figures on deaths in jails. In 1992, the jurisdictions that were the largest in 1991 were asked to indicate their policies for testing for HIV and numbers of HIV prisoners they were holding on June 30, 1992.

Prevalence of HIV Infection in U.S. Prisons

In 1991, 2.2% of Federal and State prison inmates were reported to have the human immunodeficiency virus that causes AIDS (Table 17.1). In State prisons, 2.3% of inmates were reported testing HIV-positive; in Federal prisons, 1.0%. Of the total prison population, 0.6% showed symptoms of HIV infection, including 0.2% with confirmed AIDS.

States reporting the highest percentage of prisoners infected with HIV were New York (13.8%), Connecticut (5.4%), Massachusetts (5.3%), New Jersey (4.0%), Rhode Island (3.5%), and Georgia (3.4%). Twenty-nine States reported less than 1.0%. The percentage of inmates in prison on December 31, 1991, and known to be HIV positive is related in part to the testing policies of the individual prisons or departments of corrections.

States in the Northeast led the country in the percentage of inmates known to be infected with HIV (8.1%). Five of the six States with the highest rates of HIV-positive prisoners were in the Northeast. By contrast, States in the Midwest and West had less than 1% of prisoners with HIV.

Of the inmates who tested HIV-positive, 73.0% of them were asymptomatic and 17.3% had symptoms but had not developed AIDS. The remaining 9.7% had AIDS. The West had the highest percentage of HIV-positive inmates with confirmed AIDS (21.1%), compared to the Northeast (8.8%), Midwest (11.3%), and South (6.7%).

Prison Policies for Testing for HIV

All the States, the District of Columbia, and the U.S. Bureau of Prisons tested inmates for HIV on some basis. Seventeen jurisdictions

Table 17.1. Inmates in custody of State or Federal correctional authorities known to be positive for the human Immunodeficiency virus, yearend 1991.

Jurisdiction	Total	Type of HIV infection/AIDS cases			HIV/AIDS cases as a percent of total custody population
		Asymptomatic	Symptomatic	Confirmed AIDS	
U.S. total	17,479	12,765	3,032	1,682	2.2%
Federal	630	422	91	117	1.0
State	16,849	12,343	2,941	1,565	2.3
Northeast	10,247	7,420	1,922	905	8.1%
Connecticut	574	229	264	81	5.4
Maine	1	1	0	0	.1
Massachusetts	484	100	362	22	5.3
New Hampshire	18	8	6	4	1.2
New Jersey	756	0	694	62	4.0
New York	8,000	6,833	474	693	13.8
Pennsylvania	313	247	34	32	1.3
Rhode Island	98	0	88	10	3.5
Vermont	3	2	0	1	.3
Midwest	1,128	733	268	127	.7%
Illinois	299	216	66	17	1.0
Indiana	62	60	0	2	.5
Iowa	19	17	0	2	.5
Kansas	13	1	6	6	.2
Michigan	390	124	194	72	1.1
Minnesota	14	13	1	0	.4
Missouri	127	125	0	2	.8
Nebraska	11	10	1	0	.4
North Dakota	1	1	0	0	.2
Ohio	152	129	0	23	.4
South Dakota	—	—	—	—	—
Wisconsin	40	37	0	3	.5
South	4,314	3,513	513	288	1.5%
Alabama	178	178	0	0	1.1
Arkansas	68	59	5	4	.9
Delaware	85	78	0	7	2.6
District of Columbia	—	—	—	—	—
Florida	1,105	1,015	0	90	2.4
Georgia	807	774	10	23	3.4
Kentucky	27	25	0	2	.3
Louisiana	100	100	0	0	.7
Maryland	478	324	135	19	2.5
Mississippi	106	106	0	0	1.3
North Carolina	170	116	35	19	.9
Oklahoma	74	64	0	10	.7
South Carolina	316	298	0	18	2.0
Tennessee	28	0	20	8	.3
Texas	615	251	307	57	1.2
Virginia	152	121	0	31	.9
West Virginia	5	4	1	0	.3
West	1,160	677	238	245	.7%
Alaska	9	7	0	2	.4
Arizona	84	74	0	10	.5
California	714	407	136	171	.7
Colorado	82	37	41	4	1.0
Hawaii	19	17	1	1	.8
Idaho	10	3	3	4	.5
Montana	7	7	0	0	.5
Nevada	117	72	39	6	2.0
New Mexico	10	10	0	0	.3
Oregon	24	11	12	1	.4
Utah	35	0	5	30	1.3
Washington	42	32	0	10	.5
Wyoming	7	0	1	6	.6

—Not reported.
Source: 1991 National Prisoner Statistics-1.

138

tested all prisoners, either at admission, release, or during custody. The remaining 35 jurisdictions tested at least some inmates.

Thirty-nine of the 52 jurisdictions tested if asked by an inmate and 40 if an inmate exhibited symptoms suggestive of HIV infection.

Table 17.2. Summary of prison HIV testing policies.

Testing policy	Number of Jurisdictions
All incoming inmates	16
All inmates currently in custody	3
All inmates at time of release	5
High risk groups	15
Upon inmate request	39
Upon clinical indication of need	40
Upon involvement in incident	20
Random sample	7
Other	11

Note: Detail adds to more than 52 because a jurisdiction may have more than one Policy.

Deaths in Prison

During 1991, for every 1,000 inmates, 2.5 deaths occurred in State correctional facilities. Among the 10 States with the largest prison populations, New York had the highest rate of death, about 5.6 deaths per 1,000 inmates.

Of the 1,863 deaths of prison inmates in 1991, 528—or 28%—died of AIDS. In New York and New Jersey two-thirds of the reported deaths were caused by AIDS. These two States also had the largest number of AIDS-related deaths, 210 in New York and 66 in New Jersey. Twenty-one States had no AIDS-related deaths. Of inmates who died of AIDS in prison, 3% were women. Eleven of the 15 women who died of AIDS were imprisoned in the Northeast.

Extent of HIV Testing of State Prison Inmates

Based on interviews with State prison inmates for the 1991 Survey of Inmates in State Correctional Facilities, about half of State prison inmates knew they had been tested for the HIV and reported the result of the test.

HIV Test Results, by Inmate Characteristics

Women were more likely than men to know if they had been tested and whether the results were positive or negative—as were non-Hispanics compared to Hispanics, those under age 45 compared to older prisoners, offenders imprisoned for property, drug, or public-order offenses compared to those in prison for violent offenses, and recidivists compared to first timers.

For inmates reporting test results, a higher percentage of women than men tested HIV positive (3.3% to 2.1 %). Hispanics were more likely than blacks and blacks were more likely than whites to have antibodies to HIV (3.7%, 2.6%, and 1.1%).

An estimated 6.8% of Hispanic women were HIV positive, as were 3.5% of black women and 3.5% of Hispanic men. Among white inmates, 1.9% of the women and 1% of the men were positive.

Inmates 35 to 44 years of age were more likely than those in other age groups to be HIV positive; 3.7% were positive.

Inmates in prison for drug, property, and public-order offenses were more likely than violent offenders to be HIV positive.

Table 17.3. Knowledge of HIV Testing

HIV testing	Percent of State prison inmates
Reported HIV-test results	51.2%
Had never been tested	32.2
Did not know if they had been tested	9.0
Had been tested but did not know the results	7.5
Refused to report whether they had been tested or refused to report the test results	.1
Total number of inmates	711,643

Source: Survey of Inmates in State Correctional Facilities, 1991

140

Recidivists were more likely to be HIV positive than inmates who had not previously served a sentence to either probation or a term in a correctional facility.

HIV Results, by Drug and Needle Use

About a fourth of all State prison inmates had used a needle to inject illegal drugs. (See *Survey of State Prison Inmates, 1991*, BJS report, NCJ-136949, March 1993, p. 25.) About 4 in 10 inmates who had used drugs in the month before the offense for which they were sentenced had injected drugs at some time; about 2 in 10 had ever shared a needle.

For inmates reporting test results, drug users had higher positive HIV rates than inmates who never used drugs (2.5% versus 0.8%) (Table 17.4). Needle use further increased the likelihood of being HIV positive; 4.9% of inmates who had used needles to inject drugs and 7.1 % who had shared needles were HIV positive.

Table 17.4. State prison inmates testing positive for the human immunodeficiency virus, by drug and needle use, sex, race/Hispanic origin, age, and offense.

Characteristic	Percent of State prison inmates who tested positive for HIV and who				
	Never used drugs	Ever used drugs	Used drugs in the month before offense	Used a needle to inject drugs	Shared a needle to inject drugs
All inmates	.8%	2.5%	2.8%	4.9%	7.1%
Sex					
Male	.7%	2.4%	2.7%	4.7%	6.7%
Female	.9	3.8	4.6	6.7	10.0
Race/Hispanic origin					
White non-Hispanic	.3%	1.2%	1.5%	2.4%	3.7%
Black non-Hispanic	1.1	2.9	3.2	7.2	11.1
Hispanic	.6	4.3	5.2	8.2	11.3
Age					
24 or younger	0	1.0%	.8%	.8%	2.0%
25-34	1.3	2.3	2.7	4.6	5.8
35-44	.9	4.3	5.2	7.0	10.3
45-54	.8	2.5	2.7	4.4	5.4
55 or older	.2	2.1	0	0	0
Offense					
Violent	.9%	1.5%	1.4%	2.7%	3.8%
Property	.9	3.0	3.4	5.2	5.7
Drug	.2	3.6	4.5	8.5	15.4
Public-order	1.0	2.3	2.9	4.5	9.0

Although women and men who never used drugs had the same HIV rates (less than 1 %), those women who used drugs and who used needles had higher infection rates than men with the same drug practices. Ten percent of women and 6.7% of men who had ever shared needles when using drugs were HIV positive.

Of those who reported sharing needles to inject illegal drugs, 1 in 10 black inmates, Hispanic inmates, and inmates between ages 35 and 44 were HIV positive. Over 15% of those sentenced for drug offenses and who had shared needles were HIV positive.

HIV Test Results, by Type of Prison

Maximum, medium, and minimum security level prisons had essentially the same rates of HIV infection [about 2%]. Inmates held in prisons with unclassified security levels, such as facilities for classification or reception, reported a positive rate of 11.6%.

Percentages of HIV-positive prisoners increased with the size of the prison. The HIV-positive rate in facilities holding fewer than 500 was 1.1%, compared to 2.8% in prisons with 2,500 or more.

HIV Testing Policies in the Largest Jail Jurisdictions

The jail jurisdictions that were among the 25 largest in 1991 were asked what testing policies they were following. Sixteen jurisdictions tested when ordered by a court, and 12 checked high risk groups. Two jurisdictions tested all inmates at admission in at least one facility: Philadelphia, Pennsylvania, and Fulton County (Atlanta), Georgia.

Deaths in 503 Large Jail Jurisdictions

Of the 445 deaths during the year ending June 30, 1992, in jail jurisdictions with average daily inmate populations of 100 or more, 24% were reported to be AIDS related.

Table 17.5. AIDS-related deaths in local jails, 1991-92.

Cause of death	Number
Total	445
AIDS	107
Other	338

About Bureau of Justice Statistics Special Reports

Bureau of Justice Statistics (BJS) Special Reports are written principally by BJS staff. Caroline Wolf Harlow wrote this report, under the supervision of Allen Beck. Virginia Baldau and Cheryl Crawford of the National Institute of Justice, Theodore Hammett of Abt Associates Inc. and William Darrow, Steven Jones, and Sandra Kerr of the Centers for Disease Control and Prevention gave expert advice on measurement and presentation of the HIV-related data collected. Louis Jankowski provided statistical assistance. Corrections reports are produced under the general guidance of Lawrence A. Greenfeld. Tom Hester edited the report. Marilyn Marbrook, assisted by Betty Sherman and Jayne Pugh, produced the report.

— by Caroline Wolf Harlow, Ph.D. BJS Statistician

Chapter 18

Instances of Occupational HIV Transmission to Health Care Workers

As of December 1997, CDC (Centers for Disease Control and Prevention) is aware of 54 health care workers (HCWs) in the United States who have had documented HIV seroconversion following occupational exposures, which means they tested negative for HIV infection around the time of exposure, but tested HIV positive within a year after the exposure. Another 132 HIV-infected health care workers have been classified as possible cases of occupational transmission. These 132 health care workers have a history of occupational exposure to blood, other body fluids, or HIV-infected laboratory material and report no other risk factors for HIV infection, but do not have documentation of seroconversion after the occupational exposure.

Types of Exposures and Risk for HIV Transmission

Of the 54 HCWs with documented transmission, 46 (85%) were exposed to HIV through percutaneous injuries (injuries penetrating the skin, such as from a needle stick). Another 5 had mucocutaneous exposures (they were exposed to body fluids from an HIV-infected person through the mucous membranes or skin); 2 HCWs had both percutaneous and mucocutaneous exposures; and 1 had an unknown route of exposure. Forty-nine of the 54 HCWs were exposed to the blood of an HIV-infected person, 1 to visibly bloody fluid, 1 to an unspecified fluid, and 3 to concentrated virus in a laboratory. Studies

CDC Update, National Center for HIV, STD, and TB Prevention, June 1998.

suggest that several factors may affect the risk for HIV transmission through an occupational exposure, including the quantity of blood or body fluid, the concentration of HIV in the blood or fluid, and the exposed person's underlying health and immune status.

Preventive Strategies

The primary means of preventing the HCW's occupational exposure to HIV and other bloodborne pathogens is to follow infection control precautions with the assumption that the blood and other body fluids from *all* patients are potentially infectious. These precautions include the routine use of barriers (such as gloves and/or goggles) when anticipating contact with blood or body fluids, immediately washing hands and other skin surfaces after contact with blood or body fluids, and careful handling and disposal of sharp instruments during and after use.

Table 18.1. U.S. Health Care Workers with Documented and Possible Occupationally Acquired HIV Infection and AIDS, Reported Through December 1997

Occupation	Number of Occupational Transmissions	
	Documented	Possible
Dental worker, including dentist	-	7
Embalmer/morgue technician	1	2
Emergency medical technician/paramedic	-	12
Health aide/attendant	1	15
Housekeeper/maintenance worker	1	10
Laboratory technician (clinical)	16	18
Laboratory technician (nonclinical)	3	0
Nurse	22	32
Physician (nonsurgical)	6	11
Physician (surgical)	-	6
Respiratory therapist	1	2
Technician (dialysis)	1	3
Technician (surgical)	2	2
Technician/therapist other than above	0	9
Other health care occupations	-	3
TOTAL	54	132

Safety devices have also been developed to help prevent needlestick injuries. If used properly, these types of devices may reduce the risk of exposure to HIV through percutaneous injuries. Furthermore, because many percutaneous injuries are related to sharps disposal, strategies for safer disposal, including safer design of disposal containers and placement of containers, are being developed.

Although the most important approach toward reducing the risk of occupational HIV transmission is to prevent occupational exposures, there also should be plans for post-exposure management for HCWs. One consideration in post-exposure management is the administration of antiretrovirals as post-exposure prophylaxis (PEP). The use of zidovudine as PEP has been shown to be safe and associated with decreased risk for occupationally related HIV infection. Newer antiretrovirals also may be effective, although there is less experience with their use as PEP; therefore, data are continually being collected on the use of the newer antiretrovirals. CDC recently issued guidelines for the management of HCW exposures to HIV and recommendations for PEP. These guidelines outline a number of considerations in determining whether or not an HCW should receive PEP and in choosing the type of PEP regimen.

Building Better Prevention Programs for Health Care Workers

Continued work in the following areas is needed to reduce the risk of occupational HIV transmission to health care workers:

Continue administrative efforts. All health organizations should continue to support infection control measures that prevent HCWs from becoming exposed to blood and other body fluids. The training and monitoring of HCWs and the reporting of occupational exposures are essential to prevention efforts.

Develop and promote the use of safety devices. Effective and competitively priced safety devices are needed for HCWs who frequently come into contact with potentially HIV-infected blood and other body fluids. The use of safety devices should be evaluated to determine if they are being used properly and consistently.

Monitor the effects of PEP. More data are needed on the safety and tolerability of different regimens of PEP, particularly those regimens that consist of new antiretroviral agents. Furthermore, improved communication regarding side-effects before starting treatment and close follow-up of HCWs are needed to increase compliance with the PEP.

CDC, in collaboration with hospitals and other health care organizations, will continue to promote a safe and healthy health care work environment through surveillance activities, epidemiologic and laboratory research, and the development of guidelines and recommendations for the prevention and management of occupational exposures and infections in health care workers.

Chapter 19

Report on the Global HIV/ AIDS Epidemic

HIV and AIDS: The Global Situation

The human immunodeficiency virus (HIV) continues to spread around the world, insinuating itself into communities previously little troubled by the epidemic and strengthening its grip on areas where AIDS is already the leading cause of death in adults (defined here as those aged 15-49).

Estimates by the Joint United Nations Programme on HIV/AIDS (UNAIDS) and the World Health Organization (WHO), a cosponsor of the Joint Programme, indicate that by the beginning of 1998 over 30 million people were infected with HIV, the virus that causes AIDS, and that 11.7 million people around the world had already lost their lives to the disease.

Unless a cure is found or life-prolonging therapy can be made more widely available, the majority of those now living with HIV will die within a decade.

These deaths will not be the last; there is worse to come. The virus continues to spread, causing nearly 16,000 new infections a day. During 1997 alone, that meant 5.8 million new HIV infections, despite the fact that more is known now than ever before about what works to prevent the spread of the epidemic.

Excerpted from *Report on the Global HIV/AIDS Epidemic*, Joint United National Programme on HIV/AIDS (UNAIDS) and World Health Organization (WHO), June 1998; reprinted with permission. British spellings have been Americanized. Visit UNAIDS on the World Wide Web at www.unaids.org.

It is possible that momentum for prevention will build up as the epidemic becomes more visible. Today, although one in every 100 adults in the most sexually active age bracket (15-49) is living with HIV, only a tiny fraction know about their infection. Because people can live for many years with HIV before showing any sign of illness, the virus can spread unobserved for a long time. In the face of other pressing concerns, it has been relatively easy in many parts of the world for political, religious, and community leaders to over-

Table 19.1. Global estimates of the HIV/AIDS epidemic as of end 1997

People newly infected with HIV in 1997	Total	5.8million
	Adults	5.2 million
	Women	2.1 million
	Children < 15 years	590,000
Number of people living with HIV/AIDS	Total	30.6 million
	Adults	29.4 million
	Women	12.2 million
	Children < 15 years	1.1 million
AIDS deaths in 1997	Total	2.3 million
	Adults	1.8 million
	Children < 15 years	460,000
Total number of AIDS deaths since the beginning of the epidemic	Total	11.7 million
	Adults	9.0 million
	Women	3.9 million
	Children < 15 years	2.7 million
Total number of AIDS orphans* since the beginning of the epidemic		8.2 million

Defined as children who lost their mother or both parents to AIDS when they were under the age of 15.

look the significance of the epidemic. But AIDS cases, and AIDS deaths, are growing the world over, and there are few countries where it is still possible to be ignorant of the scale of the disease. Some 2.3 million people died of AIDS during the course of 1997. In roughly the same number again HIV infection developed into symptomatic AIDS. HIV has more than doubled the adult death rate in some places, and is the single biggest cause of adult death in many others. Indeed HIV/AIDS is among the top ten killers world wide,

Table 19.2. Adults and children living with HIV/AIDS: total 30.6 million:

Region	Number
East Asia and Pacific	420,000
South and South-East Asia	5.8 million
Australia and New Zealand	12,000
Eastern Europe and Central Asia	190,000
Western Europe	480,000
North Africa and Middle East	210,000
sub-Saharan Africa	21 million
North America	860,000
Caribbean	310,000
Latin America	1.3 million

and given current levels of HIV infection, it may soon move into the top five, overtaking such well-established causes of death as diarrheal diseases.

Nearly 600,000 children were infected with HIV in 1997, mostly through their mothers before or during birth or through breastfeeding. The number of children under 15 who have lived or are living with HIV since the start of the epidemic in the late 1970s has reached around 3.8 million—2.7 million of them have already died. However, recent developments in the understanding of mother-to-child transmission and in drug research hold out a promise of reducing the number of child infections, at least in populations where pregnant women can choose to be tested for HIV.

HIV infections are concentrated in the developing world, mostly in countries least able to afford to care for infected people. In fact,

89% of people with HIV live in sub-Saharan Africa and the developing countries of Asia, which between them account for less than 10% of global Gross National Product. While in some countries HIV has remained at roughly the same low levels for a number of years, others, currently at similar absolute levels of prevalence, are experiencing a rapid spread of the virus. It is these countries that have the greatest potential to avert epidemic spread by acting quickly.

It is clear that infection rates are rising rapidly in much of Asia, Eastern Europe, and southern Africa. The picture in Latin America is mixed, with prevalence in some countries rising rapidly. In other parts of Latin America and many industrialized countries, infection is falling or close to stable. This is also the case in Uganda (one of the earliest countries to record epidemic growth in HIV infection), in Thailand (where the rapid spread of HIV has been checked by active prevention programs), and in some West African countries. Nevertheless, although the situation is improving among many groups, large numbers of new infections still occur every year in these countries.

Orphans

HIV has often caused huge increases in death rates among younger adults—just the age when people are forming families and having children. This inevitably leads to an increase in orphans. In rural areas of East Africa, four of every 10 children who have lost one of their parents by age 15 have been orphaned by HIV/AIDS. From the beginning of the epidemic until the start of 1998, some 8.2 million children around the world had lost their mother to AIDS. Many of those had lost their fathers as well. In 1997 alone, around 1.6 million children were orphaned by HIV. Over 90% of those orphans live in sub-Saharan Africa.

Extended family structures have in many countries been able to absorb some of the stress of increasing orphanhood. However, urbanization and the migration of labor, often across borders, is eating away at those structures. As the number of orphans grows and the number of potential caregivers shrinks, traditional coping mechanisms stretch to breaking point. That point may be reached much more rapidly in countries such as Thailand, where the nuclear family is increasingly the norm, and in Cambodia, where decades of war and civil strife have already taken a heavy toll on family structures and social coping mechanisms. These two countries already have the highest proportion of AIDS orphans in Asia.

The Evolving Picture Region by Region

Sub-Saharan Africa: The Epidemic Shifts South

Over two-thirds of all the people now living with HIV in the world—nearly 21 million men, women, and children—live in Africa south of the Sahara desert, and fully 83% of the world's AIDS deaths have been in this region. Since the very start of the epidemic, HIV in sub-Saharan Africa has mostly spread through sex between men and women. This means that women are more heavily affected in Africa than in other regions, where the virus initially spread most quickly among men by male-to-male sex or drug injecting. Four out of five HIV-positive women in the world live in Africa.

An even higher proportion of the children living with HIV in the world are in Africa—an estimated 87%. There are a number of reasons for this. First, more women of childbearing age are HIV-infected in Africa than elsewhere. Secondly, African women have more children on average than those in other continents, so one infected woman may pass the virus on to a higher than average number of children. Thirdly, nearly all children in Africa are breastfed. Breastfeeding is thought to account for between a third and half of all HIV transmission from mother to child. Finally, new drugs which help reduce transmission from mother to child before and around childbirth are far less readily available in developing countries, including those in Africa, than in the industrialized world.

By the early 1980s, HIV was found in a geographic band stretching from West Africa across to the Indian Ocean. The countries north of the Sahara and those in the southern cone of the continent remained apparently untouched. By 1987, the epidemic became more concentrated in the original areas, and began gradually to colonize the south. A decade later, in 1997, HIV had been recorded all over the continent.

In general, West Africa has seen its rates of infection stabilize at much lower levels than East and southern Africa. However, some of the most populous countries in West Africa are exceptions to this rule. In Côte d'Ivoire, West Africa's third most populous nation, one adult in 10 is already believed to be living with HIV. Nigeria has an estimated adult prevalence of 4.1%—relatively low by the standards of the continent, but with 118 million inhabitants (a fifth of the population of sub-Saharan Africa) this translates into 2.2 million infections. And there is no evidence that infection levels have stabilized. Clearly, if HIV prevalence in Nigeria were to approach the 20% rates all too

153

commonly seen in southern African countries, the burden would be devastating.

Today, the most severe HIV epidemics in the world are to be found in the southern countries of Africa. The virus there is still spreading rapidly, despite already high levels of infection. High-prevalence and relatively low-prevalence areas show the same pattern—a sharp rise in just four years. Some 2.9 million South Africans are thought to be living with HIV at the beginning of 1998, over 700,000 of them infected in 1997 alone.

Other countries in southern Africa face even higher rates of infection. In Botswana, the proportion of the adult population living with HIV has doubled over the last five years, with 43% of pregnant women testing HIV-positive in 1997 in the major urban center of Francistown. In Zimbabwe, one in four adults in 1997 were thought to be infected. In Harare, 32% of pregnant women were already infected in 1995. In Beit Bridge, a major commercial farming center, HIV prevalence in pregnant women shot up from 32% in 1995 to 59% in 1996. Although infection levels in Zimbabwe's cities were slightly higher than in rural areas, the difference was not great. In one town near the South African border with a large population of migrant workers, seven out of 10 women attending antenatal clinics tested HIV-positive in 1995.

The first country in Africa to respond actively to a massive national HIV/AIDS burden was Uganda. The government engaged religious and traditional leaders and other sectors of society in a vigorous debate that helped forge consensus around the need to attack the problem of HIV. Active prevention programs, focused on delaying sexual relations and negotiating safe behavior, were brought into schools. Community groups were set up to counsel people and families living with the virus. The efforts of the government and people of Uganda seem to be paying off. At both rural and urban surveillance sites infection rates are falling. The improvement has been particularly marked in the younger age groups. This is in line with behavior studies showing that young people nowadays are adopting safer sexual behavior—later sexual initiation, fewer partners, more condom use—than was common a decade ago. First signs of falling infection rates in young people are also being seen in neighboring Tanzania, in areas with active prevention programs. In women aged 15-24 in the urban area of Bukoba, prevalence fell from 28% in 1987 to 11 % in 1993. In the surrounding rural area, prevalence among women in the same age group fell from almost 10% in 1987 to 3% in 1996.

Asia: Low Infection Rates but Rapid Spread

HIV was a latecomer to Asia, but its spread has been swift. Until the late 1980s, no country in Asia experienced a major epidemic—the continent appeared practically immune. By 1992, however, a number of countries, led by Thailand, were facing increasing numbers of infections. These were generally concentrated in groups such as drug injectors and sex workers whose behavior was known to put them at risk. Although no Asian country has reached anything like the prevalence levels common in sub-Saharan Africa, HIV was by 1997 well established across the continent. The countries of South-East Asia, with the exception of Indonesia, the Philippines and Laos, are comparatively hard hit, as is India. While prevalence remains low in China, that country too has been recording an increasing number of cases.

Only a few countries in the region have developed sophisticated systems for monitoring the spread of the virus, so HIV estimates in Asia often have to be made on the basis of less information than in other regions. Because over half of the world's population lives in the region, small differences in rates can make a huge difference in the absolute numbers of people infected.

The Government of China estimated that at the end of 1996 up to 200,000 people were living with HIV/AIDS. It is now estimated that this figure had doubled by the beginning of 1998. At present, there are two major epidemics under way in China. One is among injecting drug users in the mountainous southwest of the country. The other, newer epidemic is now surfacing among heterosexuals, especially along the prosperous eastern seaboard where prostitution is re-emerging as the gap grows between rich and poor. The warning signs of high-risk behavior are worryingly clear: sexually transmitted diseases (STDs) have shot up in recent years and there are no suggestions that the upward trend will be broken.

In India, HIV infection rates, at under 1% of the total adult population, are still low by the standards of many countries, although well over 10 times higher than in neighboring China. Surveillance is patchy, but it is now estimated that about four million people in India are living with HIV. That makes India the country with the largest number of HIV-infected people in the world. Recent testing of pregnant women in Pondicherry shows infection rates of around 4%. Among truck drivers in the southern state of Madras, HIV prevalence quadrupled from 1.5% in 1995 to 6.2% just one year later. In the north-eastern state of Manipur, where the epidemic took off quickly among

155

male drug injectors, some drug clinics were registering HIV rates as high as 73% in 1996.

There is limited information about HIV infection in other parts of South Asia, but it is clear that many people are having unprotected sex with non-monogamous partners. A recent study among sex workers in Bangladesh showed that 95% had contracted genital herpes, mostly from their clients, while 60% had syphilis.

Rates of HIV infection remain low in several South and South-East Asian nations. In Bangladesh, Indonesia, Laos, Pakistan, the Philippines, and Sri Lanka, infection has not reached one adult in 1000 yet. However, other countries in the region—including Cambodia, Myanmar, Thailand, and Viet Nam—show much higher levels of HIV. The reasons for these differences are not entirely clear. Nor is there any assurance that prevalence will remain low in those areas that have seen only a modest spread so far, given the widespread occurrence of risk behavior including commercial sex and, in some places, drug injecting.

Thailand, which has experienced what is probably the best-documented epidemic in the developing world, has shown evidence of a fall in new infections, especially among sex workers and their clients. So far, the majority of the almost 800,000 people living with HIV and AIDS in Thailand—some 2.3% of the adult population—fall into these two groups, or are drug injectors. The decrease in new infections is the outcome of sustained prevention efforts aimed at increasing condom use among heterosexuals, discouraging men from visiting sex workers, and offering young women better educational and other prospects to discourage their entry into commercial sex. HIV still appears to be spreading in other groups whose behavior puts them at risk of infection but who have received less attention in prevention campaigns. HIV rates among Thailand's injecting drug users have stabilized at a relatively high level (around 40%), and a survey among men who have sex with other men in northern Thailand reported low AIDS-awareness and infrequent condom use.

Elsewhere in South-East Asia the picture is mixed. It is bleakest in Cambodia, where one in 30 pregnant women, one in 16 soldiers and policemen, and nearly one in two sex workers tested positive in sentinel HIV surveillance. While condom use has grown very rapidly (condom sales have risen from virtually nothing to around a million units a month in under three years), commercial sex remains very common: in a recent survey three-quarters of respondents in the military and the police force and two-fifths of male students said they had visited a sex worker in the last year. Viet Nam and Myanmar are also seeing a rapid spread of HIV. In Myanmar, HIV infection among sex workers rose from 4% in 1992 to over 20% in 1996, while close to two-thirds of injecting drug users are infected. Among pregnant women in six urban areas, an estimated 2.2% are infected.

Overall, about 6.4 million people are currently believed to be living with HIV in Asia and the Pacific—just over one in five of the world's total. By the end of the year 2000, that proportion is expected to grow to one in four. Around 94,000 children in Asia now live with HIV.

Latin America and The Caribbean: Most Infections Are in Marginalized Groups

In Latin America the picture is fragmented, although nearly every country in the continent now reports HIV infections. The pattern of HIV spread in Latin America is much the same as that in industrialized countries. Men who have unprotected sex with other men and drug injectors who share needles are the focal points of HIV infection in many countries in the region. Studies in Mexico suggest that up to 30% of men who have sex with men may be living with HIV. Between 3% and 11% of drug injectors in Mexico are HIV-infected, and in Argentina and Brazil the proportion may be close to half of all injectors.

Rising rates in women nevertheless show that heterosexual transmission is becoming more prominent. In Brazil in 1986, one AIDS case in 17 was a woman. Now the figure for AIDS is one in four, and a quarter of the 550,000 adults currently living with HIV in Brazil are women. In the region as a whole the proportion is around one-fifth.

In some places there is clear evidence of increasing infection among poorer and less educated members of the population. For example, in Brazil most of the early AIDS cases were in people with secondary or university education; today 60% of people living with AIDS never studied beyond primary school.

Some 1.3 million people are believed to be living with HIV in Latin America and the Caribbean. HIV prevalence is estimated at under one adult in 100 in all but a handful of the region's 44 countries and territories.

Systematic surveillance is limited. Because contraceptive use is far higher in Latin America than in Africa or Asia—and a smaller proportion of sexually active women therefore become pregnant—HIV

157

prevalence among pregnant women is likely to be less representative of rates among all sexually active women than in other parts of the developing world. That said, they are still among the best indicators of HIV in the general population. HIV has reached levels of 1% among pregnant women in Honduras and more than 3% in Porto Alegre, Brazil. Rates are substantially higher in the Caribbean. By 1993, 8% of pregnant women in Haiti were infected with the virus, and the same prevalence was reported from one surveillance site in the Dominican Republic in 1996.

Several countries in Latin America are attempting to ensure care for people living with HIV and AIDS, including providing life-prolonging antiretroviral drugs. Access to care, although better than in other areas of the developing world, remains patchy overall.

Eastern Europe: Drug Injection Drives HIV

Until the mid-1990s, most of the countries of Eastern Europe appeared to have been spared the worst of the HIV epidemic. Mass screening of blood samples from people whose behavior put them at risk of HIV showed extremely low levels of infection, right up to 1994. The whole of Eastern Europe put together had around 30,000 infections among its 450 million people at the start of 1995. At that time, Western Europe had over 15 times as many cases, while in sub-Saharan Africa over 400 times as many people were living with the virus. But in the last few years, the former socialist economies of Eastern Europe and Central Asia have seen infections increase around six-fold. By the end of 1997, some 190,000 adults in the region were living with HIV infection.

The pattern of consistently low prevalence began to change in 1995 in several of the countries of the former Soviet Union. Belarus, Moldova, the Russian Federation, and Ukraine have all registered astronomical growth in HIV infection rates over the last three years, most related to unsafe drug injecting. Now there may be nearly four times as many infections in Ukraine alone as there were in the whole Eastern European region just three years ago.

Ukraine is the worst affected country in the region. Confirmed HIV cases are rising astronomically. Only 44 people tested positive for HIV in Ukraine in 1994, roughly the same number as in 1992 and 1993. But the number of diagnoses shot up over 30-fold in 1995, and in 1996 exploded to over 12,000. In 1997, another 15,000 new infections were identified. These numbers are just the tested cases—the tip of the iceberg. The true number of infections in 1994 was probably around

1,500. Now, just four years later, over 70 times that many people— some 110,000—are estimated to be infected.

A similar pattern appears in the Russian Federation, where 158 people tested positive for HIV in 1994. Many infected men at that time reported contracting the infection from sex with other men, and only two cases were reported among injecting drug users. By the end of last year, the epidemic had taken off in the Russian Federation. Nearly 4,400 people tested positive for HIV in 1997, almost three times as many as the previous year.

The bulk of the spread has been in injecting drug users. Four of every five newly diagnosed infections are in this group. Again, the true number of infections is far higher than these figures suggest. It is estimated that in the Russian Federation there are around six people living with HIV for every one person who has actually tested HIV-positive. That means around 40,000 people may currently be living with HIV.

The sex partners of injecting drug users may provide a conduit for the virus into the general population. In some areas of Eastern Europe, there seems to be a strong overlap between drug injectors and sex workers, who will also have clients from outside the drug-injecting community. Out of a small sample of 103 sex workers arrested on the streets of the Russian city of Kaliningrad, for instance, a third were known to be injecting drug users living with HIV. The city reported that four out of every five women treated for HIV-related illness at the regional AIDS center make a living out of sex.

There is no doubt that the warning signs for a widespread sexually-transmitted epidemic of HIV exist in many areas of Eastern Europe. Although levels of HIV infection in the general population remain very low, the testing of pregnant women, blood donors, and others suggests that the virus is becoming increasingly common in society as a whole. And there has been a dramatic increase in other sexually transmitted diseases, especially syphilis. From negligible annual rates of around 10 cases per 100,000 people in the late 1980s, new syphilis infections have shot up into the hundreds. The Russian Federation, which had an annual rate in the single figures in 1987, recorded over 260 cases per 100,000 population a decade later.

The rise in new cases of sexually transmitted diseases may reflect a dramatic increase in unprotected sex, a breakdown of STD treatment services, or both. Whatever the reason, it indicates that the risk of HIV spreading rapidly throughout the general population in Eastern Europe is very real.

159

The Industrialized World: AIDS Is Falling

In general, HIV infection rates appear to be dropping in Western Europe, with new infections concentrated among drug injectors in the southern countries of the continent, particularly Greece and Portugal. It is estimated that 30,000 Western Europeans were newly infected with HIV in 1997. Antiretroviral drugs given to women during pregnancy and the availability of safe alternatives to breastfeeding kept mother-to-child transmission low; it is estimated that fewer than 500 children under the age of 15 were infected with HIV in 1997.

North America estimated it had around 44,000 new HIV infections in 1997, close to half of them among injecting drug users. As in Western Europe, transmission from mother to child was rare, with fewer than 500 new cases.

Generally, industrialized countries concentrate on following AIDS cases rather than tracking HIV. And as HIV infections continue to rise in the developing world, AIDS cases in many industrialized countries are falling.

In Western Europe, new AIDS cases (corrected for delays in reporting) fell from 23,954 in 1995 to 14,874 in 1997—a 38% drop. The fall in AIDS cases is due in part to prevention measures taken since the late 1980s by gay communities, and to a sustained rise in the proportion of young people using condoms, which led to a drop in the number of people infected with HIV. Because of the long lag time between HIV infection and symptomatic AIDS, the behavior change of the late 1980s is only now being reflected in fewer new cases of AIDS. But the downturn is probably due most of all to new antiretroviral drug therapies which postpone the development of AIDS and prolong the life of people living with HIV.

In the United States, AIDS case reports indicate that the first-ever annual decrease in new cases—6%—occurred in 1996, and an even larger reduction was expected in 1997. The biggest improvement—a drop of 11 %—was in homosexual men. In some disadvantaged sections of society, however, AIDS continues to rise. Among African-Americans, new AIDS cases rose by 19% among heterosexual men and 12% among heterosexual women in 1996. In the Hispanic community, there were 13% more cases among men and 5% more among women than a year earlier. This is partly because these communities may find it hard to access the expensive new drugs that could stave off the onset of AIDS. It is partly, too, because prevention efforts in minority communities, where transmission is often through heterosexual intercourse and drug injecting, have been less successful than in the predominantly well-educated and well-organized gay community.

North Africa and the Middle East: The Great Unknown

Less is known about HIV infection rates in North Africa or the Middle East than in other parts of the world. Some countries, particularly those with large populations of immigrant workers, carry out mass screening for the virus, but none estimates infections at more than one adult in 100. Just over 200,000 people are estimated to be living with HIV in these countries, under 1% of the world total.

Risk behavior does, however, exist. At least one country in the region has started a program to reduce risky drug-injecting practices. The generally conservative social and political attitudes in the Middle East and North Africa often make it difficult for governments to address risk behavior directly. However, in some countries in the region, governments have created elbow room for community and nongovernmental organizations to help sex workers and others whose behavior puts them at risk to protect themselves from HIV.

Understanding the Epidemic

No Simple Explanations

Since HIV first began its march across the globe, people have been trying to explain why some countries are more affected than others. Because most of the worst-hit countries are among the world's poorest, for instance, there has been a temptation to say "AIDS is a disease of poverty." Because many of the populations most affected are also among the world's least educated, there has been a temptation to say "AIDS is a disease of ignorance."

Globally, it is certainly the poorer and less educated who are feeling the brunt of the HIV epidemic. But the epidemic has spread in different ways and through different groups of people in different parts of the world. Neighboring countries often have very different epidemics. And even within a single nation, HIV can strike different populations or different geographic areas in dissimilar ways, ways that may change over the course of time.

An analysis of the relationship between education and HIV illustrates the pitfalls of drawing deceptively simple conclusions about the determinants of the epidemic. Relationships that seem clear at a global level can look very different at a regional level, and even more complex over time in a single setting.

161

It is reasonable to assume that better-educated people have better access to information about HIV, how it is transmitted, and how it can be avoided. On top of that, better-educated people are more likely to have better-paid jobs, and can afford the sorts of goods and services that allow them to act on their AIDS knowledge. If we take overall levels of literacy as an indication of educational levels in a country, we might, then, expect to find that countries with high levels of literacy have low levels of HIV. And indeed, if we compare literacy and HIV for the 161 countries in the world for which there are data on both HIV and literacy, a statistically significant pattern of just this kind emerges.

But if we look just at the region of the world worst affected by HIV, sub-Saharan Africa, a very different picture emerges. In the 44 countries of the region for which figures exist, the analysis also reveals a relationship between HIV and literacy. But the direction of the relationship is now reversed. In this region, the countries with the highest levels of HIV infection are also those whose men and women are most literate.

In this region as in all others, more-educated people are likely to be better informed about the dangers of HIV and have more disposable income than the illiterate. So why do the figures suggest they are also more likely to be HIV-infected? There are several possible explanations. It may be that social changes that accompany more schooling are also associated with behavior that increases the risk of HIV infection. This may be especially the case for women, who without education may have very much less social mobility and be exposed to a much narrower spectrum of social and sexual relationships, for instance.

Another plausible explanation may be that educated people with higher earning power use their disposable income to support behaviors that put them at risk of infection. While a rich man is more able to afford a condom than a poor man, he is also more able to afford to invite a potential partner to a night-club, to support a number of wives, or to visit sex workers. And where men tend to have at least some partners of a similar social and educational standing as themselves, higher HIV rates among educated men will translate into higher HIV prevalence among educated women. So during the early stages of the epidemic, when information about the dangers of unprotected sex is scarce, literacy may actually prove more of a liability than a protection.

This is not for a moment to suggest that cutting back on education would help reduce HIV transmission. In fact, if we break down the figures by age, we see a very different pattern. Studies among large numbers of pregnant women in various urban centers in Zambia show that in general, urban women with more years of schooling are more likely to be HIV-infected than their peers with little or no schooling. But if we look at individual age groups, we see that the pattern is far more pronounced among older women than among younger women. The most-educated women in their late 20s were twice as likely as the least-educated to be HIV-infected. But among women 10 years their junior, the difference had all but disappeared.

Why the change over time? Older women are more likely to have been infected in the earlier years of the epidemic, when little information about HIV was available. And where there is no information about HIV, more schooling makes little difference. By the time the youngest age group became sexually active, however, much more information was available. It is of course possible that in the younger age groups, extra education has not yet conferred the economic advantages that give people the means to engage in more risky behavior. The data confirm the more general pattern seen in other countries of greater self-protection in younger age groups.

The more we learn about the way HIV moves through communities, the more we understand that the relationship between HIV and other social and economic phenomena is rarely simple. Analyses that draw universal conclusions about relationships seen at the global level may be useful in pointing to general factors—such as education, economic growth or equality between men and women—which greatly influence the spread of HIV. But it should be borne in mind that global analyses may mask the important differences between regions, countries or communities which are at the core of this diverse epidemic.

Understanding Behavior

Clearly, the HIV epidemic progresses differently in different situations. It is driven by individual behaviors which put people at risk of infection. These behaviors may in turn be driven by poverty, by unequal relationships between men and women or between old and young people, or by cultural and religious norms that leave people little control over their exposure to the virus. The social, economic, and cultural situations that create this kind of vulnerability to HIV infection have not been adequately studied or explained. Perhaps more surprisingly, there is still virtually no information in many countries on the basic sexual and drug-taking behaviors and patterns of

163

sexual networking that determine how the virus spreads through a population.

Many countries have set up surveillance systems to track the spread of HIV through their populations—systems that have largely been pioneered by the countries of sub-Saharan Africa. But far fewer have collected any information on the sexual and drug-taking behaviors that are central to the spread of HIV. Since these behaviors precede infection, information about them can act as an early warning system. Such behavioral data can indicate how exposed a community may be to HIV. The information can identify groups who are especially vulnerable, and can pinpoint particular risk behaviors which threaten to drive the spread of the virus. When collected over time, it can also indicate trends in risk behavior and vulnerability, validating existing prevention approaches or suggesting what changes need to be made for greater impact.

Behavioral data can be especially crucial in the early stages of the epidemic, when the virus may be spreading largely among people with well-defined behaviors such as drug injecting or commercial sex. Only behavioral information can identify the links between such people and others in the general population, links which may, if identified early enough, suggest practical ways of preventing general epidemic spread.

Better Tracking of the Epidemic

Better behavioral surveillance is an important component of the tracking of the epidemic. It contributes to predicting trends, to planning for change and to recording success or failure. But it will always make its greatest contribution when it is used in conjunction with better monitoring of the spread of the virus itself.

The surveillance systems currently in use have in some cases failed to keep up with the needs and the development of the HIV epidemic. This is partly because of the peculiar nature of HIV infection, which on average takes many years to develop into a symptomatic disease, but which can kill people at any time from a few years after infection to more than a decade later. This means that the percentage of the population alive with HIV at a given time—the prevalence rate—reflects both newly infected individuals and those who became infected at any time over the past decade or more.

Behavioral data can help to explain this kind of serosurveillance data. But the fact remains that such prevalence rates are difficult to interpret and are slow to reflect changes in the pattern of new infections. In the early stages of the epidemic, when infections in all age groups are growing simultaneously and few HIV-infected people have yet died, all-age prevalence information is helpful in tracking the epidemic. But as the epidemic matures, and the number of people entering the HIV-infected population (by acquiring the virus) is increasingly balanced by the number leaving it (through AIDS deaths), all-age prevalence becomes less useful.

Because of these inherent difficulties, it is useful especially when tracking mature epidemics to make changes in the way serosurveillance data are collected. For example, concentrating resources on better surveillance of teenagers and people in their early 20s, who if seropositive are likely to have become infected only recently, can give a better picture of HIV incidence trends. In addition, instead of spreading precious resources very thinly—for instance, by regularly testing anonymous blood samples from all pregnant women even when infection in the general population is barely detectable—countries may find it more useful to focus on tracking the virus in groups with greater risk or vulnerability to HIV. The type of surveillance necessary will of course be dictated by the general pattern of infection in a country. Behavioral data will help identify these groups, signal possible changes in them, and pinpoint potential bridges between these and other parts of the population.

Part Three

Information for People Living with HIV/AIDS

Chapter 20

New Ways to Prevent and Treat AIDS

Preventing and treating AIDS is one of the Food and Drug Administration's top priorities. A new class of drugs, a home blood test collection kit, an oral diagnostic test, an HIV antigen test, an HIV-1 antigen test for blood supply, and an HIV viral load test are among the most recent in a long line of products FDA has approved to prevent, diagnose and treat infection with HIV, the virus that causes AIDS.

HIV Tests

The 1992 National Health Interview Survey by the Centers for Disease Control and Prevention found that only 20 percent of people at increased risk for HIV infection—such as intravenous drug users, male homosexuals, and prostitutes—agreed to be tested for HIV. More than twice that many people in the same risk group said they might use a home testing and counseling service if one were available. At the time, however, testing could only be done by a professional.

The situation changed when, on May 14, 1996, FDA approved Confide, the first HIV test system with a home-use blood collection kit. A second test kit was approved last July. It is hoped that home testing will make diagnosis easier and more accessible, especially in populations among whom the recent rise in cases of HIV is greatest, such as women, African Americans, and Hispanics. The tests are highly reliable and are designed to protect the user's anonymity.

NIH Pub. No. (FDA) 97-1268, with revisions made in May 1997.

169

FDA's approval on June 3, 1996, of OraSure Western blot, a laboratory test that does not require a blood sample, is also expected to increase participation in testing for HIV. Instead of pricking a finger—a procedure shunned by many individuals—OraSure uses a treated cotton pad to collect an oral specimen from between the gum and cheek.

The sample is tested for antibodies to HIV by a procedure that has been shown to be highly accurate. An earlier version of OraSure used a less reliable method to screen for HIV antibodies, and people who tested positive had to undergo a standard blood test to confirm the presence of the virus.

In March 1996, FDA approved the Coulter HIV-1 p24 Antigen Assay, the first blood screening test to detect antigens rather than antibodies. In screening routinely carried out since the mid-1980s, technicians check donated blood for HIV-1 antibodies by using enzyme-linked immunosorbent assay (ELISA) test kits. Since a small number of ELISA test results are nonspecific or falsely positive, the standard procedure uses a second, more specific test—the Western blot test—to validate the positive results from ELISA testing.

The Coulter test, which is used in addition to ELISA, screens blood for antigens—proteins found on the surface of the virus—that are detectable about one week earlier than HIV antibodies. The new test reduces the so-called "window" period, typically up to three months long, during which standard blood tests show no HIV antibodies, even though the donor may be infected.

The Amplicor HIV-1 Monitor Test, another new blood test approved last year, enables physicians to predict the risk of HIV disease progression by precisely measuring virus levels in blood. The test, which amplifies copies of genetic material from the virus by using polymerase chain reaction technology, is based on clinical studies showing that higher virus levels can be correlated with increased risk that the disease will progress to AIDS, and AIDS-related infection or death.

Condoms

Other than abstinence, latex-rubber condoms are the best protection against sexual transmission of HIV. Latex condoms should always be used for oral, anal and vaginal sex in any relationship that isn't mutually monogamous, and if there is any other chance that either partner may be infected. Condom manufacturers in the United States electronically test all condoms for holes and weak spots. In addition, FDA requires manufacturers to use a water test to examine samples from each batch of condoms for leakage. If the test detects a defect rate of more than 4 per 1,000, the entire lot is discarded.

The agency also encourages manufacturers to test samples of their products for breakage by using an air burst test in accordance with specifications of the International Standards Organization.

Under an FDA proposal, the labeling on latex condoms should state that "this product contains natural rubber latex." FDA has also requested manufacturers to state on the label that "[if] used properly, latex condoms will help reduce the risk of transmission of HIV infection (AIDS) and many other sexually-transmitted diseases."

Consumers should make sure the condom package is undamaged, and check each condom for damage as it is unrolled to be used. The condom should not be used if it is gummy or brittle, discolored, or has a hole. Condoms also should not be used after their expiration date or, if they don't have an expiration date, more than five years after the date of manufacture. Only water-based lubricants (for instance, glycerine or K-Y jelly) should be used with latex condoms, because oil-based lubricants such as petroleum jelly weaken natural rubber.

For people allergic to latex, FDA has approved several polyurethane condoms, which have been shown in laboratory tests to be comparable to latex condoms as a barrier to sperm and HIV virus. Each package of polyurethane condoms is labeled "For Latex Sensitive Condom Users." Natural membrane (lambskin) condoms, which are useful in preventing pregnancy, are not effective protection against HIV or other sexually transmitted diseases. Although sperm cannot pass through the lambskin material, small microorganisms, including HIV, can penetrate these condoms.

One product available for women—the polyurethane Reality Female Condom—provides limited protection against sexually transmitted diseases. FDA requires the labeling of Reality to indicate that "highly effective protection" against STDs is provided if the male partner uses a latex condom for men. Male and female condoms, however, should not be used at the same time because they won't stay in place.

Medical and Dental Equipment

To protect patients and health-care providers against exposure to potentially contaminated blood and other body liquids, FDA established quality standards for latex and synthetic rubber gloves used during surgery and patient examination. U.S. manufacturers of these products are requested to test samples from each lot to make sure they show no sign of leakage when filled for two minutes with 1,000 milliliters of water, and that they meet the standards of the American Society for Testing and Materials for stress resistance, tensile strength, materials, and dimensions. FDA also tests samples of domestic and imported surgical and patient examination gloves, using the same criteria.

FDA has joined CDC and the American Dental Association in urging dentists to autoclave—sterilize by steam under pressure—dental hand pieces and accessories between patients to remove possible contaminants. In addition, FDA requires that all such equipment must be designed to withstand autoclaving, and the labeling must include instructions for the sterilization process.

While most dentists are believed to comply with the recommendations for autoclaving, it's a good idea to ask what preventive measures the dentist follows before making an appointment.

Blood Transfusion

Each year, about 3.6 million Americans receive transfusions of blood products. FDA inspects the more than 3,000 donor centers where blood and blood components are collected and processed, and continuously updates requirements and standards designed to prevent disease transmission through transfusion.

Blood collection centers and manufacturers and distributors of blood products are responsible for maintaining five layers of overlapping safeguards.

First, potential donors must answer questions about their health and risk factors. Those whose blood may pose a health hazard are encouraged to exclude themselves. A trained and competent health professional then interviews potential donors about their medical histories.

Donors can be temporarily excluded from donating blood for such reasons as having a temperature, cold, cough, or sore throat on the day of the donation. Potential donors are permanently excluded from donating blood for reasons including evidence of HIV infection, male homosexual activity since 1977, and a history of intravenous drug abuse or viral hepatitis.

Second, blood establishments must keep current a list of deferred donors and check donor names against that list.

Third, after donation, the blood is tested for such blood-borne agents as HIV, hepatitis and syphilis.

The fourth layer of protection prevents general use of any blood products that have not been thoroughly tested.

The fifth layer of protection is FDA's requirement that blood establishments must investigate any breaches of safeguards and correct deficiencies. An error or accident can result from improper testing, incorrectly labeled components, improper interpretation of test results, improper use of equipment or failure to follow the manufacturers' directions for its use, or accepting units from donors who should have been deferred.

The system has helped reduce the risk of transfused HIV infection from 1 in 2,500 units of blood in 1985 to 1 in 440,000 to 640,000 units by the end of 1995. Since then, the Coulter test has shortened the typical window period when the HIV virus cannot be detected to less than three months. Health experts expect the use of this test to reduce the risk of transfused HIV infection even further.

Human Tissue Transplants

In December 1993, FDA issued an interim requirement that potential donors of all human tissues for transplantation—including tendons, bone, skin, and corneas—be tested for HIV-1, HIV-2, and hepatitis B and C viruses, and screened for symptoms of AIDS, hepatitis, and high-risk behaviors such as sex between males and intravenous drug abuse. Imported tissues must be accompanied by records showing that the tissues were similarly screened and tested. If such records are not available, the tissues must be shipped under quarantine.

The agency is preparing a final rule and a guideline to ensure uniformity in tissue testing and screening.

Drugs

In December 1995, a new class of drugs called protease inhibitors was added to the earlier approved class of nucleoside analogs, which included Retrovir (zidovudine, also known as AZT), Videx (didanosine, or ddI), Hivid (zalcitabine, or ddC), Zerit (stavudine, or d4t), and Epivir (lamivudine, or 3TC).

The protease inhibitors—Invirase (saquinavir), Norvir (ritonavir), and Crixivan (indinavir)—inhibit replication of HIV in a similar way as nucleoside analogs, but are active at different points in the replication process. Tested alone or in combination with the nucleoside analogs, the three protease inhibitors markedly reduced the viral load and increased the number of CD4 cells, which sharply declines in HIV infection and AIDS.

173

In June 1996, FDA approved Viramune (nevirapine), the first in a new class of drugs called non-nucleoside reverse transcriptase inhibitors. Viramune was approved for use in combination with nucleoside analogs to treat adults with HIV infection who have experienced clinical and/or immunological deterioration.

By the end of June, FDA also had approved 22 drugs for HIV- and AIDS-related conditions. Among them are NebuPent (aerosolized pentamidine isethionate) to prevent *Pneumocystis carinii* pneumonia, the most common life-threatening infection of people with AIDS, and Roferon-A (interferon alfa-2a) and Intron-A (interferon alfa-2b) for Kaposi's sarcoma, an aggressive cancer that affects primarily male homosexuals with AIDS.

Nutrition

Some patients with HIV have wasting syndrome, with symptoms that include major weight loss, chronic diarrhea or weakness, and constant or intermittent fever for at least 30 days. The syndrome is classified as an AIDS-defining illness. All people with HIV should carefully follow food safety practices, because their weakened immunity leaves them particularly vulnerable to food-borne illness. Diarrhea caused by such illness can lead to or worsen wasting syndrome.

To prevent food-borne illnesses, people with HIV should avoid nonpasteurized dairy products, wash hands and utensils with soap and hot water when preparing meals, and cook food thoroughly to kill harmful bacteria. Raw eggs and raw seafood such as oysters, clams, sushi, and sashimi should not be eaten. Additional information about food safety and HIV can be obtained from FDA.

Loss of appetite (anorexia) can be treated with two FDA-approved prescription medicines for HIV and AIDS patients. Marinol (dronabinol), a synthetic extract of marijuana, is indicated for anorexia associated with weight loss. Megace (megestrol acetate) can be used for anorexia, cachexia (emaciation), or any unexplained significant weight loss.

Unapproved Therapies

Recognizing the special needs of people with HIV infection and AIDS, FDA uses its discretion to allow them to import for their personal use unapproved but promising drugs for HIV and HIV-related life-threatening diseases. At the same time, the agency vigorously campaigns against AIDS health scams that have bilked their victims of as much as $ 10 billion a year.

As a result of FDA investigations, federal and state authorities have taken legal actions against individuals involved in hundreds of fraudulent cures for AIDS such as "energized" water, "ozone therapy," and hydrogen peroxide "treatment."

Because most of the scams are local enterprises, FDA initiated in 1989 an AIDS Health Fraud Task Force Network to monitor and counter the promotion of suspected fraudulent AIDS products. The task forces, so far established in 10 states, have built broadly based coalitions of federal, state and local authorities with the medical community and AIDS activists. They cooperate in explaining to individuals and organizations how to identify fraudulent health products and distribute general information about HIV infection.

— by Mike Kubic

Mike Kubic is a member of FDA's public affairs staff.

Chapter 21

Oral HIV-1 Antibody Tests

Q. *What is this test using oral fluid?*

A. It is an alternative to blood testing for HIV-1 antibody. The test can be used on one single oral sample. No needles or skin puncturing are required in any of the steps to detect the presence of HIV-1 antibody. A blood sample is not needed to confirm the initial results of the oral HIV rest.

Q. *Is this test as good as the blood tests that have been in use for years?*

A. Yes. A correctly performed oral specimen HIV-1 antibody test is as good as blood for testing of HIV-1 infection for diagnosis in public health and clinical settings.

Q. *How do HIV antibodies get into the mouth?*

A. Saliva contains very small amounts of HIV antibodies. Proteins can pass through the thin lining of the mouth and gums from blood vessels located close to the surface of the mouth. The collection pad, which looks like an ordinary cotton swab, encourages the flow of these proteins which are then drawn into the pad. This is why the oral test gives results that are essentially equivalent to that of a blood test for HIV antibodies.

Q. *If you can do an oral HIV antibody test on saliva, then why isn't HIV transmitted by kissing?*

Centers for Disease Control and Prevention (CDC), revised June 3, 1996.

A. This test detects HIV *antibody*, a type of protein present in oral specimens—not the virus itself. Previous studies have shown that low levels of HIV can be found in oral fluid especially when visible blood is present. However, no cases of HIV transmission are clearly attributable to saliva.

Q. *Who will be able to use this test?*

A. The device will be sold to physicians who may train non-clinicians to collect specimens from patients who consent to evaluation. Specimens must be processed in a laboratory as blood specimens are. This is not a "home test kit."

Q. *How are the results of the HIV-1 oral test interpreted?*

A. Persons who are tested for HIV antibody with this oral test should be given the same considerations as with any HIV test. They should consent to be tested and receive appropriate pre- and post-test counseling. All test results should be kept confidential. A diagnosis of HIV infection can be made with an oral HIV test after confirmation with the licensed OraSure HIV-1 Western Blot kit.* A diagnosis of HIV infection should not be made based on the results of the initial screening test alone. CDC and the Association for State and Territorial Public Health Laboratory Directors recommend that all new diagnoses of HIV infection by re-confirmed in a second (newly collected) specimen.

Q. *How much will a test cost? Will it be less than a blood test?*

A. Prices will be set by the manufacturer of this test kit, the laboratory that performs the test, and the clinician who collects the specimen or orders the test. As with other medical tests, prices are likely to vary widely. However, since the number and types of tests performed on oral fluid samples are the same as that performed on blood, the price ranges may be comparable.

Q. *When were these tests approved?*

A. On December 23, 1994, the Food and Drug Administration (FDA) approved the OraSure HIV-1 Oral Specimen Collection Device,* used to collect oral specimens for use with the Oral Fluid Vironostika HIV-1 Microelisa System.* On June 3, 1996, FDA also approved the OraSure HIV-1 Western Blot Kit,* which will be used to confirm the presence of HIV-1 antibodies in oral samples that are reactive on screening tests.

*Use of brand names is for identification only and does not imply endorsement by the Centers for Disease Control and Prevention, the U.S. Public Health Service, or the U.S. Department of Health and Human Services.

Chapter 22

Understanding Viral Load

Introduction

Measurements of HIV-RNA blood levels (viral load) are increasingly being used by health care providers to determine when to start antiretroviral therapy and when to change current therapies. This test has become very important in the management of HIV infection because studies have shown that the level of virus in the blood is a predictor of disease progression. In other words, people with high levels of HIV-RNA in their blood are more likely to rapidly progress to AIDS than people with low levels of the virus.

Because viral load testing is an integral part of the management of HIV disease, it is important to learn what this test is and how it is used. Trying to understand viral load testing isn't easy. This fact sheet was developed to help clarify information about viral load testing.

What Is Viral Load and How Is It Measured?

Viral load or viral burden is the quantity of HIV-RNA (HIV virus) that is in the blood. RNA is the genetic material of HIV that contains the information needed to make more virus. Viral load tests measure the amount of HIV-RNA in a small amount of blood (one milliliter, ml). There are three different viral load tests currently being used:

HIV/AIDS Treatment Information Service (ATIS), March 1997.

- **PCR** (polymerase chain reaction) is the most common of these tests and is the only test approved by the FDA. Test results are reported as copies/ml of plasma.

- **bDNA** (branched chain DNA assay) is also frequently used. These results are reported as units/ml of plasma.

- **NASBA** (nucleic acid sequence-based amplification) is less frequently used and reports test results as units/ml of plasma.

Because the tests do not give exactly the same results, it is important to have the same type of viral load test done each time. This will give the physician a baseline against which changes can be evaluated. Since the results of this test can vary greatly, they should be interpreted in the context of clinical management with an experienced physician.

When Should Viral Load Be Measured?

An Expert Panel for the International AIDS Society-USA[1] has issued guidelines indicating when viral load should be measured. The following is the Panel's timetable for testing:

- Take two different viral load measurements 2-3 weeks apart to determine a baseline measurement.

- Repeat every 3-6 months thereafter in conjunction with CD4 counts to monitor viral load and T-cell count.

- Repeat the test 4-6 weeks after starting or changing therapy to determine the effect on viral load.

Avoid measuring viral load in the 3-4 weeks following an immunization (including flu shots) or within one month of an infection. Temporary increases in viral load have been seen in these instances. To minimize misleading results, it's best to avoid testing at these times.

Another consideration for measuring viral load is cost. Because the test is expensive (tests can range between $63-$292 with a commonly reported cost of $200 per test), it is important to have them drawn at appropriate times.

What Prompts Changes in Viral Load?

Changes in viral load are often reported as logarithmic or "log changes." This mathematical term denotes a change in the value of what is being measured by a factor of 10. For example, if the baseline viral load by PCR were 20,000 copies/ml plasma, then a 1 log increase equals a 10-fold (10 times) increase or 200,000 copies/ml plasma. A 2 log increase equals 2,000,000 copies/ml plasma, or a 100-fold increase.

Using the same starting point of 20,000 copies/ml plasma, a 1 log decrease means that the viral load has dropped to 2,000 copies/ml. A 2 log decrease equals a viral load of 200 copies/ml plasma An easy way to figure out log changes is to either drop the last "0"or add "0" to the original number.

Any change of less than one-half log is considered insignificant. More simply, if the viral load measurement has not tripled or dropped to one-third of its previous level, the difference might be unimportant. For example, if the baseline viral load were 20,000 copies, a rise to 60,000 or a fall to 7,000 copies might just be the result of transient changes. Repeat testing of a single specimen may give two quite different results and natural biological day-to-day variability of samples from the same person may cause measurements to vary slightly. Researchers believe that clinical decisions made on the basis of changes in viral load ideally should be based on measurements taken 2-3 weeks apart.

What Does an "Undetectable" Level Mean?

Many individuals now have an "undetectable" level of virus in their blood after taking combination therapy. "Undetectable" levels do not mean that the person is "cured" or no longer infectious. "Undetectable" levels mean that current tests are not sensitive enough to measure very low levels of virus in the blood, for example less than 400 copies/ml. There are experimental assays used in research which are more sensitive and can detect levels of virus as low as 20 copies/ml but they are not generally available in clinics and doctor's offices.

Even if the measurement of virus is less than 20 copies/ml in the blood, HIV may be present and infectious in blood, genital secretions (such as semen), lymph nodes, other lymphoid tissues, and elsewhere in the body. There are insufficient data to say that individuals with "undetectable" levels of virus are no longer infectious or no longer at risk of disease progression in the future. We simply do not know yet what an "undetectable" level of virus means over the long term. Individuals with "undetectable" levels of virus still need to be monitored by their health care providers regularly and they need to practice risk free behaviors.

Is There Still a Need to Have CD4+ Levels Monitored?

Even with ongoing monitoring of viral load, it is important to monitor CD4+ levels. CD4+ levels provide information about the status of the immune system. Research has shown that when viral load is lowered, CD4+ levels usually increase. However, research is still ongoing to determine whether the increase in CD4+ levels represent normal, functioning immune cells. CD4+ levels continue to be used as the basis for deciding what type of opportunistic infection prophylaxis a patient should take. Some physicians feel decisions about prophylaxis should be based on the lowest CD4+ level recorded for a person. CD4+ cell levels are also used to measure response to an antiretroviral treatment, although most regard viral load as more important indicator. In order to provide the physician with the best possible information about a patient's disease status, it is important to have routine viral load and CD4+ levels measured.

For Additional Information

For additional information about viral load testing or other treatment issues, contact:

HIV/AIDS Treatment Information Service
1-800-448-0440 (voice)
1-800-243-7012 (TTY)
1-301-738-6616 (Fax)
atis@cdcnac.org (E-mail)
http://www.hivatis.org (Web site)

Notes

[1]Saag MS, Holodniy M, Kuritzkes DR, et al. HIV viral load markers in clinical practice: recommendations of an AIDS Society-USA Expert Panel. *Nature Medicine.* 1996;2:625-629.

ATIS would like to acknowledge the AIDS Clinical Trials Group for their contribution.

Chapter 23

Antiretroviral Therapies

Preface

The past 2 years have witnessed remarkable advances in the development of antiretroviral therapy (ART) for human immunodeficiency virus (HIV) infection, as well as measurement of HIV plasma
RNA (viral load) to guide the use of antiretroviral drugs. The use of
ART, in conjunction with the prevention of specific HIV-related
opportunistic infections (OIs), has been associated with dramatic decreases in the incidence of OIs, hospitalizations, and deaths among
HIV-infected persons.

Advances in this field have been so rapid, however, that keeping
up with them has posed a formidable challenge to health-care providers
and to patients, as well as to institutions charged with the responsibility of paying for these therapies. Thus, the Office of AIDS Research,
the National Institutes of Health, and the Department of Health and
Human Services (DHHS), in collaboration with the Henry J. Kaiser
Foundation, have assumed a leadership role in formulating the scientific principles (NIH Panel) and developing the guidelines (DHHS/
Kaiser Panel) for the use of antiretroviral drugs that are presented

This chapter contains excerpts from "Report of the NIH Panel to Define
Principles of Therapy of HIV Infection," *Morbidity and Mortality Weekly Re-
port (MMWR)*, Vol. 46. No. RR-5, April 24, 1998, "Guidelines for the Use of
Antiretroviral Agents in HIV-Infected Adults and Adolescents," *MMWR*, Vol.
46. No. RR-5, April 24, 1998; and "Antiretroviral Drugs Approved by FDA for
HIV," Office of Special Health Issues, Food and Drug Administration (FDA),
September 21, 1998.

185

in this report. CDC staff participated in these efforts, and CDC and *MMWR* are pleased to be able to provide this information as a service to its readers.

This report is targeted primarily to providers who care for HIV-infected persons, but it also is intended for patients, payors, pharmacists, and public health officials. The report comprises two articles. The first article, "Report of the NIH Panel to Define Principles of Therapy of HIV Infection," provides the basis for the use of antiretroviral drugs, and the second article, "Guidelines for the Use of Antiretroviral Agents in HIV-Infected Adults and Adolescents," provides specific recommendations regarding when to start, how to monitor, and when to change therapy, as well as specific combinations of drugs that should be considered. Both articles provide cross-references to each other so readers can locate related information. Although the principles are unlikely to change in the near future, the guidelines will change substantially as new information and new drugs become available.

Copies of this document and all updates are available from the CDC National AIDS Clearinghouse (1-800-458-5231) and are posted on the Clearinghouse World-Wide Web site (http://www.cdcnac.org). In addition, copies and updates also are available from the HIV/AIDS Treatment Information Service (1-800-448-0440; Fax 301-519-6616; TTY 1-800-243-7012) and on the ATIS World-Wide Web site (http://www.hivatis.org). Readers should consult these web sites regularly for updates in the guidelines.

Summary of the Principles of Therapy of HIV Infection

1. Ongoing HIV replication leads to immune system damage and progression to AIDS. HIV infection is always harmful, and true long-term survival free of clinically significant immune dysfunction is unusual.

2. Plasma HIV RNA levels indicate the magnitude of HIV replication and its associated rate of CD4+ T cell destruction, whereas CD4+ T cell counts indicate the extent of HIV-induced immune damage already suffered. Regular, periodic measurement of plasma HIV RNA levels and CD4+ T cell counts is necessary to determine the risk for disease progression in an HIV-infected person and to determine when to initiate or modify antiretroviral treatment regimens.

3. As rates of disease progression differ among HIV-infected persons, treatment decisions should be individualized by level of

186

risk indicated by plasma HIV RNA levels and CD4+ T cell counts.

4. The use of potent combination antiretroviral therapy to suppress HIV replication to below the levels of detection of sensitive plasma HIV RNA assays limits the potential for selection of antiretroviral-resistant HIV variants, the major factor limiting the ability of antiretroviral drugs to inhibit virus replication and delay disease progression. Therefore, maximum achievable suppression of HIV replication should be the goal of therapy.

5. The most effective means to accomplish durable suppression of HIV replication is the simultaneous initiation of combinations of effective anti-HIV drugs with which the patient has not been previously treated and that are not cross-resistant with antiretroviral agents with which the patient has been treated previously.

6. Each of the antiretroviral drugs used in combination therapy regimens should always be used according to optimum schedules and dosages.

7. The available effective antiretroviral drugs are limited in number and mechanism of action, and cross- resistance between specific drugs has been documented. Therefore, any change in antiretroviral therapy increases future therapeutic constraints.

8. Women should receive optimal antiretroviral therapy regardless of pregnancy status.

9. The same principles of antiretroviral therapy apply to HIV-infected children, adolescents, and adults, although the treatment of HIV-infected children involves unique pharmacologic, virologic, and immunologic considerations.

10. Persons identified during acute primary HIV infection should be treated with combination antiretroviral therapy to suppress virus replication to levels below the limit of detection of sensitive plasma HIV RNA assays.

11. HIV-infected persons, even those whose viral loads are below detectable limits, should be considered infectious. Therefore, they should be counseled to avoid sexual and drug-use behaviors that are associated with either transmission or acquisition of HIV and other infectious pathogens.

Guidelines for the Use of Antiretroviral Agents in HIV-Infected Adults and Adolescents

Information included in these guidelines may not represent FDA approval or approved labeling for the particular products or indications in question. Specifically, the terms "safe" and "effective" may not be synonymous with the FDA-defined legal standards for product approval.

Summary

With the development and FDA approval of an increasing number of antiretroviral agents, decisions regarding the treatment of HIV-infected persons have become complex, and the field continues to evolve rapidly. In 1996, the Department of Health and Human Services and the Henry J. Kaiser Family Foundation convened the Panel on Clinical Practices for the Treatment of HIV to develop guidelines for the clinical management of HIV-infected persons. This report includes the guidelines developed by the Panel regarding the use of laboratory testing in initiating and managing antiretroviral therapy, considerations for initiating therapy, whom to treat, what regimen of antiretroviral agents to use, when to change the antiretroviral regimen, treatment of the acutely HIV infected person, special considerations in adolescents, and special considerations in pregnant women. Viral load and CD4+ T cell testing should ideally be performed twice before initiating or changing an antiretroviral treatment regimen. All patients who have advanced or symptomatic HIV disease should receive aggressive antiretroviral therapy. Initiation of therapy in the asymptomatic person is more complex and involves consideration of multiple virologic, immunologic, and psychosocial factors. In general, persons who have <500 CD4+ T cells per mm^3 should be offered therapy; however, the strength of the recommendation to treat should be based on the patient's willingness to accept therapy as well as the prognosis for AIDS-free survival as determined by the HIV RNA copy per mL of plasma and the CD4+ T cell count. Persons who have >500

CD4+ T cells per mm^3 can be observed or can be offered therapy; again, risk of progression to AIDS, as determined by HIV RNA viremia and CD4+ T cell count, should guide the decision to treat. Once the decision to initiate antiretroviral therapy has been made, treatment should be aggressive with the goal of maximal viral suppression. In general, a protease inhibitor and two non-nucleoside reverse transcriptase inhibitors should be used initially. Other regimens may be utilized but are considered less than optimal. Many factors, including reappearance of previously undetectable HIV RNA, may indicate treatment failure. Decisions to change therapy and decisions regarding new regimens must be carefully considered; there are minimal clinical data to guide these decisions. Patients with acute HIV infection should probably be administered aggressive antiretroviral therapy; once initiated, duration of treatment is unknown and will likely need to continue for several years, if not for life. Special considerations apply to adolescents and pregnant women and are discussed in detail.

Introduction

These guidelines were developed by the Panel on Clinical Practices for Treatment of HIV Infection, convened by the Department of Health and Human Services (DHHS) and the Henry J. Kaiser Family Foundation. The guidelines contain recommendations for the clinical use of antiretroviral agents in the treatment of adults and adolescents (defined in Considerations for Antiretroviral Therapy in the HIV-Infected Adolescent) who are infected with the human immunodeficiency virus (HIV). Guidance for the use of antiretroviral treatment in pediatric HIV infection is not contained in this report. Although the pathogenesis of HIV infection and the general virologic and immunologic principles underlying the use of antiretroviral therapy are similar for all HIV-infected persons, unique therapeutic and management considerations apply to HIV-infected children. In recognition of these differences, a separate set of guidelines will address pediatric-specific issues related to antiretroviral therapy.

These guidelines are intended for use by physicians and other health-care providers who use antiretroviral therapy to treat HIV-infected adults and adolescents. The recommendations contained herein are presented in the context of and with reference to the first section of this report, "Principles of Therapy for HIV Infection," formulated by the National Institutes of Health (NIH) Panel to Define Principles of Therapy of IIIV Infection. Together, these reports provide the pathogenesis-based rationale for therapeutic strategies as well as practical guidelines for implementing these strategies. Although the guidelines represent the current state of knowledge regarding the use of antiretroviral agents, this field of science is rapidly evolving, and the availability of new agents or new clinical data regarding the use of existing agents will result in changes in therapeutic options and preferences. The Antiretroviral Working Group, a subgroup of the Panel, will meet several times a year to review new data; recommendations for changes in this document would then be submitted to the Panel and incorporated as appropriate. Copies of this document and all updates are available from the CDC National AIDS Clearinghouse (1-800-458-5231) and are posted on the Clearinghouse World-Wide Web site (http:/twww.cdcnac.org). In addition, copies and updates also are available from the HIV/AIDS Treatment Information Service (1-800448-0440; Fax 301-519-6616; TTY 1-800-243-7012) and on the ATIS World-Wide Web site (http://wwwhivatis.org). Readers should consult these web sites regularly for updates in the guidelines. These recommendations are not intended to substitute for the judgment of a physician who is expert in caring for HIV-infected persons. When possible, the treatment of HIV-infected patients should be directed by a physician with extensive experience in the care of these patients. When this is not possible, the physician treating the patient should have access to such expertise through consultations.

Each recommendation is accompanied by a rating that includes a letter and a Roman numeral, similar to the rating schemes described in previous guidelines on the prophylaxis of opportunistic infections (OIs) issued by the U.S. Public Health Service and the Infectious Diseases Society of America[1]. The letter indicates the strength of the recommendation based on the opinion of the Panel, and the Roman numeral rating reflects the nature of the evidence for the recommendation (see Table 23.1). Thus, recommendations based on data from clinical trials with clinical endpoints are differentiated from recommendations based on data derived from clinical trials with laboratory endpoints (e.g., CD4+ T cell count or plasma HIV RNA levels); when clinical trial data are not available, recommendations are based on the opinions of experts familiar with the relevant scientific literature. The majority of current clinical trial data regarding the use of antiretroviral agents has been obtained in trials enrolling predominantly young to middle-aged males. Although current knowledge indicates that women may differ from men in the absorption, metabolism, and clinical effects of certain pharmacologic agents, clinical experience and data available to date do not indicate any substantial sex differences that would modify these guidelines. However, theoretical concerns exist, and the Panel urges continuation of the current efforts to enroll more women in antiretroviral clinical trials so that the data needed to re-evaluate this issue can be gathered expeditiously.

This report addresses the following issues: the use of testing for plasma HIV RNA levels (viral load) and CD4+ T cell count; initiating therapy in established HIV infection; initiating therapy in patients who have advanced-stage HIV disease; interruption of antiretroviral therapy; changing therapy and available therapeutic options; the treatment of acute HIV infection; antiretroviral therapy in adolescents; and antiretroviral therapy in the pregnant woman.

Table 23.1. Rating system for strength of recommendation and quality of evidence supporting the recommendation

Category   Definition

Categories reflecting the strength of each recommendation

A	Strong; should always be offered
B	Moderate; should usually be offered
C	Optional
D	Should generally not be offered
E	Should never be offered

Categories reflecting the quality of evidence supporting the recommendation

I	At least one randomized trial with clinical endpoints
II	Clinical trials with laboratory endpoints
III	Expert opinion

Use of Testing for Plasma HIV RNA Levels and CD4+ T Cell Count in Guiding Decisions for Therapy

Decisions regarding either initiating or changing antiretroviral therapy should be guided by monitoring the laboratory parameters of both plasma HIV RNA (viral load) and CD4+ T cell count and by assessing the clinical condition of the patient. [For more information about viral load, see Chapter 22.] Results of these two laboratory tests provide the physician with important information about the virologic and immunologic status of the patient and the risk of disease progression to acquired immunodeficiency syndrome (AIDS) (see Principle 2 in the first section of this report). HIV viral load testing has been approved by the U.S. Food and Drug Administration (FDA) only for the RT-PCR assay (Roche) and only for determining disease prognosis. However, data presented at an FDA Advisory Committee for the Division of Antiviral Drug Products (July 14-15,1997, Silver Spring, MD) provide further evidence for the utility of viral RNA testing in monitoring therapeutic responses. Multiple analyses of more than 5,000 patients who participated in approximately 18 trials with viral load monitoring demonstrated a reproducible dose-response type association between decreases in plasma viremia and improved clinical outcome based on standard endpoints of new AIDS-defining diagnoses and survival. This relationship was observed over a range of patient baseline characteristics, including pretreatment plasma RNA level, CD4+ T cell count, and prior drug experience. The consensus of the Panel is that viral load testing is the essential parameter in decisions to initiate or change antiretroviral therapies. Measurement of plasma HIV RNA levels (viral load), using quantitative methods, should be performed at the time of diagnosis of HIV infection and every 3-4 months thereafter in the untreated patient (AIII) (Table 23.2). CD4+ T cell counts should be measured at the time of diagnosis and generally every 3-6 months thereafter (AIII). These intervals between tests are merely recommendations, and flexibility should be exercised according to the circumstances of the individual case. Plasma HIV RNA levels also should be measured immediately prior to and again at 4-8 weeks after initiation of antiretroviral therapy (AIII). This second time point allows the clinician to evaluate the initial effectiveness of therapy because in most patients, adherence to a regimen of potent antiretroviral agents should result in a large decrease (about 0.5 to 0.75 $\log_{10}$) in viral load by 4-8 weeks. The viral load should continue to decline over the following weeks, and in most persons it becomes below detectable levels (currently defined as <500 RNA copies/mL) by 12-16 weeks of therapy. The speed of viral load decline and the movement toward undetectable are affected by the baseline CD4+ T cell count, the initial viral load, potency of the regimen, adherence, prior exposure to antiretroviral agents, and the presence of any OIs. These individual differences must be considered when monitoring the effect of therapy. However, the absence of a virologic response of the magnitude previously described (i.e., about 0.5 to 0.75 $\log_{10}$ by 4-8 weeks and undetectable by 12-16 weeks) should prompt the physician to reassess patient adherence, rule out malabsorption, consider repeat RNA testing to document lack of response, and/or consider a change in drug regimen. Once the patient is on therapy, HIV RNA testing should be repeated every 3-4 months to evaluate the continuing effectiveness of therapy (AII). With optimal therapy, viral levels in plasma at 6 months should be undetectable (i.e., <500 copies of HIV RNA per mL of plasma).[2] If HIV RNA remains above 500 copies/ml in plasma after 6 months of therapy, the plasma HIV RNA test should be repeated to confirm the result, and a change in therapy should be considered according to the guidelines provided in "Considerations for Changing a Failing Regimen" (BIII). More sensitive viral load assays are in development that can quantify HIV RNA down to approximately 50 copies/mL. Preliminary data from clinical trials strongly suggest that lowering plasma HIV RNA to below 50 copies/mL is associated with a more complete and durable viral suppression, compared with reducing HIV RNA to levels between 50-500 copies/mL. However, the clinical significance of these findings is currently unclear.

When deciding whether to initiate therapy, the CD4+ T cell count and plasma HIV RNA measurement ideally should be performed on two occasions to ensure accuracy and consistency of measurement (BIII). However, in patients with advanced HIV disease, antiretroviral

Table 23.2. Indications for plasma HIV RNA testing*

Clinical indication	Information	Use
Syndrome consistent with acute HIV infection	Establishes diagnosis when HIV antibody test is negative or indeterminate	Diagnosis[†]
Initial evaluation of newly diagnosed HIV infection	Baseline viral load "set point"	Decision to start or defer therapy
Every 3–4 mos. in patients not on therapy	Changes in viral load	Decision to start therapy
4–8 wks. after initiation of antiretroviral therapy	Initial assessment of drug efficacy	Decision to continue or change therapy
3–4 mos. after start of therapy	Maximal effect of therapy	Decision to continue or change therapy
Every 3–4 mos. in patients on therapy	Durability of antiretroviral effect	Decision to continue or change therapy
Clinical event or significant decline in CD4+ T cells	Association with changing or stable viral load	Decision to continue, initiate, or change therapy

*Acute illness (e.g., bacterial pneumonia, tuberculosis, HSV, PCP) and immunizations can cause increases in plasma HIV RNA for 2–4 wks.; viral load testing should not be performed during this time. Plasma HIV RNA results should usually be verified with a repeat determination before starting or making changes in therapy. HIV RNA should be measured using the same laboratory and the same assay.

[†]Diagnosis of HIV infection determined by HIV RNA testing should be confirmed by standard methods (e.g., Western blot serology) performed 2–4 mos. after the initial indeterminate or negative test.

therapy should generally be initiated after the first viral load measurement is obtained to prevent a potentially deleterious delay in treatment. Although the requirement for two measurements of viral load may place a substantial financial burden on patients or payers, two measurements of viral load should provide the clinician with the best information for subsequent follow-up of the patient. Plasma HIV RNA levels should not be measured during or within 4 weeks after successful treatment of any intercurrent infection, resolution of symptomatic illness, or immunization (see Principle 2). Because differences exist among commercially available tests, confirmatory plasma HIV RNA levels should be measured by the same laboratory using the same technique to ensure consistent results.

A substantial change in plasma viremia is considered to be a three-fold or 0.5 $\log_{10}$ increase or decrease. A substantial decrease in CD4+ T cell count is a decrease of >30% from baseline for absolute cell numbers and a decrease of >3% from baseline in percentages of cells.[3,4] Discordance between trends in CD4+ T cell numbers and plasma HIV RNA levels can occur and was found in 20% of patients in one cohort studied.[5] Such discordance can complicate decisions regarding antiretroviral therapy and may be due to several factors that affect plasma HIV RNA testing (see Principle 2). Viral load and trends in viral load are considered to be more informative for guiding decisions regarding antiretroviral therapy than are CD4+ T cell counts; exceptions to this rule do occur, however (see Considerations for Changing a Failing Regimen); when changes in viral loads and CD4+ T cell counts are discordant, expert consultation should be considered.

Established HIV Infection

Patients who have established HIV infection are considered in two arbitrarily defined clinical categories: 1) asymptomatic infection or 2) symptomatic disease (e.g., wasting, thrush, or unexplained fever for 2 or more weeks), including AIDS, defined according to the 1993 CDC classification system.[6] All patients in the second category should be offered antiretroviral therapy. Considerations for initiating antiretroviral therapy in the first category of patients (i.e., patients who are asymptomatic) are complex and are discussed separately in the following section. However, before initiating therapy in any patient, the following evaluation should be performed:

- Complete history and physical (AII)
- Complete blood count, chemistry profile (AII)

194

- CD4+ T cell count (AI)
- Plasma HIV RNA measurement (AI)

Additional evaluation should include routine tests pertinent to the prevention of OIs, if not already performed (i.e., VDRL, tuberculin skin test, toxoplasma IgG serology, and gynecologic exam with Pap smear), and other tests as clinically indicated (e.g., chest radiograph, hepatitis C virus [HCV] serology, ophthalmologic exam) (AII). Hepatitis B virus (HBV) serology is indicated for a patient who is a candidate for the hepatitis B vaccine or who has abnormal liver function tests (AII); cytomegalovirus (CMV) serology may be useful in certain persons, as discussed in *1997 USPHS/IDSA Guidelines for the Prevention of Opportunistic Infections in Persons Infected With the Human Immunodeficiency Virus*[1] (BIII).

Considerations for Initiating Therapy in the Patient Who Has Asymptomatic HIV Infection

It has been demonstrated that antiretroviral therapy provides clinical benefit in HIV-infected persons who have advanced HIV disease and immunosuppression.[7-11] Although there is theoretical benefit to treating patients who have CD4+ T cells >500 cells/mm^3 (see Principle 3), no long-term clinical benefit of treatment has yet been demonstrated. A major dilemma confronting patients and practitioners is that the antiretroviral regimens currently available that have the greatest potency in terms of viral suppression and CD4+ T cell preservation are medically complex, are associated with several specific side effects and drug interactions, and pose a substantial challenge for adherence. Thus, decisions regarding treatment of asymptomatic, chronically infected persons must balance a number of competing factors that influence risk and benefit.

The physician and the asymptomatic patient must consider multiple risks and benefits in deciding when to initiate therapy (Table 23.3) (see Principle 3). Several factors influence the decision to initiate early therapy: the real or potential goal of maximally suppressing viral replication; preserving immune function; prolonging health and life; decreasing the risk of drug resistance due to early suppression of viral replication with potent therapy; and decreasing drug toxicity by treating the healthier patient. Factors weighing against early treatment in the asymptomatic stable patient include the following: the potential adverse effects of the drugs on quality of life, including the inconvenience of most of the maximally suppressive regimens

195

currently available (e.g., dietary change or large numbers of pills); the potential risk of developing drug resistance despite early initiation of therapy; the potential for limiting future treatment options due to cycling of the patient through the available drugs during early disease; the potential risk of transmission of virus resistant to protease inhibitors and other agents; the unknown durability of effect of the currently available therapies; and the unknown long-term toxicity of some drugs. Thus, the decision to begin therapy in the asymptomatic patient is complex and must be made in the setting of careful patient counseling and education. The factors that must be considered in this decision include the following:

1. the willingness of the individual to begin therapy;

2. the degree of existing immunodeficiency as determined by the CD4+ T cell count;

Table 23.3. Risks and benefits of early initiation of antiretroviral therapy in the asymptomatic HIV-infected patient

Potential Benefits

Control of viral replication and mutation; reduction of viral burden

Prevention of progressive immunodeficiency; potential maintenance or reconstitution of a normal immune system

Delayed progression to AIDS and prolongation of life

Decreased risk of selection of resistant virus

Decreased risk of drug toxicity

Potential Risks

Reduction in quality of life from adverse drug effects and inconvenience of current maximally suppressive regimens

Earlier development of drug resistance

Limitation in future choices of antiretroviral agents due to development of resistance

Unknown long-term toxicity of antiretroviral drugs

Unknown duration of effectiveness of current antiretroviral therapies

3. the risk for disease progression as determined by the level of plasma HIV RNA (Table 23.4)

4. the potential benefits and risks of initiating therapy in asymptomatic persons, as discussed above; and

5. the likelihood, after counseling and education, of adherence to the prescribed treatment regimen.

In regard to adherence, no patient should automatically be excluded from consideration for antiretroviral therapy simply because he or she exhibits a behavior or other characteristic judged by some to lend itself to noncompliance. The likelihood of patient adherence to a complex drug regimen should be discussed and determined by the individual patient and physician before therapy is initiated. To achieve the level of adherence necessary for effective therapy, providers are encouraged to utilize strategies for assessing and assisting adherence that have been developed in the context of chronic treatment for other serious diseases. Intensive patient education regarding the critical need for adherence should be provided, specific goals of therapy should be established and mutually agreed upon, and a long-term treatment plan should be developed with the patient. Intensive follow-up should take place to assess adherence to treatment and to continue patient counseling to prevent transmission of HIV through sexual contact and injection of drugs.

Initiating Therapy in the Patient Who Has Asymptomatic HIV Infection

Once the patient and physician have decided to initiate antiretroviral therapy, treatment should be aggressive, with the goal of maximal suppression of plasma viral load to undetectable levels. Recommendations regarding when to initiate therapy and what regimens to use are provided (Tables 23.5 and 23.6). In general, any patient who has <500 CD4+ T cells/mm^3 or >10,000 (bDNA) or 20,000 (RT-PCR) copies of HIV RNA/mL of plasma should be offered therapy (AII). However, the strength of the recommendation for therapy should be based on the readiness of the patient for treatment and a consideration of the prognosis for risk for progression to AIDS as determined by viral load, CD4+ T cell count (Table 23.4), and the slope of the CD4+ T cell count decline. The values for bDNA (Table 23.4) are the uncorrected HIV RNA values obtained from the Multicenter AIDS Cohort Study (MACS). It had previously been thought that these values, obtained on stored heparinized plasma specimens, should be multiplied by a factor of two to adjust for an anticipated twofold loss of RNA ascribed to the effects of heparin and delayed processing on the stability of RNA. However, more recent analysis suggests that the reduction ascribed to these factors is 0.2 log or less, so that no significant correction factor is necessary (Mellors J, personal communication, October 1997). RT-PCR values also are provided (Table 23.4); comparison of the results obtained from the RT-PCR and bDNA assays, using the manufacturer's controls, consistently indicates that the HIV-1 RNA values obtained by RT-PCR are approximately twice those obtained by the bDNA assay.[12] Thus, the MACS values must be multiplied by approximately 2 to be consistent with current RT-PCR values. A third

Table 23.4. Risk for progression to AIDS-defining illness in a cohort of men who have sex with men, predicted by baseline CD4+ T cell count and viral load*

CD4 ≤350 Plasma viral load (copies/mL)[§]		% AIDS (AIDS-defining complication)[†]			
bDNA	RT-PCR	No. of patients in study	3 yrs	6 yrs	9 yrs
≤500	≤1,500	—¶	—	—	—
501–3,000	1,501–7,000	30	0	18.8	30.6
3,001–10,000	7,001–20,000	51	8.0	42.2	65.6
10,001–30,000	20,001–55,000	73	40.1	72.9	86.2
>30,000	>55,000	174	72.9	92.7	95.6
CD4 351–500 Plasma viral load (copies/mL)		% AIDS (AIDS-defining complication)			
bDNA	RT-PCR	No. of patients in study	3 yrs	6 yrs	9 yrs
≤500	≤1,500	—	—	—	—
501–3,000	1,501–7,000	47	4.4	22.1	46.9
3,001–10,000	7,001–20,000	105	5.9	39.8	60.7
10,001–30,000	20,001–55,000	121	15.1	57.2	78.6
>30,000	>55,000	121	47.9	77.7	94.4
CD4 >500 Plasma viral load (copies/mL)		% AIDS (AIDS-defining complication)			
bDNA	RT-PCR	No. of patients in study	3 yrs	6 yrs	9 yrs
≤500	≤1,500	110	1.0	5.0	10.7
501–3,000	1,501–7,000	180	2.3	14.9	33.2
3,001–10,000	7,001–20,000	237	7.2	25.9	50.3
10,001–30,000	20,001–55,000	202	14.6	47.7	70.6
>30,000	>55,000	141	32.6	66.8	76.3

*Data from the Multicenter AIDS Cohort Study (MACS) (*12*).
[†]In this study, AIDS was defined according to the 1987 CDC definition and does not include asymptomatic persons who have CD4+ T cells <200/mm^3.
[§]MACS numbers reflect plasma HIV RNA values obtained by bDNA testing. RT-PCR values are consistently 2–2.5-fold higher than bDNA values, as indicated.
¶Too few subjects were in the category to provide a reliable estimate of AIDS risk.

test for HIV RNA, the nucleic acid sequence based amplification (NASBA®), is currently used in some clinical settings. However, formulas for converting values obtained from either branched DNA (bDNA) or RT-PCR assays to NASBA®-equivalent values cannot be derived from the limited data currently available.

Currently, there are two general approaches to initiating therapy in the asymptomatic patient: a) a therapeutically more aggressive approach in which most patients would be treated early in the course of HIV infection due to the recognition that HIV disease is virtually always progressive and b) a therapeutically more cautious approach in which therapy may be delayed because the balance of the risk for clinically significant progression and other factors discussed above are considered to weigh in favor of observation and delayed therapy. The aggressive approach is heavily based on the Principles of Therapy, particularly the principle (see Principle 3) that one should begin treatment before the development of significant immunosuppression and one should treat to achieve undetectable viremia; thus, all patients who have <500 CD4+ T cells/mm^3 would be started on therapy as would patients who have higher CD4+ T cell numbers and plasma viral load >10,000 (bDNA) or 20,000 (RT-PCR) (Table 23.5). The more conservative approach to the initiation of therapy in the asymptomatic person would delay treatment of the patient who has <500 CD4+ T cells/mm^3 and low levels of viremia and who has a low risk for rapid disease progression (Table 23.4); careful observation and monitoring would continue. Patients who have CD4+ T cell counts >500/mm^3 would also be observed, except those who are at substantial risk for rapid disease progression because of a high viral load. For example, the patient who has 60,000 (RT-PCR) or 30,000 (bDNA) copies of HIV RNA/mL, regardless of CD4+ T cell count, has a high probability of progressing to an AIDS-defining complication of HIV disease within 3 years (32.6% if CD4+ T cells are >500/mm^3) and should clearly be encouraged to initiate antiretroviral therapy. Conversely, a patient who has 18,000 copies of HIV RNA/mL of plasma, measured by RT-PCR, and a CD4+ T cell count of 410/mm^3, has a 5.9% chance of progressing to an AIDS-defining complication of HIV infection in 3 years (Table 23.4). The therapeutically aggressive physician would recommend treatment for this patient to suppress the ongoing viral replication that is readily detectable; the therapeutically more conservative physician would discuss the possibility of initiation of therapy but recognize that a delay in therapy because of the balance of considerations previously discussed also is reasonable. In either case, the patient should make the final decision regarding acceptance of therapy following discussion with the health-care provider regarding specific issues relevant to his/her own clinical situation.

When initiating therapy in the patient who has never been administered antiretroviral therapy, one should begin with a regimen that is expected to reduce viral replication to undetectable levels (AIII). Based on the weight of experience, the preferred regimen to accomplish this consists of two nucleoside reverse transcriptase inhibitors (NRTIs) and one potent protease inhibitor (PI) (Table 23.6). Alternative regimens have been employed; these regimens include ritonavir and saquinavir (with one or two NRTIs) or nevirapine as a substitute for the PI. Dual PI therapy with ritonavir and saquinavir (hard-gel formulation), without an NRTI, appears to be potent in suppressing viremia below detectable levels and has convenient twice-daily dosing; however, the safety of this combination has not been fully established according to FDA guidelines. Also, this regimen has not been directly compared with the proven regimens of two NRTIs and a PI; thus, the Panel recommends that at least one additional NRTI be used when the physician elects to use two PIs as initial therapy. Substituting nevirapine for the PI, or using two NRTIs alone, does not achieve the goal of suppressing viremia to below detectable levels as consistently as does combination treatment with two NRTIs and a PI and should be used only if more potent treatment is not possible.

Table 23.5. Indications for the initiation of antiretroviral therapy in the chronically HIV-infected patient

Clinical category	CD4+ T cell count and HIV RNA	Recommendation
Symptomatic (i.e., AIDS, thrush, unexplained fever)	Any value	Treat
Asymptomatic	CD4+ T Cells <500/mm^3 **or** HIV RNA >10,000 (bDNA) or >20,000 (RT-PCR)	Treatment should be offered. Strength of recommendation is based on prognosis for disease-free survival as shown in Table 4 and willingness of the patient to accept therapy.*
Asymptomatic	CD4+ T Cells >500/mm^3 **and** HIV RNA <10,000 (bDNA) or <20,000 (RT-PCR)	Many experts would delay therapy and observe; however, some experts would treat.

*Some experts would observe patients whose CD4+ T cell counts are between 350–500/mm^3 and HIV RNA levels <10,000 (bDNA) or <20,000 (RT-PCR).

Table 23.6. Recommended antiretroviral agents for treatment of established HIV infection

Preferred: Strong evidence of clinical benefit and/or sustained suppression of plasma viral load (*2, 34, 35*)
One choice each from column A and column B. Drugs are listed in random, not priority, order:

Column A	Column B
Indinavir (AI)	ZDV + ddI (AI)
Nelfinavir (AII)	d4T + ddI (AII)
Ritonavir (AI)	ZDV + ddC (AI)
Saquinavir-SGC* (AII)	ZDV + 3TC§ (AI)
Ritonavir + Saquinavir-SGC or HGC† (BII)	d4T + 3TC§ (AII)

Alternative: Less likely to provide sustained virus suppression; (*36–38*)

1 NNRTI (Nevirapine)¶ + 2 NRTIs (Column B, above) (BII)

Saquinavir-HGC + 2 NRTIs (Column B, above) (BI)

Not generally recommended: Strong evidence of clinical benefit, but initial virus suppression is not sustained in most patients (*39,40*)

2 NRTIs (Column B, above) (CI)

Not recommended**: Evidence against use, virologically undesirable, or overlapping toxicities

All monotherapies (DI)

d4T + ZDV (DI)

ddC + ddI†† (DII)

ddC + d4T†† (DII)

ddC + 3TC (DII)

---

*Virologic data and clinical experience with saquinavir-sgc are limited in comparison with other protease inhibitors.
†Use of ritonavir 400 mg b.i.d. with saquinavir soft-gel formulation (Fortovase™)400 mg b.i.d. results in similar areas under the curve (AUC) of drug and antiretroviral activity as when using 400 mg b.i.d. of Invirase™ in combination with ritonavir. However, this combination with Fortovase™ has not been extensively studied and gastrointestinal toxicity may be greater when using Fortovase™.
§High-level resistance to 3TC develops within 2–4 wks. in partially suppressive regimens; optimal use is in three-drug antiretroviral combinations that reduce viral load to <500 copies/mL.
¶The only combination of 2 NRTIs + 1 NNRTI that has been shown to suppress viremia to undetectable levels in the majority of patients is ZDV+ddI+Nevirapine. This combination was studied in antiretroviral-naive persons (*36*).
**ZDV monotherapy may be considered for prophylactic use in pregnant women who have low viral load and high CD4+ T cell counts to prevent perinatal transmission (see "Considerations for Antiretroviral Therapy in the Pregnant HIV-Infected Woman" on pages 59–62).
††This combination of NRTIs is not recommended based on lack of clinical data using the combination and/or overlapping toxicities.

Table 23.7. Characteristics of nucleoside reverse transcriptase inhibitors (NRTIs)

Generic name *Trade name*	Zidovudine (AZT, ZDV) *Retrovir*	Didanosine (ddI) *Videx*	Zalcitabine (ddC) *HIVID*	Stavudine (d4T) *Zerit*	Lamivudine (3TC) *Epivir*
Dosing recommendations	200 mg t.i.d. or 300 mg b.i.d. or with 3TC as Combivir™, 1 b.i.d.	Tablets >60kg: 200 mg b.i.d. <60 kg: 125 mg b.i.d.	0.75 mg t.i.d.	>60 kg: 40 mg b.i.d. <60 kg: 30 mg b.i.d.	150 mg b.i.d. <50 kg: 2 mg/kg b.i.d. or with ZDV as Combivir™, 1 b.i.d.
Oral bioavailability	60%	Tablet: 40% Powder: 30%	85%	86%	86%
Serum half-life	1.1 hr.	1.6 hr.	1.2 hr.	1.0 hr.	3-6 hrs.
Intracellular half-life	3 hrs.	25–40 hrs.	3 hrs.	3.5 hrs.	12 hrs.
Elimination	Metabolized to AZT glucuronide (GAZT). Renal excretion of GAZT.	Renal excretion 50%	Renal excretion 70%	Renal excretion 50%	Renal excretion unchanged
Adverse events	Bone marrow suppression: anemia and/or neutropenia. Subjective complaints: GI intolerance, headache, insomnia, asthenia.	Pancreatitis; Peripheral neuropathy; Nausea; Diarrhea	Peripheral neuropathy; Stomatitis	Peripheral neuropathy	(Minimal toxicity)

However, some experts consider that there currently are insufficient data to choose between a three-drug regimen containing a PI and one containing nevirapine in the patient who has never been administered therapy; further studies are pending. Other regimens using two PIs or a PI and a non-nucleoside reverse transcriptase inhibitor (NNRTI) as initial therapy are currently in clinical trials with data pending. Of the two available NNRTIs, clinical trials support a preference for nevirapine over delavirdine based on results of viral load assays. Although 3TC is a potent NRTI when used in combination with another NRTI, in situations in which suppression of virus replication is not complete, resistance to 3TC develops rapidly.[13,14] Therefore, the optimal use for this agent is as part of a three-or-more drug combination that has a high probability of complete suppression of virus replication. Other agents in which a single genetic mutation can confer drug

Table 23.8. Non-nucleoside reverse transcriptase inhibitors (NNRTIs)

Generic name	Nevirapine	Delavirdine
Trade name	*Viramune*	*Rescriptor*
Form	200 mg tabs	100 mg tabs
Dosing recommendations	200 mg po q.d. x 14 days, then 200 mg po b.i.d.	400 mg po t.i.d. (four 100 mg tabs in ≥3 oz. water to produce slurry)
Oral bioavailability	>90%	85%
Serum half-life	25–30 hrs.	5.8 hrs.
Elimination	Metabolized by cytochrome p450; 80% excreted in urine (glucuronidated metabolites, <5% unchanged); 10% in feces	Metabolized by cytochrome p450; 51% excreted in urine (<5% unchanged); 44% in feces
Drug interactions	Induces cytochrome p450 enzymes • The following drugs have suspected interactions that require careful monitoring if co-administered with nevirapine: rifampin, rifabutin, oral contraceptives, protease inhibitors, triazolam and midazolam.	Inhibits cytochrome p450 enzymes • Not recommended for concurrent use: terfenadine, astemizole, alprazolam, midazolam, cisapride, rifabutin, rifampin, triazolam, ergot derivatives, amphetamines, nifedipine, anticonvulsants (phenytoin, carbamazepine, phenobarbitol). • Delavirdine increases levels of clarithromycin, dapsone, quinidine, warfarin, indinavir, saquinavir. • Antacids and didanosine: separate administration by ≥1 hr.
Adverse events	Rash; increased transaminase levels; hepatitis	Rash; headaches

Table 23.9. Characteristics of protease inhibitors (PIs)

Generic name	Indinavir	Ritonavir	Saquinavir		Nelfinavir
Trade name	*Crixivan*	*Norvir*	*Invirase*™	*Fortovase*™	*Viracept*
Form	200-, 400-mg caps	100-mg caps 600 mg/7.5 mL po solution	200-mg caps	200-mg caps	250-mg tablets 50-mg/g oral powder
Dosing recommendations	800 mg q8h Take 1 hr. before or 2 hrs. after meals; may take with skim milk or low-fat meal.	600 mg q12h* Take with food if possible.	600 mg t.i.d.* Take with large meal.	1,200 mg t.i.d. Take with large meal.	750 mg t.i.d. Take with food (meal or light snack).
Oral bioavailability	65%	(Not determined)	hard-gel capsule: 4%, erratic	soft-gel capsule (not determined)	20%–80%
Serum half-life	1.5–2 hrs.	3–5 hrs.	1–2 hrs.	1–2 hrs.	3.5–5 hrs.
Route of metabolism	P450 cytochrome 3A4	P450 cytochrome 3A4>2D6	P450 cytochrome 3A4	P450 cytochrome 3A4	P450 cytochrome 3A4
Storage	Room temperature	Refrigerate capsules; refrigeration for oral solution is preferred but not required if used within 30 days.	Room temperature	Refrigerate or store at room temperature (up to 3 mos.).	Room temperature
Adverse effects	Nephrolithiasis. GI intolerance, nausea. Lab: increased indirect bilirubinemia (inconsequential). Miscellaneous: headache, asthenia, blurred vision, dizziness, rash, metallic taste, thrombocytopenia. Hyperglycemia. (¶)	GI intolerance, nausea, vomiting, diarrhea. Paresthesias (circumoral and extremities). Hepatitis. Asthenia. Taste perversion. Lab: Triglycerides increase >200%, transaminase elevation, elevated CPK and uric acid. Hyperglycemia. (¶)	GI intolerance, nausea and diarrhea. Headache. Elevated transaminase enzymes. Hyperglycemia. (¶)	GI intolerance, nausea, diarrhea, abdominal pain and dyspepsia. Headache. Elevated transaminase enzymes. Hyperglycemia. (¶)	Diarrhea. Hyperglycemia. (¶)

204

Drug interactions					
Inhibits cytochrome P450 (less than ritonavir). Contraindicated for concurrent use: terfenadine, astemizole, cisapride, triazolam, midazolam, ergot alkaloids. Indinavir levels increased by: ketoconazole§, delavirdine. Indinavir levels reduced by: rifampin, rifabutin, grapefruit juice, nevirapine. Didanosine reduces indinavir absorption unless taken >2 hrs apart. Not recommended for concurrent use: rifampin.	Inhibits cytochrome P450 (potent inhibitor). Ritonavir increases levels of multiple drugs that are not recommended for concurrent use†. Didanosine: may cause reduced absorption of both drugs; should be taken ≥2 hours apart. Ritonavir decreases levels of ethinyl estradiol, theophylline, sulfamethoxazole and zidovudine. Ritonavir increases levels of clarithromycin and desipramine.	Inhibits cytochrome P450. Saquinavir levels increased by: ritonavir, ketoconazole, grapefruit juice, nelfinavir, delavirdine. Saquinavir levels reduced by: rifampin, rifabutin, and possibly the following: phenobarbital, phenytoin, dexamethasone and carbamezepine, nevirapine. Contraindicated for concurrent use: terfenadine, astemizole, cisapride, ergot alkaloids, triazolam and midazolam.	Inhibits cytochrome P450. Saquinavir levels increased by: ritonavir, ketoconazole, grapefruit juice, nelfinavir, delavirdine. Saquinavir levels reduced by: rifampin, rifabutin, and possibly the following: phenobarbital, phenytoin, dexamethasone and carbamezepine, nevirapine. Contraindicated for concurrent use: terfenadine, astemizole, cisapride, ergot alkaloids, triazolam and midazolam.	Inhibits cytochrome P450 (less than ritonavir). Nelfinavir levels reduced by rifampin, rifabutin. Contraindicated for concurrent use: triazolam, midazolam, ergot alkaloid, terfenadine, astemizole, cisapride. Nelfinavir decreases levels of ethinyl estradiol and norethindrone. Nelfinavir increases levels of rifabutin, saquinavir, and indinavir. Not recommended for concurrent use: rifampin.	

*Dose escalation for ritonavir: Day 1-2: 300 mg b.i.d.; day 3-5: 400 mg b.i.d.; day 6-13: 500 mg b.i.d.; day 14: 600 mg b.i.d. Combination treatment regimen with saquinavir (400-600 mg po b.i.d.) plus ritonavir (400-600 mg po b.i.d.).

†Drugs contraindicated for concurrent use with ritonavir: amioderone (Cordonrone), astemizole (Hismanal), bepridil (Vascar), bupropion (Wellbutin), cisapride (Propulsid), clorazepate (Tranxene), clozapine (Clozaril), diazepam (Valium), encainide (Enkaid), estazolam (ProSom), flecainide (Tambocor), flurazepam (Dalmane), meperidine (Demerol), midazolam (Versed), piroxicam (Feldene), propoxyphene (Darvon), propafenone (Rythmol), quinidine, rifabutin, terfenadine (Seldane), triazolam (Halcion), zolpidem (Ambien), ergot alkaloids.

§Decrease indinavir to 600 mg q8h.

¶Cases of new onset hyperglycemia have been reported in association with the use of all PIs (41–43).

Table 23.10. Drugs that should not be used with protease inhibitors

			Drugs		
Drug category	Indinavir	Ritonavir*	Saquinavir (given as Invirase™ or Fortovase™)	Nelfinavir	Alternatives
Analgesics	(none)	meperidine prioxicam propoxyphene	(none)	(none)	ASA, oxycodon acetaminophen
Cardiac	(none)	amioderone encainide flecainide propafenone quinidine	(none)	(none)	limited experience
Antimycobacterial	rifampin	rifabutin†	rifampin rifabutin	rifampin	For rifabutin (as alternative for MAI treatment): clarithromycin, ethambutol (treatment, not prophylaxis), or azithromycin
Ca++ channel blocker	(none)	bepridil	(none)	(none)	limited experience
Antihistamine	astemizole terfenadine	astemizole terfenidine	astemizole terfenidine	astemizole terfenidine	loratadine
GI	cisapride	cisapride	cisapride	cisapride	limited experience
Antidepressant	(none)	bupropion	(none)	(none)	fluoxetine, desipramine
Neuroleptic	(none)	clozapine pimozide	(none)	(none)	limited experience
Psychotropic	midazolam triazolam	clorazepate, diazepam estazolam, flurazepam midazolam, triazolam zolpidem	midazolam triazolam	midazolam triazolam	temazepam, lorazepam
Ergot alkaloid (vasoconstrictor)	dihydroergot-amine (D.H.E. 45), ergotamine§ (various forms)	dihydroergot-amine (D.H.E. 45), ergotamine§ (various forms)		dihydroergotamine (D.H.E. 45), ergotamine§ (various forms)	

*The contraindicated drugs listed are based on theoretical considerations. Thus, drugs with low therapeutic indices yet with suspected major metabolic contribution from cytochrome P450 3A, CYP2D6, or unknown pathways are included in this table. Actual interactions may or may not occur in patients.
†Reduce rifabutin dose to one fourth of the standard dose.
§This is likely a class effect.

206

resistance (e.g., the NNRTIs nevirapine and delavirdine) also should be used in this manner. Use of antiretroviral agents as monotherapy is contraindicated (DI), except when no other options exist or during pregnancy to reduce perinatal transmission. When initiating antiretroviral therapy, all drugs should be started simultaneously at full dose with the following three exceptions: dose escalation regimens are recommended for ritonavir, nevirapine, and, in some cases, ritonavir plus saquinavir.

Detailed information comparing the different NRTIs, the NNRTIs, the PIs, and drug interactions between the PIs and other agents is provided (Tables 23.7-23.12). Particular attention should be paid to drug interactions between the PIs and other agents (Tables 23.9-23.12), as these are extensive and often require dose modification or substitution of various drugs. Toxicity assessment is an ongoing process; assessment at least twice during the first month of therapy and every 3 months thereafter is a reasonable management approach.

Initiating Therapy in Patients Who Have Advanced-Stage HIV Disease

All patients diagnosed as having advanced HIV disease, which is defined as any condition meeting the 1993 CDC definition of AIDS,[6] should be treated with antiretroviral agents regardless of plasma viral levels (AI). All patients who have symptomatic HIV infection without AIDS, defined as the presence of thrush or unexplained fever, also should be treated.

Special Considerations in the Patient Who Has Advanced-Stage HIV Disease

Some patients with OIs, wasting, dementia, or malignancy are first diagnosed with HIV infection at this advanced stage of disease. All patients who have advanced HIV disease should be treated with antiretroviral therapy. When the patient is acutely ill with an OI or other complication of HIV infection, the clinician should consider clinical issues (e.g., drug toxicity, ability to adhere to treatment regimens, drug interactions, and laboratory abnormalities) when determining the timing of initiation of antiretroviral therapy. Once therapy is initiated, a maximally suppressive regimen (e.g., two NRTIs and a PI) should be used (Table 23.6). Advanced-stage patients being maintained on an antiretroviral regimen should not have the therapy discontinued during an acute OI or malignancy, unless concerns exist regarding drug toxicity, intolerance, or drug interactions.

207

Table 23.11. Drug interactions between protease inhibitors and other drugs; drug interactions requiring dose modifications

	Indinavir	Ritonavir	Saquinavir*	Nelfinavir
Fluconazole	No dose change	No dose change	No data	No dose change
Ketoconazole and itraconazole	Decrease dose to 600 mg q8h	Increases ketoconazole >3-fold; dose adjustment required.	Increases saquinavir levels 3-fold; no dose change†.	No dose change
Rifabutin	Reduce rifabutin to one half dose: 150 mg q.d.	Consider alternative drug or reduce dose to one fourth of standard dose.	Not recommended with either Invirase™ or Fortovase™.	Reduce rifabutin to one half dose: 150 mg q.d.
Rifampin	Contraindicated	Unknown§	Not recommended with either Invirase™ or Fortovase™.	Contraindicated
Oral contraceptives	Modest increase in Ortho-Novum levels; no dose change.	Ethinyl estradiol levels decreased; use alternative or additional contraceptive method.	No data	Ethinyl estradiol and norethindrone levels decreased; use alternative or additional contraceptive method.
Miscellaneous	Grapefruit juice reduces indinavir levels by 26%.	Desipramine increased 145%: reduce dose; Theophylline levels decreased: increase dose.	Grapefruit juice increases saquinavir levels†.	

*Several drug interaction studies have been completed with saquinavir given as Invirase™ or Fortovase™. Results from studies conducted with Invirase™ may not be applicable to Fortovase™.
†Conducted with Invirase™.
§Rifampin reduces ritonavir 35%. Increased ritonavir dose or use of ritonavir in combination therapy is strongly recommended. The effect of ritonavir on rifampin is unknown. Used concurrently, increased liver toxicity may occur. Therefore, patients on ritonavir and rifampin should be monitored closely.

Patients who have progressed to AIDS often are treated with complicated combinations of drugs, and the clinician and patient should be alert to the potential for multiple drug interactions. Thus, the choice of which antiretroviral agents to use must be made with consideration given to potential drug interactions and overlapping drug toxicities (Tables 23.7-23.12). For instance, the use of rifampin to treat active tuberculosis is problematic in a patient who is being administered a PI, which adversely affects the metabolism of rifampin but is frequently needed to effectively suppress viral replication in these advanced patients. Conversely, rifampin lowers the blood level of PIs, which may result in suboptimal antiretroviral therapy. Although rifampin is contraindicated or not recommended for use with all of the PIs, the clinician might consider using a reduced dose of rifabutin (Tables 23.8-23.11); this topic is discussed in greater detail elsewhere.[15] Other factors complicating advanced disease are wasting and anorexia, which may prevent patients from adhering to the dietary requirements for efficient absorption of certain protease inhibitors. Bone marrow suppression associated with ZDV and the neuropathic effects of ddC, d4T and ddI may combine with the direct effects of HIV to render the drugs intolerable. Hepatotoxicity associated with certain PIs may limit the use of these drugs, especially in patients who have underlying liver dysfunction. The absorption and half life of certain drugs may be altered by antiretroviral agents, particularly the PIs and NNRTIs whose metabolism involves the hepatic cytochrome p450 (CYP450) enzymatic pathway. Some of these PIs and NNRTIs (i.e., ritonavir, indinavir, saquinavir, nelfinavir, and delavirdine) inhibit the CYP450 pathway; others (e.g., nevirapine) induce CYP450 metabolism. CYP450 inhibitors have the potential to increase blood levels of drugs metabolized by this pathway. Adding a CYP450 inhibitor can sometimes improve the pharmacokinetic profile of selected agents (e.g., adding ritonavir therapy to the hard-gel formulation of saquinavir) as well as contribute an additive antiviral effect; however, these interactions also can result in life-threatening drug toxicity (Tables 23.10-23.12). As a result, health-care providers should inform their patients of the need to discuss any new drugs, including over-the-counter agents and alternative medications, that they may consider taking, and careful attention should be given to the relative risk versus benefits of specific combinations of agents.

Initiation of potent antiretroviral therapy often is associated with some degree of recovery of immune function. In this setting, patients who have advanced HIV disease and subclinical opportunistic infections (e.g., mycobacterium avium intracellulare [MAI] or CMV) may

Table 23.12. Drug interactions: protease inhibitors and non-nucleoside reverse transcriptase inhibitors—effect of drug on levels/dose

Drug affected	Indinavir	Ritonavir	Saquinavir*	Nelfinavir	Nevirapine	Delavirdine
Indinavir (IDV)	—	No data	Levels: IDV no effect; SQV ↑4–7x§ Dose: no data	Levels: IDV ↑50%; NFV ↑80% Dose: no data	Levels: IDV ↓28% Dose: standard	Levels: IDV ↑40% Dose: IDV 600 mg q8h
Ritonavir (RTV)	No data	—	Levels: RTV no effect; SQV ↑20x†§ Dose: Invirase™ or Fortovase™ 400 mg b.i.d. + RTV: 400 mg b.i.d.	Levels: RTV no effect; NFV ↑1.5x Dose: no data	Levels: RTV ↓11% Dose: standard	Levels: RTV ↑70% Dose: no data
Saquinavir (SQV)	Levels: SQV ↑4–7x; IDV no effect§ Dose: no data	Levels: SQV ↑20x†§ RTV no effect Dose: Invirase™ or Fortovase™ 400 mg b.i.d. +RTV 400 mg b.i.d.	—	Levels: SQV ↑3–5x; NFV ↑20%§ Dose: standard NFV Fortovase™ 800 mg t.i.d.	Levels: SQV ↓25%† Dose: no data	Levels: SQV ↑5x† Dose: standard for Invirase™ Monitor transaminase levels
Nelfinavir (NFV)	Levels: NFV ↑80% IDV ↑50% Dose: no data	Levels: NFV ↑1.5x RTV no effect Dose: no data	Levels: NFV ↑20%; SQV ↑3–5x§ Dose: standard NFV Fortovase™ 800 mg t.i.d.	—	Levels: NFV ↑10% Dose: standard	Levels: NFV ↑2x DLV ↓50% Dose: standard (monitor for neutropenic complications)
Nevirapine (NVP)	Levels: IDV ↓28% Dose: standard	Levels: RTV Å11% Dose: standard	Levels: SQV ↓25%†; Dose: no data	Levels: NFV ↑10% Dose: standard	—	Do not use together
Delavirdine (DLV)	Levels: IDV ↑40% Dose: IDV 600 q8h	Levels: RTV ↑70% Dose: no data	Levels: SQV ↑5x† Dose: standard for Invirase™ Monitor transaminase levels	Levels: NFV ↑2x DLV ↓50% Dose: standard (monitor for neutropenic complications)	Do not use together	—

*Several drug interaction studies have been completed with saquinavir given as Invirase™ or Fortovase™. Results from studies conducted with Invirase™ may not be applicable to Fortovase™.
†Conducted with Invirase™.
§Conducted with Fortovase™.

develop a new immunologic response to the pathogen, and, thus, new symptoms may develop in association with the heightened immunologic and/or inflammatory response. This should not be interpreted as a failure of antiretroviral therapy, and these newly presenting OIs should be treated appropriately while maintaining the patient on the antiretroviral regimen. Viral load measurement is helpful in clarifying this association.

Interruption of Antiretroviral Therapy

There are multiple reasons for temporary discontinuation of antiretroviral therapy, including intolerable side effects, drug interactions, first trimester of pregnancy when the patient so elects, and unavailability of drug. There are no currently available studies and therefore no reliable estimate of the number of days, weeks, or months that constitute a clinically important interruption of one or more components of a therapeutic regimen that would increase the likelihood of drug resistance. If any antiretroviral medication has to be discontinued for an extended time, clinicians and patients should be aware of the theoretical advantage of stopping all antiretroviral agents simultaneously, rather than continuing one or two agents, to minimize the emergence of resistant viral strains (see Principle 4).

Changing a Failing Regimen

Considerations for Changing a Failing Regimen

The decision to change regimens should be approached with careful consideration of several complex factors. These factors include recent clinical history and physical examination; plasma HIV RNA levels measured on two separate occasions; absolute CD4+ T cell count and changes in these counts; remaining treatment options in terms of potency, potential resistance patterns from prior antiretroviral therapies, and potential for adherence/tolerance; assessment of adherence to medications; and psychological preparation of the patient for the implications of the new regimen (e.g., side effects, drug interactions, dietary requirements, and possible need to alter concomitant medications) (see Principle 7). Failure of a regimen may occur for many reasons: initial viral resistance to one or more agents, altered absorption or metabolism of the drug, multidrug pharmacokinetics that adversely affect therapeutic drug levels, and poor patient adherence to a regimen due to either poor compliance or inadequate patient education about the therapeutic agents. In regard to the last issue, the health-care provider should carefully assess patient adherence before changing antiretroviral therapy; health-care workers involved in the care of the patient (e.g., the case manager or social worker) may be helpful in this evaluation. Clinicians should be aware of the prevalence of mental health disorders and psychoactive substance use disorders in certain HIV-infected persons; inadequate mental health treatment services may jeopardize the ability of these persons to adhere to their medical treatment. Proper identification of and intervention in these mental health disorders can greatly enhance adherence to medical HIV treatment.

It is important to distinguish between the need to change therapy because of drug failure versus drug toxicity. In the latter case, it is appropriate to substitute one or more alternative drugs of the same potency and from the same class of agents as the agent suspected to be causing the toxicity. In the case of drug failure where more than one drug had been used, a detailed history of current and past antiretroviral medications, as well as other HIV-related medications, should be obtained. Optimally and when possible, the regimen should be changed entirely to drugs that have not been taken previously. With triple combinations of drugs, at least two and preferably three new drugs must be used; this recommendation is based on the current understanding of strategies to prevent drug resistance (see Principles 4 and 5). Assays to determine genotypic resistance are commercially available; however, these have not undergone field testing to demonstrate clinical utility and are not approved by the FDA. The Panel does not recommend these assays for routine use at present.

The following three categories of patients should be considered with regard to a change in therapy: 1) persons who are receiving incompletely suppressive antiretroviral therapy with single or double nucleoside therapy and with detectable or undetectable plasma viral load; 2) persons who have been on potent combination therapy, including a PI, and whose viremia was initially suppressed to undetectable levels but has again become detectable; and 3) persons who have been on potent combination therapy, including a PI, and whose viremia was never suppressed to below detectable limits. Although persons in these groups should have treatment regimens changed to maximize the chances of durable, maximal viral RNA suppression, the first group may have more treatment options because they are PI naive.

Criteria for Changing Therapy

The goal of antiretroviral therapy, which is to improve the length and quality of the patient's life, is likely best accomplished by maximal

212

suppression of viral replication to below detectable levels (currently defined as <500 copies/mL) sufficiently early to preserve immune function. However, this reduction cannot always be achieved with a given therapeutic regimen, and frequently regimens must be modified. In general, the plasma HIV RNA level is the most important parameter to consider in evaluating response to therapy, and increases in levels of viremia that are substantial, confirmed, and not attributable to intercurrent infection or vaccination indicate failure of the drug regimen, regardless of changes in the CD4+ T cell counts. Clinical complications and sequential changes in CD4+ T cell count may complement the viral load test in evaluating a response to treatment. Specific criteria that should prompt consideration for changing therapy include the following:

- *Less than a 0.5-0.75 log reduction in plasma HIV RNA by 4-8 weeks following initiation of therapy (CIII).*

- *Failure to suppress plasma HIV RNA to undetectable levels within 4-6 months of initiating therapy (BIII).* The degree of initial decrease in plasma HIV RNA and the overall trend in decreasing viremia should be considered. For instance, a patient with 10^6 viral copies/mL prior to therapy who stabilizes after 6 months of therapy at an HIV RNA level that is detectable but <10,000 copies/mL may not warrant an immediate change in therapy.

- *Repeated detection of virus in plasma after initial suppression to undetectable levels, suggesting the development of resistance (BIII).* However, the degree of plasma HIV RNA increase should be considered; the physician may consider short-term further observation in a patient whose plasma HIV RNA increases from undetectable to low-level detectability (e.g., 500-5,000 copies/mL) at 4 months. In this situation, the patient should be monitored closely. However, most patients whose plasma HIV RNA levels become detectable after having been undetectable will subsequently show progressive increases in plasma viremia that will likely require a change in antiretroviral regimen.

- *Any reproducible significant increase, defined as threefold or greater, from the nadir of plasma HIV RNA not attributable to intercurrent infection, vaccination, or test methodology except as noted above (BIII).*

- *Undetectable viremia in the patient who is being administered double nucleoside therapy (BIII).* Patients currently receiving two NRTIs who have achieved the goal of no detectable virus have the option of either continuing this regimen or modifying the regimen to conform to regimens in the preferred category (Table 23.6). Prior experience indicates that most of these patients on double nucleoside therapy will eventually have virologic failure with a frequency that is substantially greater compared with patients treated with the preferred regimens.

- *Persistently declining CD4+ T cell numbers, as measured on at least two separate occasions (see Principle 2 for significant decline) (CIII).*

- *Clinical deterioration (DIII).* A new AIDS-defining diagnosis that was acquired after the time treatment was initiated suggests clinical deterioration but may or may not suggest failure of antiretroviral therapy. If the antiretroviral effect of therapy was poor (e.g., a less than tenfold reduction in viral RNA), then a judgment of therapeutic failure could be made. However, if the antiretroviral effect was good but the patient was already severely immunocompromised, the appearance of a new opportunistic disease may not necessarily reflect a failure of antiretroviral therapy, but rather a persistence of severe immunocompromise that did not improve despite adequate suppression of virus replication. Similarly, an accelerated decline in CD4+ T cell counts suggests progressive immune deficiency providing there are sufficient measurements to ensure quality control of CD4+ T cell measurements.

A final consideration in the decision to change therapy is the recognition of the still limited choice of available agents and the knowledge that a decision to change may reduce future treatment options for the patient (see Principle 7). This consideration may influence the physician to be somewhat more conservative when deciding to change therapy. Consideration of alternative options should include potency of the substituted regimen and probability of tolerance of or adherence to the alternative regimen. Clinical trials have demonstrated that partial suppression of virus is superior to no suppression of virus. However, some physicians and patients may prefer to suspend treatment to preserve future options or because a sustained antiviral effect cannot be achieved. Referral to or consultation with an experienced HIV clinician is appropriate when the clinician is considering a change in therapy. When possible, patients who require a change in an antiretroviral regimen but without treatment options that include using currently approved drugs should be referred for consideration for inclusion in an appropriate clinical trial.

Therapeutic Options When Changing Antiretroviral Therapy

Recommendations for changes in treatment differ according to the indication for the change. If the desired virologic objectives have been achieved in patients who have intolerance or toxicity, a substitution should be made for the offending drug, preferably with an agent in the same class with a different toxicity or tolerance profile. If virologic objectives have been achieved but the patient is receiving a regimen not in the preferred category (e.g., two NRTIs or monotherapy), there is the option either to continue treatment with careful monitoring of viral load or to add drugs to the current regimen to comply with preferred treatment regimens. Most experts consider that treatment with regimens not in the preferred category is associated with eventual failure and recommend the latter tactic. At present, few clinical data are available to support specific strategies for changing therapy in patients who have failed the preferred regimens that include PIs; however, several theoretical considerations should guide decisions. Because of the relatively rapid mutability of HIV, viral strains that are resistant to one or more agents often emerge during therapy, particularly when viral replication has not been maximally suppressed. Of major concern is recent evidence of broad cross-resistance among the class of PIs. Evidence indicates that viral strains that become resistant to one PI will have reduced susceptibility to most or all other PIs. Thus, the likelihood of success of a subsequently administered PI + two NRTI regimen, even if all drugs are different from the initial regimen, may be limited, and many experts would include two new PIs in the subsequent regimen.

Some of the most important guidelines to follow when changing a patient's antiretroviral therapy are summarized (Table 23.13), and some of the treatment options available when a decision has been made to change the antiretroviral regimen are outlined (Table 23.14). Limited data exist to suggest that any of these alternative regimens will be effective (Table 23.14), and careful monitoring and consultation with an expert in the care of such HIV-infected patients is desirable. A change in regimen because of treatment failure should ideally involve complete replacement of the regimen with different drugs to which the patient is naive. This typically would include the use of two new NRTIs and one new PI or NNRTI, two PIs with one or two new NRTIs, or a PI combined with an NNRTI. Dose modifications may be required to account for drug interactions when using combinations of PIs or a PI and NNRTI (Table 23.12). In some persons, these options are not possible because of prior antiretroviral use, toxicity, or intolerance. In the clinically stable patient who has detectable viremia for whom an optimal change in therapy is not possible, it may be prudent to delay changing therapy in anticipation of the availability of newer and more potent agents. It is recommended that the decision to change therapy and design a new regimen should be made with assistance from a clinician experienced in the treatment of HIV infected patients through consultation or referral.

Table 23.13a. Guidelines for changing an antiretroviral regimen for suspected drug failure. (Continued on next page.)

- Criteria for changing therapy include a suboptimal reduction in plasma viremia after initiation of therapy, reappearance of viremia after suppression to undetectable, substantial increases in plasma viremia from the nadir of suppression, and declining CD4 + T cell numbers. Refer to the more extensive discussion of these criteria in "Criteria for Changing Therapy."

- When the decision to change therapy is based on viral load determination, it is preferable to confirm with a second viral load test.

- Distinguish between the need to change a regimen because of drug intolerance or inability to comply with the regimen versus failure to achieve the goal of sustained viral suppression; single agents can be changed or dose reduced in the event of drug intolerance.

- In general, do not change a single drug or add a single drug to a failing regimen; it is important to use at least two new drugs and preferably to use an entirely new regimen with at least three new drugs.

- Many patients have limited options for new regimens of desired potency; in some of these cases, it is rational to continue the prior regimen if partial viral suppression was achieved.

- In some cases, regimens identified as suboptimal for initial therapy are rational due to limitations imposed by toxicity, intolerance, or nonadherence. This especially applies in late-stage disease. For patients with no rational alternative options who have virologic failure with return of viral load to baseline (pretreatment levels) and a declining CD4+ T cell count, discontinuation of antiretroviral therapy should be considered.

Acute HIV Infection

Considerations for Treatment of Patients Who Have Acute HIV Infection

Various studies indicate that 50%–90% of patients acutely infected with HIV will experience at least some symptoms of the acute retroviral syndrome (Table 23.15) and can thus be identified as candidates for early therapy.[16-19] However, acute HIV infection is often not recognized in the primary-care setting because of the similarity of the symptom complex with those of the "flu" or other common illnesses. Also, acute primary infection may occur without symptoms. Physicians should maintain a high level of suspicion for HIV infection

Table 23.13b. Guidelines for changing an antiretroviral regimen for suspected drug failure. (Continued from previous page.)

- Experience is limited with regimens using combinations of two protease inhibitors or combinations of protease inhibitors with nevirapine or delavirdine; for patients with limited options due to drug intolerance or suspected resistance, these regimens provide possible alternative treatment options.

- There is limited information about the value of restarting a drug that the patient has previously received. The experience with zidovudine is that resistant strains are often replaced with "wild-type" zidovudine sensitive strains when zidovudine treatment is stopped, but resistance recurs rapidly if zidovudine is restarted. Although preliminary evidence indicates that this occurs with indinavir, it is not known if similar problems apply to other nucleoside analogues, protease inhibitors, or NNRTIs, but a conservative stance is that they probably do.

- Avoid changing from ritonavir to indinavir or vice versa for drug failure, because high-level cross- resistance is likely.

- Avoid changing from nevirapine to delavirdine or vice versa for drug failure, because high-level cross-resistance is likely.

- The decision to change therapy and the choice of a new regimen require that the clinician have considerable expertise in the care of persons living with HIV infection. Physicians who are less experienced in the care of persons with HIV infection are strongly encouraged to obtain assistance through consultation with or referral to a clinician who has considerable expertise in the care of HIV-infected patients.

in all patients with a compatible clinical syndrome (Table 23.15) and should obtain appropriate laboratory confirmation. Information regarding treatment of acute HIV infection from clinical trials is limited. There is evidence for a short-term effect of therapy on viral load and CD4+ T cell counts,[20] but there are as yet no outcome data demonstrating a clinical benefit of antiretroviral treatment of primary HIV infection. Clinical trials completed to date also have been limited by small sample sizes, short duration of follow-up, and often by the use of treatment regimens that have suboptimal antiviral activity by current standards. However, results from these studies generally support antiretroviral treatment of acute HIV infection. Ongoing clinical trials are addressing the question of the long-term clinical benefit of more potent treatment regimens.

The theoretical rationale for early intervention (see Principle 10) is fourfold:

- to suppress the initial burst of viral replication and decrease the magnitude of virus dissemination throughout the body;

- to decrease the severity of acute disease;

Table 23.14. Possible regimens for patients who have failed antiretroviral therapy: a work in progress*

Prior regimen	New regimen (not listed in priority order)
2 NRTIs +	2 new NRTIs +
Nelfinavir (NFV)	RTV; or IDV; or SQV + RTV; or NNRTI[†] + RTV; or NNRTI + IDV[§]
Ritonavir (RTV)	SQV + RTV[§]; NFV + NNRTI; or NFV + SQV
Indinavir (IDV)	SQV + RTV; NFV + NNRTI; or NFV + SQV
Saquinavir (SQV)	RTV + SQV; or NNRTI + IDV
2 NRTIs + NNRTI	2 new NRTIs + a protease inhibitor
2 NRTIs	2 new NRTIs + a protease inhibitor 2 new NRTIs + RTV + SQV 1 new NRTI + 1 NNRTI + a protease inhibitor 2 protease inhibitors + NNRTI
1 NRTI	2 new NRTIs + a protease inhibitor 2 new NRTIs + NNRTI 1 new NRTI + 1 NNRTI + a protease inhibitor

*These alternative regimens have not been proven to be clinically effective and were arrived at through discussion by the panel of theoretically possible alternative treatments and the elimination of those alternatives with evidence of being ineffective. Clinical trials in this area are urgently needed.
†Of the two available NNRTIs, clinical trials support a preference for nevirapine over delavirdine based on results of viral load assays. These two agents have opposite effects on the CYP450 pathway, and this must be considered in combining these drugs with other agents.
§There are some clinical trials that have yielded viral burden data to support this recommendation.

- to potentially alter the initial viral "set-point", which may ultimately affect the rate of disease progression;

- to possibly reduce the rate of viral mutation due to the suppression of viral replication.

The physician and the patient should be aware that therapy of primary HIV infection is based on theoretical considerations, and the potential benefits, described above, should be weighed against the potential risks (see below). Most experts endorse treatment of acute HIV infection based on the theoretical rationale, limited but supportive clinical trial data, and the experience of HIV clinicians.

The risks associated with therapy for acute HIV infection include adverse effects on quality of life resulting from drug toxicities and dosing constraints; the potential, if therapy fails to effectively suppress viral replication, for the development of drug resistance that may limit future treatment options; and the potential need for continuing therapy indefinitely. These considerations are similar to those for initiating therapy in the asymptomatic patient (see Considerations in Initiating Therapy in the Asymptomatic HIV-infected Patient).

Deciding Whom to Treat During Acute HIV Infection

Many experts would recommend antiretroviral therapy for all patients who demonstrate laboratory evidence of acute HIV infection (AII). Such evidence includes HIV RNA in plasma that can be detected by using sensitive PCR or bDNA assays together with a negative or indeterminate HIV antibody test. Although measurement of plasma HIV RNA is the preferable method of diagnosis, a test for p24 antigen may be useful when RNA testing is not readily available. However, a negative p24 antigen test does not rule out acute infection. When suspicion for acute infection is high (e.g., as in a patient who has a report of recent risk behavior in association with suggestive symptoms and signs [Table 23.15]), a test for HIV RNA should be performed (BII). (Patients diagnosed with HIV infection by HIV RNA testing should have confirmatory testing performed; see Table 23.2). Persons may or may not have symptoms of the acute retroviral syndrome. Viremia occurs acutely after infection before the detection of a specific immune response; an indeterminate antibody test may occur when a person is in the process of seroconversion.

Apart from patients who have acute primary HIV infection, many experts also would consider therapy for patients in whom seroconversion has been documented to have occurred within the previous 6 months (CIII). Although the initial burst of viremia in infected adults has usually resolved by 2 months, treatment during the 2–6-month period after infection is based on the likelihood that virus replication in lymphoid tissue is still not maximally contained by the immune system during this time. Decisions regarding therapy for patients who test antibody positive and who believe the infection is recent but for whom the time of infection cannot be documented should be made using the Asymptomatic HIV Infection algorithm mentioned previously (CIII). No patient should be treated for HIV infection until the infection is documented, except in the setting of post-exposure prophylaxis of health-care workers with antiretroviral agents[21] (or treatment of neonates born to HIV-infected mothers). All patients without a formal medical record of a positive HIV test (e.g., persons who have

Table 23.15. Acute retroviral syndrome: associated signs and symptoms and expected frequency (adapted from reference 19)

- Fever (96%)
- Lymphadenopathy (74%)
- Pharyngitis (70%)
- Rash (70%)
    Erythematous maculopapular with lesions on face and
        trunk and sometimes extremities, including palms and
        soles
    Mucocutaneous ulceration involving mouth, esophagus, or
        genitals
- Myalgia or arthralgia (54%)
- Diarrhea (32%)
- Headache (32%)
- Nausea and vomiting (27%)
- Hepatosplenomegaly (14%)
- Thrush (12%)
- Weight Loss
- Neurologic symptoms (12%)
    Meningoencephalitis or aseptic meningitis
    Peripheral neuropathy or radiculopathy
    Facial palsy
    Guillain-Barré syndrome
    Brachial neuritis
    Cognitive impairment or psychosis

tested positive by available home testing kits) should be tested by both the ELISA and an established confirmatory test (e.g., the Western Blot) to document HIV infection (AI).

Treatment Regimen for Primary HIV Infection

Once the physician and patient have decided to use antiretroviral therapy for primary HIV infection, treatment should be implemented with the goal of suppressing plasma HIV RNA levels to below detectable levels (AIII). The weight of current experience suggests that the therapeutic regimen for acute HIV infection should include a combination of two NRTIs and one potent PI (AII). Although most experience to date with PIs in the setting of acute HIV infection has been with ritonavir, indinavir or nelfinavir,[2,22-24] insufficient data are available to make firm conclusions regarding specific drug recommendations. Potential combinations of agents available are much the same as those used in established infection (Table 23.6). These aggressive regimens may be associated with several disadvantages (e.g., drug toxicity, large numbers of pills, cost of drugs, and the possibility of developing drug resistance that may limit future options); the latter is likely if virus replication is not adequately suppressed or if the patient has been infected with a viral strain that is already resistant to one or more agents. The patient should be carefully counseled regarding these potential limitations and individual decisions made only after weighing the risks and sequelae of therapy against the theoretical benefit of treatment.

Any regimen that is not expected to maximally suppress viral replication is not considered appropriate for treating the acutely HIV-infected person (EIII) because a) the ultimate goal of therapy is suppression of viral replication to below the level of detection, b) the benefits of therapy are based primarily on theoretical considerations, and c) long-term clinical outcome benefit has not been documented. Additional clinical studies are needed to delineate further the role of antiretroviral therapy in the primary infection period.

Patient Follow-up

Testing for plasma HIV RNA levels and CD4+ T cell count and toxicity monitoring should be performed as previously described in Use of Testing for Plasma HIV RNA levels and CD4+ T Cell Count in Guiding Decisions for Therapy, that is, on initiation of therapy, after 4 weeks, and every 3-4 months thereafter (AII). Some experts suggest that testing for plasma HIV RNA levels at 4 weeks is not helpful in evaluating the effect of therapy for acute infection because viral loads may be decreasing from peak viremia levels even in the absence of therapy.

Duration of Therapy for Primary HIV Infection

Once therapy is initiated, many experts would continue to treat the patient with antiretroviral agents indefinitely because viremia has been documented to reappear or increase after discontinuation of therapy (CII). However, some experts would treat for one year and then reevaluate the patient with CD4+ T cell determinations and quantitative HIV RNA measurements. The optimal duration and composition of therapy are unknown, and ongoing clinical trials are expected to provide data relevant to these issues. The difficulties inherent in determining the optimal duration and composition of therapy initiated for acute infection should be considered when first counseling the patient regarding therapy.

Considerations for Antiretroviral Therapy in the HIV-Infected Adolescent

HIV-infected adolescents who were infected through sexual contact or through injecting-drug use during adolescence appear to follow a clinical course that is more similar to HIV disease in adults than in children. In contrast, adolescents who were infected perinatally or through blood products as young children have a unique clinical course that may differ from other adolescents and long-term surviving adults. Currently, most HIV-infected adolescents were infected through sexual contact during the adolescent period and are in a relatively early stage of infection, making them ideal candidates for early intervention.

Puberty is a time of somatic growth and hormonally mediated changes, with females developing more body fat and males more muscle mass. Although theoretically these physiologic changes could affect drug pharmacology, particularly in the case of drugs with a narrow therapeutic index that are used in combination with protein-bound medicines or hepatic enzyme inducers or inhibitors, no clinically substantial impact of puberty on the use of NRTIs has been observed. Clinical experience with PIs and NNRTIs has been limited. Thus, it is currently recommended that medications used to treat HIV and OIs in adolescents should be administered in a dosage based on

Tanner staging of puberty and not specific age. Adolescents in early puberty (Tanner I-II) should receive doses as recommended in the pediatric guidelines, whereas those in late puberty (Tanner V) should receive doses recommended in the adult guidelines. Youth who are in the midst of their growth spurt (Tanner III females and Tanner IV males) should be closely monitored for medication efficacy and toxicity when choosing adult or pediatric dosing guidelines.

Considerations for Antiretroviral Therapy in the Pregnant HIV-Infected Woman

Guidelines for optimal antiretroviral therapy and for initiation of therapy in pregnant HIV-infected women should be the same as those delineated for nonpregnant adults (see Principle 8). Thus, the woman's clinical, virologic, and immunologic status should be the primary factor in guiding treatment decisions. However, it must be realized that the potential impact of such therapy on the fetus and infant is unknown. The decision to use any antiretoviral drug during pregnancy should be made by the woman following discussion with her health-care provider regarding the known and unknown benefits and risks to her and her fetus. Long-term follow-up is recommended for all infants born to women who have received antiretroviral drugs during pregnancy.

Women who are in the first trimester of pregnancy and who are not receiving antiretroviral therapy may wish to consider delaying initiation of therapy until after 10-12 weeks' gestation because this is the period of organogenesis when the embryo is most susceptible to potential teratogenic effects of drugs; the risks of antiretroviral therapy to the fetus during that period are unknown. However, this decision should be carefully considered and discussed between the health-care provider and the patient and should include an assessment of the woman's health status and the potential benefits and risks of delaying initiation of therapy for several weeks. If clinical, virologic, or immunologic parameters are such that therapy would be recommended for nonpregnant persons, many experts would recommend initiating therapy, regardless of gestational age. Nausea and vomiting in early pregnancy, which affect the ability to adequately take and absorb oral medications, may be a factor in deciding whether to administer treatment during the first trimester.

Some women already receiving antiretroviral therapy may have their pregnancy diagnosed early enough in gestation that concern for potential teratogenicity may lead them to consider temporarily stopping antiretroviral therapy until after the first trimester. Insufficient data exist that either support or refute teratogenic risk of antiretroviral drugs when administered during the first 10-12 weeks' gestation. However, a rebound in viral levels would be anticipated during the period of discontinuation, and this rebound could theoretically be associated with increased risk of early *in utero* HIV transmission or could potentiate disease progression in the woman.[25] Although the effects of all antiretroviral drugs on the developing fetus during the first trimester are uncertain, most experts recommend continuation of a maximally suppressive regimen even during the first trimester. If antiretroviral therapy is discontinued during the first trimester for any reason, all agents should be stopped simultaneously to avoid development of resistance. Once the drugs are reinstituted, they should be introduced simultaneously for the same reason.

The choice of which antiretroviral agents to use in pregnant women is subject to unique considerations (see Principle 8). Currently, minimal data are available regarding the pharmacokinetics and safety of antiretroviral agents during pregnancy for drugs other than ZDV. In the absence of data, drug choice needs to be individualized based on discussion with the patient and available data from preclinical and clinical testing of the individual drugs. The FDA pregnancy classification for all currently approved antiretroviral agents and selected other information relevant to the use of antiretroviral drugs in pregnancy is provided (Table 23.16). The predictive value of *in vitro* and animal-screening tests for adverse effects in humans is unknown. Many drugs commonly used to treat HIV infection or its consequences may have positive findings on one or more of these screening tests. For example, acyclovir is positive on some *in vitro* assays for chromosomal breakage and carcinogenicity and is associated with some fetal abnormalities in rats; however, data on human experience from the Acyclovir in Pregnancy Registry indicate no increased risk of birth defects to date in infants with *in utero* exposure to acyclovir.[26]

Of the currently approved nucleoside analogue antiretroviral agents, the pharmacokinetics of only ZDV and 3TC have been evaluated in infected pregnant women to date.[27,28] Both drugs seem to be well tolerated at the usual adult doses and cross the placenta, achieving concentrations in cord blood similar to those observed in maternal blood at delivery. All the nucleosides except ddI have preclinical animal studies that indicate potential fetal risk and have been classified as FDA pregnancy category C (see Table 23.16); ddI has been classified as category B. In primate studies, all the nucleoside analogues seem to cross the placenta, but ddI and ddC apparently have

Table 23.16. Preclinical and clinical data relevant to use of antiretrovirals during pregnancy

Antiretroviral drug	FDA-defined pregnancy category*	Placental passage [Newborn: maternal drug]	Long-term animal carcinogenicity studies	Rodent teratogen
Zidovudine†	C	Yes (human) [0.85]	Positive (rodent, vaginal tumors)	Positive (near lethal dose)
Zalcitabine	C	Yes (rhesus) [0.30–0.50]	Positive (rodent, thymic lymphomas)	Positive (hydrocephalus at high dose)
Didanosine	B	Yes (human) [0.5]	Negative (no tumors, lifetime rodent study)	Negative
Stavudine	C	Yes (rhesus) [0.76]	Not completed	Negative (but sternal bone calcium decreases)
Lamivudine	C	Yes (human)[~1.0]	Negative (no tumors, lifetime rodent study)	Negative
Saquinavir	B	Unknown	Not completed	Negative
Indinavir	C	Yes (rats) ("Significant" in rats; low in rabbits)	Not completed	Negative (but extra ribs in rats)
Ritonavir	B	Yes (rats) [mid-term fetus, 1.15; late-term fetus, 0.15–0.64]	Not completed	Negative (but cryptorchidism in rats)§
Nelfinavir	B	Unknown	Not completed	Negative
Neviparine	C	Yes (human) [~1.0]	Not completed	Negative
Delavirdine	C	Yes (rats) [late-term fetus, blood, 0.15; late-term fetus, liver 0.04]	Not completed	Ventricular septal defect

*Food and Drug Administration-defined pregnancy categories are: A = Adequate and well-controlled studies of pregnant women fail to demonstrate a risk to the fetus during the first trimester of pregnancy (and there is no evidence of risk during later trimesters); B = Animal reproduction studies fail to demonstrate a risk to the fetus, and adequate but well-controlled studies of pregnant women have not been conducted; C = Safety in human pregnancy has not been determined, animal studies are either positive for fetal risk or have not been conducted, and the drug should not be used unless the potential benefit outweighs the potential risk to the fetus; D = Positive evidence of human fetal risk based on adverse reaction data from investigational or marketing experiences, but the potential benefits from the use of the drug in pregnant women may be acceptable despite its potential risks; X = Studies in animals or reports of adverse reactions have indicated that the risk associated with the use of the drug for pregnant women clearly outweighs any possible benefit.

†Despite certain animal data indicating potential teratogenicity of ZDV when near-lethal doses are given to pregnant rodents, considerable human data are available to date indicating that the risk to the fetus, if any, is extremely small when given to the pregnant mother beyond 14 weeks' gestation. Follow-up for up to age 6 years for 734 infants born to HIV-infected women who had in utero exposure to ZDV has not demonstrated any tumor development (44). However, no data are available with longer follow-up to evaluate for late effects.

§These are effects seen only at maternally toxic doses.

significantly less placental transfer (fetal to maternal drug ratios of 0.3 to 0.5) than do ZDV, d4T, and 3TC (fetal to maternal drug ratios >0.7).[29]

Of the NNRTIs, only nevirapine administered once at the onset of labor has been evaluated in pregnant women. The drug was well tolerated after a single dose and crossed the placenta and achieved neonatal blood concentrations equivalent to those in the mother. The elimination of nevirapine administered during labor in the pregnant women in this study was prolonged (mean half-life following a single dose, 66 hours) compared with nonpregnant persons (mean half-life following a single dose, 45 hours). Data on multiple dosing during pregnancy are not yet available. Delavirdine has not been studied in Phase I pharmacokinetic and safety trials in pregnant women. In premarketing clinical studies, outcomes of seven unplanned pregnancies were reported. Three of these were ectopic pregnancies, and three resulted in healthy live births. One infant was born prematurely, with a small ventricular septal defect, to a patient who had received approximately 6 weeks of treatment with delavirdine and ZDV early in the course of pregnancy.

Although studies of combination therapy with protease inhibitors in pregnant HIV-infected women are in progress, no data are currently available regarding drug dosage, safety and tolerance during pregnancy. In mice, indinavir has substantial placental passage; however, in rabbits, little placental passage was observed. Ritonavir has been demonstrated to have some placental passage in rats. There are some special theoretical concerns regarding the use of indinavir late in pregnancy. Indinavir is associated with side effects (hyperbilirubinemia and renal stones) that theoretically could be problematic for the newborn if transplacental passage occurs and the drug is administered shortly before delivery. These side effects are particularly problematic because the immaturity of the metabolic enzyme system of the neonatal liver would likely be associated with prolonged drug half-life leading to extended drug exposure in the newborn that could lead to potential exacerbation of physiologic neonatal hyperbilirubinemia. Because of immature neonatal renal function and the inability of the neonate to voluntarily ensure adequate hydration, high drug concentrations and/or delayed elimination in the neonate could result in a higher risk for drug crystallization and renal stone development than observed in adults. These concerns are theoretical and such effects have not been reported; because the half-life of indinavir in adults is short, these concerns may only be relevant if drug is administered near the time of labor. Gestational diabetes is a pregnancy-related complication that can develop in some women; administration of any of the four currently available protease inhibitors has been associated with new onset diabetes mellitus, hyperglycemia, or exacerbation of existing diabetes mellitus in HIV-infected patients.[30] Pregnancy is itself a risk factor for hyperglycemia, and it is unknown if the use of protease inhibitors will exacerbate this risk for hyperglycemia. Health-care providers caring for infected pregnant women who are being administered PI therapy should be aware of the possibility of hyperglycemia and closely monitor glucose levels in their patients and instruct their patients on how to recognize the early symptoms of hyperglycemia.

To date, the only drug that has been shown to reduce the risk of perinatal HIV transmission is ZDV when administered according to the following regimen: orally administered antenatally after 14 weeks' gestation and continued throughout pregnancy, intravenously administered during the intrapartum period, and administered orally to the newborn for the first 6 weeks of life.[31] This chemoprophylactic regimen was shown to reduce the risk for perinatal transmission by 66% in a randomized, double-blind clinical trial, pediatric ACTG 076.[32] Insufficient data are available to justify the substitution of any antiretroviral agent other than ZDV to reduce perinatal HIV transmission; further research should address this question. For the time being, if combination antiretroviral drugs are administered to the pregnant woman for treatment of her HIV infection, ZDV should be included as a component of the antenatal therapeutic regimen whenever possible, and the intrapartum and neonatal ZDV components of the chemoprophylactic regimen should be administered to reduce the risk for perinatal transmission. If a woman is not administered ZDV as a component of her antenatal antiretroviral regimen (e.g., because of prior history of nonlife-threatening ZDV-related severe toxicity or personal choice), intrapartum and newborn ZDV should continue to be recommended; when use of ZDV is contraindicated in the woman, the intrapartum component may be deleted, but the newborn component is still recommended. ZDV and d4T should not be administered together due to potential pharmacologic antagonism. When d4T is a preferred nucleoside for treatment of a pregnant woman, it is recommended that antenatal ZDV not be added to the regimen; however, intrapartum and neonatal ZDV should still be given.

The time-limited use of ZDV alone during pregnancy for chemoprophylaxis of perinatal transmission is controversial. The potential benefits of standard combination antiretroviral regimens for treatment of HIV infection should be discussed with and offered to all pregnant

HIV-infected women. Some women may wish to restrict exposure of their fetus to antiretroviral drugs during pregnancy but still wish to reduce the risk of transmitting HIV to their infant. For women in whom initiation of antiretroviral therapy for treatment of their HIV infection would be considered optional (e.g., CD4+ count >500/mm^3 and plasma HIV RNA <10,0000-20,000 RNA copies/mL), time-limited use of ZDV during the second and third trimesters of pregnancy is less likely to induce the development of resistance due to the limited viral replication existing in the patient and the time-limited exposure to the antiretroviral drug. For example, the development of resistance was unusual among the healthy population of women who participated in Pediatric (P)-ACTG 076.[33] The use of ZDV chemoprophylaxis alone during pregnancy might be an appropriate option for these women. However, for women who have more advanced disease and/or higher levels of HIV RNA, concerns about resistance are greater and these women should be counseled that a combination antiretroviral regimen that includes ZDV for reducing transmission risk would be more optimal for their own health than use of ZDV chemoprophylaxis alone.

Monitoring and use of HIV-1 RNA for therapeutic decision making during pregnancy should be performed as recommended for nonpregnant persons. Transmission of HIV from mother to infant can occur at all levels of maternal HIV-1 RNA. In untreated women, higher HIV-1 RNA levels correlate with increased transmission risk. However, in ZDV-treated women this relationship is markedly attenuated.[32] ZDV is effective in reducing transmission regardless of maternal HIV RNA level. Therefore, the use of the full ZDV chemoprophylaxis regimen, including intravenous ZDV during delivery and the administration of ZDV to the infant for the first 6 weeks of life, alone or in combination with other antiretrovirals, should be discussed with and offered to all infected pregnant women regardless of their HIV-1 RNA level. Health-care providers who are treating HIV-infected pregnant women are strongly encouraged to report cases of prenatal exposure to antiretroviral drugs (either administered alone or in combinations) to the Antiretroviral Pregnancy Registry. The registry collects observational, nonexperimental data regarding antiretroviral exposure during pregnancy for the purpose of assessing potential teratogenicity. Registry data will be used to supplement animal toxicology studies and assist clinicians in weighing the potential risks and benefits of treatment for individual patients. The registry is a collaborative project with an advisory committee of obstetric and pediatric practitioners, staff from CDC and NIH, and staff from pharmaceutical manufacturers. The registry allows the anonymity of patients, and birth outcome follow-up is obtained by registry staff from the reporting physician. Referrals should be directed to Antiretroviral Pregnancy Registry, Post Office Box 13398, Research Triangle Park, NC 27709-3398; telephone (800) 258-4263.

Conclusion

The Panel has attempted to use the advances in current understanding of the pathogenesis of HIV in the infected person to translate scientific principles and data obtained from clinical experience into recommendations that can be used by the clinician and patient to make therapeutic decisions. The recommendations are offered in

Table 23.17. Antiretroviral Drugs Approved by FDA for HIV (as of September 21, 1998)

Brand Name	Generic Name	Firm Name	Approval Date
Retrovir Capsules	zidovudine, AZT	Glaxo Wellcome	19 March 87
Retrovir Syrup	zidovudine, AZT	Glaxo Wellcome	28 September 89
Retrovir Injection	zidovudine, AZT	Glaxo Wellcome	02 February 90
Videx	didanosine, ddl	Bristol Meyers-Squibb	09 October 91
Hivid	zalcitabine, ddC	Hoffman-La Roche	19 June 92
Zerit	stavudine, d4T	Bristol Myers-Squibb	24 June 94
Epivir	lamivudine, 3TC	Glaxo Wellcome	17 November 95
Invirase	saquinavir	Hoffman-La Roche	06 December 95
Norvir	ritonavir	Abbott Laboratories	01 March 96
Crixivan	indinavir	Merck & Co., Inc.	13 March 96
Viramune	nevirapine	Boehringer Ingelheim Pharmaceuticals, Inc.	21 June 96
Viracept	nelfinavir	Agouron Pharmaceuticals	14 March 97
Rescriptor	delavirdine	Pharmacia & Upjohn	04 April 97
Combivir	zidovudine and lamivudine	Glaxo Wellcome	26 September 97
Fortovase	saquinavir	Hoffman-La Roche	07 November 97
Sustiva	efavirenz	DuPont Pharmaceuticals	17 September 98

the context of an ongoing dialogue between the patient and the clinician after having defined specific therapeutic goals with an acknowledgment of uncertainties. It is necessary for the patient to receive a continuum of medical care and services, including social, psychosocial, and nutritional services, with the availability of expert referral and consultation. To achieve the maximal flexibility in tailoring therapy to each patient over the duration of his or her infection, it is imperative that drug formularies allow for all FDA-approved NRTI, NNRTI, and PI as treatment options. The Panel strongly urges industry and the public and private sectors to conduct further studies to allow refinement of these guidelines. Specifically, studies are needed to optimize recommendations for first-line therapy; to define second-line therapy; and to more clearly delineate the reason(s) for treatment failure. The Panel remains committed to revising their recommendations as such new data become available.

Acknowledgment

The Panel extends special appreciation to Charles Carpenter (Brown University School of Medicine, Providence, RI) for his advice in the development of this document and to Gerry Bally (Health Canada) and Anita Rachlis (Sunnybrook Health Science Centre, University of Toronto, Toronto, Canada) for their participation. The Panel acknowledges the special contributions of Sharilyn Stanley, Barbara Brady, and Elaine Daniels in the preparation of this document.

References

1. USPHS/IDSA Prevention of Opportunistic Infections Working Group. 1997 USPHS/IDSA guidelines for the prevention of opportunistic infections in persons infected with human immunodeficiency virus. *MMWR* 1997;46(No. RR-12).

2. Perelson AS, Essunger P, Cao Y, *et al*. Decay characteristics of HIV-1-infected compartments during combination therapy. *Nature* 1997;387:188-91.

3. Stein DS, Korvick JA, Vermund SH. CD4+ lymphocyte cell enumeration for prediction of clinical course of human immunodeficiency virus disease: a review. *J Infect Dis* 1992;165:352-63.

4. Carpenter CC, Fischl MA, Hammer SM, *et al*. Antiretroviral therapy for HIV infection in 1997: Updated recommendations

of the international AIDS Society-USA panel. *JAMA* 1997;277:1962-9.

5. Raboud JM, Montaner JSG, Conway B, *et al.* Variation in plasma RNA levels, CD4 cell counts, and p24 antigen levels in clinically stable men with human immunodeficiency virus infection. *J Infect Dis* 1996;174:191-4.

6. CDC. 1993 revised classification system for HIV infection and expanded surveillance case definition for AIDS among adolescents and adults. *MMWR* 1992;41(No. RR-17).

7. Fischl MA, Richman DD, Grieco MH, *et al.* The efficacy of azidothymidine (AZT) in the treatment of patients with AIDS and AIDS-related complex: a double-blind, placebo-controlled trial. *N Engl J Med* 1987;317:185-91.

8. Fischl MA, Richman DD, Hansen N, *et al.* The safety and efficacy of zidovudine (AZT) in the treatment of subjects with mildly symptomatic human immunodeficiency virus type 1 infection: a double-blind, placebo-controlled trial. *Ann Intern Med* 1990;112:727-37.

9. Volberding PA, Lagakos SW, Koch MA, *et al.* Zidovudine in asymptomatic human immunodeficiency virus infection: a controlled trial in persons with fewer than 500 CD4-positive cells per cubic millimeter. *N Engl J* Med 1990;322:941-9.

10. Volberding PA, Lagakos SW, Grimes JM, *et al.* The duration of zidovudine benefit in persons with asymptomatic HIV infection: prolonged evaluation of protocol 019 of the AIDS Clinical Trials Group. *JAMA* 1994;272:437-42.

11. Hammer SM, Katzenstein DA, Hughes MD, *et al.* A trial comparing nucleoside monotherapy with combination therapy in HIV-infected adults with CD4 cell counts from 200 to 500 per cubic millimeter. *N Engl J Med* 1996;335:1081-90.

12. Mellors JW, Munoz A, Giorgi JV, *et al.* Plasma viral load and CD4+ lymphocytes as prognostic markers of HIV-1 infection. *Ann Intern Med* 1997;126:946-54.

13. Schuurman R, Nijhuis M, van Leeuwen R, et al. Rapid changes in human immunodeficiency virus type 1 RNA load and appearance of drug-resistant virus populations in persons treated with lamivudine (3TC). *J Infect Dis* 1995;171:1411-9.

14. Keulen W, Back NKT, van Wijk A, *et al.* Initial appearance of the 184IIe variant in lamivudine-treated patients is caused by the mutational bias of human immunodeficiency virus type 1 reverse transcriptase. *J Virol* 1997;71:3346-50.

15. CDC. Clinical update-impact of HIV protease inhibitors on the treatment of HIV-infected tuberculosis patients with rifampin. *MMWR* 1996;45:921-5.

16. Schacker T, Collier AC, Hughes J, *et al.* Clinical and epidemiologic features of primary HIV infection. *Ann Intern Med* 1996;125:257-64.

17. Kinloch-de Loës S, de Saussure P, Saurat J, Stalder H, Hirschel B, Perrin, LH. Symptomatic primary infection due to human immunodeficiency virus type 1: review of 31 cases. *Clin Infect Dis* 1993;17:59-65.

18. Tindall B, Cooper D. Primary HIV infection: host responses and intervention strategies. *AIDS* 1991;5:1-14.

19. Niu MJ, Stein D, Schnittman SM. Primary human immunodeficiency virus type 1 infection: review of pathogenesis and early treatment intervention in humans and animal retrovirus infections. *J Infect Dis* 1993;168:1490-501.

20. Lafeuillade A, Poggi C, Tamalet C, Profizi N, Tourres C, Costes O. Effects of a combination of zidovudine, didanosine, and lamivudine on primary human immunodeficiency virus type 1 infection. *J Infect Dis* 1997;175:1051-5.

21. CDC. Update: provisional public health service recommendations for chemoprophylaxis after occupational exposure to HIV. *MMWR* 1996;45:468-72.

22. Hoen B, Harzic M, Fleury HF, *et al.* ANRS053 trial of zidovudine (ZDV), lamivudine (3TC), and ritonavir combination in patients with symptomatic primary HIV-1 infection: preliminary results [Abstract 232]. In: *Program and abstracts of the 4th Conference on Retroviruses and Opportunistic Infections.* Washington, DC: January 22-26, 1997.

23. Tamalet C, Poizot Martin IP, Lafeuillade A, *et al.* Viral load and genotypic resistance pattern in HIV-1 infected patients treated by a triple combination therapy including nucleoside and protease inhibitors (NIs and PIs) initiated at primary infection

[Abstract 592]. In: *Program and abstracts of the 4th Conference on Retroviruses and Opportunistic Infections*. Washington, DC: January 22-26, 1997.

24. Perrin L, Markowitz M, Calandra G, Chung M, and the MRL Acute HIV Infection Study Group. An open treatment study of acute HIV infection with zidovudine, lamivudine and indinavir sulfate [Abstract 238]. In: *Program and abstracts of the 4th Conference on Retroviruses and Opportunistic Infections*. Washington, DC: January 22-26, 1997.

25. Minkoff H, Augenbraun M: Antiretroviral therapy for pregnant women. *Am J Obstet Gynecol* 1997; 176:478-89.

26. CDC. Pregnancy outcomes following systemic prenatal acyclovir exposure—June 1, 1984–June 30, 1993. *MMWR* 1993;42:806-9.

27. O'Sullivan MJ, Boyer PJJ, Scott GB, *et al.* The pharmacokinetics and safety of zidovudine in the third trimester of pregnancy for women infected with human immunodeficiency virus and their infants: Phase I Acquired Immunodeficiency Syndrome Clinical Trials Group study (protocol 082). *Am J Obstet Gynecol* 1993;168:1510-6.

28. Moodley J, Moodley D, Pillay K, et al: Antiviral effect of lamivudine alone and in combination with zidovudine in HIV-infected pregnant women [Abstract 607]. In: *Proceedings of the 4th Conference on Retroviruses and Opportunistic Infections*. Washington, DC: January 22-26, 1997.

29. Sandberg JA, Slikker W: Developmental pharmacology and toxicology of anti-HIV therapeutic agents: dideoxynucleosides. *FASEB J.* 1995;9:1157-63.

30. FDA Public Health Advisory: Reports of diabetes and hyperglycemia in patients receiving protease inhibitors for the treatment of human immunodeficiency virus (HIV). *JAMA* 1997;278:379.

31. CDC. Public Health Service Task Force recommendations for the use of antiretroviral drugs in pregnant women infected with HIV-1 for maternal health and for reducing perinatal HIV-1 transmission in the United States. *MMWR* 1998;47(RR-2).

32. Sperling RS, Shapiro DE, Coombs RW, *et al.* Maternal viral load, zidovudine treatment, and the risk of transmission of human immunodeficiency virus type 1 from mother to infant. *N Engl J Med* 1996;335:1621-9.

33. Eastman PS, Shapiro DE, Coombs RW, *et al*. Maternal genotypic zidovudine (ZDV) resistance and failure of ZDV therapy to prevent mother-child HIV-1 transmission [Abstract 516]. In: *Program and abstracts of the 4th Conference on Retroviruses and Opportunistic Infections*. Washington, DC: January 22-26, 1997.

34. Hammer SM, Squires KE, Hughes MD, *et al*. A controlled trial of two nucleoside analogues plus indinavir in persons with human immunodeficiency virus infection and CD4 cell counts of 200 per cubic millimeter or less. *N Engl J Med* 1997;337:725-33.

35. Gulick RM, Mellors JW, Havlir D, *et al*. Treatment with indinavir, zidovudine, and lamivudine in adults with human immunodeficiency virus infection and prior antiretroviral therapy. *N Engl J Med* 1997;337:734-9.

36. de Jong MD, Vella S, Carr A, *et al*. High-dose nevirapine in previously untreated human immunodeficiency virus type-1-infected persons does not result in sustained suppression of viral replication. *J Infect Dis* 1997;175:966-70.

37. Schapiro JM, Winters MA, Stewart F, *et al*. The effect of high-dose saquinavir on viral load and CD4+ T-cell counts in HIV-infected patients. *Ann Intern Med* 1996;124:1039-50.

38. Bartlett JG: Protease inhibitors for HIV infection. *Ann Intern Med* 1996;124:1086-8.

39. Eron JT, Benoit SL, Jemsek J, *et al*. Treatment with lamivudine, zidovudine, or both in HIV-positive patients with 200 to 500 CD4+ cells per cubic millimeter. *N Engl J Med* 1995; 333:1662-9.

40. Staszewski S, Loveday C, Picazo JJ, *et al*. Safety and efficacy of lamivudine-zidovudine combination therapy in zidovudine-experienced patients. *JAMA* 1996;276:111-7.

41. Dubé MP, Johnson DL, Currier JS, Leedom JM. Protease inhibitor-associated hyperglycaemia (letter). *Lancet* 1997;350:713-4.

42. Visnegarwala F, Krause KL, Musher DM. Severe diabetes associated with protease inhibitor therapy (letter). *Ann Intern Med* 1997;127:947.

43. Eastone JA, Decker CE New-onset diabetes mellitus associated with use of protease inhibitor (letter). *Ann Intern Med* 1997;127:948.

44. Hanson C, Cooper E, Antonelli T, et al: Lack of tumors in infants with perinatal HIV exposure and fetal/neonatal exposure to zidovudine (AZT) [Abstract 304.3]. In: *Proceedings of the National Conference on Women and HIV.* Pasadena, CA: May 4-7, 1997.

Chapter 24

HIV Protease Inhibitors and You

Introduction

This chapter will give you information about new drugs to treat HIV infection, called protease inhibitors. Since these are new medicines, you may have questions about how they work and what to expect when taking them. No book can answer all of your questions, or take the place of a doctor in helping you make the important decisions you are facing, but this information will help you understand the basics about HIV protease inhibitors.

The six Department of Health and Human Services agencies that co-sponsor the HIV/AIDS Treatment Information Service (ATIS) provided support for this text. (ATIS is co-sponsored by: Agency for Health Care Policy and Research, Centers for Disease Control and Prevention, Health Resources and Services Administration, Indian Health Service, National Institutes of Health, and Substance Abuse and Mental Health Services Administration.) ATIS is a free telephone reference service for people who need information about HIV and AIDS treatment. Reference specialists at ATIS answer questions and provide information on federally approved treatments for HIV and AIDS.

You can contact the HIV/AIDS Treatment Information Service at:

1-800-448-0440 (Voice)   1-800-243-7012 (TTY)
1-301-519-6616 (Fax)   www.hivatis.org (Web site)
atis@cdcnac.org (E-mail)

HIV/AIDS Treatment Information Service (ATIS), December 1997.

How do protease inhibitors work?

Protease inhibitors are antiviral drugs. They interrupt the way HIV uses a healthy cell to make more virus. When HIV enters a healthy cell, its only goal is to make more viruses to infect other healthy cells. It does this by making the cell produce certain proteins the virus can use to copy itself. Two of the proteins used by the virus are reverse transcriptase and protease. The goal of the protease inhibitor is to stop the protease from helping to assemble a new virus. Figure 24.1 shows the virus entering the cell (1), the cell making new proteins (2-3), the proteins forming a new virus (4), and the cell releasing the new virus to infect other cells (5). It also shows some steps in the process that can be interrupted by protease inhibitors and other antiviral drugs (reverse transcriptase inhibitors) that are taken along with protease inhibitors.

What can protease inhibitors do?

Protease inhibitors are the most powerful anti-HIV drugs available so far. Although many different factors affect how well any drug

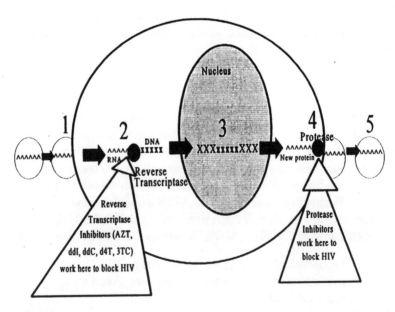

Figure 24.1.

will work for an individual, some people who have taken protease inhibitors have had the following benefits:

* increase in CD4 (t cell) counts, which can help fight infections
* decrease in the amount of virus in the blood (viral load), which may slow down the disease process
* feeling of improved overall health and ability to do more of their usual activities (i.e., work, travel, socialize)

Researchers are not sure how long protease inhibitors will work in a person infected with HIV, but they have seen promising results in studies. They are hopeful that people will live longer, healthier lives because of the benefits of these new drugs.

Is this a cure?

Protease inhibitors are not called a cure because researchers do not yet know how well they will work in different people. Some people have had their viral load drop to a level that is too low for current tests to measure. Even though the virus cannot be found in their blood, doctors believe HIV is still in their bodies and that it would reproduce quickly if they stop taking the protease inhibitor. In other people, protease inhibitors may not work as well or the benefits might not last. Clinical trials are going on to help answer questions about where HIV "hides" and why people have different results with protease inhibitors.

Which protease inhibitor will I take?

There are five approved HIV protease inhibitors: *ritonavir* (Norvir) and *nelfinavir* (Viracept) are for use by adults and children, while *indinavir* (Crixivan) and the two forms of *saquinavir* (Invirase and Fortovase) are approved for adults only. Invirase was approved in 1995, and Fortovase, a new, stronger form of *saquinavir*, was approved in 1997. The company that makes both drugs will continue to make Invirase available to people who already take that form of *saquinavir* through Spring 1998. After that, it will be available to them under a limited distribution program. A decision about which drug to take should be made with a doctor who knows your individual condition, and has medical knowledge of HIV disease. By finding out about the available treatment options, you can talk to your doctor about the risks and benefits of different drug combinations.

Will I need other medications?

If you take *saquinavir* (Invirase or Fortovase) you will also need to take one or two other antiviral medications, called reverse transcriptase inhibitors. Reverse transcriptase inhibitors such as *AZT* (Retrovir), *ddI* (Videx), *ddC* (Hivid), *d4T* (Zerit), or *3TC* (Epivir) are antiviral drugs that block HIV at a different point in its life cycle than protease inhibitors (see Figure 24.1). Although *indinavir* (Crixivan), *ritonavir* (Norvir), and *nelfinavir* (Viracept) may be taken by themselves, most doctors will also prescribe one or two reverse transcriptase inhibitors along with the protease inhibitor. Research shows that combining two or more antiviral drugs is more effective than taking one drug alone. The HIV/AIDS Treatment Information Service can give you information on all of these anti-HIV drugs.

How often will I take my protease inhibitor? For how long?

Each of the approved protease inhibitors is taken in a different way. You may take your protease inhibitor two or three times every day, depending on which one you take. It is important to take the protease inhibitor on schedule so the drug will stay at the same level in your body. **Taking a "drug holiday" or skipping doses is dangerous.** Missing one or more doses can allow the virus to become resistant, meaning the virus changes itself to avoid the medication and keep making copies of itself.

You should take the protease inhibitor for as long as your tests show it is helpful; your doctor will keep track of your progress based on blood tests that you will have on a regular basis.

How will I take my protease inhibitor?

You will take the protease inhibitor orally (by mouth). Whichever protease inhibitor you take, it is important to set a medication routine and stick to it. Some medications work best if taken on an empty stomach, while others must be taken with food, or with a large amount of water. Your doctor or pharmacist should give you specific instructions for taking your medication. The charts on the following pages have information about dosage and special instructions for each of the approved protease inhibitors.

NELFINAVIR (VIRACEPT) DOSAGE INFORMATION FOR CHILDREN	
Body Weight	**Dosage**
15.5 lb to <18.5 lb	4 scoops or 1 teaspoon
18.5 lb to <23 lb	5 scoops or 1¼ teaspoons
23 lb to <26.5 lb	6 scoops or 1½ teaspoons
26.5 lb to <31 lb	7 scoops or 1¾ teaspoons
31 lb to <35 lb	8 scoops or 2 teaspoons
35 lb to <39.5 lb	9 scoops or 2¼ teaspoons
39.5 lb to <50.5 lb	10 scoops or 2½ teaspoons
≥50.5 lb	15 scoops or 3¾ teaspoons

RITONAVIR (NORVIR) DOSAGE INFORMATION FOR CHILDREN	
Body Surface Area [1]	**Liquid Dosage**
0.25 m²	1.25 mL
0.50 m²	2.5 mL
1.00 m²	5 mL
1.25 m²	6.25 mL
1.50 m²	7.5 mL

[1] — *Calculated with the following equation:*

$$bsa(m^2) = \sqrt{(Ht[cm] x Wt[kg])/3600}$$

PROTEASE INHIBITOR	ADULT DOSAGE	SPECIAL INSTRUCTIONS
nelfinavir [1,2,3] (Viracept)	3 tablets, 3 times a day *(9 total tablets each day)*	Take with a meal or a snack Keep at room temperature
saquinavir[4] (Fortovase)	6 capsules, 3 times a day *(18 total capsules each day)*	Take within 2 hours of a full meal Keep refrigerated until the expiration date printed on the label. If capsules reach room temperature, they should be used within 3 months
saquinavir[4] (Invirase)	3 capsules, 3 times a day *(9 total capsules each day)*	Take within 2 hours of a full meal Keep at room temperature
indinavir (Crixivan)	2 capsules, 3 times a day *(6 total capsules each day)*	Take on an empty stomach 1 hour before or 2 hours after a meal *Drink at least 1½ liters of liquid every day* Keep at room temperature in original bottle

PROTEASE INHIBITOR	ADULT DOSAGE	SPECIAL INSTRUCTIONS
ritonavir[3] (Norvir)	6 capsules, 2 times a day *(12 total capsules each day)* **OR** 7.5 mL liquid, 2 times a day	Take with meals Keep refrigerated

[1]—*Phenylketonurics: Viracept oral powder contains 11.2 mg phenylalanine per gram.*

[2]—*Persons with hemophilia should be monitored for increased bleeding.*

[3]—*Interferes with effectiveness of birth control pills; a different method or backup should be used.*

[4]—*The two forms of saquinavir (Invirase and Fortovase) require different doses and handling. Please refer to the appropriate instructions for each drug.*

Remember that you may be taking other antiviral drugs with the protease inhibitor. Planning when to take several different medications can be tricky, so review the instructions carefully and ask for some help from your doctor or pharmacist if you have trouble staying on schedule.

Are there medications I should not take with protease inhibitors?

Some drugs can cause problems (interactions) when they are taken together. Interactions might make your drugs less effective, or they could make you sick. Even some of the drugs that you might be taking to treat an infection or to keep you from getting an opportunistic illness (prophylaxis) should not be taken with a protease inhibitor. Your doctor may say that taking those drugs together is contraindicated. For example, rifamycin drugs (rifampin and rifabutin) which are used to treat TB (tuberculosis) or MAC (Mycobacterium avium complex) can interact with protease inhibitors. In this interaction, the rifamycin makes the protease inhibitor less effective, and the protease inhibitor increases the chances of rifamycin side effects.

If you have HIV and you also have either TB or MAC, you should talk to you doctor about these options:

- stopping the protease inhibitor during treatment including rifampin and other anti-TB/anti-MAC drugs;

- stopping the protease inhibitor during treatment including rifampin and other anti-TB/anti-MAC drugs, then stopping the rifampin, but continuing the other anti-TB/anti-MAC drugs and the protease inhibitor;

- taking the anti-TB/anti-MAC treatment with rifabutin instead of rifampin (**only** if the protease inhibitor is *indinavir* (Crixivan);

- taking one-half the usual dose of rifabutin (**only** if the protease inhibitor is *nelfinavir* (Viracept).

Also, if you have not yet started a protease inhibitor, the recommendation is to finish treatment with rifampin and other anti-TB/anti-MAC drugs before starting the protease inhibitor.

Check the tables at the end of this chapter to make sure you are not taking drugs together that are contraindicated. **Be sure to talk to your doctor before stopping or starting any drug.** Usually, your doctor can prescribe a different drug that will help you avoid an illness or treat a symptom.

How will I know if my protease inhibitor is working?

Your doctor will schedule you for checkups to monitor your blood tests and see how well your treatment plan is working. Some of the tests might include a CD4+ (T cell) count and a test to measure the amount of HIV in your blood (viral load) so that your doctor can tell if the medication is working against the virus. You may also have tests to check how well your liver and kidneys are working, and other measures of your overall health.

Will I have side effects?

People react to medications in different ways. Some people have mild effects or no symptoms at all, while others may have many side effects or severe symptoms. Even when side effects occur, they can be temporary, or get better over time.

Some of the common side effects are listed on the following pages, but please remember that you may have only some of these or none at all.

Abdominal Pain

Some medicines can cause pain or discomfort in your abdomen (belly). If you have severe pain, if the pain is also in your back, or if your skin or eyes look yellow (jaundiced) let your doctor know.

Bleeding Problems

Some people with hemophilia type A or B have reported increased bleeding problems. It is not known whether this is related to protease inhibitors, but these problems should be reported to the doctor immediately so they can be treated.

Blood Sugar Problems

Some people taking protease inhibitors have had problems with their blood sugar levels, or have developed diabetes. Symptoms such as increased thirst, hunger, urination or weight loss should be reported to the doctor immediately.

People with diabetes who are considering protease inhibitor therapy should talk with their doctors about carefully monitoring their glucose (blood sugar) level.

Diarrhea

Medications may cause you to have diarrhea (loose bowel movements). If you have severe cramping, or the problem lasts more than a day, call your doctor to ask about medicines that might help.

Fatigue

You may have less energy or feel tired more often. This may be the result of the drug reducing the number of red blood cells in your body, which carry oxygen to your tissues and organs. A condition called anemia can occur if there are not enough red blood cells to carry oxygen throughout your body. Let your doctor know if you become dizzy or short of breath. Some of your blood tests will also let the doctor know if the drug is causing anemia.

Headache

If you get severe or long-lasting headaches, ask your doctor which pain reliever you can take to help relieve them.

Kidney/Bladder Problems

This can especially be a problem if you are taking *indinavir* (Crixivan). Making sure you drink enough liquids can help avoid some kidney or bladder effects. You should watch for signs that might signal a problem, such as:

- urinating, or feeling that you need to, more than usual
- pain or burning feeling when you urinate
- blood or reddish color in urine
- fever or chills
- pain in the back or side

Mouth Problems

Some medications may cause mouth ulcers or sores. If it becomes difficult to eat or brush your teeth, or if you think you have signs of an infection, such as dark red or white patches, you should call your doctor.

Nausea/Vomiting

There may be occasional nausea or vomiting after taking medication, or it may be severe or long-lasting. If you vomit for more than a day, or have trouble keeping down liquids, call your doctor.

Numbness/Tingling Sensations

Some common areas that can feel numb or tingle are the fingers/ hands, toes/feet and around the mouth. You may also feel some pain in these areas. Your doctor may call it neuropathy. Call your doctor if you have these side effects. Sometimes they get better with time, but they may get worse and may last even after you stop taking the medication.

Your doctor can help you decide how to handle these side effects.

Skin Problems

You may have a rash or dry, itchy skin with some drugs. If your skin breaks out in hives or if you have sudden or intense itching, it may mean you are allergic to a drug. Call your doctor immediately to get treatment.

You should also ask your doctor or pharmacist if your medicine can make you more sensitive to sunlight, since you may sunburn more easily.

Taste Changes

Medication can sometimes leave a taste in your mouth, or make foods or liquids taste odd. You may need to try different foods, or vary your diet if you find that things taste unpleasant.

How long do side effects last?

Sometimes side effects get worse over time, and other times they get better as your body adjusts to the medication. Any side effects should be reported to your doctor right away, especially if they are sudden, severe or seem to be getting worse. Your doctor may know ways to help ease the problem, or may suggest a change in treatment if it is too bad.

Side effects will often go away after you stop taking a drug, but sometimes they can be long lasting or even permanent after stopping the drug. Also, since protease inhibitors are fairly new, there may be delayed effects that are not yet known.

People taking medications for HIV may get discouraged if they feel sicker after they start a drug treatment than they did before. They may feel that the quality of their life was better before starting their drug.

Talk to your doctor if you feel this way so you can make an informed decision about your treatment. Many experts recommend treating HIV early, before symptoms start to make you feel sick. Your doctor may suggest that you stay on the drug for a certain length of time to see if the side effects improve.

Side effects are a risk of taking any drug that you must weigh against possible benefits.

What if I still have questions?

You will want to talk about your options with your doctor or other health care provider. It is important to get all of the information you need to make you feel comfortable with your decisions about medical treatment.

Talking to a family member, a friend or a support group might also help in making a decision about treatment. They can help you think of questions to ask your doctor.

Also, reference specialists at the HIV/AIDS Treatment Information Service may be able to answer some of your questions. You can call Monday through Friday from 9 a.m. to 7 p.m. Eastern time at 1-800-448-0440.

If you have specific questions about one of the protease inhibitors, you may want to call the company that makes the drug, listed below:

Crixivan (*indinavir sulfate*)
approved for marketing by FDA: 3/14/96
Merck Research Laboratories
1-800-379-1332

Fortovase & Invirase (*saquinavir mesylate*)
Fortovase approved for marketing by FDA: 11/7/97
lnvirase approved for marketing by FDA: 12/7/95
Hoffmann-LaRoche Incorporated
1-800-526-6367

Norvir (*ritonavir*)
approved for marketing by FDA: 3/1/96 (adults), 3/14/97 (children)
Abbott Laboratories
1-800-441-4987

Viracept (*nelfinavir*)
approved for marketing by FDA: 3/14/97 (adults and children)
Agouron Pharmaceuticals
1-888-847-2237

Medications That Should Not Be Used with:

Medications That Should Not Be Used with Saquinavir *(Invirase, Fortovase)*

DRUG CATEGORY	POTENTIAL ALTERNATIVES
Antimycobacterial (anti-TB or anti-MAC): rifampin (Rifadin, others) rifabutin	azithromycin (Zithromax) ethambutol (Myambutol)
Sedative/hypnotic: midazolam (Versed) triazolam (Halcion)	very limited clinical experience
Ergot deriavatives (anti-migraine)	very limited clinical experience
Cold and allergy antihistamines: astemizole (Hismanal), terfenadine (Seldane)	loratadine (Claritin)
Gastrointestinal: cisapride (Propulsid)	very limited clinical experience

Medications That Should Not Be Used with Indinavir *(Crixivan),* Nelfinavir *(Viracept)*

DRUG CATEGORY	POTENTIAL ALTERNATIVES
Antimycobacterial (Anti-TB or anti-MAC): rifampin (Rifadin, others)	clarithromycin (Biaxin) azithromycin (Zithromax) ethambutol (Myambutol)
Cold and allergy antihistamines: astemizole (Hismanal), terfenadine (Seldane)	loratadine (Claritin)
Gastrointestinal: cisapride (Propulsid)	very limited clinical experience
Sedative/hypnotic	midazolam (Versed) triazolam (Halcion)

249

Medications That Should Not Be Used with Ritonavir *(Norvir)*
(Continued on next page.)

DRUG CATEGORY	POTENTIAL ALTERNATIVES
Analgesic (pain reliever): meperidine (Demerol) piroxicam (Feldene) propoxyphene (Darvon, others)	acetaminophen (Tylenol, others) aspirin (Bayer, others) oxycodone (Percocet, others)
Cardiovascular (for the heart): amiodarone (Cordarone) flecainide (Tambocor) propafenone (Rythmol) quinidine (various)	very limited clinical experience
Antimycobacterial (Anti-TB or anti-MAC): rifabutin (Mycobutin)	clarithromycin (Biaxin) azithromycin (Zithromax) ethambutol (Myambutol)
Calcium Channel Blocker (for the heart): bepridil (Vascor)	very limited clinical experience
Ergot Alkaloid (vasoconstrictor): dihydroergotamine (D.H.E. 45) Ergotamine (various)	
Cold and allergy antihistamines: astemizole (Hismanal), terfenadine (Seldane)	loratadine (Claritin)

Medications That Should Not Be Used with Ritonavir *(Norvir)*
(Continued from previous page.)

DRUG CATEGORY	POTENTIAL ALTERNATIVES
Gastrointestinal: cisapride (Propulsid)	very limited clinical experience
Psychotropic (antidepressant): bupropion (Wellbutrin)	fluoxetine (Prozac) desipramine (Norpramin)
Psychotropic (neuroleptic): clozapine (Clozaril) pimozide (Orap)	very limited clinical experience
Sedative/hypnotic: alprazolam (Xanax) clorazepate (Tranxene) diazepam (Valium) estazolam (ProSom) flurazepam (Dalmane) midazolam (Versed) triazolam (Halcion) zolpidem (Ambien)	Temazepam (Restoril) Lorazepam (Ativan)

— Please note that alternatives may not be therapeutically equivalent
References: Product Labeling
Invirase™ (December 6, 1995)
Norvir™ (March 1, 1996)
Drug Interactions: *Physician Guide*
Crixivan™ (March 13, 1996)
Fortovase™ (November 7, 1997)

Drugs That May Interact with:

Drugs That May Interact with Ritonavir *(Norvir). The following is a list of medications that may potentially interact with ritonavir therapy.* (Continued on next page.)

DRUG CATEGORY	DRUGS THAT MAY INTERACT
Analgesics, Narcotics (pain relievers)	alfentanil (Alfenta) fentanyl (Sublimaze)
Antiarrhythmics (for the heart)	disopyramide (Norpace) lidocaine (Xylocaine, others)
Anticoagulants (for the blood)	R-warfarin (Coumadin)
Anticonvulsants	carbamazepine (Tegretol) clonazepam (Klonopin) ethosuximide (Zarontin)
Antidepressants, other	nefazodone (Serzone) sertraline (Zoloft) trazodone (Desyrel)
Antiemetics	dronabinol (Marinol) ondansetron (Zofran)
Antihistamine	loratadine (Claritin)
Anti-HIV protease inhibitors	nelfinavir (Viracept)
Antimycobacterial (anti-TB or anti-MAC)	rifampin (Rifadin, others)
Antiparasitics	quinidine (various)

***Drugs That May Interact with* Ritonavir *(Norvir).** The following is a list of medications that may potentially interact with ritonavir therapy.* (Continued from previous page.)

DRUG CATEGORY	DRUGS THAT MAY INTERACT
Calcium Channel Blockers	amlodipine (Norvasc) diltiazem (Cardizem, Diltiazem) felodipine (Plendil) isradipine (DynaCirc) nicardipine (Cardene) nifedipine (Adalat, Procardia) nimodipine (Nimotop) nisoldipine (Sular) verapamil (Calan, Isoptin)
Cancer chemotherapeutic agents	etoposide (VePesid) paclitaxel (Taxol) tamoxifen (Nolvadex, others) vinblastine (Velban) vincristine (Oncovin)
Corticosteriods	dexamethasone (Decadron, others) prednisone (various)
Hypolipidemics	lovastatin (Mevacor) pravastatin (Pravachol)
Immunosuppressants	cyclosporine (Sandimmune, Neoral) tacrolimus (Prograf)

References: Norvir™ Prescribing information (March 1, 1996)

Drugs That May Interact with Nelfinavir *(Viracept).* *The following is a list of medications that may potentially interact with nelfinavir therapy.*

DRUG CATEGORY	DRUGS THAT MAY INTERACT
Anticonvulsants	carbamazepine (Tegretol) phenobarbital phenytoin (Dilantin)
Anti-HIV protease inhibitors	indinavir (Crixivan) ritonavir (Norvir)
Oral contraceptives (birth control pills)	ethinyl estradiol norethindrone

References: Viracept® Prescribing information,
(March 14, 1997)

Chapter 25

Protease Inhibitors and Risks Associated with Diabetes and Hyperglycemia

Reports of Diabetes and Hyperglycemia in Patients Receiving Protease Inhibitors

The Food and Drug Administration would like to call to your attention recent post marketing reports of new onset diabetes mellitus, hyperglycemia or exacerbation of existing diabetes mellitus occurring in HIV-infected patients receiving protease inhibitor therapy. At the present time there exists no conclusive evidence establishing a definite causal relationship between protease inhibitor therapy and the incidence of diabetes and hyperglycemia. Based on present reporting, we believe the occurrence of this event is relatively infrequent. As such, patients for whom these products are indicated should not discontinue therapy without consulting their health care professional. However, given the potential seriousness of this complication, we believe that patients and health care professionals should be notified of this information.

Summary of Reports

- As of May 12, 1997, there have been 83 cases reported to FDA of diabetes mellitus or hyperglycemia in HIV-infected patients who were receiving anti-retroviral protease inhibitor therapy; 27of the 83 cases were reported to require hospitalization. Fourteen

U.S. Food and Drug Administration (FDA) Public Health Advisory, January 1998.

patients were known to be diabetic at baseline; for these patients, there was a loss of glucose control. The average time of onset was approximately 76 days after initiating protease inhibitor therapy, but occurred as early as four days after starting therapy. Five cases of diabetic ketoacidosis occurred, including patients who were not reported to be diabetic at baseline; however, the baseline status of these patients is not well characterized.

- Some patients required either initiation or dose adjustments of insulin or oral hypoglycemic agents for the treatment of these events. On an average, fifty percent of patients discontinued their protease inhibitor therapy as a result of this acute adverse event. Hyperglycemia persisted in some patients after protease inhibitor therapy was withdrawn including patients not known to be diabetic at baseline; however a causal relationship between protease inhibitor therapy and these events has not been established.

- Many of these reports occurred in patients with confounding medical conditions, some of which required therapy with agents that have been associated with the development of diabetes mellitus or hyperglycemia.

- Diabetes and hyperglycemia have been reported to varying degrees for Crixivan® (indinavir), Invirase® (saquinavir), Norvir® (ritonavir) and Viracept® (nelfinavir).

The FDA will continue close monitoring for additional events. We encourage all health care professionals to report any cases of diabetes or hyperglycemia, or any other serious toxicity associated with the use of protease inhibitors, to the FDA's MEDWATCH program at 1-800-FDA-1088/fax 1-800-FDA-0178; or to the respective pharmaceutical manufacturers:

- Crixivan® (indinavir), Merck Research Laboratories, 1-800-672-6372

- Invirase® (saquinavir), Hoffman-La Roche, 1-800-526-6367

- Norvir® (ritonavir), Abbott Laboratories, 1-800-633-9110

- Viracept® (nelfinavir), Agouron Pharmaceuticals, 1-888-847-2237

Chapter 26

Caring for Someone with AIDS at Home

Introduction

One of the best places for people with AIDS to be cared for is at home, surrounded by the people who love them. Many people living with AIDS can lead an active life for long periods of time. Most of the time, people with AIDS do not need to be in a hospital. Being at home is often cheaper, more comfortable, more familiar, and gives them more control of their life. In fact, people with AIDS-related illnesses often get better faster and with less discomfort at home with the help of their friends and loved ones.

If you are caring for someone with AIDS at home, remember that each person living with AIDS is different and is affected by HIV, the virus that causes AIDS, in different ways. You should get regular updates from the person's doctor or nurse on what kind of care is needed. Many times what is needed is not medical care, but help with the normal chores of life: shopping, getting the mail, paying bills, cleaning the house, and so on.

Also remember that AIDS causes stress on both the person who is sick and on you as you care for them. Caring for someone with AIDS is a serious responsibility. You will have to work with the person with AIDS to decide what needs to be done, how much you can do, and when additional help is needed. But, by rising to the challenges of caring for someone with HIV infection and AIDS, you can share emotionally

American Red Cross and America Responds to AIDS, HIV/DHAP/9-95-05D, CDC NAC Inventory number D817, 1995; reprinted with permission.

satisfying experiences, even joy, with those you love. You can also find new strengths within yourself. But you need to take care of yourself as well as the person with AIDS.

How to Get Ready to Take Care of Someone at Home

Every situation is different, but here are some tips to get you started.

First, read this guide. Have the person living with HIV or AIDS read it. Have other people living in the same house as the person with AIDS read it. The information in this chapter is for both people with diagnosed AIDS and people with HIV infection who are sick and need care.

Take a home care course, if possible. Learn the skills you need to take care of someone at home and how to manage special situations. Your local Red Cross chapter, Visiting Nurses Association, State health department, or HIV/AIDS service organization can help you find a home care course. See the "Places To Call For Help" section at the end of this chapter or consult "Additional Help and Information" at the end of this book.

Talk with the person you will be caring for. Ask them what they need. If you are nervous about caring for them, say so. Ask if it is OK for you to talk to their doctor, nurse, social worker, case manager, other heath care professional or lawyer when you need to. Together you can work out what is best for both of you.

Talk with the doctor, nurse, social worker, case manager, and other health care workers who are also providing care. They may need the patient's permission, sometimes in writing, to talk to you, but you need to talk to these people to find out how you can help. Work with them and the person you are caring for to develop a plan for who does what.

- Get clear, written information about medicines and other care you'll give. Ask what each drug does and what side effects to look out for.

- Ask the doctor or nurse what changes in the person's health or behavior to watch for. For example, a cough, fever, diarrhea, or confusion may mean an infection or problem that needs a new medicine or even putting the person in the hospital.

- You also need to know whom to call for help or information and when to call them. Make a list of doctors, nurses, and other people you might need to talk to quickly, their phone numbers, and when they are available. Keep this list by the phone.

Talk to a lawyer or AIDS support organization. For some medical care or life support decisions, you may need to be legally named as the care coordinator. If you are going to help file insurance claims, apply for government aid, pay bills, or handle other businesses for the person with AIDS, you may also need a power of attorney. There are many sources of help for people with AIDS, and you can help the person with AIDS get what they are entitled to.

Think about joining a support group or talking to a counselor. Taking care of someone who is sick can be hard emotionally as well as physically. Talking about it with people with the same kind of worries helps sometimes. You can learn how other people cope and realize that you are not alone.

Take care of yourself. You can't take care of someone else if you are sick or upset. Get the rest and exercise you need to keep going. You also need to do some things you enjoy, such as visit your friends and relatives. Many AIDS service organizations can help with "respite care" and send someone to be with the person you're caring for while you get out of the house awhile.

What You Need to Know about HIV and AIDS

If you are going to be caring for someone with HIV infection, you need to understand the basic facts about HIV and AIDS. AIDS (acquired immunodeficiency syndrome) is caused by HIV (human immunodeficiency virus). People who are infected with HIV can look and feel healthy and may not know for years that they are infected. However, they can infect other people no matter how healthy they seem. HIV slowly wipes out parts of the body's immune system; then the HIV-infected person gets sick because the body can't fight off diseases. Some of these diseases can kill them.

Signs of HIV infection are like those of many other common illnesses, such as swollen glands, tiring easily, losing weight, fever, or diarrhea. Different people have different symptoms.

IIIV is in people's blood, semen, vaginal fluid, and breast milk. The only way to tell if someone is infected with HIV is with a blood test.

259

There is no vaccine to prevent HIV infection and no cure for AIDS. There are treatments that can keep infected people healthy longer and prevent some diseases that people with AIDS often get. Research is ongoing.

HIV slowly makes an infected person sicker and sicker. Diseases and infections will cause serious illness, but people often get better— until the next illness. Sometimes, HIV can damage the brain and cause changes in feelings and moods, even make it hard to think clearly. Someone with AIDS can feel fine in the morning and be very sick in the afternoon. It can seem like riding a roller coaster, slowly climbing up to feeling good, then plunging down into another illness.

How HIV Is Spread

The most common ways HIV is spread are:

- By having unprotected anal, vaginal, or oral sex with someone who is infected with HIV

- By sharing needles or syringes ("works") with someone who is infected with HIV

- From mothers to their babies before the baby is born, during birth, or through breast-feeding. Taking the drug AZT during pregnancy and birth can reduce the chances of infecting the baby by two-thirds, but will not prevent all babies from becoming infected with HIV.

Earlier in the AIDS epidemic some people became infected through blood transfusions, blood products (such as clotting factors given to people with hemophilia), or organ or tissue transplants. This has been very rare in the United States since 1985, when the test for HIV was licensed. Since then, all donated blood and donors of organs or tissue are tested for HIV.

Health care workers, such as nurses, risk getting infected if they are stuck with a needle containing infected blood or splashed with infected blood in the eyes, nose, mouth, or on open cuts or sores. In a few cases, a person sharing a house with a person with HIV infection or taking care of a person with AIDS has become infected themselves. These infections may have been caused by sharing a razor, getting blood from the infected person into open cuts or sores, or some other way of having contact with blood from the infected person. If you are taking care of a person with HIV infection, carefully follow the steps on protecting yourself from infection discussed later in this chapter.

How HIV Is _Not_ Spread

You don't get HIV from the air, food, water, insects, animals, dishes, knives, forks, spoons, toilet seats, or anything else that doesn't involve blood, semen, vaginal fluids, or breast milk. You don't get HIV from feces, nasal fluid, saliva, sweat, tears, urine, or vomit, unless these have blood mixed in them. You can help people with HIV eat, dress, even bathe, without becoming infected yourself, as long as you follow the steps described in the section on "Protecting Yourself" later in this chapter. You do get other germs from many of the things listed above, so do use common sense.

Giving Care

People living with AIDS should take care of themselves as much as they can for as long as they can. They need to be and feel as independent as possible. They need to control their own schedules, make their own decisions, and do what they want to do as much as they are able. They should develop their own exercise program and eating plan. In addition to regular visits to the doctor, many people with AIDS work at staying healthy by eating properly, sleeping regularly, doing physical exercises, praying or meditating, or other things. If the person you are caring for finds something that helps them, encourage them to keep it up. An exercise program can help maintain weight and muscle tone and can make a person feel better if it is tailored to what the person can do. Well-balanced, good-tasting meals help people feel good, give them energy, and help their body fight illness. People with HIV infection are better off if they don't drink alcoholic drinks, smoke, or use illegal drugs. Keeping up-to-date on new treatments and understanding what to expect from treatments the person is taking are also important.

There are some simple things you can do to help someone with AIDS feel comfortable at home.

- Respect their independence and privacy.

- Give them control as much as possible. Ask to enter their room, ask permission to sit with them, etc. Saying "Can I help you with that?" lets them keep control.

- Ask them what you can do to make them comfortable. Many people feel shy about asking for help, especially help with things like using the toilet, bathing, shaving, eating, and dressing.

- Keep the home clean and looking bright and cheerful.

- Let the person with AIDS stay in a room that is near a bathroom.

- Leave tissues, towels, a trash basket, extra blankets and other things the person might need close by so these things can be reached from the bed or chair.

If the person you are caring for has to spend most of their time in bed, be sure to help them change position often. If possible, a person with AIDS should get out of bed as often as they can. A nurse can show you how to help someone move from a bed to a chair without hurting yourself or them. This helps prevent stiff joints, bedsores, and some kinds of pneumonia. They may also need your help to turn over or to adjust the pillows or blankets. A medical "trapeze" over the bed can help the person shift position by themselves if they are strong enough. If they are so weak they can't turn over, have a nurse show you how to use a sheet to help roll the person in bed from side to side. Usually a person in bed needs to change position at least every 4 hours.

Bedsores

Bedsores or other broken skin can be serious problems for someone with AIDS. In addition to changing position in bed often, to help keep skin healthy, put extra-soft material (sheepskin, "egg crate" foam, or water mattresses) under the person, keep the sheets dry and free from wrinkles, and massage the back and other parts of the body (like hips, elbows, and ankles) that press down on the bed. Report any red or broken areas on the skin to the doctor or nurse right away.

Exercises

Even in bed, a person can do simple arm, hand, leg, and foot exercises. These are usually called "range of motion" exercises. These exercises help prevent stiff, sore joints and help keep the blood moving. A doctor, nurse, or physical therapist can show you how to help.

Breathing

If someone is having trouble breathing, sitting them up may help. Raise the head of a hospital-type bed or use extra pillows or some other soft back support. If they have severe trouble breathing, they need to see a doctor.

Comfort

A good back rub can help a person relax as well as help their circulation. A nurse, physical therapist, or book on massage can give you some tips on how to give a good back rub. Put books, remote controls, water, tissues, and a bell to call for help within easy reach. If the person can't get up, put a urinal or bedpan within easy reach.

Providing Emotional Support

You are caring for a person, not just a body; their feelings are important too. Since every person is different, there are no rules about what to do or say, but here are some ideas that may help.

* Keep them involved in their care. Don't do everything for them or make all their decisions. Nobody likes feeling helpless.

* Have them help out around the house if they can. Everybody likes to feel useful. They want to be part of the group, contributing what they can.

* Include them in the household. Make them part of normal talk about books, TV shows, music, what is going on in the world, and so on. Many people will want to feel involved in the things that are happening around them. But you don't always have to talk, just being there is sometimes enough. Just watching TV together or sitting and reading in the same room is often comforting.

* Talk about things. Sometimes they may need to talk about AIDS or talk through their own situation as a way to think out loud. Having AIDS can make a person angry, frustrated, depressed, scared, and lonely, just like any other serious illness. Listening, trying to understand, showing you care, and helping them work through their emotions is a big part of home care. A support group of other people with AIDS can also be a good place for them to talk things out. Contact the National Association of People With AIDS for information about support groups in your area. If they want professional counseling, help them get it.

* Invite their friends over to visit. A little socializing can be good for everyone.

* Touch them. Hug them, kiss them, pat them, hold their hands to show that you care. Some people may not want physical closeness, but if they do, touch is a powerful way of saying you care.

- Get out together. If they are able, go to social events, shopping, riding around, walking around the block, or just into the park, yard, or porch to sit in the sun and breathe fresh air.

Guarding Against Infections

People living with AIDS can get very sick from common germs and infections. Hugging, holding hands, giving massages, and many other types of touching are safe for you, and needed by the person with AIDS. But you have to be careful not to spread germs that can hurt the person you are caring for.

Wash Your Hands

Washing your hands is the single best way to kill germs. Do it often! Wash your hands after you go to the bathroom and before you fix food. Wash your hands again before and after feeding them, bathing them, helping them go to the bathroom, or giving other care. Wash your hands if you sneeze or cough; touch your nose, mouth, or genitals; handle garbage or animal litter; or clean the house. If you touch anybody's blood, semen, urine, vaginal fluid, or feces, wash your hands immediately. If you are caring for more than one person, wash your hands after helping one person and before helping the next person. Wash your hands with warm, soapy water for at least 15 seconds. Clean under your fingernails and between your fingers. If your hands get dry or sore, put on hand cream or lotion, but keep washing your hands frequently.

Cover Your Sores

If you have any cuts or sores, especially on your hands, you must take extra care not to infect the person with AIDS or yourself. If you have cold sores, fever blisters, or any other skin infection, don't touch the person or their things. You could pass your infection to them. If you have to give care, cover your sores with bandages and wash your hands before touching the person. If the rash or sores are on your hands, wear disposable gloves. Do not use gloves more than one time; throw them away and get a new pair. If you have boils, impetigo, or shingles, if at all possible, stay away from the person with AIDS until you are well.

Keep Sick People Away

If you or anybody else is sick, stay away from the person with AIDS until you're well. A person with AIDS often can't fight off colds, flu, or other common illnesses. If you are sick and nobody else can do what needs to be done for the person with AIDS, wear a well-fitting, surgical-type mask that covers your mouth and nose and wash your hands before coming near the person with AIDS.

Watch Out for Chickenpox

Chickenpox can kill a person with AIDS. If the person you are caring for has already had chickenpox, they probably won't get it again. But, just to be on the safe side:

- Never let anybody with chickenpox in the same room as a person with AIDS, at least not until all the chickenpox sores have completely crusted over.

- Don't let anybody who recently has been near somebody with chickenpox in the same room with a person who has AIDS. After 3 weeks, the person who was exposed to chickenpox can visit, if they aren't sick. Most adults have had chickenpox, but you have to be very careful about children visiting or living in the house if they have not yet had chickenpox. If you are the person who was near somebody with chickenpox and you have to help the person with AIDS, wear a well-fitting, surgical-type mask, wash your hands before doing what you have to do for the person with AIDS, and stay in the room as short a time as you can. Tell the person with AIDS why you are staying away from them.

- Don't let anybody with shingles (herpes zoster) near a person with AIDS until all the shingles have healed over. The germ that causes shingles can also cause chickenpox. If you have shingles and have to help the person with AIDS, cover all the sores completely and wash your hands carefully before helping the person with AIDS.

- Call the doctor as soon as possible if the person with AIDS does get near somebody with chickenpox or shingles. There is a medicine that can make the chickenpox less dangerous, but it must be given very soon after the person has been around someone with the germ.

Get Your Shots

Everybody living with or helping take care of a person with AIDS should make sure they took all their "childhood" shots (immunizations). This is not only to keep you from getting sick, but also to keep you from getting sick and accidentally spreading the illness to the person with AIDS. Just to be sure, ask your doctor if you need any shots or boosters for measles, mumps, or rubella since these shots may not have been available when you were a child. Discuss any vaccinations with your doctor and the doctor of the person with AIDS before you get the shot. If the person with AIDS is near a person with measles, call the doctor that day. There is a medicine that can make the measles less dangerous, but it has to be given very soon after the person is around the germ.

Children or adults who live with someone with AIDS and who need to get vaccinated against polio should get an injection with "inactivated virus" vaccine. The regular oral polio vaccine has weakened polio virus that can spread from the person who got the vaccine to the person with AIDS and give them polio.

Everyone living with a person with AIDS should get a flu shot every year to reduce the chances of spreading the flu to the person with AIDS. Everyone living with a person with AIDS should be checked for tuberculosis (TB) every year.

Be Careful with Pets and Gardening

Pets can give love and companionship. Having a pet around can make a person with AIDS feel better and enjoy life more. However, people with HIV or AIDS should not touch pet litter boxes, feces, bird droppings, or water in fish tanks. Many pet animals carry germs that don't make healthy people sick, but can make the person with AIDS very sick. A person with AIDS can have pets, but must wash their hands with soap and water after handling the pet. Someone who does not have HIV infection must clean the litter boxes, cages, fish tanks, pet beds, and other things. Wear rubber gloves when you clean up after pets and wash your hands before and after cleaning. Empty litter boxes every day, don't just sift. Just like the people living with a person with AIDS, pets need yearly checkups and current vaccinations. If the pet gets sick, take it to the veterinarian right away. Someone with AIDS should not touch a sick animal.

Gardening can also be a problem. Germs live in garden or potting soil. A person with AIDS can garden, but they must wear work gloves while handling dirt and must wash their hands before and after handling dirt. You should do the same.

Food

Someone with AIDS can eat almost anything they want; in fact, the more the better. A well-balanced diet with plenty of nutrients, fiber, and liquids is healthy for everybody. Fixing food for a person with AIDS takes a little care, although you should follow these same rules for fixing food for anybody.

- Don't use raw (unpasteurized) milk.

- Don't use raw eggs. Be careful; raw eggs may be in homemade mayonnaise, hollandaise sauce, ice cream, fruit drinks (smoothies), or other homemade foods.

- All beef, pork, chicken, fish, and other meat should be cooked well done, with no pink in the middle.

- Don't use raw fish or shellfish (like oysters).

- Wash your hands before handling food and wash them again between handling different foods.

- Wash all utensils (knives, spatulas, mixing spoons, etc.) before reusing them with other foods. If you taste food while cooking, use a clean spoon every time you taste; do not stir with the spoon you taste with.

- Don't let blood from uncooked beef, pork, or chicken or water from shrimp, fish, or other seafood touch other food.

- Use a cutting board to cut things on and wash it with soap and hot water between each food you cut.

- Wash fresh fruits and vegetables thoroughly. Cook or peel organic fruits and vegetables because they may have germs on the skins. Don't use organic lettuce or other organic vegetables that cannot be peeled or cooked.

A person living with AIDS does not need separate dishes, knives, forks, or spoons. Their dishes don't need special cleaning either. Just wash all the dishes together with soap or detergent in hot water.

A person with AIDS can fix food for other people. Just like everybody else who fixes food, people with AIDS should wash their hands first and not lick their fingers or the utensils while they are cooking. However, no one who has diarrhea should fix food.

To keep food from spoiling, serve hot foods hot and cold foods cold. Cover leftover food and store it in the refrigerator as soon as possible.

Personal Items

A person with HIV infection should not share razors, toothbrushes, tweezers, nail or cuticle scissors, pierced earrings or other "pierced" jewelry, or any other item that might have their blood on it.

Laundry

Clothes and bed sheets used by someone with AIDS can be washed the same way as other laundry. If you use a washing machine, either hot or cold water can be used, with regular laundry detergent. If clothes or sheets have blood, vomit, semen, vaginal fluids, urine, or feces on them, use disposable gloves and handle the clothes or sheets as little as possible. Put them in plastic bags until you can wash them. You can but you don't need to add bleach to kill HIV; a normal wash cycle will kill the virus. Clothes may also be dry cleaned or hand-washed. If stains from blood, semen, or vaginal fluids are on the clothes, soaking them in cold water before washing will help remove the stains. Fabrics and furniture can be cleaned with soap and water or cleansers you can buy in a store; just follow the directions on the box. Wear gloves while cleaning.

Cleaning House

Cleaning kills germs that may be dangerous to the person with AIDS. You may want to clean and dust the house every week. Clean tubs, showers, and sinks often; use household cleaners, then rinse with fresh water. You may want to wet mop floors at least once a week. Clean the toilet often; use bleach mixed with water or a commercial toilet bowl cleaner. You may clean urinals and bedpans with bleach after each use. Replace plastic urinals and bedpans every month or so. About ¼ cup of bleach mixed with 1 gallon of water makes a good disinfectant for floors, showers, tubs, sinks, mops, sponges, etc. (or 1 tablespoon of bleach in 1 quart of water for small jobs). Make a new batch each time because it stops working after about 24 hours. Be sure to keep the bleach and the bleach and water mix, like other dangerous chemicals, away from children.

Protect Yourself

A person who has AIDS may sometimes have infections that can make you sick. You can protect yourself, however. Talk to the doctor or nurse to find out what germs can infect you and other people in the house. This is very important if you have HIV infection yourself. For example, diarrhea can be caused by several different germs. Wear disposable gloves if you have to clean up after or help a person with diarrhea and wash your hands carefully after you take the gloves off. Do not use disposable gloves more than one time.

Another cause of diarrhea is the *cryptosporidiosis* parasite. It is spread from the feces of one person or animal to another person or animal, often by contaminated water, raw food, or food that isn't cooked well enough. Again, wash your hands after using the bathroom and before fixing food. You can check with your local health department to see if *cryptosporidiosis* is in the water. If you hear that the water in your community may have *cryptosporidiosis* parasites, boil your drinking water for at least 1 minute to kill the parasite, then let the water cool before drinking it. You may want to buy bottled (distilled) water for cooking and drinking if the *cryptosporidiosis* parasite or other organisms that might make a person with HIV infection sick could be in the tap water.

If the person with AIDS has a cough that lasts longer than a week, the doctor should check them for TB. If they do have TB, then you and everybody else living in the house should be checked for TB infection, even if you aren't coughing. If you are infected with TB germs, you can take medicine that will prevent you from developing TB.

If the person with AIDS gets yellow jaundice (a sign of acute hepatitis) or has chronic hepatitis B infection, you and everybody else living in the house and any people the person with AIDS has had sex with should talk to their doctor to see if anyone needs to take medicine to prevent hepatitis. All children should get hepatitis B vaccine whether or not they are around a person with AIDS.

If the person with AIDS has fever blisters or cold sores (*herpes simplex*) around the mouth or nose, don't kiss or touch the sores. If you have to touch the sores to help the person, wear gloves and wash your hands carefully as soon as you take the gloves off. This is especially important if you have eczema (allergic skin) since the *herpes simplex* virus can cause severe skin disease in people with eczema. Throw the used gloves away; never use disposable gloves more than once.

Many persons with or without AIDS are infected with a virus called *cytomegalovirus* (CMV), which can be spread in urine or saliva. Wash your hands after touching urine or saliva from a person with AIDS. This is especially important for someone who may be pregnant because a pregnant woman infected with CMV can also infect her unborn child. CMV causes birth defects such as deafness.

Remember, to protect yourself and the person with AIDS from these diseases and others, be sure to wash your hands with soap and water before and after giving care, when handling food, after taking gloves off, and after going to the bathroom.

Gloves

Because the virus that causes AIDS is in the blood of infected persons, blood or other body fluids (such as bloody feces) that have blood in them could infect you. You can protect yourself by following some simple steps. Wear gloves if you have to touch semen, vaginal fluid, cuts or sores on the person with AIDS, or blood or body fluids that may have blood in them. Wear gloves to give care to the mouth, rectum, or genitals of the person with AIDS. Wear gloves to change diapers or sanitary pads or to empty bedpans or urinals. If you have any cuts, sores, rashes, or breaks in your skin, cover them with a bandage. If the cuts or sores are on your hands, use bandages and gloves. Wear gloves to clean up urine, feces, or vomit to avoid all the germs, HIV and other kinds, that might be there.

There are two types of gloves you can use. Use disposable, hospital-type latex or vinyl gloves to take care of the person with AIDS if there is any blood you might touch. Use these gloves one time, then throw them away. Do not use latex gloves more than one time even if they are marked "reusable." You can buy hospital-type gloves by the box at most drug stores, along with urinals, bedpans, and many other medical supplies. Many insurance companies and Medicaid will pay for these gloves if the doctor writes a prescription for them. For cleaning blood or bloody fluids from floors, bed, etc., you can use household rubber gloves, which are sold in any drug or grocery store. These gloves can be cleaned and reused. Clean them with hot, soapy water and with a mixture of bleach and water (about ¼ cup bleach to 1 gallon of water). Be sure not to use gloves that are peeling, cracked, or have holes in them. Don't use the rubber gloves to take care of a person with AIDS; they are too thick and bulky.

To take gloves off, peel them down by turning them inside out. This will keep the wet side on the inside, away from your skin and other people. When you take the gloves off, wash your hands with soap and water right away. If there is a lot of blood, you can wear an apron or smock to keep your clothes from getting bloody. (If the person with AIDS is bleeding a lot or very often, call the doctor or nurse.) Clean up spilled blood as soon as you can. Put on gloves, wipe up the blood with paper towels or rags, put the used paper towels or rags in plastic bags to get rid of later, then wash the area where the blood was with a mix of bleach and water.

Since HIV can be in semen, vaginal fluid, or breast milk just as it can be in blood, you should be as careful with these fluids as you are with blood.

If you get blood, semen, vaginal fluid, breast milk, or other body fluid that might have blood in it in your eyes, nose, or mouth, immediately pour as much water as possible over where you got splashed, then call the doctor, explain what happened, and ask what else you should do.

Needles and Syringes

A person with AIDS may need needles and syringes to take medicine for diseases caused by AIDS or for diabetes, hemophilia, or other illnesses. If you have to handle these needles and syringes, you must be careful not to stick yourself. That is one way you could get infected with HIV.

Use a needle and syringe only one time. Do not put caps back on needles. Do not take needles off syringes. Do not break or bend needles. If a needle falls off a syringe, use something like tweezers or pliers to pick it up; do not use your fingers. Touch needles and syringes only by the barrel of the syringe. Hold the sharp end away from yourself.

Put the used needle and syringe in a puncture-proof container. The doctor, nurse, or an AIDS service organization can give you a special container. If you don't have one, use a puncture-proof container with a plastic top, such as a coffee can. Keep a container in any room where needles and syringes are used. Put it well out of the reach of children or visitors, but in a place you can easily and quickly put the needle and syringe after they are used. When the container gets nearly full, seal it and get a new container. Ask the doctor or nurse how to get rid of the container with the used needles and syringes.

If you get stuck with a needle used on the person with AIDS, don't panic. The chances are very good (better than 99%) that you will not be infected. However, you need to act quickly to get medical care. Put the needle in the used needle container, then wash where you stuck yourself as soon as you can, using warm, soapy water. Right after washing, call the doctor or the emergency room of a hospital, no matter what time it is, explain what happened, and ask what else you should do. Your doctor may want you to take medicine, such as AZT. If you are going to take AZT, you should begin taking it as soon as possible, certainly within a few hours of the needlestick.

Wastes

Flush all liquid waste (urine, vomit, etc.) that has blood in it down the toilet. Be careful not to splash anything when you are pouring liquids into the toilet. Toilet paper and tissues with blood, semen, vaginal fluid, or breast milk may also be flushed down the toilet.

Paper towels, sanitary pads and tampons, wound dressings and bandages, diapers, and other items with blood, semen, or vaginal fluid on them that cannot be flushed should be put in plastic bags. Put the items in the bag, then close and seal the bag. Ask the doctor, nurse, or local health department about how to get rid of things with blood, urine, vomit, semen, vaginal fluid, or breast milk on them. If you don't have plastic bags handy, wrap the materials in enough newspaper to stop any leaks. Wear gloves when handling anything with blood, semen, vaginal fluids, or breast milk on it.

Sex

If you used to or still do have sex with a person with HIV infection, and you didn't use latex condoms the right way every time you had sex, you could have HIV infection too. You can talk to your doctor or a counselor about taking an HIV antibody test. Call the CDC National AIDS Hotline at 1-800-342-AIDS for information about HIV antibody testing and referrals to places in your area that you can get confidential or anonymous HIV testing. The idea of being tested for HIV may be scary. But, if you are infected, the sooner you find out and start getting medical care, the better off you will be.

Talk to your sex partner about what will need to change. It is very important that you protect yourself and your partner from transmitting HIV infection and other sexually transmitted diseases. Talk about types of sex that don't risk HIV infection. If you do decide to have sexual intercourse (vaginal, anal, or oral), use condoms. Latex condoms can protect you from HIV infection if they are used the right way every time you have sex. Ask your doctor, counselor, or call the CDC National AIDS Hotline at 1-800-342-AIDS for more information about safer sex.

Other Help You Can Give

Dealing with hospitals or insurance companies, filling out forms, and looking up records can be difficult even if you are well. Many people with AIDS need help with these tasks.

- Getting a ride to the doctor's office, clinic, drug store, or other places can be a problem. Don't wait to be asked, offer to help.

- Keeping a diary of medical events and other information for the person you are taking care of can help them and any other people who are helping. Be sure the person you are caring for knows what you are writing and helps keep the diary if they can.

- Keeping a record of medicine and other care for the doctor or the other people providing care can help a lot. Make sure you know what drugs the person is taking, how often they should take them, and what side effects to watch out for. The doctor, nurse, or pharmacist can tell you what to do. People who are sick sometimes forget to take medicine or take too much or too little. Divided pill boxes or a chart showing what medicines to take, when to take them, and how much of each to take can help.

- If the person you are caring for has to go into the hospital, you can still help. Take a special picture or other favorite things to the hospital. Tell the hospital staff of any special needs or habits the person has or if you see any problems. Most of all, visit often.

Children with AIDS

Infants and children with HIV infection or AIDS need the same things as other children—lots of love and affection. Small children need to be held, played with, kissed, hugged, fed, and rocked to sleep. As they grow, they need to play, have friends, and go to school, just like other kids. Kids with HIV are still kids, and need to be treated like any other kids in the family.

Kids with AIDS need much of the same care that grown-ups with AIDS need, but there are a few extra things to look out for.

- Watch for any changes in health or the way the child acts. If you notice anything unusual for that child, let the doctor know. For a child with AIDS, little problems can become big problems very quickly. Watch for breathing problems, fever, unusual sleepiness, diarrhea, or changes in how much they eat. Talk to the child's doctor about what else to look for and when to report it.

- Talk to the doctor before the child gets any immunizations (including oral polio vaccine) or booster shots. Some vaccines could make the child sick. No child with HIV or anyone in the household should ever take oral polio vaccine.

- Stuffed and furry toys can hold dirt and might hide germs that can make the child sick. Plastic and washable toys are better. If the child has any stuffed toys, wash them in a washing machine often and keep them as clean as possible.

- Keep the child away from litter boxes and sandboxes that a pet or other animal might have been in.

- Ask the child's doctor what to do about pets that might be in the house.

- Try to keep the child from getting infectious diseases, especially chickenpox. If the child with HIV infection gets near somebody with chickenpox, tell the child's doctor right away. Chickenpox can kill a child with AIDS.

- Bandage any cuts or scrapes quickly and completely after washing with soap and warm water. Use gloves if the child is bleeding.

Taking care of a child who is sick is very hard for people who love that child. You will need help and emotional support. You are not alone. There are people who can help you get through this. See the section on "Places To Call For Help" in this chapter or the resources listed at the end of this book.

Changing Symptoms

People with AIDS seem to get very sick, then get better, then get very sick, then better, and so on. Sometimes they get sicker and sicker. You can't always tell if they are going to live through a particular illness or not. These times are very rough on everyone involved. If you know what to expect, you can deal with these rough times better.

Dementia

Dementia (having trouble thinking) can be a problem for a person with AIDS. AIDS can affect the brain and cause poor memory; short attention span; trouble moving, speaking, or thinking; less alertness; loss of interest in things; and wide mood swings. These problems can upset the person with AIDS as well as the people around them. Mental problems can make it hard to follow the planned routines for care and make it difficult to protect the person with AIDS from infections. Be prepared to recognize these problems, understand what is happening, and talk to the doctor, nurse, social worker, or mental health worker about what to do.

If the person you are caring for does develop mental problems, you can help:

- Keep important things in the same place all the time, a place that is easy to reach and easy to see.

- If you need to, remind the person you are caring for where they are and who you are.

- Put a clock and a calendar where the person you are caring for can see them. Mark off the days on the calendar. Write in what will happen each day.

- Put up pictures of people who might be in the house with their names on the pictures where the person with AIDS can see them.

- Speak in short, simple sentences.

- Don't be afraid to be firm. Remove things like dangerous objects from reach.

- Keep the sound from TVs, radios, and other noises down so the person doesn't get confused by unexpected sounds.

- Talk to a health care worker who deals with people with dementia about how to handle problems.

As AIDS Progresses

Here are some of the things to expect as AIDS enters its final stages and ways to try to cope. Like other people nearing death, a person with AIDS who is near death:

- Sleeps more and more and is hard to wake up. Try to talk to them and do things during those times when they do seem alert.

- Becomes confused about where they are, the time or date, or who people are. Tell them where they are, what time and day it is, and who people are. Don't scold them for forgetting, just tell them.

- Begins to wet their pants or lose bowel control. Clean them, using gloves, and use powder or lotion to prevent rashes. A catheter for passing urine may become necessary.

- Has skin that feels cool to the touch and may turn darker on the side of their body touching the bed as the circulation slows down. Keep them covered with warm blankets, but don't use electric blankets because they can burn a person with poor circulation.

275

- May have trouble seeing or hearing. Even so, never talk to other people as if the person with AIDS can't hear you. Always talk to the person with AIDS or anyone else in the room as if the person with AIDS hears you.

- May seem restless, pulling at the sheets on the bed or acting as if they see things that you don't. Stay calm, speak slowly, and reassure the person. Comfort them with gentle reminders about who you are and where they are.

- May stop eating and drinking. Wipe their mouth often with a wet cloth. Keep their lips wet with lip moisturizer.

- May almost stop urinating. If there is a catheter, it may need to be rinsed or flushed to keep it from getting blocked. A nurse can show you how to do this.

- Has noisy breathing because they can't cough up the fluids that collect in the back of their throat. Talk to their doctor; the doctor may suggest raising the head of the bed or putting extra pillows under their head. Turning them on their side may also help. If they can swallow, feed them some ice chips. If they have trouble swallowing, a cool, wet washcloth on the lips can keep their mouth and lips moist and may satisfy their thirst. If they begin to have irregular breathing or seem to stop breathing for a minute, call the doctor.

Hospice Care

Many people have found hospice care (programs for people who are dying and their caregivers) for adults and children a big help. Others feel that hospice care isn't right for them. Hospice services can help caregivers, family, and other loved ones, as well as help the dying person deal with the concerns and fears that may come near the end of their life. You should be able to find hospice organizations listed in your local phone book.

Final Arrangements

A person with AIDS, like every other adult, should have a will. This can be a difficult subject to discuss, but a will may need to be written before there is any question of the mental competence of the person with AIDS. You may want to be sure the person you are caring for has a will and that you know where it is.

Living wills, which specify what medical care the person with AIDS wants or does not want, also have to be written before their mental competence could be questioned. You, as the caregiver, may be the person asked to see that the doctors follow the wishes of the person with AIDS. This can be a very hard experience to deal with, but is another way of showing respect for a dying person. You may want to be sure the person you are caring for knows that they can control their medical care through living wills.

Often, people who know that they will die soon choose to make their own funeral or memorial arrangements. This helps make sure that the funeral will be done the way they want it done. It also makes things easier for those left behind. They no longer have to guess what their friend or loved one would have wanted. You may be asked to help the person with AIDS plan the funeral, make arrangements with the funeral home, and select a cemetery plot or mausoleum. You may be able to help the person with AIDS decide how they wish to be buried or if they want to be cremated.

After the death, there will still be things to do. Programs that have been providing help, such as Supplemental Security Income, will have to be officially informed of the death. Some money already sent or received may have to be returned. The will may name you, a relative, or another person as the one to handle these tasks.

Dying at Home

Whether or not to die at home is a big decision, but it may not have to be made right away. As the health of the person with AIDS changes, you and they may change your minds several times. However, it is something you should talk about with the person with AIDS ahead of time. Plans should be made; legal papers may need to be signed. What the dying person wants and needs, the needs and abilities of the caregivers and other loved ones, the advice of the doctors and other medical professionals, the advice of clergy or other spiritual leaders, may all need to be considered in deciding what is best. Consideration must be given to everyone living in the home. Small children and others may not be ready to cope with death in their home. Others in the home may prefer to face the final moments of the person with AIDS in familiar surroundings. Just be sure the person with AIDS knows that they will not die alone, that the people they love will try to be with them, wherever they choose to die. You also should get help to deal with your own grief after the death.

Help for You

Taking care of someone who is very sick is hard. It wears you down physically and emotionally and creates stress. You can get very angry watching a person you love get sicker and sicker no matter how hard you work or how much you care. You have to do something with this anger. Many people can talk out their anger with other people who have the same problems or with counselors, ministers, rabbis, friends, family, or health workers. Many AIDS service organizations can help you find people to talk to.

You should not try to be the only person taking care of someone with AIDS. You need some time for yourself. The sicker the person you are taking care of becomes, the more important this is. If you try to do everything yourself, you will wear yourself out and not be able to go on. You are not alone. Other people have done this before. Learn from them. Call the places listed below for help.

Places to Call for Help

Call the CDC National AIDS Hotline for answers to questions about HIV infection or AIDS, materials on sex and AIDS, or referrals to local organizations in your community. One of the referrals you should ask for is the telephone number of your local Red Cross chapter. The telephone number of the Hotline is 1-800-342-AIDS (1-800-342-2437). If you want to speak in Spanish, call 1-800-344-7432. If you have hearing problems and have a TTY machine, call 1-800-243-7889.

The CDC National AIDS Clearinghouse can provide copies of this text and other materials about HIV and AIDS. The Clearinghouse can also check computer records for organizations in your area dealing with AIDS or materials about HIV or AIDS from health departments, the American Red Cross, or other community-based organizations. The telephone number is 1-800-458-5231. The international number is 00-301-217-0023. The fax number is 1-301-738-6616.

The National HIV/AIDS Treatment Service can answer questions about treatments for AIDS and diseases linked to AIDS. The telephone number in the United States and Canada is 1-800-448-0440. The international number is 00-301-217-0023. If you have a hearing problem and have a TTY machine, call 1-800-243-7012.

The AIDS Clinical Trials Information Service can provide information about current trials of new drugs for AIDS or diseases linked to AIDS. The telephone number is 1-800-TRIALS-A (1-800-874-2572).

The National Association of People With AIDS (NAPWA) is an association of people who have HIV infection or AIDS. To contact them, call 1-202-898-0414.

Your local phone book should have listings for the local American Red Cross chapter, nursing homes, hospice organizations, the state and local health departments, local HIV or AIDS service organizations, and local medical organizations or referral agencies.

Your local American Red Cross chapter may have special programs on HIV infection and AIDS for African-Americans, Hispanics, and managers and workers on the job. Some Red Cross chapters may offer other training or help with transportation. Both the CDC National AIDS Clearinghouse and the American Red Cross can provide brochures and other materials about HIV and AIDS intended for women, young people, parents, teachers, and those at high risk for or infected with HIV.

Chapter 27

HIV Wasting Syndrome

A common problem among HIV-infected people is the HIV wasting syndrome, defined as unintended and progressive weight loss often accompanied by weakness, fever, nutritional deficiencies and diarrhea. The syndrome, also known as cachexia, can diminish the quality of life, exacerbate illness and increase the risk of death for people with HIV.

Wasting can occur as a result of HIV infection itself but also is commonly associated with HIV-related opportunistic infections and cancers. HIV wasting syndrome is diagnosed in HIV-infected people who have unintentionally lost more than 10 percent of their body weight. Most patients with advanced HIV disease and AIDS eventually experience some degree of wasting.

The National Institute of Allergy and Infectious Diseases (NIAID) supports basic and clinical research aimed at better understanding and improving treatments for this debilitating condition. Several studies of therapies and nutrition for HIV wasting are being conducted in NIAID's AIDS clinical trials research network. The AIDS Clinical Trials Group (ACTG), one component of this network, has established the Wasting Pathogen Study Group. Monthly, this group of preclinical and clinical investigators discusses research ideas and priorities as well as ongoing and planned clinical trials.

Many approaches have been used to reverse weight loss in HIV-infected people, including appetite stimulants, anabolic agents,

National Institute of Allergy and Infectious Diseases (NIAID), Fact Sheet, May 1997.

cytokine inhibitors, and hormones. Goals of therapy include both increase in body weight and increase in lean body mass (muscle).

Currently, the precise causes of the HIV wasting syndrome are not well known, and probably vary among individuals. However, a growing body of evidence suggests that many factors may contribute to wasting including inadequate dietary intake, malabsorption of nutrients, abnormalities in metabolism and energy expenditure, and HIV-related infections.

Reduced caloric intake among HIV-infected people is often the result of a loss of appetite, frequently because of nausea. A number of agents to enhance dietary intake have been evaluated in NIAID clinical trials; two of them—megestrol acetate (megace) and dronabinol (marinol, which contains the active ingredient of marijuana, THC)—are currently approved by the U.S. Food and Drug Administration (FDA) for the treatment of HIV wasting syndrome. Nutritional supplements also have a role in boosting caloric intake and currently are being assessed in NIAID's clinical trials research network.

Many HIV-infected people suffer from aphthous ulcers of the mouth or esophagus that make eating difficult. A recent NIAID-supported study demonstrated that the drug thalidomide can safely and effectively heal these ulcers. This finding promises to remove a major impediment to adequate nutrition for HIV-infected people who suffer from these painful sores.

Despite ingesting sufficient calories, many people with HIV lose nutrients because of diarrhea, vomiting or malabsorption of nutrients in their intestines. Malabsorption may be caused by HIV itself as well as by enteric infections associated with HIV disease. Research into HIV's effects on the gastrointestinal tract and into diseases such as cryptosporidiosis and microsporidiosis may help explain the causes of HIV-associated diarrhea and wasting.

Increased calorie usage, and in some cases the breakdown of muscle and other tissues, also contributes to HIV wasting. Agents that reverse metabolic abnormalities, such as testosterone and growth hormones, have been studied by NIAID-supported investigators and others. One such drug, a growth factor known as somatropin (Serostim), was approved by the FDA in 1996 for the treatment of HIV-associated wasting. Researchers also have found that increased levels of immune-signaling molecules (cytokines) such as interleukin-6 and tumor necrosis factor-alpha (TNF-alpha) are associated with HIV wasting. Drugs that block TNF-alpha may have a role in the treatment of this condition.

A number of clinical trials of potential therapies for HIV wasting syndrome are ongoing or imminent in the NIAID-supported ACTG and Terry Beirn Community Programs for Clinical Research on AIDS (CPCRA).

• CPCRA investigators are comparing the effectiveness of three nutritional regimens in increasing lean body mass and improving absorption of nutrients:

— whole protein and long-chain triglycerides plus a multivitamin;
— partially hydrolyzed protein and medium-chain triglycerides plus a multivitamin;
— a multivitamin alone.

• Another CPCRA trial compares:

— an oral anabolic agent, oxandrolone;
— an anabolic agent plus an appetite stimulant (megace);
— megace alone. As part of this study, some patients will take part in an exercise regimen. The investigators anticipate that this study will provide insights into the impact of increases in lean body mass and weight on survival and disease progression.

• In the ACTG, protocol 892 will attempt to correlate changes in viral load with changes in body composition and total body weight.

• ACTG 313 is comparing a regimen of megace and testosterone enenthate vs. megace alone. The primary objective of this study is to assess whether treatment with megace and testosterone leads to increased lean body mass, rather than the accrual of fat seen with megace alone.

• ACTG 329, a study enrolling women with HIV wasting syndrome, is assessing whether treatment with nandrolone results in weight gain and increases in lean body mass. Nandrolone is a male hormone called androgen with minimal masculinizing effects.

For enrollment information about AIDS-related clinical trials, call 1-800-TRIALS-A from 9 a.m. to 7 p.m. Eastern Time, Monday through Friday.

Chapter 28

Maintaining Nutritional Health

Introduction

Ever since you discovered that you are infected with human immunodeficiency virus (HIV), everyone seems to be telling you how you should be living your life. You may have read stacks of self-help books and pamphlets. Maybe you've gone to an HIV or AIDS support group meeting. You've probably heard all kinds of conflicting advice about diets, nutritional supplements, exercise, and other therapies to fight the virus. You want to do the right thing, but you're not sure what that might mean for you.

Is this the time to be concerned about your diet? Yes, it is. How, when, and what you eat can affect your health. Specific foods or nutrients will not destroy the virus, but following sound eating habits can make you feel better, look better, and stay healthy longer. If you always have wanted to eat better, now is the time to do it. This text presents information that you can use to plan a healthful diet and deal with HIV-related symptoms.

Managing Symptoms

Maintaining your nutritional health is an important part of your total treatment plan. The symptoms that you experience during an infection or as a side effect to treatment may determine how you feel about eating.

Eating healthy, combined with keeping your weight at a proper level, will help strengthen your body and its ability to fight infection. Weight loss is a warning signal that means you're not providing your body with enough calories. Never ignore weight loss, even if it happens gradually. Talk with your doctor or dietitian to determine possible causes of weight loss. Here are some common problems that can lead to weight loss, along with tips for dealing with them.

I Get Too Full Too Fast

Eat often during the day. Three meals a day may not be enough for you, especially if you can't eat a full meal at one sitting. Eating five to six times per day seems to work best for most people with H IV infection, particularly those who do not feel well. Make what you eat count: Choose foods with lots of calories and protein to help meet your need for these important nutrients. Pack more calories and protein into your food with the ideas show in Table 28.1.

Table 28.1. To Increase Calories and Protein

Add...	To...
dried fruits or nuts, honey, jam, sugar, cream, half and half	hot or cold cereal
butter, margarine, sour cream	vegetables,cooked cereal, potatoes, noodles, or rice
bacon, avocado, olives, mayonnaise	sandwiches, salads, or casseroles
cream or sour cream	soups, fruit, or puddings
cream cheese	fruit or crackers
peanut butter	sauces, shakes, toast, crackers, waffles, or celery
extra chopped meat, shredded cheese, hard-cooked eggs, egg substitute	Soups, sauces, vegetables, salads, and casseroles
dry milk powder	regular milk, scrambled eggs, soups, gravies, or desserts

I Don't Feel Like Eating

This is a common problem that can be caused by medication, fatigue, concern about your illness, or an infection. On days when your appetite is good, be sure to eat plenty to make up for days when you don't feel like eating as much. On days when your appetite is not as good, the following suggestions also may be helpful:

- Eat your favorite foods as often as you like.

- Eat smaller amounts more frequently if you don't feel like having a large meal.

- Eat in a relaxing setting, with a friend, or while listening to your favorite music.

- Add more flavor to your foods with spices and herbs, lemon wedges, mustard, barbecue sauce, catsup, or hot sauce.

- Order take-out food delivered to your home, or check with your dietitian for home food delivery services such as Meals on Wheels.

- Keep a snack supply of high-calorie, high-protein foods such as crackers, cheese, peanut butter, and ice cream. Eat them whenever you feel like it.

- Liquid foods or foods that do not take a lot of energy to chew or cook are perfect for times like this. When you don't feel like eating much, make a milkshake or have a supplement drink. (Ask your doctor or dietitian to recommend one.)

- Try not to fill up on liquids before you eat. Drink small amounts when you eat, and sip fluids between your eating times.

- Keep easy-to-prepare foods on hand for quick fixing. Examples are canned food, frozen meals, or frozen leftovers.

It's important to consume enough calories and nutrients to avoid weight loss. If you find that you can't regain your appetite, consult your doctor. He or she can prescribe appetite stimulants, and a dietitian can help you plan meals that maximize the value of what you eat. Be sure to mention this to your doctor if you are losing weight.

I Feel Like I'm Going to Throw Up

This can be a side effect to an infection or medication, and foods may not seem appealing at this time. The following suggestions may be helpful to keep you on track nutritionally:

- Salty foods or dry foods such as crackers may help to calm your stomach.

- Cold foods such as ice cream, frozen yogurt, sherbet, gelatin, pudding or custard, cottage cheese and fruit, ice pops, juice, cold cereal, or a sandwich may be easier to eat.

- Eating small, frequent meals is a good idea. Often, nausea is worse when there is nothing in your stomach.

- Rest between your meals, but do not lie completely flat. Elevate your upper body or sit up for at least 2 hours after eating.

- If the smell of food bothers you, ask someone to cook for you or make sure that the cooking area is well ventilated so that food smells don't linger.

- Spicy foods, high-fat foods, and caffeine may be hard to tolerate and also can be irritating to your stomach or intestines.

- If your medication seems to cause nausea, check with your doctor or pharmacist to time your doses so that you can take them when you are eating or right after you eat.

Diarrhea Is a Problem for Me

This symptom can be caused by many things, including medications, stress, infections, or severe weight loss. Whatever the cause, diarrhea means that your body is not getting the important nutrients from foods you are eating. It is also critical to pay attention to your intake of fluids to prevent dehydration. Use the following tips to help deal with and lessen your diarrhea.

- Drink plenty of liquids such as juices, clear carbonated beverages, broth, fruit drinks, sports beverages, or water. It is best to avoid drinks containing caffeine or alcohol; they are stimulating to the intestines, and alcohol can cause further dehydration. Try frozen liquids such as ice pops or sherbet. Gelatin counts as a liquid and may be a food that is easy to eat.

288

- Potassium is a vital mineral that is lost when you have diarrhea, and depletion can lead to muscle cramping and fatigue. Replace potassium with bananas, sports drinks, fruit juices (especially orange juice and nectars), mashed potatoes, or canned fruits without seeds or skins.

- You may not feel like eating much, but skipping meals is not a good idea. Foods you may be able to tolerate are plain white rice, noodles, mashed potatoes, crackers, white toast, eggs, hot cereal, applesauce or other canned fruits without seeds or skins, bananas, gelatin, ice cream, sherbet, or broth-type soups.

- To be avoided are greasy or fatty foods with excessive amounts of butter, margarine, or oils, and foods that are fried. For more tips, see the section on fat intolerance below.

- Foods that are high in fiber or that have skins or seeds can be irritating and are also hard to digest. Avoid raw fruits and vegetables and whole-grain breads or cereals. Cooked vegetables, canned fruits without skins and seeds, and white bread are better choices when diarrhea is a problem.

- You can eat low-fat milk and lean meats if you can tolerate them. Dairy aids containing lactase can help you digest and absorb milk sugar without causing bloating and diarrhea (see the section on lactose intolerance below). Stick to plain boiled, baked, or broiled meats and stay away from spicy foods or sauces.

- Cramps often accompany diarrhea and can be a sign of gas or air in your intestines. Drinking carbonated beverages can worsen this problem and should be avoided. Foods that cause gas, such as beans, cabbage, broccoli, cauliflower, or brussels sprouts also should be avoided if they seem to cause these problems.

Note: If your diarrhea increases in frequency or lasts for more than a week, consult your doctor immediately. Unchecked diarrhea can cause further problems, and medications to help you get it under control are available. Dehydration and potassium loss are the serious problems that must be prevented or corrected.

I Have Lactose Intolerance, So It's Difficult to Eat Dairy Products

If you notice that milk, cheese, and ice cream cause cramping, gas, bloating, or diarrhea, your body may be having trouble digesting lactose, a type of sugar found in milk and milk products. You may find that suddenly you cannot tolerate dairy products of any kind, but with time it may subside and you can add these protein-rich foods back into your diet. Check with your dietitian for recipes or other recommendations.

If you experience problems with milk or other dairy products, the following suggestions should help:

- Beware of foods containing milk, such as pudding, custard, ice cream, cream soups, cream pies, gravies, or sauces, as they may also cause problems.

- Products are available that can help you digest lactose. These lactase pills and drops should be taken before you eat something that contains large amounts of lactose. Some milk and dairy food items already have these products in them and are found in the regular dairy section of your supermarket.

- Some dairy products that contain less lactose may be easier to tolerate. Buttermilk, cottage cheese, sour cream, aged cheeses, sherbet, and yogurt are examples. In place of milk, try nondairy products like enriched soy milk, nondairy cream, or other milk substitutes.

- Kosher foods labeled pareve or parve are acceptable because they are milk-free.

Mouth Sores, Dry Mouth, and Swallowing Difficulty Make It Hard to Eat Anything

Infections in your mouth and throat can cause painful sores, making it difficult to eat or swallow. And some medications can cause your mouth to feel dry. Taking care of your teeth and gums is important and often can help you manage these symptoms. The following suggestions also can help:

- Soft foods that are smooth in consistency and easy to swallow are usually the easiest to eat. Using a blender, adding gravies or sauces to finely cut meat, eating casseroles or stews, or eating foods of the same consistency can make swallowing easier. Adding liquids to foods or dunking foods in liquids can make them less irritating to your mouth and throat.

- Avoid spicy foods, extremely hot foods, or foods with a high acid content such as orange juice or tomatoes; they can make mouth sores more painful. Cold foods such as ice pops, ice cream, sherbet, frozen yogurt, or thick milkshakes can numb your mouth and can be easy to swallow as well.

- If you find that you gag easily, avoid sticky foods such as peanut butter and slippery foods such as gelatin.

- Sometimes food that is neither too hot nor too cold is easier to handle. Try puddings, custard, eggs, canned fruits, cottage cheese, yogurt, bananas, and creamed cereals. Or try dipping toast, cookies, or crackers in milk or another beverage.

- Avoid foods that require a lot of chewing or are tough and fibrous.

- Rinse your mouth frequently and drink lots of fluid to help with dryness. If dryness continues to be a problem even when you moisten your foods, your doctor or dentist may prescribe artificial saliva for you.

What Should I Do When I Have a Fever?

Your needs for both fluid and calories are higher when you have a fever. For some, fevers or "night sweats" do not affect how you feel about eating. If you are experiencing fevers or night sweats, remember to increase your intake of fluids to more than 8 cups per day and eat frequently, up to six or more times daily if you can. This is also an important time to watch your weight closely, as it can signal whether you're getting enough nutrients from your food.

I Have Trouble Digesting Fat

Fats are an excellent source of calories, they can also be hard to digest at times. Fat intolerance—difficulty digesting and absorbing fats—can be a problem for people with HIV infection and AIDS. If you feel discomfort after eating a meal or a food that was high in fat, you may need to reduce the amount of fat you eat. You usually do not have to cut it completely from your diet. In fact, this is not usually recommended unless you are experiencing prolonged and severe diarrhea. If fat intolerance becomes a problem, it is best to avoid foods such as:

- Fried foods
- Hot dogs
- Sausages
- Bacon
- Pepperoni
- Luncheon meats

- Tuna in oil
- Cheeses
- Chips
- French fries
- Cream sauces
- Gravies
- Salad dressing
- Mayonnaise
- Peanut butter

- Doughnuts
- Ice cream
- Chocolate
- Rich desserts
- Whole milk
- Cream or half & half
- Too much butter, oils, or margarine

Products with a special form of fat that is more easily digested and products that contain no fat but have extra calories and protein are also available. These products may be helpful to keep your intake and weight at appropriate levels. Consult your dietitian or doctor to help choose a product that best fits your needs.

A Few More Words

Eating healthy should be near the top of your treatment plan. Health care professionals such as registered dietitians, your doctor, and nurses can help you make food choices that are right for you, and they can discuss nutrition options with you. Because the symptoms you experience can be varied and can change over time, regular visits with your health care providers are important. As new treatments and therapies emerge, good nutrition will help to support your treatment and provide you with the strength you need to fight HIV disease.

If you need more information about food and nutrition related to HIV disease, talk to a registered dietitian, the expert on diet, health, and nutrition. To find a registered dietitian, ask a doctor or nurse to refer you to one. Or call The American Dietetic Association at (800) 366-1655, and ask for the name of a registered dietitian in your area.

Chapter 29

You Can Prevent Cryptosporidiosis

What Is Cryptosporidiosis?

Cryptosporidiosis (krip-to-spo-rid-e-O-sis), often called "crypto," is a disease caused by a one-celled parasite, *Cryptosporidium parvum* also known as crypto." Crypto, which cannot be seen without a very powerful microscope, is so small that over 10,000 of them would fit on the period at the end of this sentence.

What Are the Symptom of Crypto?

Although sometimes persons infected with crypto do not get sick, when they do get sick they can have watery diarrhea, stomach cramps, an upset stomach, or a slight fever. In some cases, persons infected with crypto can have severe diarrhea and lose weight. The first symptoms of crypto may appear 2 to 10 days after a person becomes infected.

How Does Crypto Affect You If Your Immune System Is Severely Weakened?

In people with AIDS and in others whose immune system is weakened, crypto can be serious, long-lasting, and sometimes fatal. If your

An undated brochure produced by the Centers for Disease Control and Prevention (CDC), included in current list of available publications, inventory no. D080.

CD4+ cell count is below 200, crypto is more likely to cause diarrhea and other symptoms for a long time. If your CD4+ count is above 200, your illness may not last more than 1 to 3 weeks or slightly longer. However, you could still carry the infection, which means that the crypto parasites are living in your intestines, but are not causing illness. If your CD4+ count later drops below 200, your symptoms may reappear.

How Is Crypto Spread?

You can get crypto by putting anything in your mouth that has touched the "stool" (bowel movement) of a person or animal with crypto. You can also get crypto by touching your mouth after touching the stool of infected persons or animals or touching soil or objects contaminated with stool. Drinking contaminated water or eating contaminated food can also give you crypto. Cryptosporidiosis is *not* spread by contact with blood.

Can Crypto Be Treated?

Yes, but no drug has been found yet to cure it. Some drugs, such as paromomycin, may reduce the symptoms of crypto, and new drugs are being tested. If you think you have crypto, or if you just have diarrhea, talk with your health care provider about testing and treatment. Diarrhea can cause dehydration. You should drink plenty of fluids to prevent dehydration. Oral rehydration powders and sportsade drinks can also help prevent dehydration.

How Can I Protect Myself from Crypto?

You can reduce your risk of getting crypto. The more steps you take, the less likely you are to get crypto. These actions will also help protect you against other diseases.

1. **Wash your hands.** Washing your hands often with soap and water is probably the single most important step you can take to prevent crypto and other illnesses. Always wash your hands before eating and preparing food. Wash your hands well after touching children in diapers; after touching clothing, bedding, toilets, or bed pans soiled by someone who has diarrhea; after gardening; any time you touch pets or other animals; and after touching anything that might have had contact with even the smallest amounts of human or animal

stool, including dirt in your garden and other places. Even if you wear gloves when you do these activities you should still wash your hands well when you finish. Children should be supervised by adults to make sure they wash their hands well.

2. **Practice safer sex.** Infected people may have crypto on their skin in the anal and genital areas, including the thighs and buttocks. However, since you cannot tell if someone has crypto, you may want to take these precautions with any sex partner:

   - Rimming (kissing or licking the anus) is so likely to spread infection that you should avoid it, even if you and your partner wash well before.

   - Always wash your hands well after touching your partners anus or rectal area.

3. **Avoid touching farm animals.** If you touch a farm animal, particularly a calf, lamb, or other young animal, or visit a farm where animals are raised, wash your hands well with soap and water before preparing food or putting anything in your mouth. Do not touch the stool of *any* animal. After you visit a farm or other area with animals, have someone who is not HIV infected clean your shoes, or if you clean them yourself, wear disposable gloves. Wash your hands after taking off the gloves.

4. **Avoid touching the stool of pets.** Most pets are safe to own. However, someone who is not HIV infected should clean their litter boxes or cages, and dispose of the waste. If you must clean up after a pet, use disposable gloves. Wash your hands afterwards. The risk of getting crypto is greatest from pets that are less than 6 months old, animals that have diarrhea, and stray animals. Older animals can also have crypto, but they are less likely to have it than younger animals. If you get a puppy or kitten that is less than 6 months old, have the animal tested for crypto before bringing it home. If any pet gets diarrhea have it tested for crypto.

5. **Be careful when in lakes, rivers, or pools, and when using hot tubs.** When swimming in lakes, rivers, or pools, and when using hot tubs, avoid swallowing water. Several outbreaks of crypto have been traced to swallowing contaminated water while swimming. Crypto is not killed by the amount of chlorine normally used in swimming pools and water parks.

Crypto also can remain alive in fresh and salt water for several days, so swimming in polluted lake or ocean water may also be unsafe.

6. **Wash and/or cook your food.** Fresh vegetables and fruits may be contaminated with crypto. Therefore, wash well all vegetables or fruit you will eat uncooked. If you take extra steps to make your water safe (see below for ways to do so), use this safe water to wash your fruits and vegetables. When you can, peel fruit that you will eat raw, after washing it. Do not eat or drink unpasteurized milk or dairy products. Cooking kills crypto. Therefore, cooked food and processed or packaged foods are probably safe if, after cooking or processing, they are not handled by someone infected with crypto.

7. **Drink safe water.** Do not drink water directly from lakes, rivers, streams, or springs. Because you cannot be sure if your tap water contains crypto, you may wish to avoid drinking tap water, including water and ice from a refrigerator ice-maker, which are made with tap water. Because public water quality and treatment vary throughout the United States, always check with the local health department and water utility to see if they have issued any special notices about the use of tap water by HIV infected persons. You may also wish to take some additional measures: boiling your water, filtering your water with certain home filters, or drinking certain types of bottled water. Processed carbonated (bubbly) drinks in cans or bottles are probably safe, but drinks made at a fountain might not be because they are made with tap water. If you choose to take these extra measures, use them all the time, not just at home. If the public health department advises boiling the water, do not drink tap water unless you boil it. You could also use one of the bottled waters described below.

A. *Boiling water:* Boiling is the best extra measure to ensure that your water is free of crypto and other germs. Heating water at a rolling boil for 1 minute kills crypto, according to Centers for Disease Control and Prevention (CDC) and Environmental Protection Agency (EPA) scientists. After the boiled water cools, put it in a clean bottle or pitcher with a lid and store it in the refrigerator. Use the water for drinking, cooking, or making ice. Water bottles and ice trays should be cleaned with soap and water before

296

use. Do not touch the inside of them after cleaning. If you can, clean water bottles and ice trays yourself.

B. ***Filtering tap water:*** Not all available home water filters remove crypto. All filters that have the words "reverse osmosis" on the label protect against crypto. Some other types also work, but not all filters that are supposed to remove objects 1 micron or larger from water are the same. Look for the words "absolute 1 micron." Some "1 micron" and most "nominal 1 micron" filters will not work against crypto. Also look for the words "Standard 53" and the words "cyst reduction" or "cyst removal" for an NSF-tested filter that works against crypto.

To find out if a particular filter removes crypto, contact NSF International (3475 Plymouth Road, P.O. Box 130140, Ann Arbor, MI 48113-0140; telephone 1-800-673-8010; fax 734-769-0109), an independent testing group. Ask NSF for a list of "Standard 53 Cyst Filters." Check the model number on the filter you intend to buy to make sure it is *exactly* the same as the number on the NSF list. Look for the NSF trademark on filters, but be aware that NSF tests filters for many different things. Because NSF testing is expensive, many filters that may work against crypto have not been tested. Reverse osmosis filters work against crypto whether they have been tested by NSF or not. Many other filters not tested by NSF also work if they have an absolute pore size of 1 micron or smaller.

Filters collect germs from your water, so someone who is not HIV infected should change the filter cartridges for you; if you do it yourself, wear gloves and wash your hands afterwards. Filters may not remove crypto as well as boiling does because even good brands of filters may sometimes have manufacturing flaws that allow small numbers of crypto to get past the filter Also, poor filter maintenance or failure to replace filter cartridges as recommended by the manufacturer can cause your filter to fail.

C. ***Bottled water:*** If you drink bottled water read the label and look for this information:

Bottled water labels reading "well water," "artesian well water," "spring water," or "mineral water" do not guarantee that the water does not contain crypto. However, water that comes from protected well or protected spring water sources is less likely to contain crypto than bottled water or tap water from less protected sources, such as rivers and lakes. Any bottled water (no matter what the source) that has been treated by one or more of the methods listed in the top part of the water filters table (below) is considered safe.

Table 29.1. If you choose to buy a filter, look for this information on the label:

Filters designed to remove crypto (any of the four messages below on a package label indicate that the filter should be able to remove crypto)

- Reverse osmosis (with or without NSF testing)
- Absolute pore size of 1 micron or smaller (with or without NSF testing)
- Tested and certified by NSF Standard 53 for cyst removal
- Tested and certified by NSF Standard 53 for cyst reduction

Filters labeled only with these words may **not** be designed to remove crypto

- Nominal pore size of 1 micron or smaller
- One micron filter
- Effective against giardia
- Effective against parasites
- Carbon filter
- Water purifier
- EPA approved—Caution: EPA does not approve or test filters.
- EPA registered—Caution: EPA does not register filters for crypto removal.
- Activated carbon
- Removes chlorine
- Ultraviolet light
- Pentiodide resins
- Water softener

D.*Home distillers:* You can remove crypto and other germs from your water with a home distiller. If you use one, you need to carefully store your water as recommended for storing boiled water.

E.*Other drinks:* Soft drinks and other beverages may or may not contain crypto. You need to know how they were prepared to know if they might contain crypto.

Table 29.2. If you choose to buy water look for this information on the label:

Water labeled as follows has been processed by method effective against crypto

- Reverse osmosis treated
- Distilled
- Filtered through an *absolute* 1 micron or smaller filter
- "One micron absolute"

Water labeled as follows may **not** have been processed by method effective against crypto

- Filtered
- Micro-filtered
- Carbon-filtered
- Particle-filtered
- Multimedia-filtered
- Ozonated
- Ozone-treated
- Ultraviolet light-treated
- Activated carbon-treated
- Carbon dioxide-treated
- Ion exchange-treated
- Deionized
- Purified
- Chlorinated

Juices made from fresh fruit can also be contaminated with crypto. Recently several people became ill after drinking apple cider made from apples contaminated with crypto. You may wish to avoid unpasteurized juices or fresh juices if you do not know how they were prepared.

8. **Take extra care when traveling.** If you travel to developing nations you may be at a greater risk for crypto because of poorer water treatment and food sanitation. Warnings about food, drinks, and swimming are even more important when visiting developing countries. Avoid raw fruits and vegetables, tap water or ice made from tap water, unpasteurized milk or dairy products, and items purchased from street vendors. These items may be contaminated with crypto. Steaming-hot foods, fruits you peel yourself, bottled and canned processed drinks, and hot coffee or tea are probably safe. Talk with your health care provider about other guidelines for travel abroad.

Table 29.3. If you drink prepared drinks, look for drinks prepared to remove crypto:

Crypto killed or removed in preparation

- Canned or bottled soda, seltzer and fruit drinks
- Steaming hot (175 degrees F or hotter) tea or coffee

Crypto may **not** be killed or removed in preparation

- Fountain drinks
- Fruit drinks you mix with tap water from frozen concentrate
- Iced tea or coffee

Chapter 30

Thrush: What You Need to Know about Yeast Infections

What is thrush?

Thrush most commonly refers to yeast (*Candida*) infections of the mouth, throat and esophagus. This same yeast can affect the vagina (causing a type of vaginitis) which is sometimes referred to as vaginal thrush.

Yeast is an organism that is normally present in the body. However, for people with weakened immune systems, yeast can grow out of control and lead to thrush, a serious health problem. For people with HIV disease, thrush often develops when CD4 counts drop below 400. In addition, thrush can occur when taking antibiotics (ex. azithromycin and clarithromycin) regardless of CD4 count.

What are the symptoms of thrush?

Symptoms can vary widely—but thrush usually shows up as whitish spots or plaque (large patches of white build-up) inside the mouth, throat and/or esophagus. Red ulcers or patches may also indicate oral thrush infections. Vaginal yeast infections commonly have a thick yellowish/whitish discharge and harsh odor accompanied by mild to severe itching.

Complications from thrush can include trouble with eating, painful swallowing, chest pain and, if left untreated, possible additional infections of the skin and internal organs. Thrush is not dangerous but it can greatly affect the quality of a person's life. Malnutrition and systemic infections are some of the severe complications that can result from untreated thrush.

What can I do to prevent thrush?

Because yeast is normally found in the body, it is difficult to prevent thrush once the immune system becomes weakened. Diet and nutrition may play a role in preventing thrush. Decreasing sugar intake and adding "good" bacteria to a diet such as acidophilus found in yogurt may help prevent thrush. Good oral hygiene is also important, such as brushing the teeth, tongue and gums after meals and flossing once a day. Most dentists are very knowledgeable about oral thrush, and can provide additional information. For people with recurrent thrush, care providers may recommend a steady course of anti-fungal medication to prevent further infections.

What should I do if I think I have thrush?

Seek medical attention immediately. Severe thrush can make it difficult to eat or take medication, which can lead to poor nutrition and weight loss or contribute to additional medical complications.

Currently, effective treatments for thrush are only available with a prescription. Some people try to treat thrush at home, and although some home remedies may help the symptoms—they cannot treat the infection.

What treatments are available?

There is a wide range of antifungal medications used to treat thrush. Care providers often try topical treatments as their first line of therapy. (creams, oral rinses, suppositories and troches (lozenges) are common forms of topical treatment.

Medications in this category include:

- clotrimazole (Lotrimin, Mycelex)

- amphotericin B (Fungizone)

- miconazole (Monistat) (Miconazole cream or suppositories are used to treat yeast infections of the vagina. It is not used for treatment of oral thrush.)

- nystatin (Mycostatin)

Recurring infections, the inability of topical agents to completely clear up symptoms or the presence of thrush in more than one place in the body are signs of more severe thrush. In these cases systemic therapy is required. Systemic medications come in oral, injectable and intravenous formulas.

Medications in this category include:

- itraconazole (Sporanox Oral Solution)

- ketoconazole (Nizoral)

- fluconazole (Diflucan)

- amphotericin B (Fungizone) (Intravenous amphotericin B is commonly used only when resistance to other systemic agents is found.)

Any treatment of thrush should be closely monitored, because antifungal medications can have several side effects. These side effects include fever, nausea, abdominal pain and rash.

Is drug resistance a problem with antifungal treatments?

Drug-resistance is a growing concern with regard to fungal infections. Many strains of fungus that cause thrush are naturally resistant or have developed resistance due to repeat exposure to some therapies.

One important consideration is that many antifungal medications are indicated for the treatment of other more serious and life threatening fungal infections that may occur during the course of HIV disease. If resistance develops to a treatment being used for thrush, the treatment may also be ineffective in treating other fungal infections in the body. It is recommended that resistance be discussed with a care provider prior to choosing a treatment.

—text edited by Dr. Bruce S. Rashbaum, Washington, D.C

Chapter 31

Fluconazole Prevents Yeast Infections in Women with HIV

In a multicenter clinical trial sponsored by the National Institute of Allergy and Infectious Diseases (NIAID), weekly doses of the drug fluconazole safely prevented certain common yeast infections and was not associated with adverse events or drug resistance. This is the first large, long-term study of HIV-infected women to evaluate whether fluconazole, which is used to treat yeast infections, can prevent them as well.

Paula Schuman, M.D., from Wayne State University, Detroit Medical Center, will present the research findings today [July 10, 1996] at the XIth International Conference on AIDS in Vancouver, British Columbia.

"This study is part of NIAID's concentrated effort to develop better prevention and treatment strategies specifically targeted to HIV-infected women," says Steven Schnittman, M.D., assistant director for clinical research, NIAID Division of AIDS. "Fluconazole appears to safely and effectively prevent mucosal candidiasis, the most common fungal infection affecting women with HIV. In addition, the effectiveness of the drug is not at the expense of clinical resistance."

Vaginal yeast infections are common and easily treated in most women. They usually are caused by *Candida albicans*, a yeast that normally lives in the body. HIV-infected women, however, frequently develop yeast infections of the mouth, vagina and throat that are particularly persistent and difficult to treat, often increasing in severity as their immune systems weaken.

National Institute of Allergy and Infectious Diseases (NIAID), July 10, 1996.

"The study proves that fluconazole has a useful role in the clinical management of HIV-infected women at risk for recurrent yeast infections," says Dr. Schuman. "As more and more women become infected with HIV and strategies of how best to use this class of drugs continue to be debated, this research provides some needed answers."

In the NIAID trial, called the Women's Fungal Study or CPCRA 010, 323 HIV-infected women with CD4+ T cell counts of less than 300 cells/mm3 of blood were randomly assigned to receive 200 mg of fluconazole once a week or placebo. After a median follow-up period of 29 months, fluconazole reduced the risk of at least one yeast infection of the mouth and vagina by 44 percent. The drug reduced the risk of oral candidiasis by 50 percent and vaginal candidiasis by 38 percent. During the study, 41 patients on fluconazole and 23 on placebo experienced at least one adverse event; however, no serious toxicities were seen. The researchers also looked at the effect of fluconazole on yeast infections of the throat and on invasive fungal disease, but too few cases occurred in each arm of the study to determine with statistical certainty if fluconazole prevented these conditions.

In a substudy, researchers investigated *Candida* resistance to fluconazole both clinically and in the test tube. Of those women who developed yeast infections, only 13, six in the fluconazole group and seven in the placebo group, developed clinical resistance to the drug after treatment. "This finding demonstrates that the resistance rates did not differ between the two groups, indicating that the regimen of fluconazole used was not associated with clinical resistance," says Dr. Schuman. "The *in vitro* resistance results currently are being analyzed.

The fluconazole study was conducted at 14 sites of the Terry Beirn Community Programs for Clinical Research on AIDS (CPCRA), one of three national AIDS clinical trials networks supported by NIAID.

NIAID, a component of the National Institutes of Health (NIH), conducts and supports research to prevent, diagnose and treat such illnesses as AIDS and other sexually transmitted diseases, tuberculosis, asthma and allergies. NIH is an agency of the U.S. Public Health Service, U.S. Department of Health and Human Services.

Chapter 32

You Can Prevent Toxoplasmosis

Introduction

- Toxoplasmosis is caused by a parasite.
- Infection with the parasite causing toxoplasmosis can be prevented by taking several precautions.
- People with HIV infection should be tested for toxoplasmosis.
- The most effective drug for preventing toxoplasmosis among patients with a CD4+ count *below* 100 is TMP-SMX.

What is toxoplasmosis?

Toxoplasmosis [tok-so-plaz-MO-sis], or "toxo," is a common opportunistic infection among people with AIDS. The parasite *Toxoplasma gondii* [tok-so-PLAZ-ma GON-de] causes the disease toxo, which usually affects the brain. Most people infected with this parasite have no symptoms. However, people whose immune systems are severely weakened often get toxo. Toxo can also occur in infants whose mothers become infected with *Toxoplasma* during pregnancy. Toxo is called an opportunistic infection because it uses the "opportunity" presented by a weakened immune system to develop in the body.

An undated fact sheet produced by the Centers for Disease Control and Prevention; listed in current catalog of publications as Inventory No. D238. *Use of trade names and commercial sources is for identification only and does not imply endorsement by the Public Health Service or the U.S. Department of Health and Human Services.

How is toxo spread?

Toxo can be spread in two ways:

1.Through contact with infected cat stool

Toxoplasma can grow and complete its life cycle only in cats and other felines. For about 2 weeks after a cat becomes infected, the cat passes millions of parasites in its stool every day. The parasites mature and can infect humans from 2 to 5 days after they are passed in the cats stool. No veterinary treatment can prevent cats from being infected or from passing the parasite. People most often become infected by eating food, drinking water, or having contact with soil that contains infected cat stool.

2. By eating undercooked meats

Toxoplasma infects several hundred kinds of birds and mammals. They get toxo in the same way that humans do—by eating food or drinking water that contains infected cat stool. After the parasite infects an animal, it spreads throughout the animal's body. As a result, people can become infected by eating raw or undercooked meat. However, the parasite cannot spread from one person to another except from an infected mother to her child during pregnancy.

How does toxo develop in a person with a weakened immune system?

The immune system responds when a person is infected with *Toxoplasma*. This response causes the parasite to hide in an inactive form (a cyst) within *tissues* — usually in the brain or skeletal muscle. These cysts remain inactive as long as the infected person's immune system is strong. However, when the immune system becomes weak, the parasite can become active again and cause illness.

In the United States, from 15 percent to 40 percent of people with HIV infection have antibodies to *Toxoplasma*. The presence of antibodies to *Toxoplasma* in these people means that they have been infected with the parasite and probably have tissue cysts. People with HIV infection are at greatest risk of developing toxo because these cysts may become active again as the immune system becomes weaker. Having low numbers of CD4+ T lymphocytes (the cells that help the body fight off infections) indicates that a person with HIV infection has a weakened immune system. Without preventive treatment, up to half of all AIDS patients with *Toxoplasma* antibodies and low CD4+ lymphocyte counts become ill with toxo.

What are the symptoms of toxo?

The most common symptoms of toxo in AIDS patients are headache, confusion, and fever. Other symptoms include seizures, poor coordination, and nausea or vomiting.

How can you prevent infection with Toxoplasma?

Five important practices can reduce your risk of being infected with the parasite:

1. Do not eat undercooked or raw red meat. Red meat is a common source of *Toxoplasma* in the United States. The parasites in meat can be killed by cooking the meat until the temperature inside the meat reaches 165° F. If you don't have a meat thermometer, cook meat until it is no longer pink in the center. Red meat is also safe from toxo if it has been frozen for at least 24 hours, smoked, or cured. Chicken, other fowl, and eggs almost never contain *Toxoplasma* tissue cysts. However, you should still cook these foods until they are well done because of the risk for other infections.

2. Take special precautions if you have a cat. You do not need to give up your cat. However, the cat's stool should be removed from the litter box every day to get rid of any parasites before they mature and become infectious. It is best if someone who is not infected with HIV and not pregnant cleans the litter box. However, if you must clean the box yourself, wear gloves and wash your hands with soap and water immediately afterwards. Keep your cat indoors to prevent it from hunting. Feed your cat only commercial cat food or cook all meat products thoroughly before giving them to your cat. Do not give your cat raw or undercooked meat.

   If you choose to adopt or buy a cat, get a healthy cat that is at least 1 year old.

3. Avoid handling stray cats and kittens. They are more likely than other cats to be infected with *Toxoplasma*.

4. Wash your hands with soap and water after touching raw meat and after gardening, yard work, and other outdoor activities.

This will lower your chances of possible hand-to-mouth contact with meat and soil that may contain the parasites.

5. Wash all fruits and vegetables well before eating them raw.

What should I do to prevent inactive infection from becoming active again?

Nearly all cases of toxo among AIDS patients occur because inactive tissue cysts become active again. This happens only when the immune system is severely weakened, and almost never before a person's CD4+ count falls below 100. Therefore, all HIV-infected people should get tested for antibody to *Toxoplasma* soon after their HIV infection is diagnosed.

If you have a positive *Toxoplasma* antibody test, you should receive drugs to prevent toxo when your CD4+ lymphocyte count falls below 100. The drug recommended for preventing toxo is trimethoprim-sulfamethoxazole [tri-METH-o-prim sul-feh-meth-OK-seh-zol), or TMP-SMX (e.g., Bactrim or Septra).* This drug is also recommended for preventing *Pneumocystis carinii* (noo-mo-SIS-tis ka-RIN-e-i),pneumonia (PCP), another common opportunistic infection. Dapsone [DAP-son] with pyrimethamine [pir-i-METH-eh-men] is recommended for preventing toxo and PCP in the few patients who cannot take TMP-SMX.

Can a person who has had toxo get it again?

Yes. If you have had toxo, you should take drugs to prevent infection from happening again for the rest of your life. The combination of pyrimethamine with sulfadiazine (sul-feh-DI-eh-zen) and leucovorin [loo-ko-VO-rin] is very effective in preventing additional episodes of both toxo and PCP. These drugs are also used to treat toxo after someone becomes ill. Pyrimethamine plus clindamycin [klin-deh-MI-sin] is often used for patients who cannot take sulfa drugs. However, this last combination of two drugs does not also protect against PCP Patients who take this combination should take other medicines to prevent PCP.

Chapter 33

Pneumocystis Carinii
Pneumonia (PCP)

Pneumocystis carinii pneumonia (PCP) is a life-threatening lung infection that can affect people with weakened immune systems, such as those infected with HIV, the virus that causes AIDS. More than three-quarters of all people with HIV disease will develop PCP if they do not receive treatment to prevent it.

PCP is caused by a tiny parasite. In addition to the lungs, the parasite can infect the eyes, ears, skin, liver and other organs. The organism probably infects most people during childhood, but it usually does not cause illness in healthy people. Because the parasite remains in the body for life, it can cause disease at any time if the immune system becomes severely damaged, as in HIV infection, or is suppressed by drugs. People with HIV infection are particularly prone to PCP when their CD4+ T-cell levels fall below 200. CD4+ T cells (also called T4 cells or T helper cells) are important immune system cells targeted by HIV.

Symptoms and Diagnosis

The respiratory symptoms of PCP include a dry cough, chest tightness and difficulty breathing. People with this infection can experience fever, fatigue and weight loss for weeks or even months before

National Institute of Allergy and Infectious Diseases, Fact Sheet, November 1994; and, *"Pneumocystis carinii* Pneumonia," from Centers for Disease Control and Prevention, "1997 USPHS/IDSA guidelines for the prevention of opportunistic infections in persons infected with human immunodeficiency virus," *Morbidity and Mortality Weekly Report (MMWR)* 1997:46(No.RR-12):4-6.

having any respiratory symptoms. If a person with PCP is not treated, the infection can seriously impair the lungs' ability to transport oxygen from inhaled air into the blood, which can lead to death. People with respiratory symptoms usually undergo a chest x-ray to determine if signs of pneumonia are present. Doctors diagnose PCP itself by detecting the organism in sputum or in fluid removed from the lung by bronchoscopy, a procedure in which a tiny tube is threaded through the patient's airways. Rarely, doctors may have to surgically remove a sample of lung tissue for examination.

Treatment

Acute

The standard treatment for people with PCP is either a combination of trimethoprim and sulfamethoxazole (TMP/SMX, also called Bactrim or Septra), or pentamidine. Both treatments are highly effective and their widespread use for both the treatment and prevention of PCP has made the likelihood of dying from a PCP infection less than ten percent.

Patients take TMP/SMX orally or through a vein for at least three weeks. More than half of the patients who receive the combination drug experience such side effects as skin rashes, a decrease in the number of red or white blood cells, nausea, vomiting or kidney impairment. Some of these side effects may be severe enough to discontinue treatment.

Pentamidine is given intravenously and, like TMP/SMX, is likely to prompt side effects in more than half the patients who receive it. These side effects include low blood sugar, low blood pressure, a depletion of red or white blood cells and inflammation of the pancreas. Most of these side effects stop once patients discontinue the drug, although pentamidine can permanently damage the pancreas.

Pentamidine and TMP/SMX are equally effective in the treatment of people with PCP, but TMP/SMX is generally preferred because it tends to cause less severe side effects. If the side effects of either treatment are intolerable, or if patients fail to improve within a reasonable time, doctors may treat them with other drugs such as atovaquone, dapsone or trimetrexate.

Maintenance

Most people with AIDS will experience another bout with PCP if they do not continue to take medication to prevent its recurrence. This is called maintenance therapy. Doctors recommend that people with AIDS who have recovered from PCP take oral TMP/SMX daily for the rest of their lives, at a lower dose than that prescribed for treatment. For people who cannot tolerate TMP/SMX, an aerosolized form of pentamidine inhaled into the lungs monthly is effective in preventing PCP recurrence. People who cannot tolerate the side effects of either TMP/SMX or aerosolized pentamidine may be given other drugs whose effectiveness at preventing PCP and side effects are not well known. These drugs include dapsone, pyrimethamine-sulfadoxine (Fansidar) or intravenous pentamidine.

Guidelines for Preventing PCP Infections

The following guidelines are excerpted from the U.S. Public Health Service (USPHS) and the Infectious Diseases Society of America (IDSA) recommendations for the prevention of PCP. Single copies of the complete report, *1997 USPHS/IDSA Guidelines for the Prevention of Opportunistic Infections in Persons Infected with Human Immunodeficiency Virus* are available from the Centers for Disease Control and Prevention, National AIDS Clearinghouse, P.O. Box 6003, Rockville, MD 20846-6003. Telephone: (800) 458-5231.

Prevention of Exposure

Although some authorities recommend that HIV-infected persons at risk for PCP not share a hospital room with a patient who has PCP, data are insufficient to support this recommendation as standard practice.

Prevention of Disease

Adults and adolescents who have HIV infection (including those who are pregnant) should be administered chemoprophylaxis against PCP if they have a CD4+ T-lymphocyte count of $<200/\mu L$, unexplained fever ($>100°$ F [$37.7°$ C]) for 2 weeks or more, or a history of oropharyngeal candidiasis.

Trimethoprim-sulfamethoxazole (TMP-SMX) is the preferred prophylactic agent. One double-strength tablet/day is the preferred regimen. However, one single-strength tablet/day also appears to be highly effective and may be better tolerated. TMP-SMX may confer cross-protection against toxoplasmosis and many bacterial infections. For patients who have an adverse reaction that is not life-threatening, treatment with TMP-SMX should be continued if clinically feasible; for those who have discontinued such therapy, its reinstitution should be strongly considered. Whether it is best to reintroduce the drug at the original dose or at a lower and gradually increasing dose or to try a desensitization regimen is unknown.

If TMP-SMX cannot be tolerated, alternative prophylactic regimens include dapsone, dapsone plus pyrimethamine plus leucovorin, and aerosolized pentamidine administered by the Respirgard II™ nebulizer (Marquest, Englewood, CO). Regimens that include dapsone plus pyrimethamine also are protective against toxoplasmosis but not against most bacterial infections. Because data regarding their efficacy for PCP prophylaxis are insufficient for a firm recommendation, the following regimens generally cannot be recommended for this purpose: aerosolized pentamidine administered by other nebulization devices currently available in the United States, intermittently administered parenteral pentamidine, oral pyrimethamine/sulfadoxine, oral clindamycin plus primaquine, oral atovaquone, and intravenous trimetrexate. However, the use of these agents may be considered in unusual situations in which the recommended agents cannot be administered.

Prevention of Recurrence

Adults and adolescents who have a history of PCP should be administered chemoprophylaxis with the regimens indicated above to prevent recurrence.

Notes

Pediatric Notes

Children born to HIV-infected mothers should be administered prophylaxis with TMP-SMX beginning at 4-6 weeks of age. Prophylaxis should be discontinued for children who are subsequently found not to be infected with HIV. HIV-infected children and children whose infection status remains unknown should continue to receive prophylaxis for the first year of life. The need for subsequent prophylaxis should be determined on the basis of age-specific CD4+ T-lymphocyte count thresholds.

Children who have a history of PCP should be administered lifelong chemoprophylaxis to prevent recurrence.

Note Regarding Pregnancy

Chemoprophylaxis for PCP should be administered to pregnant women as well as to other adults and adolescents. TMP-SMX is the recommended prophylactic agent. Because of theoretical concerns regarding possible teratogenicity associated with drug exposures during the first trimester, providers may choose to withhold prophylaxis with TMP-SMX during the first trimester. In such cases, aerosolized pentamidine may be considered because of its lack of systemic absorption and the resultant lack of exposure of the developing embryo to the drug.

Chapter 34

Tuberculosis (TB) and HIV

Tuberculosis (TB) is a disease that is spread from person-to-person through the air, and it is particularly dangerous for people infected with HIV. Worldwide, TB is the leading cause of death among people infected with HIV.

An estimated 10-15 million Americans are infected with TB bacteria, with the potential to develop active TB disease in the future. About 10 percent of these infected individuals will develop TB at some point in their lives. However, the risk of developing TB disease is much greater for those infected with HIV and living with AIDS. Because HIV infection so severely weakens the immune system, people dually infected with HIV and TB have a 100 times greater risk of developing active TB disease and becoming infectious compared to people not infected with HIV. CDC estimates that 10 to 15 percent of all TB cases and nearly 30 percent of cases among people ages 25 to 44 are occurring in HIV-infected individuals.

This high level of risk underscores the critical need for targeted TB screening and preventive treatment programs for HIV-infected people and those at greatest risk for HIV infection. All people infected with HIV should be tested for TB, and, if infected, complete preventive therapy as soon as possible to prevent TB disease.

CDC Update, National Center for HIV, STD, and TB Prevention, June 1998; and "Tuberculosis," from Centers for Disease Control and Prevention, "1997 USPHS/IDSA guidelines for the prevention of opportunistic infections in persons infected with human immunodeficiency virus," *Morbidity and Mortality Weekly Report (MMWR)* 1997:46(No.RR-12):10-12.

Intersection of Two Global Epidemics

- Approximately 2 billion people (one-third of the world's population) are infected with *Mycobacterium tuberculosis*, the cause of TB.

- TB is the cause of death for one out of every three people with AIDS worldwide.

- The spread of the HIV epidemic has significantly impacted the TB epidemic—one-third of the increase in TB cases over the last five years can be attributed to the HIV epidemic (Source: Joint United Nations Programme on HIV/AIDS).

The Continued Threat of Multidrug-Resistant TB

Every nation must face the challenge of combating multidrug-resistant (MDR) TB. People infected with HIV and living with AIDS are at greater risk for developing MDR TB. MDR TB is extremely difficult to treat and can be fatal. While the number of cases has remained stable in the United States over the past few years, people with MDR TB have now been reported from 43 states and the District of Columbia.

To prevent the continued emergence of drug-resistant strains of TB, treatment for TB must be improved in the United States and across the globe. Inconsistent or partial treatment is the main cause of TB that is resistant to available drugs (MDR-TB). The most effective strategy for ensuring completion of treatment is Directly Observed Therapy, and its use must be expanded.

Another challenge that individuals co-infected with HIV and TB face is the possible complications that can occur when taking HIV treatment regimens along with drugs commonly used to treat TB. Physicians prescribing these drugs must carefully consider all potential interactions.

Addressing the Dangers of the Interconnected TB/HIV Epidemics Requires Expanded Efforts

TB control is an exercise in vigilance; the goal of controlling and eventually eliminating TB requires a targeted and continuous effort to address the prevention and treatment needs for those most at risk, including HIV-infected individuals. Efforts to eliminate TB are therefore essential to reducing the global toll of HIV.

Guidelines for Preventing TB

The following guidelines are excerpted from the U.S. Public Health Service (USPHS) and the Infectious Diseases Society of America (IDSA) recommendations for the prevention of TB. Single copies of the complete report, *1997 USPHS/IDSA Guidelines for the Prevention of Opportunistic Infections in Persons Infected with Human Immunodeficiency Virus* are available from the Centers for Disease Control and Prevention, National AIDS Clearinghouse, P.O. Box 6003, Rockville, MD 20846-6003. Telephone: (800) 458-5231.

Prevention of Exposure

HIV-infected persons should be advised that certain activities and occupations may increase the likelihood of exposure to tuberculosis. These include volunteer work or employment in health-care facilities, correctional institutions, and shelters for the homeless, as well as in other settings identified as high risk by local health authorities. Decisions about whether to continue with activities in these settings should be made in conjunction with the health-care provider and should be based on factors such as the patient's specific duties in the workplace, the prevalence of tuberculosis in the community, and the degree to which precautions are taken to prevent the transmission of tuberculosis in the workplace. Whether the patient continues with such activities may affect the frequency with which screening for tuberculosis needs to be conducted.

Prevention of Disease

When HIV infection is first recognized, the patient should receive a tuberculin skin test (TST) by administration of intermediate-strength (5-TU) purified protein derivative (PPD) by the Mantoux method. Routine evaluation for anergy is not recommended. However, there are selected situations in which anergy evaluation may assist in guiding individual decisions about preventive therapy (e.g., for TST-negative persons in populations at high risk for *M. tuberculosis* infection).

All HIV-infected persons who have a positive result in the TST (5 mm or more of induration) should undergo chest radiography and clinical evaluation for the exclusion of active tuberculosis. HIV-infected persons who have symptoms suggestive of tuberculosis should undergo chest radiography and clinical evaluation regardless of their TST status.

All HIV-infected persons who have a positive TST result yet have no evidence of active tuberculosis and no history of treatment or prophylaxis for tuberculosis should be administered 12 months of preventive chemotherapy with isoniazid (INH). Because HIV-infected persons are at risk for peripheral neuropathy, those receiving INH should also receive pyridoxine. The decision to use alternative antimycobacterial agents for chemoprophylaxis should be based on the relative risk of exposure to resistant organisms and may require consultation with public health authorities. Rifamycin/protease inhibitor interactions need to be taken into account when non-INH preventive therapy is considered. The need for direct observation as a means of documenting adherence to chemoprophylaxis should be considered on an individual basis.

HIV-infected persons who are close contacts of persons who have infectious tuberculosis should be administered preventive therapy—regardless of TST results or prior courses of chemoprophylaxis—after the diagnosis of active tuberculosis has been excluded. In addition to household contacts, such persons might also include contacts in the same drug treatment or health-care facility, coworkers, and other contacts if transmission of TB is demonstrated. Such persons should be tested with 5-TU PPD. If the TST result is initially negative, the person should be evaluated again 3 months after the discontinuation of contact with the infectious source, and the information obtained should be considered in decisions about whether chemoprophylaxis should continue).

TST-negative, HIV-infected persons from risk groups or geographic areas with a high prevalence of *M. tuberculosis* infection may be at increased risk of primary or reactivation tuberculosis. Some experts recommend preventive therapy for some persons in this category. However, the efficacy of preventive therapy in this group has not been demonstrated, and such prophylaxis cannot be routinely recommended. Decisions concerning the use of chemoprophylaxis in these situations must be considered individually.

Although the reliability of the TST may diminish as the CD4+ T-lymphocyte count declines, annual repeat testing should be considered for HIV-infected persons who are TST-negative on initial evaluation and who belong to populations in which there is a substantial risk of exposure to *M. tuberculosis*. In addition to documenting tuberculous infection, TST conversion in an HIV-infected person should alert health-care providers to the possibility of recent *M. tuberculosis* transmission and should prompt notification of public health officials for investigation to identify a possible source case.

The administration of BCG vaccine to HIV-infected persons is contraindicated because of its potential to cause disseminated disease.

Prevention of Recurrence

Chronic suppressive therapy for a patient who has successfully completed a recommended regimen of treatment for tuberculosis is not necessary.

Notes

Pediatric Note

Infants born to HIV-infected mothers should have a TST (5-TU PPD) at or before age 9-12 months and should be retested at least every 2-3 years. Children living in households with *M. tuberculosis*-infected (TST-positive) persons should be evaluated for tuberculosis; children exposed to a person who has active tuberculosis should be administered preventive therapy after active tuberculosis has been excluded. Decisions to discontinue prophylaxis for children who remain uninfected after removal from exposure to a source case can be made as for adults (see "Prevention of Disease" above).

Note Regarding Pregnancy

Chemoprophylaxis for tuberculosis is recommended during pregnancy for HIV-infected patients who have either a positive TST or a history of exposure to active tuberculosis, after active tuberculosis has been excluded. A chest radiograph should be obtained before treatment and appropriate abdominal/pelvic lead apron shields should be used to minimize radiation exposure to the embryo/fetus. In the absence of exposure to drug-resistant TB, INH is the prophylactic agent of choice. Because of theoretical concerns regarding possible teratogenicity associated with drug exposures during the first trimester, providers may choose to initiate prophylaxis after the first trimester. Preventive therapy with INH should be accompanied by pyridoxine to reduce the risk of neurotoxicity. Experience with rifampin or rifabutin during pregnancy is more limited, but anecdotal experience with rifampin has not been associated with adverse pregnancy outcomes.

Chapter 35

Mycobacterium Avium
Complex (MAC)

Mycobacterium avium complex, also known as MAC, is a bacterial infection that can be localized (limited to a specific organ or area of the body) or disseminated throughout the body. It is a life-threatening disease, although new treatments offer promise for both prevention and treatment. MAC disease is extremely rare in people who are not infected with HIV, the virus that causes AIDS.

Symptoms and Diagnosis

Disseminated MAC can affect almost any organ of the body. It can cause symptoms of fever, weight loss, night sweats, fatigue, loss of appetite, loose stools or diarrhea, abdominal pain, anemia (low numbers of red blood cells) and enlargement of the liver or spleen.

The symptoms of MAC resemble those of many other conditions in people with AIDS. The diagnosis of MAC is made by identifying the organism in blood samples or tissue from affected organs such as bone marrow or liver tissue.

National Institute of Allergy and Infectious Diseases, Fact Sheet, November 1994; and, "Disseminated Infection with *Mycobacterium avium* Complex," from Centers for Disease Control and Prevention, "1997 USPHS/IDSA guidelines for the prevention of opportunistic infections in persons infected with human immunodeficiency virus," *Morbidity and Mortality Weekly Report (MMWR)* 1997:46(No.RR-12):12-13.

Treatment

Acute Therapy

Doctors use a number of different drug combinations to treat MAC. A special task force of the U.S. Public Health Service recommended that at least two drugs be used, one of which should be either azithromycin or clarithromycin.

Guidelines for Preventing MAC Infections

The following guidelines are excerpted from the U.S. Public Health Service (USPHS) and the Infectious Diseases Society of America (IDSA) recommendations for the prevention of MAC. Single copies of the complete report, *1997 USPHS/IDSA Guidelines for the Prevention of Opportunistic Infections in Persons Infected with Human Immunodeficiency Virus* are available from the Centers for Disease Control and Prevention, National AIDS Clearinghouse, P.O. Box 6003, Rockville, MD 20846-6003. Telephone: (800) 458-5231.

Prevention of Exposure

Organisms of the *M. avium* complex (MAC) are common in environmental sources such as food and water. Current information does not support specific recommendations regarding avoidance of exposure.

Prevention of Disease

Adults and adolescents who have HIV infection should receive chemoprophylaxis against disseminated MAC disease if they have a CD4+ T-lymphocyte count of <50 cells/μL. Clarithromycin or azithromycin are the preferred prophylactic agents. The combination of clarithromycin and rifabutin is no more effective than clarithromycin alone for chemoprophylaxis and is associated with a higher rate of adverse effects than either drug alone; this combination should not be used. The combination of azithromycin with rifabutin is more effective than azithromycin alone; however, the additional cost, increased occurrence of adverse effects, and absence of a difference in survival when compared with azithromycin alone do not warrant a routine recommendation for this regimen. In addition to their preventive activity for MAC disease, clarithromycin and azithromycin confer protection against respiratory bacterial infections. If clarithromycin or azithromycin cannot be tolerated, rifabutin is an alternative prophylactic agent for MAC disease. Before prophylaxis is initiated, disseminated MAC disease should be ruled out by clinical assessment, which may include obtaining a blood culture for MAC if warranted. Because treatment with rifabutin could result in the development of resistance to rifampin in persons who have active tuberculosis, the latter condition should also be excluded before rifabutin is used for prophylaxis. Tolerance, cost, and drug interactions are among the issues that should be considered in decisions regarding the choice of prophylactic agents for MAC disease. Particular attention to interactions of antiretroviral protease inhibitors with rifabutin and, to a lesser extent, clarithromycin, is warranted (see Drug Interaction Note).

Although the detection of MAC organisms in the respiratory or gastrointestinal tract may be predictive of the development of disseminated MAC infection, no data are available on the efficacy of prophylaxis with clarithromycin, azithromycin, rifabutin, or other drugs in patients with MAC organisms at these sites and a negative blood culture. Therefore, routine screening of respiratory or gastrointestinal specimens for MAC cannot be recommended at this time.

Prevention of Recurrence

Patients who are treated for disseminated MAC disease should continue to be administered full therapeutic doses of antimycobacterial agents for life. The choice of the drug regimen should be made in consultation with an expert. Unless there is good clinical or laboratory evidence of macrolide resistance, the use of a macrolide (clarithromycin or azithromycin) is recommended in combination with at least one other drug (i.e., ethambutol or rifabutin). Treatment of MAC disease with clarithromycin in a dose of 1,000 mg twice a day is associated with decreased survival compared with clarithromycin administered 500 mg twice a day; thus, the higher dose should not be used. Clofazimine has been demonstrated not to be effective in the treatment of MAC disease and should not be used.

Notes

Drug Interaction Note

Patients concurrently being administered protease inhibitor antiretroviral therapy generally should not be administered rifabutin. However, if co-administration of rifabutin and a protease inhibitor is necessary, indinavir and nelfinavir are the preferred protease inhibitors, and the dose of rifabutin should be reduced by 50% with cither of these drugs. Although protease inhibitors may also increase clarithromycin levels, no recommendation for dose adjustment of either clarithromycin or protease inhibitors can be made based on existing data.

Pediatric Note

HIV-infected children aged <13 years who have advanced immunosuppression may also develop disseminated MAC infections, and prophylaxis should be offered to high-risk children according to the following CD4+ thresholds: children aged 6 years or older, <50 cells/μL; children aged 2-6 years, <75 cells/μL; children aged 1-2 years, <500 cells/μL; and children aged <12 months, <750 cells/μL. For the same reasons that clarithromycin and azithromycin are the preferred prophylactic agents for adults, they should also be considered for children; oral suspensions of both are commercially available in the United States. A liquid formulation of rifabutin suitable for pediatric use is under development but currently is not commercially available in the United States.

Note Regarding Pregnancy

Chemoprophylaxis for MAC disease should be administered to pregnant women as well as to other adults and adolescents. However, because of general concern about administering drugs during the first trimester of pregnancy, some providers may choose to withhold prophylaxis during the first trimester. Of the available agents, the safety profile in animal studies and anecdotal safety in humans suggest that azithromycin is the drug of choice. Experience with rifabutin is limited. Clarithromycin has been demonstrated to be a teratogen in animals and should be used with caution during pregnancy.

Chapter 36

Cytomegalovirus Infection (CMV)

People rarely hear about cytomegalovirus (CMV) because, even though it's very common, it seldom causes illness. Most people become infected before they reach three years of age, and by the time they reach adulthood, up to 85% of the U.S. population may be infected. The immune system of a healthy person may not prevent CMV from infecting the body, but it normally does inactivate the virus and confine it to a dormant state throughout a person's life. If CMV is acquired for the first time later in a person's life, it can cause a brief mononucleosis-like illness. CMV's greatest threat is to immune-deficient patients and to babies whose mothers are infected during early pregnancy.

Transmission

CMV is present in nearly all human body fluids, particularly urine, saliva, semen, breast milk, and blood. It is commonly transmitted in day-care centers, where the children and staff members come into contact with infected children's saliva or urine-soaked diapers. The virus then can be carried from unwashed hands or shared toys to the mucosal tissue of the mouth or nose. CMV also can be transmitted from one sexual partner to another. A woman can transmit the virus

National Institute of Allergy and Infectious Diseases, Fact Sheet, March 1995; and, "Cytomegalovirus Disease," from Centers for Disease Control and Prevention, "1997 USPHS/IDSA guidelines for the prevention of opportunistic infections in persons infected with human immunodeficiency virus," *Morbidity and Mortality Weekly Report (MMWR)* 1997:46(No.RR-12):22-24.

327

to her baby before it is born or at delivery, through contact with cervical fluids. In addition, it is possible to acquire CMV from transfused blood or transplanted organs.

In Immune-Deficient Patients

A person undergoing organ transplantation or cancer chemotherapy must take drugs that suppress the immune system. If the patient had become infected with CMV earlier in life, the now weakened immune system allows the previously dormant virus to reactivate, resulting in life-threatening illness. In someone who is already taking immune-suppressant drugs when first exposed to the virus, the new infection can cause severe illness. Similarly, in patients with immune-deficiency diseases such as AIDS, CMV can cause pneumonia, hepatitis, encephalitis (brain inflammation), colitis, and a serious eye infection called retinitis.

Effects on Babies

CMV infection is of concern if a woman is in early pregnancy when she is first infected with the virus. Some of the babies born to these women may eventually develop minor impairments affecting hearing, vision, or mental capacity. A small percentage of the babies are born with severe neurologic damage, including mental retardation or profound hearing loss. Prenatal tests of amniotic fluid can offer some evidence that fetal infection may have occurred.

CMV Mononucleosis

While CMV infection occurs uneventfully in most people, it can sometimes cause an acute form of mononucleosis. The symptoms include fever that lasts 2 to 3 weeks, hepatitis, and occasionally a rash. CMV mono is a self-limiting disease and, for people who do not have a serious immune deficiency, the prognosis is excellent.

Diagnosis

Results of tests for CMV can be misleading. The current tests, which detect immune cells in the blood called antibodies, indicate only that a person has been infected at some point in life. If a patient has symptoms that suggest a recently acquired CMV infection, a doctor may do sequential tests, in which changes in antibody levels may indicate active infection. Since those changes can be hard to distinguish from normal fluctuations, researchers are working to develop tests that will be more specific. However, in immune-deficient patients, the tests can be useful for measuring the effectiveness of therapy, and CMV screening in newborns can identify potential problems, such as a hearing defect. Researchers are now refining rapid and inexpensive tests that screen for CMV in saliva.

Treatment

Two antiviral drugs, ganciclovir and foscarnet, now are available for treating CMV infection (such as retinitis) in immune-deficient patients. Such treatment is not recommended for people with healthy immune systems because the risk from disease is small compared with the side-effects of the drugs.

Prevention

Good hygienic practices such as handwashing, especially in day-care settings, can reduce the risk of transmission. However, intensive infection-control measures generally are not practical in dealing with a virus as common as CMV. A preventive vaccine is in early stages of development.

Guidelines for Preventing CMV Infections

The following guidelines are excerpted from the U.S. Public Health Service (USPHS) and the Infectious Diseases Society of America (IDSA) recommendations for the prevention of CMV. Single copies of the complete report, *1997 USPHS/IDSA Guidelines for the Prevention of Opportunistic Infections in Persons Infected with Human Immunodeficiency Virus* are available from the Centers for Disease Control and Prevention, National AIDS Clearinghouse, P.O. Box 6003, Rockville, MD 20846-6003. Telephone: (800) 458-5231.

Prevention of Exposure

HIV-infected persons who belong to risk groups with relatively low rates of seropositivity for cytomegalovirus (CMV) and who anticipate possible exposure to CMV (e.g., through blood transfusion or employment in a child-care facility) should be tested for antibody to CMV. These groups include patients who have not had male homosexual contact and those who are not injecting-drug users.

HIV-infected adolescents and adults should be advised that CMV is shed in semen, cervical secretions, and saliva and that latex condoms must always be used during sexual contact to reduce the risk of exposure to CMV and to other sexually transmitted pathogens.

HIV-infected adults and adolescents who are child-care providers or parents of children in child-care facilities should be informed that they—like all children at these facilities—are at increased risk of acquiring CMV infection. Parents and other caretakers of HIV-infected children should be advised of the increased risk to children at these centers. The risk of acquiring CMV infection can be diminished by good hygienic practices such as hand washing.

HIV-exposed infants and HIV-infected children, adolescents, and adults who are seronegative for CMV and require blood transfusion should be administered only CMV antibody-negative or leukocyte-reduced cellular blood products in nonemergency situations.

Prevention of Disease

Prophylaxis with oral ganciclovir may be considered for HIV-infected adults and adolescents who are CMV seropositive and who have a CD4+ T-lymphocyte count of <50 cells/μL. Neutropenia, anemia, limited efficacy, lack of improvement in survival, and cost are among the issues that should be considered in decisions about whether to institute prophylaxis in individual patients. Acyclovir is not effective in preventing CMV disease, and valaciclovir is not recommended because of an unexplained trend toward increased mortality observed in persons who have AIDS and who were administered this drug for CMV prophylaxis. Therefore, neither acyclovir nor valaciclovir should be used for this purpose. The most important method for preventing severe CMV disease is recognition of the early manifestations of the disease. Early recognition of CMV retinitis is most likely when the patient has been educated on this topic. Patients should be made aware of the significance of increased "floaters" in the eye and should be advised to assess their visual acuity regularly by simple techniques such as reading newsprint. Regular funduscopic examinations performed by a health-care provider or specifically by an ophthalmologist are recommended by some experts for patients with low (e.g., <100 cells/μL) CD4+ T-lymphocyte counts.

Prevention of Recurrence

CMV disease is not cured with courses of the currently available antiviral agents (i.e., ganciclovir, foscarnet, or cidofovir). Chronic suppressive or maintenance therapy is indicated. Effective regimens include parenteral or oral ganciclovir, parenteral foscarnet, combined parenteral ganciclovir and foscarnet, parenteral cidofovir, and (for retinitis only) ganciclovir administration via intraocular implant. The intraocular implant does not provide protection to the contralateral eye or to other organ systems. In spite of maintenance therapy, recurrences develop routinely and require reinstitution of high-dose induction therapy or replacement of the implant.

Notes

Pediatric Note

Some experts recommend obtaining a CMV urine culture on all HIV-infected (or exposed) infants at birth or at an early postnatal visit to identify those infants with congenital CMV infection. In addition, beginning at 1 year of age, CMV antibody testing on an annual basis may be considered for CMV-seronegative (and culture-negative) HIV-infected infants and children who are severely immunosuppressed. Annual testing will allow identification of children who have acquired CMV infection and might benefit from screening for retinitis.

HIV-infected children who are CMV-infected and severely immunosuppressed may benefit from a dilated retinal examination performed by an ophthalmologist every 4-6 months. In addition, older children should be counseled to be aware of "floaters" in the eye, similar to the recommendation for adults.

Oral ganciclovir is currently under investigation in CMV-infected children, and no recommendation about its use can be made at this time.

Note Regarding Pregnancy

Because of the lack of recommendation for its routine use in nonpregnant adults and the lack of experience with this drug during pregnancy, ganciclovir is not recommended for primary prophylaxis against CMV disease during pregnancy. Ganciclovir should be discontinued for patients who conceive while being administered primary prophylaxis. Because of the risks to maternal health, prophylaxis against recurrent CMV disease is indicated during pregnancy. The choice of agents to be used in pregnancy should be individualized after consultation with experts.

Chapter 37

Opportunistic Infections and Your Pets

If I'm infected with HIV, should I have pets?

Most people living with HIV infection can and should keep their pets because there are benefits from having pets. However, people with HIV infection should know the health-related risks from owning a pet or caring for animals. Animals may carry opportunistic infections that may be harmful to you. An infection is "opportunistic" because an HIV-infected person's weakened immune system gives the infection an opportunity to develop. Your decision to own or care for pets should be made with certain precautions in mind. If you plan to own a pet, you should also be educated about the type of pet you want.

- Although the risks are low, you are at increased risk of getting an opportunistic infection from handling pets or other animals.
- Several simple precautions are all you need to take while handling pets or other animals.
- You can enjoy the many benefits of owning a pet.

What can I do to protect myself from opportunistic infections spread by animals?

General Precautions

To protect your pet and yourself from infection, be careful about what your pet eats and drinks. Feed your pet only commercial pet food,

An undated fact sheet produced by the Centers for Disease Control and Prevention (CDC), listed in current catalog of materials, inventory number D154.

333

or cook all egg, poultry, and meat products thoroughly before giving to your pet. Do not let pets drink from toilet bowls or get into garbage. Pets should not be allowed to scavenge, hunt, or eat another animal's stool.

Do not handle animals that have diarrhea. If the diarrhea lasts for more than 1 or 2 days, have a friend or relative take your pet to your veterinarian. Ask the veterinarian to specifically check for infections such as cryptosporidiosis, salmonellosis, and campylobacteriosis.

Avoid getting a pet that is younger than 6 months old—especially if it has diarrhea.

If you are getting a pet from a pet store, animal breeder, or animal shelter (pound), look into the sanitary conditions and licensing of these sources. If you are not sure about the animal's health, have it checked out by your veterinarian.

Do not touch stray animals because you could get scratched or bitten. Stray animals may carry opportunistic infections—or even rabies (a deadly virus transmitted by animal bites).

Table 37.1. Infections carried by animals include the following:

Disease	Type of organism	Transmission	Illness
bartonellosis (bahr-te-nel-0-sis)	bacteria	cat scratch	skin lesions
campylobacteriosis (kamp-pe-lo-bak-ter-e-O-sis)	bacteria	animal stool	diarrhea/blood infection
cryptosporidiosis (krip-to-spo-rid-e-O-sis)	parasite	animal stool	severe diarrhea
mycobacteriosis (mi-ko-bak-ter-e-O-sis)	bacteria	aquarium water	skin lesions
salmonellosis (sal-mu-nel-O-sis)	bacteria	animal stool	diarrhea/blood infection
toxoplasmosis (tok-so-plaz-MO-sis)	parasite	cat stool	brain infection

Do not touch the stool of your pet. Always wash your hands after playing with or caring for animals. This is especially important before eating or handling food.

Specific Precautions

Cats: You should be aware of the risks of certain infections such as toxoplasmosis and bartonellosis and of diarrheal illnesses caused by *Salmonella* or *Campylobacter* that can be spread by cats. If you choose to adopt or buy a cat, get one that is at least 1 year old and in good health. Older cats are less likely to carry infections that are harmful to you.

Clean litter boxes every day to further lower the risk for toxoplasmosis and diarrheal illnesses. Someone who is not infected with HIV and is not pregnant should change the litter box. If you must clean the box, wear gloves and wash your hands immediately after changing the litter.

Keep your cat indoors to prevent it from hunting. These precautions will reduce your risk for toxoplasmosis and diarrheal illnesses.

To avoid being scratched or bitten by your cat, have its nails clipped. There may be other scratch prevention alternatives, such as the attachment of soft toenail tips, that you can discuss with your veterinarian. If you do get scratched or bitten, wash the wounds immediately to avoid *Bartonella* infection.

Birds: Buy only healthy birds to reduce the risk for infection.

Other pets: Avoid owning reptiles such as snakes, lizards, and turtles. Many are carriers of *Salmonella*. If you do touch any reptile, immediately wash your hands thoroughly with soap and water to reduce the risk of salmonellosis.

Aside from rabies, little is known about the risk of infections from these animals. Avoid handling exotic pets such as monkeys, ferrets, or non-domesticated animals such as raccoons, lions, bats, and skunks.

Wear gloves (such as vinyl or household cleaning gloves) for the following activities:

- when you clean aquariums to lower the risk for infection with the organism *Mycobacterium marinum* [Mi-ko-bak-ter-eam mahr-E-num]

- when you clean animal cages to lower the risk of salmonellosis and other bacterial infections.

335

I have a job that involves contact with animals. Should I quit?

Jobs that involve working with animals (such as jobs in pet stores, veterinary clinics, farms, and slaughterhouses) may carry a risk for infections. Whether you should work in this type of job should be decided by you and your doctor. People who work in animal-related jobs should take these additional precautions:

- Be familiar with and follow the worksite's policies to remain safe and reduce any risk of infection. Use or wear personal protective gear, such as coveralls, boots, and gloves as recommended.

- Do not clean chicken coops or dig in areas where birds roost if histoplasmosis [his-to-plaz-MO-sis] is found in the area.

- Do not touch young farm animals—especially if they have diarrhea—because of the risk of cryptosporidiosis and of illnesses caused by *Salmonella.*

Can someone with HIV infection spread it to their pets?

No. HIV is not transmitted to or by cats, dogs, birds, or other pets.

There are several viruses that cause AIDS-like disease in different animals, such as cats (feline leukemia virus or FeLV is an example), sheep, and cows. Each of these viruses causes illness in a certain species only and does not affect other species or humans. Just as HIV does not infect dogs or cats, FeLV does not infect humans or dogs.

Are there any tests a pet should have before I bring it home?

A pet should be in overall good health. However, no specific tests are necessary unless the animal has diarrhea or appears sick. If your pet is sick, your veterinarian can help you choose the necessary tests.

What precautions, if any, should I take when visiting friends or relatives who have animals?

When visiting anyone with pets, you should take the same precautions as you would in your own home. Do not touch animals that may not be healthy. You may want to tell your friends and family about the need for these precautions before you plan any visits.

Should HIV-infected children handle pets?

In handling pets, the same precautions apply for children as for adults. Moreover, children may want to snuggle more with their pets. Some pets (cats, for example) may bite or scratch to get away from children. Adults should be extra watchful and supervise an HIV-infected child's handwashing to prevent the possible spread of infections.

Given all the precautions needed, should I have a pet?

Studies have shown that owning a pet can be rewarding. Pets can help a sick person feel psychologically and even physically better. Many people feel that pets are more than just animals—they are companions and part of the family! If a pet gives you pleasure, with common sense precautions, the benefits usually outweigh the risks.

Chapter 38

Kaposi's Sarcoma

What Is Kaposi's Sarcoma?

Kaposi's sarcoma (KS) is a disease in which cancer (malignant) cells are found in the tissues under the skin or mucous membranes that line the mouth, nose, and anus. KS causes red or purple patches (lesions) on the skin and/or mucous membranes and spreads to other organs in the body, such as the lungs, liver, or intestinal tract.

Until the early 1980's, Kaposi's sarcoma was a very rare disease that was found mainly in older men, patients who had organ transplants, or African men. With the acquired immunodeficiency syndrome (AIDS) epidemic in the early 1980's, doctors began to notice more cases of Kaposi's sarcoma in Africa and in gay men with AIDS. Kaposi's sarcoma usually spreads more quickly in these patients.

If there are signs of KS, a doctor will examine the skin and lymph nodes carefully (lymph nodes are small bean-shaped structures that are found throughout the body; they produce and store infection-fighting cells). The doctor also may order other tests to see if the patient has other diseases.

The chance of recovery (prognosis) depends on what type of Kaposi's sarcoma the patient has, the patient's age and general health, and whether or not the patient has AIDS.

National Cancer Institute, PDQ Database at cancernet.nci.nih.gov; last updated February 1998.

339

Stages of Kaposi's Sarcoma

There is no accepted staging system for Kaposi's sarcoma. Patients are grouped depending on which type of Kaposi's sarcoma they have. There are three types of Kaposi's sarcoma:

Classic

Classic Kaposi's sarcoma usually occurs in older men of Jewish, Italian, or Mediterranean heritage. This type of Kaposi's sarcoma progresses slowly, sometimes over 10 to 15 years. As the disease gets worse, the lower legs may swell and the blood may not be able to flow properly. After some time, the disease may spread to other organs. Many patients with classic Kaposi's sarcoma may develop another type of cancer later on in their lives.

Immunosuppressive Treatment Related

Kaposi's sarcoma may occur in people who are taking drugs to make their immune systems weaker (immunosuppressants). The immune system helps the body fight off infection. People who have had an organ transplant (such as a liver or kidney transplant) have to take drugs to prevent their immune system from attacking the new organ.

Epidemic

Kaposi's sarcoma in patients who have acquired immunodeficiency syndrome (AIDS) is called epidemic Kaposi's sarcoma. AIDS is caused by a virus called the human immunodeficiency virus (HIV), which attacks and weakens the immune system. Infections and other diseases can then invade the body, and the immune system cannot fight against them. Kaposi's sarcoma in people with AIDS usually spreads more quickly than other kinds of Kaposi's sarcoma and often is found in many parts of the body.

Recurrent

Recurrent disease means that the KS has come back (recurred) after it has been treated. It may come back in the area where it first started or in another part of the body.

How Kaposi's Sarcoma Is Treated

There are treatments for all patients with Kaposi's sarcoma. Four kinds of treatment are used:

- surgery (taking out the cancer)

- chemotherapy (using drugs to kill cancer cells)

- radiation therapy (using high-dose x-rays to kill cancer cells)

- biological therapy (using the body's immune system to fight cancer)

Radiation therapy is a common treatment of Kaposi's sarcoma. Radiation therapy uses high-dose x-rays or other high-energy rays to kill cancer cells and shrink tumors. Radiation for Kaposi's sarcoma comes from a machine outside the body (external beam radiation therapy).

Surgery means taking out the cancer. A doctor may remove the cancer using one of the following:

- Local excision cuts out the lesion and some of the tissue around it.

- Electrodesiccation and curettage burns the lesion and removes it with a sharp instrument.

- Cryotherapy freezes the tumor and kills it.

Chemotherapy uses drugs to kill cancer cells. Chemotherapy may be taken by pill, or it may be put into the body by a needle in a vein or muscle. Chemotherapy is called a systemic treatment because the drug enters the bloodstream, travels through the body, and can kill cancer cells outside the original site. Chemotherapy for Kaposi's sarcoma also may be injected into the lesion (intralesional chemotherapy).

Biological therapy tries to get the body to fight the cancer. It uses materials made by the body or made in a laboratory to boost, direct, or restore the body's natural defenses against disease. Biological therapy is sometimes called biological response modifier (BRM) therapy or immunotherapy.

Treatment by Stage

Treatment of Kaposi's sarcoma depends on the type of Kaposi's sarcoma the patient has, and the patient's age and general health.

Standard treatment may be considered because of its effectiveness in patients in past studies, or participation in a clinical trial may be considered. Not all patients are cured with standard therapy and some standard treatments may have more side effects than are desired. For these reasons, clinical trials are designed to find better ways to treat cancer patients and are based on the most up-to-date information. Clinical trials are ongoing in most parts of the country for most stages of Kaposi's sarcoma. To learn more about clinical trials, call the Cancer Information Service at 1-800-4-CANCER (1-800-422-6237); TTY at 1-800-332-8615.

Classic Kaposi's Sarcoma

Treatment may be one of the following:

1. Radiation therapy.
2. Local excision.
3. Systemic or intralesional chemotherapy.
4. Chemotherapy plus radiation therapy.

Immunosuppressive Treatment Related Kaposi's Sarcoma

Depending on the patient's condition, the cancer may be controlled if immunosuppressive drugs are stopped. If the patient cannot stop taking these drugs or if this does not work, treatment may be one of the following:

1. Radiation therapy.
2. A clinical trial of chemotherapy.

Epidemic Kaposi's Sarcoma

Treatment may be one of the following:

1. Surgery (local excision, electrodesiccation and curettage, or cryotherapy).
2. Intralesional chemotherapy.
3. Systemic chemotherapy. Clinical trials are testing new drugs and drug combinations.
4. A clinical trial of biological therapy.

Recurrent Kaposi's Sarcoma

Treatment of recurrent Kaposi's sarcoma depends on the type of Kaposi's sarcoma, and the patient's general health and response to earlier treatments. The patient may want to take part in a clinical trial.

To Learn More

To learn more about Kaposi's sarcoma, call the National Cancer Institute's Cancer Information Service at 1-800-4-CANCER (1-800-422-6237); TTY at 1-800-332-8615. By dialing this toll-free number, trained information specialists can answer your questions.

The Cancer Information Service also has booklets about cancer that are available to the public and can be sent on request. The following general booklets on questions related to cancer may be helpful:

- *What You Need To Know About Cancer*
- *Taking Time: Support for People with Cancer and the People Who Care About Them*
- *What Are Clinical Trials All About?*
- *Chemotherapy and You: A Guide to Self-Help During Treatment*
- *Radiation Therapy and You: A Guide to Self-Help During Treatment*
- *Eating Hints for Cancer Patients*
- *Advanced Cancer: Living Each Day*
- *When Cancer Recurs: Meeting the Challenge Again*

There are other places where people can get material and information about cancer treatment and services. The social service office at a hospital can be checked for local and national agencies that help with getting information about finances, getting to and from treatment, getting care at home, and dealing with problems.

What Is PDQ?

PDQ is a computer system that gives up-to-date information on cancer and its prevention, detection, treatment, and supportive care. It is a service of the National Cancer Institute (NCI) for people with cancer and their families and for doctors, nurses, and other health care professionals.

To ensure that it remains current, the information in PDQ is reviewed and updated each month by experts in the fields of cancer treatment, prevention, screening, and supportive care. PDQ also provides information about research on new treatments (clinical trials), doctors who treat cancer, and hospitals with cancer programs. The treatment information in this summary is based on information in the PDQ summary for health professionals on this cancer.

How to use PDQ

PDQ can be used to learn more about current treatment of different kinds of cancer. You may find it helpful to discuss this information with your doctor, who knows you and has the facts about your disease. PDQ can also provide the names of additional health care professionals who specialize in treating patients with cancer. The PDQ database can be accessed through the National Cancer Institute's website at: www.cancernet.nci.nih.gov.

Before you start treatment, you also may want to think about taking part in a clinical trial. PDQ can be used to learn more about these trials. A clinical trial is a research study that attempts to improve current treatments or finds information on new treatments for patients with cancer. Clinical trials are based on past studies and information discovered in the laboratory. Each trial answers certain scientific questions in order to find new and better ways to help patients with cancer. Information is collected about new treatments, their risks, and how well they do or do not work. When clinical trials show that a new treatment is better than the treatment currently used as "standard" treatment, the new treatment may become the standard treatment. Listings of current clinical trials are available on PDQ. Many cancer doctors who take part in clinical trials are listed in PDQ.

To learn more about cancer and how it is treated, or to learn more about clinical trials for your kind of cancer, call the National Cancer Institute's Cancer Information Service. The number is 1-800-4-CAN-CER (1-800-422-6237); TTY at 1-800-332-8615. The call is free and a trained information specialist will be available to answer cancer-related questions.

PDQ is updated whenever there is new information. Check with the Cancer Information Service to be sure that you have the most up-to-date information.

For more information from the National Cancer Institute, please write to this address:

National Cancer Institute
Office of Cancer Communications
31 Center Drive, MSC 2580
Bethesda, MD 20892-2580

Chapter 39

Managing Pain in HIV Disease

For some it can be a raging headache that comes from nowhere and goes in a snap, for others the constant tingling sensation in the feet or fingers caused by peripheral neuropathy and for still others it can be a severe burning in a throat coated with thrush. Each of these experiences of pain commonly occur in people with advanced HIV disease, or AIDS. Studies suggest that 40% to 60% of people with AIDS are likely to be in pain and that this condition also affects about one third of people with early stage HIV disease.

Pain in people with HIV is similar to, and occasionally stronger than, pain in people with cancer. Clinicians should follow the same core principles for the management and treatment of pain in both groups. The World Health Organization (WHO) guidelines for management of cancer pain have been endorsed by the U.S. Public Health Service (PHS)'s Agency for Health Care Policy and Research (AHCPR) and by clinical experts in AIDS care. Treatment should be based on WHO's analgesic ladder, and the selection of analgesics (pain relievers) should be based on the severity and mechanism of pain. Opioid analgesics are the most powerful and effective pain relievers for treating severe pain. The most common side effects of pain medication are constipation, nausea, vomiting, drowsiness and slowed breathing. Counter-measures can be taken to prevent or treat these side effects in order to ease unnecessary pain in people with HIV/AIDS.

From *Medical Alert*, issue one, © 1998 The National Association of People with AIDS, 1413 K Street NW, 7th Floor, Washington DC 20005 (202) 898-0435; reprinted with permission.

The American Pain Society 16th Annual Scientific Meeting held in New Orleans, October 23-26, 1997 offered participants current information about the diagnosis, treatment, and management of acute pain, chronic cancer and noncancer pain, and recurrent pain.

Pain Is Undertreated in Most People with HIV

According to William Breithart, MD of Memorial Sloan-Kettering Cancer Center in New York (212-639-2000) pain in AIDS is much less adequately treated than cancer pain. Recent studies cited by Dr. Breithart, during his keynote address, suggest that "only 6% of AIDS patients with severe pain are prescribed a strong opioid like morphine, despite the fact that the WHO Analgesic Ladder suggests that clinicians consider using strong opioids in all patients with severe pain." Using the Pain Management Index as a measure of adequacy of analgesic therapy, only 15% of AIDS patients with pain receive adequate analgesic therapy, compared to almost 60% of cancer pain patients. Dr. Breithart has also found that women with AIDS-related pain are twice as likely to be undertreated than men. People with less formal education and those who contracted HIV through injection drug use are also more undertreated for pain.

The Women, Suffer...

April Hazard Vallerand, Ph.D., R.N., University of Pennsylvania School of Nursing in Philadelphia (732-780-6224) reported the findings of a pilot study to assess the relationship of pain to functional status and quality of life in women with HIV/AIDS. A sample of 25 women with HIV infection or AIDS with pain complaints in a primary care clinic dedicated to the care of people with HIV were asked to complete several assessment tools including the Brief Pain Inventory (BPI), the Inventory of Functional Status—Chronic Pain (IFS-CP), the Functional Assessment of HIV Infection (FAHI) quality of life instrument, and a demographic data sheet. The majority of participants had severe pain in the past week. Adequacy of analgesic therapy was assessed using the Pain Management Index and the type and frequency of analgesics prescribed for pain. Based on the PMI, 79% of the women reporting severe pain were receiving inadequate pain relief therapy. Of the 12 participants reporting severe pain, 7 were receiving no analgesic therapy, while only 2 were prescribed a strong opioid. The women with pain were found to have decreased functional status. Lower quality of life scores were also found in those women with lower functional status.

Dr. Vallerand acknowledges in her conclusion a need for more information on the effects of pain and its relationship to function status in women. But given previous data on the lack of effective pain medication being offered to women, improving the management of pain in women should be a priority for clinicians.

...While Drug Users Struggle

In a poster session Dr. Gayle Newshan, Ph.D., NP, St. Vincent's Hospital in New York City (212-604-7465) reported on her study designed to increase understanding of the lived experience of pain in hospitalized people with AIDS using a qualitative perspective (Is Anybody Listening? A Phenomenological Study of Pain in Hospitalized Persons with AIDS). For this study, data was gathered from audiotape, open-ended interviews with eleven hospitalized people, film, literature, first-person accounts and clinical observations. The evaluative criteria of trustworthiness was applied to assure rigor. The participants interviewed were a mixed group: 8 men and 3 women, ages 28-44. Of these 7 were white, 2 black, and 2 Latino. Eight individuals had a history of chemical dependence (either alcohol and/or cocaine and/or heroin).

From the interviews and other data five themes were identified, four of which were common among all participants: knowing pain, battling pain, pain's influence and having AIDS. The fifth theme, being a drug user, was found only among the chemically dependent.

Theme 1 ("Knowing Pain") is focused on the difficult task of describing pain and its impact on the body. According to the study, participants often described pain using metaphors, such as "It feels like someone poking you with needles." Theme 2 (Battling Pain) centers on the strategies adopted by individuals for addressing pain and the barriers to pain relief. Barriers include nurses, family members, friends and patients themselves who do not take episodes of pain seriously, especially among those with histories drug addiction. Interestingly, Dr. Newshan reports that participants both fought for and feared 'the big guns,' or strong opiates. One participant described the experience of opiates for pain management as "It's like pulling teeth to get them" while another said the morphine caused him/her "to feel like a zombie—it was scary." Under theme 3 (Pain's Influence) all of the participants described the limitations placed on their lives due to pain and, often, the greater spirituality they gained.

Theme 4 (Having AIDS) related pain to the "uckky" experience of having AIDS. And theme 5 (Being a drug user) captures the very real experience of people living with AIDS who have histories of drug use. For these individuals pain management is made especially hard because of the high tolerance to the effects of opiates that their bodies have developed and the bias of many healthcare providers in prescribing pain medication to current or former drug users.

The participants of the study who all experience multiple sources of pain which influences all of their lives, and often feel unheard recommended the following for clinicians:

1. Listen to me.

2. Do not abandon me.

3. Keep trying.

4. Keep me informed.

5. Do not judge me.

Dr. Newshan concludes, "as healthcare givers, we must ask [ourselves], 'Am I listening?'"

Duragesic: Another Route to Pain Relief

In another study conducted by Dr. Newshan with Matthew Lefkowitz, MD, State University of New York, Health Science Center at Brooklyn, New York (718-625-4244) the authors compared the analgesic efficacy of at least 15 days of a stable dose of oral opioids with the analgesic efficacy of at least 15 consecutive days of therapy with fentanyl transdermal system (Duragesic) in patients with AIDS related chronic pain. Side effects, quality of life, and patient satisfaction were also evaluated.

Fentanyl transdermal system (FTS) is delivered by a noninvasive transdermal system (a skin patch) which allows continuous delivery of a potent opioid providing pain relief for up to 72 hours. While the FTS is approved for the treatment of chronic pain in people requiring opioid analgesia and research has shown its effectiveness for treating cancer, the product had not been evaluated for its effectiveness in treating chronic pain in people with AIDS.

The study, supported by Janssen Research Foundation, was an open-label, pre-treatment vs. Post-treatment trial of outpatients at one site in the United States. All patients had experienced at least moderate pain control with a stable daily dose of a potent oral opioid for the 3 days preceding enrollment. On enrollment (visit 1), patients completed a pain questionnaire and underwent a history and physical examination. For 15 days, participants remained on a stable dose of the oral opioid analgesic that had been prescribed previously. At The end of 15 days (visit 2) patients' medication was titrated to a stable dose of FTS according to the package insert instructions. After the participants had received a stable dose of FTS for a least 15 consecutive days, the end of study (visit 3) assessments were made. The assessments included the Brief Pain Inventory before (visit 2) and after (visit 3) 15 days of treatment with FTS.

Among the exclusion criteria were use of ritonavir (Norvir) during the trial, life expectancy of less than 3 months, active substance abuse, and the inability to speak, read or understand English.

A total of 35 individuals were enrolled in the study. Of the group 74% were men, 26% were women; 37% were Latino, 34% were black, 23% were white and 6% were of unknown racial origin. Nearly 70% of the participants had completed high school, including 17% who had also completed college. The participants were divided among those who were former intravenous drug users (43%), those who had never used intravenous drugs (49%) and those who were enrolled in a methadone treatment program (8%). At study start, most patients were taking more than one medication for chronic pain: 71 % were taking strong oral opioids and 45.7% were taking nonsteroidal anti-inflammatory drugs, such as aspirin or ibuprofen. Of those taking a strong opioid, the majority (63%) were taking oxycodone plus acetaminophen (Percocet) before beginning treatment with the FTS.

The participants reported that the major impediments to pain management were the difficulty of assessing pain (74.3%), the belief that pain was part of their condition (62.9%), and the fear of becoming addicted to pain medication (54.3%).

The participants received therapy with FTS for a mean of 22.5±1.9 days, and the mean dose administered was 50±4.6mcg. During the FTS period, 32.4% of participants reported adverse events. The most frequently reported side effects were headache, somnolence, and bronchitis, reported by 2 persons each. Additionally, one participant died during the oral opioid phase and one withdrew because of excessive somnolence during the FTS phase.

The investigators report their study shows Duragesic effectively alleviates chronic pain in patients with AIDS. On a scale of 0% to 100% relief, the mean pain relief score increased from 77.1% with oral opioids to 87.5% with FTS (Figure 39.1). The Fentanyl transdermal system provided an overall improvement in general activity, mood, walking ability, normal work, relationships, and enjoyment of life over oral opioids (Figure 39.2). There was no difference in adherence to therapy or frequency of side effects in the two groups (Figure 39.3).

For More Information

An informational brochure on pain in HIV/AIDS is available on NAPWAFax (Document No.1901) at (202) 789-2222. For additional information contact Cancer Care at (212) 221-3300 or wwwcancercareinc.org.

—by A. Cornelius Baker

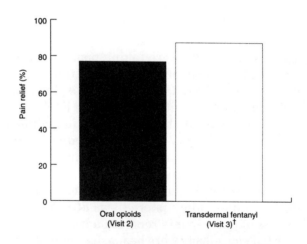

Figure 39.1. *Change in percent of pain relief by visit**

* A mean increase in score from visit 2 to visit 3 (visit 3 - visit 2 >0) indicates improvement. Item was scored as follows: 0% = no relief, to 100% = complete relief.

† P < 0.001 (Wilcoxon's signed rand test).

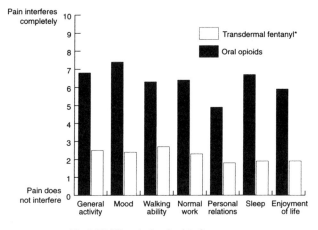

* P < 0.001 (Wilcoxn's signed rank test).

Figure 39.2. Pain interference by type of activity*

* P < 0.001 (Wilcoxon's signed rand test).

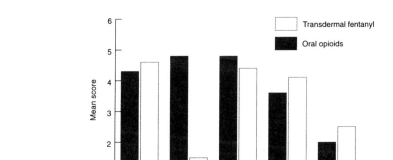

* P=0.03
† P=0.001 (Wilcoxon's signed rand test).

Figure 39.3. Satisfaction with pain medication

* P = 0.03
† P = 0.001 (Wilcoxon's signed rand test).

Chapter 40

Social Security Benefits for People with HIV Infection

Background Information

Acquired immunodeficiency syndrome (AIDS) is characterized by the inability of the body's natural immunity to fight infection. It is caused by a retrovirus known as human immunodeficiency virus, or HIV. Generally speaking, people with HIV infection fall into two broad categories:

1. those with symptomatic HIV infection, including AIDS; and

2. those with HIV infection but no symptoms.

Although thousands of people with HIV infection are receiving Social Security or SSI disability benefits, we believe there may be others who might be eligible for these benefits. Social Security is committed to helping all men, women and children with HIV infection learn more about the disability programs we administer. And if you qualify for benefits, we are just as committed to ensuring that you receive them as soon as possible.

You should also be aware that the Social Security Administration's criteria for evaluating HIV infection are not linked to the Center for Disease Control's (CDC) definition of AIDS. This is because the goals of the two agencies are different. The CDC defines AIDS primarily for surveillance purposes, not for the evaluation of disability.

Social Security Administration SSA Pub. No. 05-10020, May 1997.

What Benefits Are You Eligible for?

We pay disability benefits under two programs: Social Security Disability Insurance, sometimes referred to as SSDI, and Supplemental Security Income, often called SSI. The medical requirements are the same for both programs, and your disability is determined by the same process. However, there are major differences in the nonmedical factors, which are explained in the next two sections.

Social Security Disability Insurance Benefits: The Nonmedical Rules of Eligibility

Here are examples of how people qualify for SSDI:

- Most people qualify for Social Security disability by working, paying Social Security taxes, and in turn, earning "credits" toward eventual benefits. The maximum number of credits you can earn each year is four. The number of credits you need to qualify for disability depends on your age when you become disabled. Nobody needs more then 40 credits and younger people can qualify with as few as six credits.

- Disabled widows and widowers age 50 or older could be eligible for a disability benefit on the Social Security record of a deceased spouse.

- Disabled children age 18 or older could be eligible for dependent's benefits on the Social Security record of a parent who is getting retirement or disability benefits or on the record of a parent who has died. (The disability must have started before age 22.)

- Children under the age of 18 qualify for dependents benefits on the record of a parent who is getting retirement or disability benefits or on the record of a parent who has died, merely because they are under age 18.

For more information about Social Security disability benefits in general, ask Social Security for a copy of the booklet *Disability* (Publication No. 05-10029).

How Much Will Your Benefits Be?

How much your Social Security benefit will be depends on your earnings history. Generally, higher earnings translate into higher

Social Security benefits. You can find out how much you will get by contacting Social Security and asking for an estimate of your benefits. We'll give you a form you can use to send for a free statement that contains a record of your earnings and an estimate of your benefits.

In addition to checking your benefit, we encourage you to use this statement to verify that your earnings have been properly recorded in our files. It's important that you do this because any missing or unreported wages could lower your Social Security benefit or even prevent you from qualifying for disability benefits. If you find a problem, contact your local Social Security office right away, show them proof of your actual wages, and the record will be corrected. **This can be particularly important for people who have tested positive for HIV but have not developed symptoms, so that any potential benefits will not be delayed by wage correction efforts.**

Disabled widows, widowers and children eligible for benefits as a dependent on a spouse's or parent's Social Security record receive an amount that is a percentage of the worker's Social Security benefit.

Supplemental Security Income: The Nonmedical Rules of Eligibility

SSI is a program that pays monthly benefits to people with low incomes and limited assets who are 65 or older, or blind or disabled.

As its name implies, Supplemental Security Income **supplements** a person's income up to a certain level that can go up every year based on cost-of-living adjustments. The level varies from one state to another, so check with your local Social Security office to find out more about SSI benefit levels in your state.

We don't count all the income you have when we figure out if you qualify for SSI. And if you work, there are special rules we use for counting your wages. Again, check with Social Security to find out if you can get SSI.

In addition to rules about income, people on SSI must have limited assets. Generally, individuals with assets under $2,000, or couples with assets under $3,000, can qualify for SSI. However, when we figure your assets, we don't count such items as your home, your car (unless it's an expensive one) and most of your personal belongings.

Your Social Security office can tell you more about the income and asset limits. For more general information, ask for a copy of the booklet *SSI* (Publication No. 05-11000).

355

How Does Social Security Define Disability?

In this section, we'll explain the criteria you must meet in order to be considered "disabled." First, we'll explain in general terms how Social Security defines and determines disability. Then we'll discuss how it applies to people with HIV infection.

The General Definition of Disability

Disability under Social Security is based on your inability to work because of a medical condition. You will be considered disabled if you are unable to do any kind of "substantial" work for which you are suited. (Usually, monthly earnings of $500 or more are considered substantial.) Your inability to work must be expected to last at least a year. Or, the condition that keeps you from working must be so severe that you are not expected to live.

For children, we decide if the condition results in marked and severe functional limitations. The condition must have lasted or be expected to last for at least 12 months or be so severe that the child is not expected to live.

How This Definition of Disability Applies to People with HIV Infection

A person with symptomatic HIV infection is often severely limited in his or her ability to work. In other words, if the evidence shows that you have symptomatic HIV infection that severely limits your ability to work, and if you meet the other eligibility factors, the chances are very good that you will be able to receive Social Security or SSI benefits.

On the other hand, some people with HIV infection may be less impaired and able to work, so they may not be eligible for disability.

How Does Social Security Evaluate Your Disability?

Social Security works with an agency in each state, usually called a Disability Determination Service (DDS), to evaluate disability claims. At the DDS, a disability evaluation specialist and a doctor follow a step-by-step process that applies to all disability claims, thus assuring a consistent national approach to evaluating disability.

First, the DDS specialists decide whether your impairment is "severe." This simply means the evidence must show that your disability interferes with your ability to work.

The next step in the process is deciding whether the disability is included in a list of impairments. This list describes, for each of the major body systems, impairments that are considered severe enough to prevent an adult from doing any substantial work, or in the case of children under the age of 18, impairments that result in marked and severe functional limitations.

Recently we published a list of impairments for HIV infections. In this list, we have included many conditions associated with symptomatic HIV infection, including some that specifically apply to women and children with HIV infection.

Some of the HIV-related conditions included in the HIV list of impairments are shown below. The level of severity that an impairment must meet to be found disabling are also specified in the regulations.

- Pulmonary tuberculosis resistant to treatment

- Kaposi's sarcoma

- *Pneumocystis carinii* pneumonia (PCP)

- Carcinoma of the cervix

- Herpes Simplex

- Hodgkin's disease and all lymphomas

- HIV Wasting Syndrome

- Syphilis and Neurosyphilis

- Candidiasis

- Histoplasmosis

Remember: these are just a few examples. You can see a complete list of HIV-related impairments at any Social Security office. The complete list will also include the findings necessary for listed impairments to be considered disabling by Social Security.

If you have symptoms of HIV infection that are not specifically included in (or equal in severity to) the impairments on our list, then DDS disability specialists will look at how frequently these conditions occur and how they affect your ability to function.

The DDS team will evaluate how well you function in three general areas: daily activities; social functioning; and the ability to complete tasks in a timely manner, which requires the ability to maintain concentration, persistence and pace.

If you have "marked limitations" in any one of these functional areas and repeated manifestations of HIV meeting the criteria in the listings, you may be found disabled. A marked limitation is one that seriously interferes with your ability to function independently, appropriately and effectively. It does not mean that you must be confined to bed, hospitalized or in a nursing home.

If the specialists decide that you are not disabled at this point because you do not have a condition that exactly matches or is equal in severity to one on our list and you are an adult, then they will look to see if your condition prevents you from doing the work you normally do. If it does not, your claim will be denied. If it does' your claim will be considered further. We then look to see if you can do any other type of work based on your age, education, past work experience and transferable skills. If you cannot do any other kind of work, your claim will be approved. If you can, your claim will be denied.

Remember, at all steps in the process, your impairment must be documented. Documentation includes medical records from your doctors, as well as laboratory test results, X-ray reports etc. The HIV infection itself—that is, the presence of the virus—must be documented as well as any HIV-related manifestations. At all steps in the process it is important that we have evidence of signs, symptoms and laboratory findings associated with HIV infection, as well as information on how well you are able to function day-to-day. The signs and symptoms may include: repeated infections; fevers/night sweats; enlarged lymph nodes, liver or spleen; lower energy or generalized weakness; dyspnea on exertion; persistent cough; depression/anxiety; headache; anorexia; nausea and vomiting; and side effects of medication and/or treatment, as well as how your treatment affects your daily activities.

Evaluation of HIV Infection in Women

Statistics show that there is an increasing number of women with HIV diseases. Social Security's guidelines for the immune system recognize that HIV infection can show up differently in women than in men. In addition to following the criteria outlined in the previous section, DDS disability evaluators consider specific criteria for diseases common in women. These include: vulvovaginal candidiasis (yeast infection); genital herpes; pelvic inflammatory disease (PID); invasive cervical cancer; genital ulcerative disease; and condyloma (genital warts caused by the human papillomavirus). Again, the level of severity necessary for these impairments to be considered disabling is included in the list of impairments.

Evaluation of HIV Infection in Children

We also have separate listings for children with HIV infection. These guidelines recognize the fact that the course of the disease in children can differ from adults. In order to be found disabled, a child must have a condition that exactly matches or is equal in severity to either the adult or childhood HIV listing or another impairment found in the list of impairments.

For more information about disability benefits for children, ask Social Security for a copy of the booklet *Social Security And SSI Benefits For Children With Disabilities* (Publication No. 05-10026).

How Do You File for Disability Benefits?

You apply for Social Security and SSI disability benefits by calling or visiting any Social Security office. All Social Security files are kept strictly confidential. It would help if you have certain documents with you when you apply. But don't delay filing because you don't have all the information you need. We'll help you get the rest of it after you sign up. The information you'll need may include:

- your Social Security number and birth certificate;

- the Social Security numbers and birth certificates for family members signing up on your record; and

- a copy of your most recent W-2 form (or your tax return if you're self-employed).

If you're signing up for SSI, you will need to provide records that show that your income and assets are below the SSI limits. This might include such things as bank statements, rent receipts, car registration, etc.

You'll also need to give us information about how your condition affects your daily activities, the names and addresses of your doctors and clinics where you've received treatment and a summary of the kind of work you've done in the last 15 years. If you have medical evidence such as reports of blood tests, laboratory work or a physical, it would be helpful if you brought them with you. Below we give you some guidelines for providing us with medical and vocational information that will help speed up your claim. But first we want you to know what Social Security does to make the process work as smoothly as possible.

359

What Steps Has Social Security Taken to Ensure Prompt Processing and Payment of Disability Benefits?

All HIV infection claims are given prompt attention and priority handling. For many people applying for SSI with a medical diagnosis of symptomatic HIV infection, the law allows us to **presume** they are disabled. This permits us to pay up to six months of benefits pending a final decision on the claim. You will qualify for this immediate payment if:

- a medical source confirms that the HIV infection is severe enough to meet SSA's criteria;

- you meet the other SSI nonmedical eligibility requirements; and

- you are not doing "substantial" work.

If you have symptomatic HIV infection but the local Social Security office cannot provide immediate payment, a disability evaluation specialist at the DDS may still make a "presumptive" disability decision at any point in the process where the evidence suggests a high likelihood that your claim will be approved. (If we later decide you are not disabled, you will **not** have to pay back the money you received.)

Special arrangements have been made with a number of AIDS service organizations, advocacy groups and medical facilities to help us get the evidence we need to streamline the claims process. And many DDS's have Medical/Professional Relations Officers who work directly with these organizations to make this process work smoothly.

What You Can Do to Expedite the Processing of Your Claim

You can play an active and important role in ensuring that your claim is processed accurately and quickly. The best advice we can give you is to keep thorough records that document the symptoms of your illness and how it affects your daily activities, and then to provide all of this information to Social Security when you file your claim.

- **Document the symptoms of your illness early and often.**
  Use a calendar to jot down brief notes about how you feel on each day. Record any of your usual activities you could not do on any given day. Be specific. And don't forget to include any psychological or mental problems.

- **Help your doctor help you.** Not all doctors may be aware of all the kinds of information we need to document your disability. Ask your doctor or other health care professional to track the course of your symptoms in detail over time and to keep a thorough record of any evidence of fatigue, depression, forgetfulness, dizziness and other hard-to-document symptoms.

- **Keep records of how your illness affected you on the job.** If you were working, but lost your job because of your illness, make notes that describe what it is about your condition that forced you to stop working.

- **Give us copies of all these records when you file.** In addition to these records, be sure to list the names, addresses and phone numbers of all the doctors, clinics and hospitals you have been to since your illness began. Include your patient or treatment identification number if you know it. Also include the names, addresses and phone numbers of any other people who have information about your illness.

Helping You Return to Work

If you return to work, Social Security has a number of special rules, called "work incentives," that provide cash benefits and continued Medicare or Medicaid coverage while you work. They are particularly important to people with HIV disease who, because of the recurrent nature of HIV-related illnesses, may be able to return to work following periods of disability.

The rules are different for Social Security and SSI beneficiaries. For people getting Social Security disability benefits, they include a nine-month "trial work period" during which earnings, no matter how much, will not affect benefit payments; and a three-year guarantee that, if benefits have stopped because a person remains employed after the trial work period, a Social Security check will be paid for any month earnings are below the "substantial" level (generally $500). In addition, Medicare coverage extends through the three-year timeframe after the trial work period, even if your earnings are substantial.

SSI work incentives include continuation of Medicaid coverage even if earnings are too high for SSI payments to be made, help with setting up a "plan to achieve self-support" (PASS), and special consideration for pay received in a sheltered workshop so that SSI benefits may continue even though the earnings might normally prevent payments.

These and other work incentives are explained in detail in the publication *Working While Disabled...How We Can Help* (Publication No. 05-10095). For a free copy, just call or visit your nearest Social Security office.

What You Need to Know about Medicaid and Medicare

Medicaid and Medicare are our country's two major government-run health insurance programs. Generally, people on SSI and other people with low incomes qualify for Medicaid, while Medicare coverage is earned by working in jobs covered by Social Security, for a railroad or for the federal government. Many people qualify for both Medicare and Medicaid.

Medicaid Coverage

In most states, Social Security's decision that you are eligible for SSI also makes you eligible for Medicaid coverage. (Check with your local Social Security or Medicaid office to verify the requirements in your state.)

State Medicaid programs are required to cover certain services, including inpatient and outpatient hospital care and physician services. States have the option to include other services, such as intermediate care, hospice care, private duty nursing and prescribed drugs.

For more information about Medicaid, contact your local Medicaid agency.

Medicare Coverage

If you get Social Security disability, you will qualify for Medicare coverage 24 months after the month you became entitled to those benefits. Medicare helps pay for:

- inpatient and outpatient hospital care;

- doctor's services;

- diagnostic tests;

- skilled nursing care;

- home health visits;

- hospice care;

- and other medical services.

For more information about Medicare, call or visit your local Social Security office to ask for the booklet *Medicare* (Publication No. 05-10043).

Help for Low-Income Medicare Beneficiaries

If you get Medicare and have low income and few resources, your state may pay your Medicare premiums and, in some cases, other "out-of-pocket" Medicare expenses such as deductibles and coinsurance. Only your state can decide if you qualify. To find out if you do, contact your state or local welfare office or Medicaid agency. For more general information about the program, contact Social Security and ask for the leaflet *Medicare Savings For Qualified Beneficiaries* (HCFA Publication No. 02184).

For More Information

You can get recorded information about Social Security coverage 24 hours a day, including weekends and holidays, by calling Social Security's toll-free number, **1-800-772-1213**. You can speak to a service representative between the hours of 7 a.m. and 7 p.m. on business days. Our lines are busiest early in the week and early in the month so, if your business can wait, it's best to call at other times. Whenever you call, have your Social Security number handy.

People who are deaf or hard of hearing may call our toll-free "TTY" number, 1-800-325-0778, between 7 a.m. and 7 p.m. on business days.

Social Security information also is available to users of the Internet. Type http://www.ssa.gov to access Social Security information.

The Social Security Administration treats all calls confidentially — whether they're made to our toll-free numbers or to one of our local offices. We also want to ensure that you receive accurate and courteous service. That is why we have a second Social Security representative monitor some incoming and outgoing telephone calls.

Chapter 41

Viatical Settlements

If you have a terminal illness—or if you are caring for someone who is terminally ill—chances are you're giving a great deal of thought to time and money. You may be thinking about life insurance, too. It's in that context that you may hear the phrases *accelerated benefits* and *viatical settlements*.

Accelerated benefits sometimes are called "living benefits." They are the proceeds of life insurance policies that are paid by the insurer to policyholders before they die. Occasionally, these benefits are included in policies when they are sold, but usually, they are offered as riders or attachments to new or existing policies.

Viatical settlements involve the sale of a life insurance policy. If you have a terminal illness, you may consider selling your policy to a viatical settlement company for a lump sum cash payment. In a viatical settlement transaction, people with terminal illnesses assign their life insurance policies to viatical settlement companies in exchange for a percentage of the policy's face value. The viatical settlement company, in turn, may sell the policy to a third-party investor. The viatical settlement company or the investor becomes the beneficiary to the policy, pays the premiums, and collects the face value of the policy after the original policyholder dies.

The fact is that any decisions affecting life insurance benefits can have a profound financial and emotional impact on dependents, friends, and care-givers. Before you make any major changes regarding your

An undated publication of the Federal Trade Commission (FTC); included in the FTC's current "Best Sellers," Public Reference publication list.

policy, talk to someone whose advice and expertise you can count on—
a lawyer, an accountant, or a good friend.

Investigate Your Options

Options exist for people with terminal illnesses when financial
needs are critical. For example, you may consider a loan from the original beneficiary of your life insurance policy, accelerated benefits on
your life insurance policy, or a viatical settlement.

Many life insurance policies in force nationwide now include an
accelerated benefits provision. Companies offer anywhere from 25 to
100 percent of the death benefit as early payment, but policyholders
can collect these payments only under very specific circumstances.
The amount and the method of payment vary with the policy.

Indeed, if you own a life insurance policy, call your insurance agent
or company to find out about your alternatives. Ask whether your life
insurance policy allows for accelerated benefits or loans, and how much
it will cost. Some insurers add accelerated benefits to life insurance
policies for an additional premium, usually computed as a percentage of the base premium. Others offer the benefits at no extra premium, but charge the policyholder for the option if and when it is used.
In most cases, the insurance company will reduce the benefits advanced to the policyholder before death to compensate for the interest it will lose on its early payout. There also may be a service charge.

In addition, you may consider selling your life insurance policy to
a viatical settlement company, a private enterprise that offers a terminally ill person a percentage of the policy's face value. It is not considered an insurance company.

The viatical settlement company becomes the sole beneficiary of
the policy in consideration for delivering a cash payment to the policyholder and paying the premiums. When the policyholder dies, the
viatical settlement company collects the face value of the policy.

Viatical settlements are complex legal and financial transactions.
They require time and attention from physicians, life insurance
companies, lawyers, and accountants or financial planners. The entire transfer process can take up to four months to complete.

Eligibility for Viatical Settlements

Each viatical settlement company sets its own rules for determining which life insurance policies it will buy. For example, viatical
settlement companies may want to know that:

- you've owned your policy for at least two years;
- your policy has a reasonably large face value;
- you have a waiver from current or potential beneficiaries; and
- you are terminally ill. Usually, this means that death is expected to occur within two years.

Investors may insist that your policy be from a company that is large or well-known and one that will be able to pay the death benefit. If your life insurance policy was provided by your employer, investors also will want to know if it can be converted into an individual policy or otherwise be guaranteed to remain in force before it can be assigned. Finally, investors probably will ask you to release all your medical records to them.

Financial Implications

If you sell your policy to a viatical settlement company, you may owe federal capital gains tax on the difference between the payment you receive and the amount you've paid in premiums. You also may owe state tax, although several states, including California and New York, have made these settlements tax-free.

Collecting accelerated benefits or making a viatical settlement also may affect your eligibility for public assistance programs based on financial need, such as Medicaid. The federal government does not require policyholders either to choose accelerated benefits or cash in their policies before qualifying for Medicaid benefits. But once the policyholder cashes in the policy and receives a payment, the money may be counted as income for Medicaid purposes and may affect eligibility.

The Congress is currently considering a proposal to change the tax code so that accelerated benefits and viatical settlements would be excluded from taxes. Your lawyer or accountant will be able to tell you the tax status of these payments. Up to now, payments of accelerated benefits from an insurance company have been tax-exempt in some states. Because viatical settlement companies are not considered insurance companies, viatical payments generally have not been exempt from taxes in most states.

Guidelines for Consumers

The daily physical and emotional demands of a terminal illness can be overwhelming, and financial burdens can seem insurmountable.

367

If you are considering making a viatical settlement on your life insurance policy—or if you are helping someone with this decision—these consumer guidelines should help you avoid costly mistakes and make the choice that's right.

- Contact two or three viatical settlement companies to make sure offers are competitive, and be aware of prevailing discount rates. A viatical settlement company may pay 60 percent of the face value of a policy to a person whose life expectancy is two years or less, and 80 percent to someone whose life expectancy is six months or less.

- Check with your state insurance department to see if viatical settlement companies or brokers must be licensed. If so, check the status of the companies with whom you are considering doing business.

- Don't fall for high pressure tactics. You don't have to accept an offer, and you can change your mind. Some states require a 15-day cooling off period before any viatical settlement transaction is complete.

- Verify that the investor or the company has the money for your payout readily available. Large companies may have cash on hand; smaller ones may have uneven cash flows or may be "shopping" the policy to third parties.

- Ask the company to set up an escrow account with a reputable financial institution at the beginning of the transfer so you can be sure the funds are available to cover the offer.

- Insist on a timely payment. No more than a few months should elapse from the initial contact with the company to closing. Check with your state attorney general's office or department of insurance to see if there are complaints against the company *before* you do business.

- Ask the company about possible tax consequences and implications for public assistance benefits. Some states require viatical settlement companies to make these disclosures and tell you about other options that may be available from your life insurance company.

- Ask about privacy. Some companies may not protect a policyholder's privacy when they act as brokers for payouts from potential investors.

- Contact a lawyer to check on the possible probate and estate considerations. If you make a viatical settlement, there will be no life insurance benefits for the person you originally designated as beneficiary.

For More Information

Any decision that affects your life insurance benefits can affect the people who care for and about you. Before you make a decision, talk to someone you trust—a lawyer, an accountant, or a good friend. You also may want to contact the following organizations for more information.

Affording Care
429 E. 52nd Street, Unit 4-G
New York City, NY 10022-6431

American Council of Life Insurance
1001 Pennsylvania Avenue, N.W.
Washington, D.C. 20004-2599

National Association of Insurance Commissioners
444 North Capitol Street, N.W.
Washington, D.C. 20001

National Association of People With AIDS
1413 K Street, N.W.
Washington, D.C. 20005

National Viatical Association
7910 Woodmont Ave., Suite 1430
Bethesda, MD 20814

North American Securities Administrators Association
555 New Jersey Avenue, N.W.
Washington, D.C. 20001

Viatical Association of America
1200 19th Street, N.W., Suite 300
Washington, D.C. 20036

Your State Attorney General
Office of Consumer Protection
Your State Capital

Your State Insurance Commissioner
Department of Insurance
Your State Capital

The Federal Trade Commission

(FTC) is an independent agency that seeks to protect the public against unfair, deceptive, and fraudulent advertising and marketing practices through law enforcement and education efforts. For a complete list of free FTC publications, write:

Best Sellers, Public Reference
Federal Trade Commission
Washington, D.C. 20580
(202) 326-2222
For TDD, call (202) 326-2502

Or use the Internet for on-line access to FTC consumer and business publications. The FTC ConsumerLine is located on the Internet at CONSUMER. FTC.GOV or through the World Wide Web at http://www.ftc.gov.

Part Four

HIV/AIDS Prevention

Chapter 42

HIV Infection: Progress Review

Highlights

* Perinatally-acquired AIDS cases decreased by 27 percent from 1992 to 1995.

* the number of deaths from AIDS decreased 19 percent overall in the first nine months of 1996 compared with the some period of 1995.

* AIDS is now the leading cause of death for people aged 25-44.

* Use of a triple drug treatment regimen including protease inhibitors has had a dramatic effect in prolonging the lives of some AIDS patients. However, application of this regimen has not been uniform in all communities.

* The cost of this combination antiretroviral therapy is conservatively estimated at $10,000-$12,000 per year per patient.

* Early in the decade, women made up 10 percent of the population infected with HIV; the proportion has now risen to 20 percent. In 1990, approximately 30 percent of new cases of HIV infection occurred in blacks; this increased to 41 percent in 1996.

* Injecting drug use is directly or indirectly associated with one-third of AIDS cases in the U.S.

Healthy People 2000, "Progress Review: HIV Infection," U.S. Department of Health and Human Services (DHHS), Public Health Service, July 8, 1997.

- An estimated 40 percent of people at risk for HIV/AIDS have not been tested for infection.

- Approximately 70 percent of people in prison today have a history of injecting drug use or substance abuse, factors which place them at high risk of having contracted HIV infection.

Review

The Acting Assistant Secretary for Health chaired a review of progress on Healthy People 2000 objectives related to preventing and controlling HIV infection. The Centers for Disease Control and Prevention (CDC), as lead agency for this priority area, presented a report on trends, surveillance, prevention, care and treatment, as well as research issues. The status of objectives for which there have been recent updates is as follows:

18.1. The incidence of AIDS cases per 100,000 in the total population declined from 29.8 in 1994 to 28.6 in 1995, continuing a downward trend which began in 1993. Among targeted sub-groups, a decline in incidence was recorded for blacks (from 102.9 in 1994 to 100.5 in 1995) and for Hispanics (from 49.4 to 47.1.) In women, however, the incidence rose from 10.9 in 1994 to 11.2 in 1995. The number of new AIDS cases reported in men who have sex with men declined from 34,146 in 1994 to 30,696 in 1995. Among injecting drug users, the number of new cases declined from 20,734 in 1994 to 19,100 in 1995. These data are by year of diagnosis, adjusted for delays in reporting and under-reporting.

18.3. Among 15-year old adolescents, the proportion of females who reported having had sexual intercourse declined from 27 percent in 1988, to 22 percent in 1995; the proportion of males declined from 33 percent in 1988 to 27 percent in 1995. The year 2000 target is 15 percent. Among 17-year olds, the proportion of females remained much the same—50 percent in 1988 and 51 percent in 1995. The target is 40 percent. Supplemental data for in-school adolescents show mixed trends.

18.4. Condom use at last sexual intercourse has increased. Among sexually active unmarried females aged 15-44, use increased from 19 percent in 1988 to 25 percent in 1995. The target is 50 percent. Among black females, use doubled from 12.4 percent in 1988 to 25 percent in 1995. The target is 75 percent. Among sexually active young women aged 15-19 in grades 9-12, use increased from 40 percent in 1990 to

49 percent in 1995. The target is 60 percent. Among sexually active males aged 15-19 in grades 9-12, use increased from 49 percent in 1990 percent in 1990 to 61 percent in 1995. The target is 75 percent. It is understood that condom use is by the partner in the percentages reported for females.

18.5. In 1995, 34.1 percent of injecting drug users were in treatment, a decline from 47.8 percent in 1994. The target is 50 percent.

18.6. The percentage of injecting drug users in treatment in 1992-96 who did not share needles was estimated as 60 percent. The target is 75 percent.

18.8. For 83 percent of all positive HIV tests in 1995, the people tested returned for counseling. Some people may have been tested more than once. This exceeds the target of 80 percent.

18.10. In 1994, 86 percent of middle and senior high schools provided instruction about HIV prevention in required courses; 84 percent provided instruction about STD prevention in required courses. The target is to have 95 percent of schools offer at least one STD class.

18.11. In 1995, 49.1 percent of students at colleges and universities were given AIDS or HIV infection prevention information; 43.4 percent received STD prevention information; and 41.4 percent were taught about AIDS or HIV in a college class. The target is 90 percent in each category.

18.13. In 1994, 81.8 percent of Title X funded family planning clinics provided pretest counseling on HIV to their clients, an increase from 66 percent in 1990. HIV testing for clients was provided by 73.5 percent of these clinics, compared with 60 percent in 1990.

18.15. The proportion of sexually active females aged 15-17 who, in 1995, reported abstaining from sexual intercourse for 3 months prior to the interview was 27 percent. Supplemental data indicate that 23 percent of in-school sexually active females aged 15-17 reported such abstention, as did 34 percent of in-school sexually active males aged 15-17. The target for males and females is 40 percent.

18.16. In 1995, 2 percent of small businesses (15-49 employees) and 25 percent of large businesses (750 or more employees) had comprehensive HIV/AIDS workplace programs that included policies, management training and employee education. The targets are 10 percent and 50 percent, respectively. The proportion of businesses having policies on HIV/AIDS in 1995 was as follows: small businesses, 18 percent; medium businesses (50-749 employees), 42 percent; large businesses, 79 percent. Management training in HIV/AIDS was provided in the following proportions: small businesses,18 percent; medium businesses, 41 percent; large businesses, 77 percent. The proportion offering employee education in HIV/AIDS was as follows: small businesses, 6 percent; medium businesses, 16 percent; large businesses, 32 percent.

Follow-up

- Focus efforts to prevent and control HIV/AIDS on population groups most at risk—adolescents, people in prison, women, injecting drug users, and racial/ethnic groups.

- Seek to increase the number of people who know their serostatus by encouraging those at high risk to be tested.

- Develop better linkages between prevention and care.

- Strengthen the public health infrastructure capacity to test for HIV infection and counsel and treat patients.

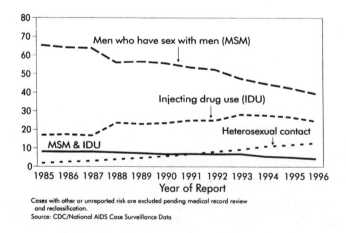

Cases with other or unreported risk are excluded pending medical record review and reclassification.
Source: CDC/National AIDS Case Surveillance Data

Figure 42.1. AIDS Cases by Exposure Category and Year of Report 1985-1996, United States (Percentage of Cases)

- Expand research efforts to develop less expensive AIDS medications that can be taken less frequently.

- Establish a comprehensive vaccine development strategy which takes account of genetic variability and provides for accelerated trials in the U.S. and abroad.

- Increase the availability and acceptability of female-controlled methods of HIV/AIDS prevention.

- Explore ways to demystify and destigmatize HIV/AIDS.

- Seek to implement a national HIV surveillance system which adequately addresses issues related to the use of identifiers in reporting of cases and, at the same time, ensures confidentiality.

- Pursue global collaboration in research on HIV/AIDS and dissemination of information about advances in methodologies of prevention and treatment.

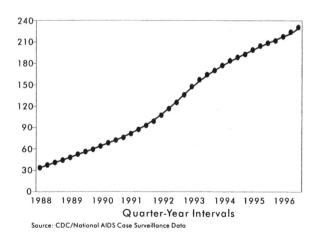

Source: CDC/National AIDS Case Surveillance Data

Figure 42.2. Adults and Adolescents Living with AIDS January 1988–September 1996. Adjusted For Reporting Delays, United States (Number In Thousands)

Chapter 43

Preparing for a New Era in HIV/AIDS Prevention

We have entered a new era in the HIV epidemic—both in terms of treatment and prevention. Dramatic progress has been made in preventing new infections and in slowing the progression of disease for those infected. From January through September 1996, the estimated number of deaths dropped 19%, from 37,900 to 30,700, versus the comparable 1995 period.

The decline in deaths likely reflects the impact of new combination therapies in lengthening the healthy lifespan of infected individuals and the slowing of the epidemic overall. HIV prevention efforts have contributed to a slowing in the spread of the disease, with annual increases in new AIDS cases in the U.S. dropping from over 85% in the mid-1980's to a current rate of less than 5% each year. In 1995, the increase in AIDS incidence slowed to only 2%. With sustained prevention and continued improvements in treatment for HIV infection, we may soon begin to see measurable declines in AIDS incidence.

The greatest successes have been seen among those at highest risk—gay and bisexual men—particularly those affected by the first wave of HIV infection. We saw signs of behavior change in this group in the late 1980's. Now we are seeing a slowing in the rate of new AIDS cases among gay men overall, and declines in new infections in some areas.

HIV prevention efforts are having an impact in many diverse areas of prevention. Communities across the U.S. are demonstrating

Statement from the Director, Centers for Disease Control and Prevention (CDC), July 14, 1997.

success in a number of areas. Condom use is increasing among some sexually-active young people, injecting drug users (IDUs) in some areas are reducing risky behaviors, and we have seen dramatic progress in preventing perinatal transmission.

But at least 40,000 new infections are occurring each year, and much work is left to be done. Nationwide, AIDS cases are now increasing most rapidly among women—particularly minorities. AIDS incidence in women now outpaces men, and heterosexual transmission is the fastest growing mode of transmission. Heterosexual AIDS cases are now growing at 15-20% a year, compared to increases of 5% or less among men-who-have-sex-with-men (MSM) and injecting drug users (IDUs).

Other troubling trends point to the need for increased efforts among young and minority gay and bisexual men—who remain at high risk. Recent studies have found that as many as 5-9% of young gay and bisexual men ages 15-22 may be infected in many areas.

HIV has evolved from a period of explosive growth in a few geographic areas, primarily among gay and bisexual men and IDUs, to the development of diverse local subepidemics, where the dynamics of HIV vary by community and region. So, while communities will face many of the same concerns, programs must be locally designed to be relevant and effective. CDC's challenge will be to ensure each community has the tools to address the evolving epidemic and the unique challenges facing the community.

This is a time of renewed optimism in the fight against AIDS. Yet with these prevention and treatment advances, we also face new challenges—challenges that must be met, if we are to preserve the progress made.

First, AIDS prevalence has increased 10% since mid-1995. If the number of new HIV infections each year remains stable or increases, and HIV-related deaths continue to decrease, there will be an increasing number of people living with HIV and AIDS. Consequently, additional resources will be needed to provide these individuals quality services, treatment, and care.

Second, to continue to provide the necessary data to plan, direct, and evaluate HIV prevention efforts, HIV/AIDS surveillance systems must adapt to changes in medical practices which increase survival following diagnosis of HIV or AIDS. If progression to AIDS is successfully delayed for an increasing number of individuals, AIDS case reports may no longer provide a reliable indication of trends in the epidemic and will underrepresent the need for treatment services and care. Surveillance systems will therefore need to improve methods to monitor the number of individuals with living with HIV infection.

And finally, as we continue to work to develop better treatment options, we must not lose sight of the fact that preventing HIV infection is the only way to reduce the burden of this disease. Targeted, sustained prevention reduces the number of people who need to undergo complex, costly treatment regimens.

To this point, as the epidemic has evolved, so must prevention. Prevention in this era of continuous and incremental advances in science will become more complex than ever before. After 15 years of planning, implementing, and evaluating efforts to stem the HIV epidemic, we know that preventing HIV infection depends not only on studying and implementing biomedical interventions to thwart the virus, but even more upon influencing millions of individuals in diverse populations to adopt or maintain safe behaviors. As we move forward scientifically, we must be attuned to how these advances are communicated and influence people's perceptions of risk and their attendant behaviors.

It is essential that individuals at risk for HIV infection continue to protect themselves through safer behaviors. Available therapies are complex, and a great deal of uncertainties remain about long-term effectiveness, safety, and the possibility of resistance. New options offer great hope for those already infected, but HIV remains a life-threatening infection that can and should be prevented.

Progress in both treatment and prevention will be incremental during the next era of this epidemic. While we have made significant progress in fighting this disease, a great deal remains unknown about the specific mechanisms of infection, and disease progression from the time of HIV infection to development of illness. As our understanding advances, the public must receive accurate and timely information. But both scientists and the media must be careful to communicate these advances along with the cautionary notes.

For example, the next communication challenge in this era of prevention will stem from the possibility of a medical regimen to reduce the chance of HIV infection after a sexual or drug-related exposure to HIV (post-exposure prophylaxis or PEP). While no data currently exist about the effectiveness of PEP for these types of exposures, scientists and medical experts are now discussing the possibilities. At this point, there are more questions than answers. As these discussions evolve, communication must be clear, so that people do not see PEP as a means of primary prevention. While such a therapy may reduce infections in isolated situations, taking a chance on a complex and costly drug regimen after exposure should not take the place of adopting and maintaining behaviors that can prevent HIV exposure in the first place.

We hope that progress in this and other areas of HIV prevention and treatment over the next decade will be dramatic, and that advances will continue to be made. To meet this challenge, CDC is committed to maintaining a comprehensive approach to HIV prevention, including providing the best available epidemiological and behavioral data, conducting prevention research to develop new tools and methods for prevention, and working with communities to ensure that scientific advances and lessons learned are applied to designing effective prevention programs. And as we enter a new era in combating this epidemic, we must fight the disease on multiple levels—but remember that it is always better to prevent than to treat this disease.

—Statement from Helene Gayle, M.D., M.P.H. Director,
National Center for HIV, STD, and TB Prevention,
Centers for Disease Control and Prevention (CDC).

Chapter 44

Combating Complacency in HIV Prevention

In the United States, complacency about the need for HIV prevention may be among the strongest barriers communities face as they plan to meet the next century's prevention needs. The great success that many people, but not all, have had with new highly active antiretroviral therapies (HAART, also known as drug "cocktails") and the resulting decline in the number of newly reported AIDS cases and deaths are indeed good news. The underlying reality, however, is that the HIV epidemic in our country is far from over. This is true not only for the nation, but for the continuing number of HIV-infected individuals who now must face years—perhaps a lifetime—of multiple daily medications, possible unpleasant or severe side effects, and great expense associated with the medicines needed to suppress HIV and prevent opportunistic infections.

The success of HAART is good news for the people living longer, better lives because of it, but the availability of treatment may lull people into believing that preventing HIV infection is no longer important. This complacency about the need for prevention adds a new dimension of complexity for both program planners and individuals at risk.

- While the number of AIDS cases is declining, the number of people *living* with HIV infection is growing. This increased prevalence of HIV in the population means that even more prevention efforts are needed, not fewer. For individuals at risk, increased

CDC Update, National Center for HIV, STD, and TB Prevention, June 1998.

prevalence means that each risk behavior carries an increased risk for infection. This makes the danger of relaxing preventive behaviors greater than ever.

- Past prevention efforts have resulted in behavior change for many individuals and have helped slow the epidemic overall. However, many studies find that high-risk behaviors, especially unprotected sex, are continuing at far too high a rate. This is true even for some people who have been counseled and tested for HIV, including those found to be infected.

- The long-term effectiveness of HAART is unknown. Further, HIV may develop resistance to these drugs. The powerful treatments are complicated and involve taking large numbers of pills. Even the most motivated patients may forget to take all their medications or skip doses. Some patients have been known to take "drug holidays," completely stopping their medications for a number of days or weeks. These drug treatments are less effective when treatment schedules are not followed. Diversions from the prescribed treatment regimen increase the possibility of drug resistance developing, which would greatly narrow future treatment options for those infected with a drug-resistant strain of HIV. And, if the development of drug-resistance is coupled with a relaxation in preventive behaviors, resistant strains could be transmitted to others and spread widely.

- Research among gay and bisexual men suggests that some individuals are less concerned about becoming infected than in the past and may be inclined to take more risks. This may be equally true in other groups at risk who might believe they no longer need to use condoms because protease inhibitors are so effective in treating HIV disease. The truth is, despite medical advances, HIV remains a serious and usually fatal disease that requires complex, costly, and difficult treatment regimens. These treatments don't work for everyone. Sometimes when they do work, they have unpleasant or intolerable side effects. Some people can't take them because the interaction with their other drugs causes serious problems. Still others find it extremely difficult to maintain the drug treatment schedules. As we continue working to develop better treatment options, we must not lose sight of the fact that preventing HIV infection in the first place precludes the need for people to follow these difficult regimens.

The Challenge of Monitoring the HIV/AIDS Epidemic

The "treatment effect" on trends in the AIDS epidemic not only increases our need for combating complacency, but means that we have never been closer to losing our ability to monitor the epidemic.

• Until recently, AIDS cases provided a reliable picture of trends in the HIV epidemic. Before highly effective treatments were available, researchers could take into account the time between HIV infection and progression to AIDS and estimate where and how many new infections were occurring based on observed cases of disease. Today, trends in AIDS cases and deaths may provide a valuable measure of groups for whom highly effective treatment is not available or has not succeeded. However, they no longer tell us enough about where and how many new infections are occurring—information critical for addressing the increasing need for prevention and treatment services. To allow the U.S. to target programs and resources most effectively, we must be able to keep pace with where the epidemic is going. This means we need to improve our ability to track early HIV infections, *before* they progress to AIDS.

Pay Attention to Prevention! It works...

Sustained, comprehensive prevention efforts begun in the 1980s have had a substantial impact on slowing the HIV/AIDS epidemic in our country. While it is difficult to measure prevention—or how many thousands of infections did not occur as a result of efforts to date—we know the epidemic was growing at rate of over 80% each year in the mid-1980s and has now stabilized. While the occurrence of approximately 40,000 new infections annually is deeply troubling, we have made tremendous progress. We also have more scientific evidence than ever before on which prevention programs are most effective. There is no question that prevention works and remains the best and most cost-effective approach for bringing the HIV/AIDS epidemic under control and saving lives.

HIV Prevention Programs Have Been Proven Effective

• Many studies indicate that prevention programs can contribute to changes in personal behavior that reduce risks of infection, and these changes are sustained over time. A 1997 scientific consensus conference sponsored by the National Institutes of

385

Health that reviewed existing data on the effectiveness of HIV behavioral interventions concluded that "behavioral interventions to reduce risk for HIV/AIDS are effective and should be disseminated widely."

- Comprehensive school-based HIV and sex education programs have been shown to delay the initiation of sexual intercourse, reduce the frequency of intercourse, reduce the number of sex partners, or increase the use of condoms or other contraceptives.

- Efforts to reduce risks of injection drug users through policy changes also have been evaluated and found to be very effective. For example, both New York and Connecticut reported significant reductions in the sharing of drug injection equipment after implementation of programs and policies that increased access to sterile injection equipment.

- Perinatal prevention programs that identify and treat pregnant women who are HIV infected have shown dramatic success in reducing HIV transmission to their babies.

- Screening the blood supply for HIV and heat-treating blood products for the treatment of hemophilia have nearly eliminated HIV transmission through these early transmission routes.

- Postexposure prophylaxis for health care workers has shown some success in reducing HIV transmission rates among those with occupational exposure to HIV-infected blood.

- Numerous HIV prevention programs have been shown to be cost-effective when compared against the resources required to treat and deliver HIV medical care to a person over the remaining years of their life. With the rising costs of lifetime treatment of HIV, effective prevention has become even more cost effective. New CDC estimates find that if only 1,255 infections are prevented each year, CDC's federally funded HIV prevention efforts in the United States are cost effective. If only 3,995 infections are prevented, our nation's investment in HIV prevention has actually saved money.

Comprehensive HIV Prevention Programs Work Best

- People with HIV risk behaviors need an array of prevention messages, skills, and support to help them reduce sexual and drug-related risks. Drug injectors, for example, not only need strategies to help them stop using drugs or sharing needles, but also need to learn ways to protect themselves from sexual transmission if their partner has ever injected drugs and may have shared needles.

- Substance use is a major problem in this country, and the intersection of substance use and sexual HIV transmission cannot be overlooked. Ideally, everyone who abuses any drug (including alcohol) should be offered counseling and treatment to help them stop using drugs and prevent HIV infection. HIV prevention interventions for the vast majority of substance users who are not in treatment also must address the sexual risks that are common among people who use drugs, including "crack" cocaine, marijuana, and alcohol.

- Each and every generation of young people needs comprehensive, sustained health information and interventions that help them develop life-long skills for avoiding behaviors that could lead to HIV infection. Such comprehensive programs should include the involvement of parents as well as educators. The most effective programs start at an early age and are designed to encourage the adoption of healthy behaviors, such as exercising and eating a healthy diet, and to prevent the initiation of unhealthy ones, such as drug use, excessive alcohol consumption, smoking, and premature sexual activity, before they start.

- Scientific studies show that treatment of other sexually transmitted diseases can greatly reduce the risk of transmitting and acquiring HIV.

The Many Dimensions of Prevention Provide Multiple Opportunities for Intervention

- *Primary HIV prevention* means keeping people from becoming infected with HIV in the first place. Interventions must focus not only on uninfected populations—there also is a major role for preventing further infections by focusing on infected individuals and helping them develop skills for reducing the risk of infecting others.

- *Secondary HIV prevention* means keeping people who already are HIV-infected safe and healthy by helping them avoid opportunistic infections and stopping the infection from progressing to AIDS.

- In all prevention efforts, there is a growing need to address the link between HIV treatment and prevention. In some cases, such as preventing perinatal transmission to infants by providing antiretroviral drugs to the mother, treatment is prevention. We also know that the treatment of other STDs can greatly reduce a person's risk for sexually acquired HIV infection. And, scientists even now are exploring the possibility that combination drug therapies may reduce infectivity. With the lines between prevention and treatment beginning to fade, ongoing services for people who are HIV positive must balance medical advances with the behavioral and social support needed to preserve their quality of life and prevent the spread of infection.

- We must maintain a focus on behavioral strategies. Even a vaccine doesn't stop a disease unless people use it—and in the case of HIV, a vaccine is unlikely to confer 100% lifelong immunity. Because no medical advance can succeed on its own, people must adapt their behaviors to work in tandem with it. To do this, they need several things:

  —*Access* to prevention services and new medical treatments. For example, pregnant women who may not know they are infected with HIV cannot reduce the risk of transmission to their children unless they first get prenatal care that includes routine HIV counseling and voluntary testing. Those found to be infected then must have access to antiretroviral drugs.

  —*Assistance in developing skills* to use new medical treatments. HAART, for example, involves complex treatment regimens and may require the development of compliance-related skills. For example, people may need to learn how to deal with side effects, what drug interactions might occur, how to lessen the risk of developing drug resistance, or how to cope with complicated schedules.

  —*Support and encouragement* from family, friends, care providers, and the community at large will help people make and sustain behavioral changes in their lives.

Today, more than ever, we must recognize that medical advances do not negate the need for preventing disease—in fact, the availability of newer and better treatments often *increases* the need for prevention. How well we continue our work to develop integrated approaches to prevention and treatment may well define the future course of the HIV pandemic.

Chapter 45

Condoms and Their Use in Preventing HIV Infection

With nearly 1 million Americans infected with HIV, most of them through sexual transmission, and an estimated 12 million cases of other sexually transmitted diseases (STDs) occurring each year in the United States, effective strategies for preventing these diseases are critical.

Refraining from having sexual intercourse with an infected partner is the best way to prevent transmission of HIV and other STDs. But for those who have sexual intercourse, latex condoms are highly effective when used consistently and correctly.

The correct and consistent use of latex condoms during sexual intercourse—vaginal, anal, or oral—can greatly reduce a person's risk of acquiring or transmitting STDs, including HIV infection. In fact, recent studies provide compelling evidence that latex condoms are highly effective in protecting against HIV infection when used for every act of intercourse.

This protection is most evident from studies of couples in which one member is infected with HIV and the other is not, i.e., "discordant couples." In a 2-year study of discordant couples in Europe, among 124 couples who reported consistent use of latex condoms, none of the uninfected partners became infected. In contrast, among the 121 couples who used condoms inconsistently, 12 (10 percent) of the uninfected partners became infected.

HIV/AIDS Prevention, Centers for Disease Control and Prevention (CDC), February 1996.

In another study, among a group of 134 discordant couples who did not use condoms at all or did not use them consistently, 16 partners (12 percent) became infected. This contrasts markedly with infections occurring in only 3 partners (2 percent) of the 171 couples in this study who reported consistently using condoms over the 2-year period.

What Is Consistent and Correct Condom Use?

Condoms must be used consistently and correctly to provide maximum protection. Consistent use means using a condom with each act of intercourse. Correct condom use includes all of the following steps:

- Use a new condom for each act of vaginal, anal, or oral intercourse.

- Put on the condom as soon as erection occurs and before any vaginal, anal, or oral contact with the penis.

- Hold the tip of the condom and unroll it onto the erect penis, leaving space at the tip of the condom, yet ensuring that no air is trapped in the condom's tip.

- Adequate lubrication is important to prevent condom breakage, but use only water-based lubricants, such as glycerine or lubricating jellies (which can be purchased at any pharmacy). Oil-based lubricants, such as petroleum jelly, cold cream, hand lotion, or baby oil, can weaken the condom.

- Withdraw from the partner immediately after ejaculation, holding the condom firmly to the base of the penis to keep it from slipping off.

Myths about Condoms

Misinformation and misunderstanding persist about condom effectiveness. The Centers for Disease Control and Prevention (CDC) provides the following updated information to address some common myths about condoms. This information is based on findings from recent epidemiologic, laboratory, and clinical studies.

Myth #1: Condoms Don't Work

Some persons have expressed concern about studies that report failure rates among couples using condoms for pregnancy prevention.

Analysis of these studies indicates that the large range of efficacy rates is related to incorrect or inconsistent use. In fact, latex condoms are highly effective for pregnancy prevention, but only when they are used properly. Research indicates that only 30 to 60 percent of men who claim to use condoms for contraception actually use them for every act of intercourse. Further, even people who use condoms every time may not use them correctly. Incorrect use contributes to the possibility that the condom could leak at the base or break.

Myth #2: Condoms Frequently Break

Some have questioned the quality of latex condoms. Condoms are classified as medical devices and are regulated by the Food and Drug Administration. Every latex condom manufactured in the United States is tested for defects before it is packaged. During the manufacturing process, condoms are double-dipped in latex and undergo stringent quality control procedures. Several studies clearly show that condom breakage rates in this country are less than 2 percent. Most of the breakage is likely due to incorrect usage rather than poor condom quality. Using oil-based lubricants can weaken latex, causing the condom to break. In addition, condoms can be weakened by exposure to heat or sunlight or by age, or they can be torn by teeth or fingernails.

Myth #3: HIV Can Pass through Condoms

A commonly held misperception is that latex condoms contain "holes" that allow passage of HIV. Laboratory studies show that intact latex condoms provide a highly effective barrier to sperm and microorganisms, including HIV and the much smaller hepatitis B virus.

Myth #4: Education about Condom Efficacy Promotes Sexual Activity

Five U.S. studies of specific sex education programs have demonstrated that HIV education and sex education which included condom information either had no effect upon the initiation of intercourse or resulted in delayed onset of intercourse; four studies of specific programs found that HIV/sex education did not increase frequency of intercourse, and a program that included resistance skills actually resulted in a decrease in the number of youth who initiated sex. In addition, a World Health Organization (WHO) review cited 19 studies of sex education programs that found no evidence that sex education leads to earlier or increased sexual activity in young people. In fact, five of the studies cited by WHO showed that such programs can lead to a delay or decrease in sexual activity.

In a recent study of youth in Switzerland, an AIDS prevention program focusing on condom use did not increase sexual activity or the number of sex partners. But condom use did increase among those who were already sexually active. A 1987 study of young U.S. men who were sent a pamphlet discussing STDs with an offer of free condoms did not find any increase in the youths' reported sexual activity.

Preventing HIV Infection and Other STDs

Recommended Prevention Strategies

Abstaining from sexual intercourse is the most effective HIV prevention strategy.

For individuals who are sexually active, the following are highly effective:

- Engaging in sexual activities that do not involve vaginal, anal, or oral intercourse

- Having intercourse only with one uninfected partner

- Using latex condoms correctly from start to finish with each act of intercourse

Other HIV Prevention Strategies

Condoms for Women

The female condom or vaginal pouch has recently become available in the United States. A small study of this condom as a contraceptive indicates a failure rate of 21-26 percent in 1 year among typical users; for those who use the female condom correctly and consistently, the rate was approximately 5 percent. Although laboratory studies indicate that the device serves as a mechanical barrier to viruses, further clinical research is necessary to determine its effectiveness in preventing transmission of HIV. If a male condom cannot be used, consider using a female condom.

Plastic Condoms

A polyurethane male condom was approved by FDA in 1991 and is now available in the United States. It is made of the same type of plastic as the female condom. The lab studies show that the new polyurethane condoms have the same barrier qualities as latex. Lab testing has shown that particles as small as sperm and HIV cannot pass through this polyurethane material. A study of the effectiveness of this polyurethane condom for prevention of pregnancy and STDs is underway. The new polyurethane condoms offer an alternative for condom users who are allergic to latex. Also, polyurethane condoms can be made thinner than latex, have no odor, and are safe for use with oil-based lubricants.

Spermicides

Although studies indicate that nonoxynol-9, a spermicide, inactivates HIV in laboratory testing, it is not clear whether spermicides used alone or with condoms during intercourse provide protection against HIV. Therefore, latex condoms with or without spermicides should be used to prevent sexual transmission of HIV.

Making Responsible Choices

In summary, sexually transmitted diseases, including HIV infection, are preventable. The effectiveness of responsible prevention strategies depends largely on the individual. Whatever strategy one chooses, its effectiveness will depend primarily on consistent adherence to that choice.

Chapter 46

The Role of Sexually Transmitted Disease Detection and Treatment in HIV Prevention

Testing and treatment of sexually transmitted diseases (STDs) can be an effective tool in preventing the spread of HIV, the virus that causes AIDS. Consequently, HIV programs and STD testing and treatment programs should develop strong linkages. This is especially important for programs targeting sexually active young women, who represent one of the fastest growing populations with AIDS.

What Is the Link between HIV and other STDs?

In the United States, the spread of HIV infection among women through sexual transmission has followed in the footsteps of other STD epidemics. For example, the geographic distribution of heterosexual HIV transmission in the South closely parallels that of syphilis. Most of the health districts with the highest rates of syphilis and gonorrhea are concentrated in the South, where HIV prevalence among childbearing women also is high.

Individuals who are infected with STDs are at least two to five times more likely than uninfected individuals to acquire HIV if exposed to the virus through sexual contact. In addition, if an HIV-infected individual also is infected with another STD, that person is substantially more likely than other HIV-infected persons to transmit HIV through sexual contact (Wasserheit, 1992).

CDC Update, National Center for HIV, STD, and TB Prevention, July 1998.

How Do STDs Facilitate HIV Infection?

There is substantial biological evidence demonstrating that the presence of other STDs increases the likelihood of both transmitting and acquiring HIV.

Increased Susceptibility

STDs probably increase susceptibility to HIV infection by two mechanisms. Genital ulcers (e.g., syphilis, herpes, or chancroid) result in breaks in the genital tract lining or skin. These breaks create a "portal of entry" for HIV. Non-ulcerative STDs (e.g., chlamydia, gonorrhea, and trichomoniasis) increase the concentration of cells in genital secretions that can serve as targets for HIV (e.g., CD4+ cells).

Increased Infectiousness

Studies have shown that when HIV-infected individuals are also infected with other STDs, they are more likely to have HIV in their genital secretions. For example, men who are infected with both gonorrhea and HIV are more than twice as likely to shed HIV in their genital secretions than are those who are infected only with HIV. Moreover, the median concentration of HIV in semen is as much as 10 times higher in men who are infected with both gonorrhea and HIV than in men infected only with HIV.

How Can STD Treatment Slow the Spread of HIV Infection?

New evidence from intervention studies indicates that detecting and treating STDs can substantially reduce HIV transmission at the individual and community levels.

STD Treatment Reduces an Individual's Ability to Transmit HIV

Studies have shown that treating STDs in HIV-infected individuals decreases both the amount of HIV they shed and how often they shed the virus.

STD Treatment Reduces the Spread of HIV Infection in Communities

Two community-level randomized trials have examined the role of STD treatment in HIV transmission. Together, their results have begun to clarify conditions under which STD treatment is likely to be most successful in reducing HIV transmission. First, *continuous* interventions to improve access to effective STD treatment services are likely to be more effective in reducing HIV transmission than *intermittent* interventions through strategies such as periodic mass treatment. Second, STD treatment is likely to be most effective in reducing HIV transmission where STD rates are high and the heterosexual HIV epidemic is young. Third, treatment of symptomatic STDs may be particularly important. The first trial, conducted in a rural area of Tanzania, demonstrated a decrease of about 40% in new heterosexually transmitted HIV infections in communities with continuous access to improved treatment of symptomatic STDs, as compared to communities with minimal STD services, where incidence remained about the same (Grosskurth et al., 1995). However, in the second trial conducted in Uganda, a reduction in HIV transmission was not demonstrated when the STD control approach was community-wide mass treatment administered to everyone every 10 months in the absence of ongoing access to improved STD services (Wawer, 1998).

What Does This Mean for HIV Prevention Programs?

Strong STD prevention, testing, and treatment can play a vital role in comprehensive programs to prevent sexual transmission of HIV. Furthermore, STD trends can offer important insights into where the HIV epidemic may grow, making STD surveillance data helpful in forecasting where HIV rates are likely to increase. Better linkages are needed between HIV and STD prevention efforts nationwide in order to control both epidemics.

In the context of persistently high prevalence of STDs in many parts of the United States and with emerging evidence that the U.S. HIV epidemic increasingly is affecting population groups with the highest rates of curable STDs, CDC's Advisory Committee on HIV and STD Prevention (ACHSP) has recommended the following:

- Early detection and treatment of curable STDs should become a major, explicit component of comprehensive HIV prevention programs at national, state, and local levels.

- In areas where STDs that facilitate HIV transmission are prevalent, screening and treatment programs should be expanded.

- HIV and STD prevention programs in the United States, along with private and public sector partners, should take joint responsibility for implementing this strategy.

The ACHSP also notes that early detection and treatment of STDs should be only one component of a comprehensive HIV prevention program, which also must include a range of social, behavioral, and biomedical interventions.

References

CDC. 1998. HIV prevention through early detection and treatment of other sexually transmitted diseases—United States Recommendations of the Advisory Committee for HIV and STD Prevention.

Grosskurth H, et al. 1995. "Impact of improved treatment of sexually transmitted diseases on HIV infection in rural Tanzania: randomized controlled trial." In: *The Lancet*, 346:530-36.

Kassler W, et al. STD control for HIV prevention in the U.S.: Is there likely to be an impact? [Abstract No. 33238]. In: *Conference Supplement of the 12th World AIDS Conference*. Geneva, Switzerland, June 28-July 3, 1998.

Wawer MJ. The Rakai randomized, community-based trial of STD control for AIDS prevention: no effect on HIV incidence despite reductions in STDs [Abstract No. 12473]. In: *Conference Supplement of the 12th World AIDS Conference*. Geneva, Switzerland, June 28-July 3, 1998.

Institute of Medicine. 1997. *The Hidden Epidemic: Confronting Sexually Transmitted Diseases*. Washington, DC: National Academy Press.

Wasserheit JN. 1992. "Epidemiologic synergy: Interrelationships between human immunodeficiency virus infection and other sexually transmitted diseases. " *Sexually Transmitted Diseases* 9:61-77.

Chapter 47

Interventions to Prevent
HIV Risk Behaviors

Abstract

Objective

To provide health care providers, patients, and the general public with a responsible assessment of behavioral intervention methods that may reduce the risk of HIV infection.

Participants

A non-Federal, nonadvocate, 12-member panel representing the fields of psychiatry, psychology, behavioral and social science, social work, and epidemiology. In addition, 15 experts in psychiatry, psychology, behavioral and social science, social work, and epidemiology presented data to the panel and a conference audience of 1,000.

Evidence

The literature was searched through Medline and an extensive bibliography of references was provided to the panel and the conference audience. Experts prepared abstracts with relevant citations from the literature. Scientific evidence was given precedence over clinical anecdotal experience.

Interventions to Prevent HIV Risk Behaviors. NIH Consensus Statement 1997 Feb. 11-13; 15(2):1-28.

Consensus Process

The panel, answering predefined questions, developed its conclusions based on the scientific evidence presented in open forum and the scientific literature. The panel composed a draft statement that was read in its entirety and circulated to the experts and the audience for comment. Thereafter, the panel resolved conflicting recommendations and released a revised statement at the end of the conference. The panel finalized the revisions within a few weeks after the conference.

Conclusions

Behavioral interventions to reduce risk for HIV/AIDS are effective and should be disseminated widely. Legislative restriction on needle exchange programs must be lifted because such legislation constitutes a major barrier to realizing the potential of a powerful approach and exposes millions of people to unnecessary risk. Legislative barriers that discourage effective programs aimed at youth must be eliminated. Although sexual abstinence is a desirable objective, programs must include instruction on safer sex behaviors. The erosion of funding for drug abuse treatment programs must be halted because research data clearly show that such programs reduce risky drug abuse behavior and often eliminate drug abuse itself. Finally, new research must focus on emerging risk groups such as young people, particularly those who are gay and who are members of ethnic minority groups, and women, in whom transmission of the HIV virus to their children remains a major public health problem.

Introduction

One in 250 people in the United States is infected with the human immunodeficiency virus (HIV), which causes AIDS; AIDS is the leading cause of death among men and women between the ages of 25 and 44. Every year, an additional 40,000–80,000 Americans become infected with HIV, mostly through behaviors that are preventable. In the United States, unsafe sexual behavior among men who have sex with men and unsafe injection practices among drug users still account for the largest number of cases. However, the rate of increase is greater for women than men, and there have been larger annual increases from heterosexual HIV transmission than among men who have sex with men.

The purpose of this conference was to examine what is known about behavioral interventions that are effective with different populations in different settings for the two primary modes of transmission: unsafe sexual behavior and nonsterile injection practices. Experts also provided the international and national epidemiology of HIV and a review of AIDS prevention efforts.

An extensive body of research has led to significant information on how to help individuals change their HIV-related risk behaviors. The interventions studied were based on a variety of models of behavior change, including social learning theory and related health and substance abuse models. The interventions begin with HIV and substance abuse education, but also include skill acquisition, assertiveness training, and behavioral reinforcement components. Recent research leads to the conclusion that aggressive promotion of safer sexual behavior and prevention and treatment of substance abuse could avert tens of thousands of new HIV infections and potentially save millions of dollars in health care costs. To date, however, there has not been widespread agreement among health professionals as to which interventions are most effective, in which settings, and among which populations.

Because behavioral interventions are currently the only effective way of slowing the spread of HIV infection, recommendations coming from this conference have immediate implications for service delivery in health care and educational settings, including schools; substance abuse treatment programs; community-based organizations; sexually transmitted disease clinics; inner-city health programs reaching disenfranchised high-risk women, men, and adolescents; rural health programs; and mental health programs that serve high-risk people with chronic mental illness. Knowing which behavior change interventions are most effective will assist public health personnel in allocating resources.

The conference brought together behavioral and social scientists, prevention researchers, statisticians and research methodologists, clinicians, physicians, nurses, social workers, mental health professionals, other health care professionals, and members of the public.

Following 1½ days of presentations and audience discussion, an independent, non-Federal consensus panel weighed the scientific evidence and developed a draft consensus statement that addressed the following five questions:

- How can we identify the behaviors and contexts that place individuals/communities at risk for HIV?

- What individual-, group-, or community-based methods of intervention reduce behavioral risks? What are the benefits and risks of these procedures?

- Does a reduction in these behavioral risks lead to a reduction in HIV?

- How can risk-reduction procedures be implemented effectively?

- What research is most urgently needed?

How Can We Identify the Behaviors and Contexts That Place Individuals/ Communities at Risk for HIV?

Major Behavioral Risks

Research to date has identified the key risk behaviors for HIV transmission to be unprotected anal and vaginal intercourse, having multiple sex partners, and using nonsterile drug injection equipment. Although there are some documented cases of transmission through oral-genital sexual contact, methodological issues make it difficult to precisely determine risk. At the present time, oral-genital sexual contact is considered to be a somewhat less risky behavior for contracting HIV than anal or vaginal intercourse.

Contexts That Influence Risk

Important social and biological contexts and cofactors increase or decrease the likelihood of risk behaviors. A major contextual influence is the prevalence of HIV itself in the local population, which greatly influences the impact of any risk behavior. Other contextual influences include: individual factors such as age and developmental stage, early initiation of sexual behavior, sexual identity, self-esteem, untreated sexually transmitted diseases, use of alcohol, and use of other drugs; interpersonal factors such as sex with a partner of unknown HIV status, partner commitment, and negotiation of safe sex; social norms and values such as cultural and religious beliefs, gender role norms, and social inclusion versus marginalization of gay men, ethnic minorities, people of color, sex workers, women, and drug users; and political, economic, and health policy factors such as laws and regulations, employment opportunities, poverty, sexism, racism, homophobia, and availability of basic public health tools for protective behavior, such as condoms and sterile injection equipment.

Although many of the behavioral risk factors are quite well known, the contextual risk factors are only beginning to be understood. For example, intervention programs with younger gay men need to address the fact that some of them consider HIV to be a threat mainly to older men. Negotiation about safe sex practices is much more difficult for women in populations where there are cultural barriers to doing so. Programs targeting sex workers have been highly efficacious in other countries, but in this country would encounter cultural and political barriers. The impact of poverty on seeking treatment for sexually transmitted diseases is much greater in countries without access to universal medical care. These contextual factors combine in dynamic ways to increase behavioral risk.

Means of Identifying Behaviors and Contexts

Behavioral risks have been identified by combining data from epidemiological studies and data from studies of homosexual and heterosexual couples with only one HIV-positive partner. Ongoing measurement of biomedical transmission factors will continue to be important as the epidemic changes. Because contextual factors are more numerous and more difficult to measure than biomedical factors, a wide variety of methods have been used to identify and measure them, including qualitative, ethnographic, and observational techniques. This work is multidisciplinary and requires ongoing consultation with local community groups. Contextual information is essential for designing tailored interventions that respond to the needs and preferences of people in particular communities. In addition, if a particular intervention is not effective for some participants, this information could guide development of the next generation of interventions.

Changing Trends in Specific Behaviors and Community Contexts That Produce Elevated Risk for HIV Infection

A number of established and several new and emerging behaviors and community contexts increase risk for HIV infection. In general, youth in school are showing an increase in condom use at last contact, but a trend for decreased condom use as they get older. Among gay men, the infection rate is increasing among African-American, Latino, and younger men. Injecting drug users are at increased risk because of conditions in their communities, including unavailability of sterile injecting equipment, dealer provision of infected needles, and social situations that encourage multiperson reuse of needles and other drug paraphernalia. Women, particularly women of color, recently increased dramatically as a risk group in the United States and constitute 50 percent of those infected worldwide. Much of the growth in their risk is caused by sexual contact with partners whose sexual or drug use behavior put the women at risk. Vertical transmission from infected mother to infant continues to be a source of high risk for the infant, even with the treatment for mothers and infants that is now available. In addition, a variety of other special settings and subpopulations at increased risk, including incarcerated youth and adults and individuals with chronic mental illnesses, deserve greater attention.

What Individual-, Group-, or Community-Based Methods of Intervention Reduce Behavioral Risks? What Are the Benefits and Risks of These Procedures?

When we consider the available knowledge from the entire body of literature, we can reach a clear conclusion: Prevention programs significantly reduce HIV risk behaviors. This is true across a variety of risk behaviors and in a variety of populations at risk.

Do Prevention Programs Reduce Behavioral Risk?

Experts in the field have used different designs for evaluating prevention programs. The most rigorous design used in some areas of research, the randomized controlled trial, has been used in HIV prevention research but is more appropriate for testing some questions than others. For example, evaluating the effects of legislative changes would rarely be possible with randomized research. To draw its conclusions, the panel examined the body of literature in a given area by considering all existing approaches to research, the strength of a given design for addressing a specific question, the number and strength of existing studies, and the convergence of effects.

Men Who Have Sex with Men

Considerable research has focused on risk reduction in men who have sex with men. Descriptive studies and nonrandomized studies with control groups show positive behavioral effects, as do randomized studies. The studies with random assignment to groups are clustered in two areas: individual interventions delivered in small group

404

settings and programs aimed at changing community norms (e.g., using peer leaders in community settings to deliver programs). These intervention programs focus on information, skills building, self-management, problem solving, and psychological factors such as self-efficacy and intentions. Studies with clearly defined interventions, retention of samples to allow followup periods as long as 18 months, and reasonable sample sizes show substantial effects for intervention over minimal intervention or control conditions. More intensive interventions (e.g., more sessions) boost efficacy.

Heterosexual Transmission

Adult Women at Risk From Sexual Transmission. Data from a variety of settings demonstrate the ability to prevent HIV risk behaviors in women. A randomized trial involving a cognitive behavioral intervention aimed at inner-city women with high risk of acquiring HIV through heterosexual contact provides some of the strongest evidence of impact. Three months after intervention, women in the intervention reported a slightly greater than doubling of condom use from 26 percent to 56 percent for all intercourse occasions; no such change occurred for women in the comparison group. A second randomized trial, targeted at pregnant women, shows similar results at a 6-month followup. Results from a third randomized study yet to be published show reductions in unprotected sex and sexually transmitted diseases. A study in rural Tanzania involving treatment for sexually transmitted diseases, condom distribution, and health education found more than a 50 percent reduction in HIV seroconversion incidence over a 2-year period in women ages 15–24. Seroconversion also diminished in counseling programs for women attending a clinic in Kigali, Rwanda, and for sex workers in Bombay, India.

Couples. There is evidence that consistent and correct condom use reduces HIV seroconversion to nearly zero in both male and female heterosexual partners. Counseling of couples in a European study was associated with large increases in protected sexual behavior.

Adolescents. The strongest support for reductions in a broad array of risky sexual behaviors comes from rigorous studies. Five randomized controlled trials used cognitive and behavioral skills training and targeted male and female, African-American, Latino, and European-American adolescents in health clinics and inner-city schools. Studies varied in sample size, and followups were limited to

405

1 year or less, but results were consistently positive, with outcomes such as condom acquisition, condom use, and reduced number of partners.

Injecting Drug Users

Prevention for injecting drug users has involved drug abuse treatment in some cases, and outreach focused on both drug use and HIV risk behavior in others. Both approaches have been effective. Programs aimed specifically at treating drug abuse show positive effects on risk behavior and have the additional benefit of affecting drug use. These have shown minimal effects on high-risk sex. Community studies training outreach workers or using an educational media campaign to reduce the use of nonsterile needles show increased protected sexual behavior and slowing of seroconversion rates, along with impressive reductions in drug use.

Needle Exchange Programs

An impressive body of evidence suggests powerful effects from needle exchange programs. The number of studies showing beneficial effects on behaviors such as needle sharing greatly outnumber those showing no effects. There is no longer doubt that these programs work, yet there is a striking disjunction between what science dictates and what policy delivers. Data are available to address three central concerns:

1. Does needle exchange promote drug use? A preponderance of evidence shows either no change or decreased drug use. The scattered cases showing increased drug use should be investigated to discover the conditions under which negative effects might occur, but these can in no way detract from the importance of needle exchange programs. Additionally, individuals in areas with needle exchange programs have increased likelihood of entering drug treatment programs.

2. Do programs encourage non-drug users, particularly youth, to use drugs? On the basis of such measures as hospitalizations for drug overdoses, there is no evidence that community norms change in favor of drug use or that more people begin using drugs. In Amsterdam and New Haven, for example, no increases in new drug users were reported after introduction of a needle exchange program.

3. Do programs increase the number of discarded needles in the community? In the majority of studies, there was no increase in used needles discarded in public places.

There are just over 100 needle exchange programs in the United States, compared with more than 2,000 in Australia, a country with less than 10 percent of the U.S. population. Can the opposition to needle exchange programs in the United States be justified on scientific grounds? Our answer is simple and emphatic—no. Studies show reduction in risk behavior as high as 80 percent in injecting drug users, with estimates of a 30 percent or greater reduction of HIV. The cost of such programs is relatively low. Needle exchange programs should be implemented at once.

Policy and Large-Scale Interventions

As in other areas (e.g., smoking, injury control), policy interventions can remove barriers to protective behavior. In the United States and other countries, such interventions have resulted in dramatic reductions in risk behavior. In Connecticut, for example, a single legislative action legalizing over-the-counter purchase of sterile injection equipment led to an immediate and profound reduction in the sharing of nonsterile needles. A national campaign in Switzerland to promote the use of condoms dramatically reduced risky sexual behavior. Regulations on the use of condoms by sex workers in Thailand also led to fewer unprotected sex acts. The results thus far have been impressive. Given the potential benefit of policy changes, these should be implemented as local circumstances allow and, once implemented, should be evaluated as often and thoroughly as possible.

Issues in Need of Further Work

Populations and Settings

A promising start has been made to reduce risk in persons often marginalized. Homeless, chronically mentally ill, runaway, incarcerated, HIV-positive, and physically and developmentally challenged persons face obstacles that affect their ability to initiate and maintain behavior change. In addition, little is known about the risk behaviors of lesbians and bisexual women, heterosexual men, persons over 50 years old, and sexually active youth.

African-American and Latino communities experience disproportionate rates of infection. The application of culturally appropriate

407

strategies demands ethnographic research to understand values, attitudes, behaviors, and factors such as socioeconomic status in different communities. Cultural factors may affect the ability of individuals to change behavior. Researchers from different ethnic or cultural backgrounds may help address this issue. Language and cultural barriers to delivery of interventions must be addressed, with special consideration for individuals whose physical or other impairments limit access to most programs.

Prenatal care and sexually transmitted disease clinics are proven to be effective settings for delivery of HIV intervention. Further research is needed in these and other medical settings. In addition, individuals in institutions such as prisons and mental health facilities, and those in remote areas, require special attention.

Maintenance, Generalizability, and Theory

Understanding and evaluating the maintenance of behavior change requires multivariate, longitudinal studies. In this way, changes in patterns of behavior and causal associations can be estimated. Long-term followup of subjects is necessary. Similarly, more attention to generalizability is needed. An intervention proven effective in one city may not be applicable in another city with a similar population but with different community norms. Methodological issues in need of additional attention include research strategies that measure and enhance validity of self-report, standardization of risk behavior questions and questioning techniques, comparability of intervention conditions across different studies, examining participants and nonresponders to an intervention, and measuring changes in multiple risk profiles over time.

A developmental framework may be helpful for considering the origins of HIV risk behavior. Efforts are needed to incorporate knowledge of childhood antecedents of HIV risk behaviors in adolescents. Can early intervention that alters these antecedents reduce or delay HIV risk behaviors? The body of research now being done to reduce already existing risk behaviors such as unprotected sex and drug use needs to be linked with other research traditions that target antecedents of HIV risk behaviors.

Impact and Cost-Effectiveness

Reviews on HIV prevention conclude that programs produce significant effects, but a statistical advantage may not necessarily equate to meaningful change. An example comes from a study on condom use in more than 13,000 injecting drug users. An intervention nearly doubled consistent condom use, from a baseline level of 10 percent to 19 percent. Although the change was significant from a public health perspective, 81 percent of this high-risk population still engaged in high-risk sexual behavior. This highlights the importance of examining and improving impact as well as assessing statistical significance. Impact is assessed by understanding the efficacy of an intervention, the magnitude of behavior change, and the influence of this change on seroconversion.

A key issue is the degree to which the field has confronted the issue of efficacy (impact of interventions in controlled circumstances) versus effectiveness (effects in real-world setting). Little effectiveness research has been done. This limits the ability to estimate the impact likely to occur if the current generation of risk-reduction strategies, proven useful in efficacy trials, were applied on a large scale outside the research setting. The panel concluded that HIV prevention research is mature enough that some, but not all interventions, are ready for tests of effectiveness. This will require different research strategies and the involvement of professionals from additional disciplines beyond those used for efficacy trials.

The cost-effectiveness of interventions is an important issue in decisions about resource allocation. Research thus far has been positive, but more research is needed to examine the costs and benefits of HIV risk prevention programs.

Behavioral Issues Arising from Biomedical Advances

Important advances in medicine have created new and pressing behavioral issues. Pharmacologic treatment of HIV-positive individuals may increase longevity, but it is not known how such successfully treated individuals will alter their recreational drug use or sexual behavior. Complicated medical regimens raise issues of adherence, with the possibility that incomplete adherence will lead to resistant strains of the virus. Studies of biochemical preventive treatment after sexual exposure to HIV raise questions about risk-reduction counseling. For example, will individuals feel free to engage in risky sex as post-exposure treatment becomes more an option?

Pharmacologic treatment profiles now exist to reduce transmission of HIV from mother to newborn child. This demonstrated preventive intervention offers new opportunities to study behavioral issues and barriers to access in a new and important context.

409

Policy

Current evidence suggests that some of the most powerful positive effects on HIV risk behavior have been produced by legislative and regulatory changes. One need look no further than to the experience in Connecticut, where one legislative action permitting the purchase of sterile injection equipment had an immediate and pronounced effect on behavior. Here we see the potentially low cost and high effectiveness of intervention at the policy level. Policymaking can be conceptualized as behavior, and as such can and should be studied. Social policy, legal change, and community mobilization are powerful means of intervention and must be a legitimate area of inquiry at the National Institutes of Health and the Centers for Disease Control and Prevention.

Several examples beyond the Connecticut experience show the power of policy changes. Australia, for instance, has a low rate of HIV despite population profiles in some areas similar to profiles in areas in the United States that have high HIV seroconversion rates. Cities such as Tacoma, Toronto, Sydney, Glasgow, and Lund have kept the HIV infection rate low, coincident with policies making sterile needles available for injecting drug users, boosting education aimed at risk reduction, making condoms more available, and enhancing programs for the treatment of sexually transmitted diseases. Impressive results have been reported from around the world on government action to reduce risk and infection in many populations at risk.

Little qualitative and quantitative research has been done in HIV prevention policy, and no body of evidence exists to inform the field about the factors that influence policy, where policy intervention is most likely to be effective, and how best to encourage policy and legislative changes. We believe that funding should be devoted to the study of policy and legislative changes and that National, State, and local levels be considered.

Of utmost importance is that HIV prevention policy be based, whenever possible, on scientific information. This occurs too little — the behavior placing the public health at greatest risk may be occurring in legislative and other decisionmaking bodies. The Federal ban on funding for needle exchange programs as well as restrictions on selling injection equipment are absolutely contraindicated and erect formidable barriers to implementing what is known to be effective. Many thousands of unnecessary deaths will occur as a result.

The single greatest increase in HIV prevention funding occurred with 1996 Federal legislation in the United States providing $50 million within block grant entitlements for programs teaching adolescents abstinence from sexual behavior. Among the criteria for programs funded through the block grant program are the following two requirements: (1) "has as its exclusive purpose, teaching the social, psychological, and health gains to be realized by abstaining from sexual activity" and (2) "teaches that a mutually faithful monogamous relationship in the context of marriage is the expected standard of human sexual activity" (Public Health Service Act, Public Law 104-193, Sec. 912). Some programs based on an abstinence model propose that approaches such as the use of condoms are ineffective. This model places policy in direct conflict with science because it ignores overwhelming evidence that other programs are effective. Abstinence-only programs cannot be justified in the face of effective programs and given the fact that we face an international emergency in the AIDS epidemic.

Another instance of policy conflicting with knowledge is in providing treatment for drug abuse. Research shows that treatment of drug abusers with methadone maintenance, outpatient drug-free treatments, residential treatment, or detoxification not only decreases drug use but has a substantial effect on risk behaviors (use of shared needles and unprotected sex). At the same time that this knowledge has reached a critical mass, funding of drug treatment programs has been reduced in many localities. This tragic trend must be reversed.

Policy and legislative change can have rapid, powerful, and positive results. This key area of the field has been given little attention, a problem that needs remedy. A coordinated effort is needed, and the Government must take strong and immediate steps to protect its citizens. Drawing together legal and policy changes and program implementation occurring at international, National, and local levels offers great promise. Strong political leadership is necessary to direct this effort. The United States has much to learn from other countries where political leaders have taken this issue seriously and, by supporting vigorous prevention strategies, have prevented even more tragedy from occurring from AIDS.

Does a Reduction in These Behavioral Risks Lead to a Reduction in HIV?

The evidence is unequivocal that consistent and effective use of condoms and of sterile injecting equipment on the part of injection drug users is nearly 100 percent effective in protecting against HIV.

411

Reduction in risky behavior leads to reduction in HIV to a degree that depends on context, particularly the local prevalence of HIV infection.

It is important to keep HIV seroincidence in mind as the ultimate outcome of interest for HIV prevention efforts. Seroincidence estimates also allow us to compare effectiveness and cost of different programs. Direct measurement of HIV infection is a feasible and desirable outcome variable for some programs. However, practical, ethical, and fiscal barriers often make reliance on measured seroconversion undesirable. In these instances, proxy indices—including other biological markers or modeled estimates of seroincidence based on behavioral outcomes—can be used to estimate the effects of prevention programs on seroincidence.

Study Designs That Lend Themselves to Using Seroconversion as an Outcome

To find reliable differences between intervention and control or comparison samples, one must expect a minimum number of seroconversions in the control sample within the timeframe of the study. These are found in populations where seroconversion rates are high, in large samples, or in studies with long followup. Only a limited number of situations have lent themselves to clinical trials and other studies on this scale.

Many studies using seroincidence as a measure of outcome were conducted in developing countries where HIV incidence is high and policy interventions or community-level programs have been implemented. Among these are studies from Tanzania and Bombay with comparison populations and from Thailand, where an historical comparison was employed. Few studies in the United States have used HIV or any biological measure as an endpoint for the reasons cited above. In the United States and elsewhere, seroconversion has been used to measure the effect of sterile injection equipment availability, bleach cleaning interventions, and methadone treatment with injecting drug users.

Constraints on Using Seroconversion Outcomes

Although seroconversion is a preferred standard for intervention efficacy, there are practical and ethical obstacles to its use. For example, there is a potential selective dropout of research participants who will not agree to repeated HIV testing. Furthermore, research costs can be greatly increased by pre- and post-test counseling and followup or referral for research subjects who are identified as HIV-positive in the study. Counseling and referral are, of course, required by ethical research practice. Nevertheless, where possible and feasible, it is important that behavioral and policy interventions be validated using seroincidence as an outcome.

Transmission Models to Estimate Effects of Behavioral Outcomes on HIV Infection Rates

When HIV seroconversion outcomes are not feasible, well-designed self-report behavioral outcomes have shown indications of being valid and reliable. These behavioral outcomes can be employed in transmission models to estimate the number of averted cases. The models have been developed from studies of HIV-discordant couples and epidemiological studies. Although use of these models requires assumptions about future prevalence and about relationships among variables being studied, a reasonable range of estimates about the probable impact of the intervention on HIV can thus be generated. In theory, estimates of HIV seroconversion during the study may be extended into the future under varying estimates of the maintenance of positive behavioral outcome. The models may also be extended to estimate the potential impact were the program more widely implemented in similar contexts. Finally, potential effects on seroconversion in field settings may be estimated, using these models, from data on behavioral outcomes from studies done in research settings. These models can estimate the impact on seroconversion using reasonable assumptions that the interventions will have less effectiveness in field settings.

Estimates of the effects of behavioral outcomes on HIV seroconversion are still relatively few and mostly retrospective. It should be possible to produce such estimates in advance of prevention trials, contingent on the targeted magnitude of behavioral outcomes and the expected prevalence of HIV infection in the local population. We recommend that such estimates be employed as an additional outcome measure for trials with behavioral endpoints whenever possible. Ongoing work on these models is needed to update and improve the database used to produce and validate them. Furthermore, there is a need to validate, by use of empirical data, the assumption that transmission rates based on naturally occurring behaviors are equivalent to transmission rates based on behavioral changes in response to prevention efforts. These models can also be used to estimate the validity of self-reports.

Other Biological Markers as Surrogates for HIV Seroconversion

Incidence of certain sexually transmitted diseases has been used as a plausible surrogate for HIV seroconversion. The same sexual behaviors are risks for HIV and some sexually transmitted diseases. Sexually transmitted diseases are a powerful potentiator of HIV seroconversion in exposed persons. The higher incidence of sexually transmitted diseases also makes detection of program effects more sensitive. Two ongoing multicenter randomized controlled trials for heterosexual populations have chosen incidence of sexually transmitted diseases as a biologic marker to study the efficacy of HIV prevention interventions, as have international studies such as the study in Tanzania. Unpublished results of a Centers for Disease Control and Prevention project show a decrease in the rate of sexually transmitted diseases to be correlated with a decrease in HIV-related risk behavior. Hepatitis C has been used effectively as a biological marker in studies involving injecting drug user populations, because of overlapping transmission routes. Sexually transmitted disease incidence, hepatitis C incidence, and other infectious disease incidence are reasonable markers for expected HIV exposure.

How Can Risk-Reduction Procedures Be Implemented Effectively?

Studies Ready for Implementation

A number of interventions have been evaluated in current research and are ready to be implemented within communities. Indeed, some are already being implemented by health departments and community-based organizations. Interventions at the *individual level* include the following:

- Outreach, needle exchange activities, treatment programs, and face-to-face counseling programs for substance abusing populations

- Cognitive-behavioral small group, face-to-face counseling, and skills-building (i.e., proper condom use, negotiation, refusal) programs for men who have sex with men

- Cognitive-behavioral small group, face-to-face counseling, and skills building (i.e., proper condom use, negotiation, refusal) programs for women that pay special attention to their concerns (e.g., child care, transportation, and relationships with significant others)

• Condom distribution and testing and treatment for sexually transmitted diseases for sex workers and other sexually active individuals at high risk for sexually transmitted diseases

• Cognitive-behavioral educational and skills-building groups for youth and adolescents in various settings.

At the *family or dyad level*, interventions include counseling for couples (including HIV-serodiscordant couples) in both the United States and other countries. Within the community, interventions include changing community norms through community outreach and opinion leaders for men who have sex with men as well as injection drug-using networks.

At the *policy level* there are a number of strategies:

• Lifting government restrictions on needle exchange programs

• Providing increased government funding for drug and alcohol treatment programs, including methadone maintenance

• Support for sex education interventions that focus beyond abstinence

• Lifting constraints on condom availability (e.g., in correctional facilities).

Implementation Considerations

Several factors may influence implementation of HIV risk behavior interventions within the United States.

First, compliance with interventions is improved when targeted individuals are involved at every phase of the process of conceptualization, development, and implementation of the programs. Input of these individuals is needed to help solve this health crisis.

Second, programs need to be culturally sensitive. This requires attention not only to ethnicity and language but also to other factors including social class, age, developmental stage, and sexual orientation.

Third, an appropriate intervention dosage must be selected for the population; this includes the number, length, and intensity of the intervention. Studies demonstrate that numerous intervention points over extended periods of time are more efficacious than once-only approaches for most populations. Almost all reported studies have short followup (3–18 months), which suggests that attention must be paid to maintenance efforts. It may be necessary to include additional, periodic intervention points for subsets of the population; longer term followup would assist in determining this fact.

Fourth, when HIV risk behavior interventions are being introduced, it is important to address community myths. For example, scientifically derived results do not support assertions that needle exchange programs will lead to increased needle-injecting behavior among current users or an increase in the number of users. Nor do the data indicate that sex education programs result in earlier onset of sexual behavior or more sexual partners, or that condom distribution fosters more risky behavior. To the contrary, outcomes of these programs are quite consistent with the values of most communities. For example, behavioral interventions lead injecting drug users to inject less frequently, and the number of users in a community may decrease; after interventions, young people tend to delay initiation of intercourse or, if they are sexually active, have fewer partners; and adults, following intervention, engage in fewer incidents of risky sexual behavior. Armed with this knowledge, those who implement programs should confidently solicit the support and involvement of local government, educational, and religious leaders.

Despite notable gains relevant to implementation of prevention programs, very little cost analysis information has been available to guide community-based organizations, State and local health departments, and other practitioners. These analyses are important in determining the most cost-effective interventions for implementation. In addition, communities lack fiscal resources to support such interventions once they are proven successful. Finally, there are social and cultural barriers to implementation of programs; these include homophobia, gender inequality, and racism.

Sufficient training of personnel, monitoring of procedures to ensure fidelity to key components and established methods, and strong evaluation plans are essential components of any implementation strategy. When training and local capacity building are necessary for implementation, training and technical assistance should be available to facilitate prevention programs at State and local levels. Evaluation results should be reported and widely disseminated so as to advance both science and practice. Newly implemented programs yielding results different from established findings should be carefully compared with original designs in order to explain the variance in outcomes.

The Next Step

Just as the Food and Drug Administration conditionally approves experimental drugs in emergency situations, so should policymakers support active dissemination of the most promising programs at this time based on the urgency of the AIDS epidemic. A critical issue that must be addressed involves the criteria for choosing interventions most ready for implementation in the community. The most obvious is evidence of strong program effects observed under rigorous, controlled research conditions. Among programs with strong effects, priority should be given to interventions that can be delivered with high reliability and fidelity to the original program model. Usually such programs do not require significant new demands or elaborate training at the delivery site.

At this next stage there will nevertheless be programs that show promise but still require additional research to ensure their effectiveness. At least two criteria should be considered in choosing promising programs for further evaluation. First, programs that show strong short-term effects but lack long-term results should be studied to estimate their long-term effectiveness. Second, programs that have shown promising effects for only a very narrowly defined range of settings or conditions of implementation should be studied to assess the generalizability of their effectiveness in other settings and contexts.

Numerous other interventions developed solely by community organizations were not described during the consensus development conference by the researchers, yet were brought to the attention of the panel by the public statements at the conference by community activists and practitioners. The efficacy of these approaches has not been demonstrated through careful evaluation. However, because community workers have developed a number of innovative and promising programs, there is a great need for them to work together with researchers to further HIV risk behavior intervention science and practice.

What Research Is Most Urgently Needed?

The most urgently needed research is that which is essential for containing the HIV/AIDS epidemic. In particular, we need to track emerging behavioral risk factors and to aim preventive procedures at these risk factors with as much precision as possible.

Tracking Emerging Risk

A most urgent area for research is in developing improved methods of identifying emerging risks within large populations. For example, in the United States we need to know as early as possible what settings, regions, and subpopulations are likely to show increases in seroconversion to HIV. The best strategy for this identification is to track increases in known behavioral risks, which when combined with sufficiently high HIV prevalence predicts regions of particular vulnerability. Regional strategies are needed for regularly tracking increases in these behaviors in order to effectively offer known prevention strategies before seroconversion occurs. These regional strategies must be coordinated with the National HIV tracking system. Research is needed on how to collect this information regionally. How can studies collect representative data/behavioral information from regional populations in ways that are fully acceptable to the local communities involved? This regional strategy of risk tracking can draw on two areas of established research. First, clearly established risky behaviors serve as reliable harbingers of seroconversion. These include behaviors that directly increase the likelihood of HIV transmission, such as unprotected sex and needle sharing and practices that make these behaviors more likely, such as alcohol abuse in adolescents. Second, methods for inquiring about these risky behaviors have been established and validated. Careful evaluation of the most cost-efficient approaches to regional tracking is needed, as well as approaches to ensure that strategies used are compatible with community values and maximum effectiveness.

Young People

The epidemic in the United States is currently shifting to young people, particularly those who are gay, members of racial and ethnic minorities, and out-of-school adolescents. Because adolescents may be at risk for HIV infection in their early to mid teens, it is important to establish interventions for youth at an earlier age before the onset of risk behavior (sexual activity and drug use). Thus, the U.S. program of research must give highest priority to providing effective prevention programs for these subpopulations. Programs already shown to be effective for these subpopulations must be improved to

418

ensure long-term maintenance of the reduction in risky behavior. Current interventions should be widely disseminated, and improved interventions, as they become available, should quickly replace those that have been less effective. Dissemination should include careful training of providers, monitoring to ensure fidelity of delivery, continuous evaluation of effectiveness, and modification where required by community and cultural needs and circumstances.

HIV-Positive Individuals

Effective interventions with people who are HIV-positive can enable them to practice safer sex and safer needle use and thus help to contain the HIV epidemic. There is a startling paucity of well-developed interventions specifically designed for HIV-positive persons. Moreover, as biological treatment for those who are HIV-positive improves, the need for these preventive services will become even more pressing.

Women

It is essential to continue development of interventions to reduce heterosexual transmission of HIV to women as well as their risk of drug abuse behavior. These interventions should focus on the effect of community expectations of women and power differentials in their relationships with men. Moreover, additional research with female condoms and microbicides may facilitate preventive interventions that enhance women's control of exposure to HIV risk.

Linking Scientific Findings to Law and Policy

Most urgent is the need to rapidly bridge the serious gap that is widening between clear scientific results and the law and policies of the United States. As this statement has noted forcefully, there is clear scientific evidence supporting needle exchange programs, drug abuse treatment, and interventions with adolescents as essential components of our National program to contain the AIDS epidemic. Even as evidence rapidly accumulates on the success of these programs, however, legislation has been passed to make provision of these interventions extremely difficult. There is no more urgent need than to remedy this dangerous chasm. National leaders, legislators, scientists, and service providers must unite to understand fully this growing catastrophe. Why are voters unaware of these issues? What pressures and circumstances of government make it unresponsive to these compelling public health needs and effective programs? What are the limits in scientific communication that may obscure the legislative import of these scientific findings?

Conclusions and Recommendations

1. Preventive interventions are effective for reducing behavioral risk for HIV/AIDS and must be widely disseminated. Their application in practice settings may require careful training of personnel, close monitoring of the fidelity of procedures, and ongoing monitoring of effectiveness. Results of this evaluation must be reported, and where effectiveness in field settings is reduced, program modifications must be undertaken immediately.

   Three approaches are particularly effective for risk reduction in drug abuse behavior: needle exchange programs, drug abuse treatment, and outreach programs for drug abusers not enrolled in treatment. Several programs were deemed effective for risky sexual behavior. These programs include (1) information about HIV/AIDS and (2) building skills to use condoms and to negotiate the interpersonal challenges of safer sex. Effective safer sex programs have been developed for men who have sex with men, for women, and for adolescents.

2. The epidemic in the United States is shifting to young people, particularly those who are gay and who are members of ethnic minority groups. New research must focus on these emerging risk groups. Interventions must be developed and perfected, and special attention must be given to long-term maintenance of effects. In addition, AIDS is steadily increasing in women, and transmission of HIV virus to their children remains a major public health problem. Interventions focused on their special needs are essential.

3. Regional tracking of changes in behavioral risk will be necessary to identify settings, subpopulations, and geographical regions with special risk for seroconversion to HIV-positive status as the epidemic continues to change. This effort, if properly coordinated with National tracking strategies, could play a critical part in a U.S. strategy to contain the spread of HIV.

4. Programs must be developed to help individuals already infected with HIV to avoid risky sexual and substance abuse

behavior. This National priority will become more pressing as new biological treatments prolong life. Thus, prevention programs for HIV-positive people must have outcomes that can be maintained over long periods of time, in order to slow the spread of infection.

5. Legislative restriction on needle exchange programs must be lifted. Such legislation constitutes a major barrier to realizing the potential of a powerful approach and exposes millions of people to unnecessary risk.

6. Legislative barriers that discourage effective programs aimed at youth must be eliminated. Although sexual abstinence is a desirable objective, programs must include instruction in safe sex behavior, including condom use. The effectiveness of these programs is supported by strong scientific evidence. However, they are discouraged by welfare reform provisions, which support only programs using abstinence as the only goal.

7. The erosion of funding for drug and alcohol abuse treatment programs must be halted. Research data are clear that the programs reduce risky drug and alcohol abuse behavior and often eliminate drug abuse itself. Drug and alcohol abuse treatment is a central bulwark in the Nation's defense against HIV/AIDS.

8. The catastrophic breach between HIV/AIDS prevention science and the legislative process must be healed. Citizens, legislators, political leaders, service providers, and scientists must unite so that scientific data may properly inform legislative process. The study of policy development, the impact of policy, and policy change must be supported by Federal agencies.

Additional Information

For a list of Consensus Development Panel members, speakers, Planning Committee members, Conference sponsors and co-sponsors, and a bibliography of references provided by the speakers, please consult a copy of the original document available by writing to the NIH Consensus Program Information Center, P.O. Box 2577, Kensington, MD 20891; by calling toll free 1-888-NIH-Consensus (888-644-2667); or by visiting the NIH Consensus Development Program home page on the World Wide Web at http://consensus.nih.gov.

Chapter 48

Pregnancy and HIV: Is AZT the Right Choice for You and Your Baby?

Take Good Care of Yourself

You can improve your chances of having a healthy baby. Here are some steps you can take while you are pregnant that will help both you and your baby.

- Get prenatal care early in your pregnancy.
- Get tested for HIV.
- Practice safer sex.
- Exercise regularly if your health care provider says it's okay.
- Eat healthy meals.
- Get enough rest.
- Do not use alcohol or other drugs not prescribed by your doctor.
- Do not smoke.
- Tell your health care provider about any medicine you are already taking.
- Check with your health care provider before taking any new medicine.

If you know that you have HIV infection, you also should:

- Tell your health care provider that you have HIV.

U.S. Department of Health and Human Services, Public Health Service, Pub. No. 96-0007, December 1997.

- Talk with your doctor or nurse about the risks and benefits for you and your baby if you take AZT.

If You Have HIV You Should Know

If you are pregnant and have HIV or AIDS, you may pass the virus to your baby. Taking AZT can lessen the chance that HIV will pass to your baby.

AZT is a medicine used to treat HIV infection. AZT is also called zidovudine or ZDV.

This chapter talks about the choice you have to take or not take AZT while you are pregnant. It also gives questions to ask your doctor, nurse, or other health care provider. Then you can make up your own mind about what is best for you and your baby.

Babies and HIV Infection

HIV stands for human immunodeficiency virus. HIV causes AIDS. As yet, there is no cure for either HIV or AIDS. Some babies who have HIV become very sick and die in their first year. Others live longer but may still get sick.

A baby can get HIV from an HIV-infected mother in three ways:

1. During pregnancy.
2. During delivery.
3. After delivery through breast feeding.

The chances are about one in four that HIV will pass from a mother to her baby before or during birth. This is only an average. No one can tell you for sure what your baby's chances are.

After delivery, your health care provider will ask for your consent to test your baby for HIV. Many babies can be diagnosed as either HIV-infected or not infected by 6 months of age. In some cases, it takes up to 18 months to know for sure if a baby has HIV.

If you have HIV and are pregnant, the most important thing you can do is to see your health care provider early and often during your pregnancy.

What You Should Know about AZT

AZT is one of the medicines that work against HIV. AZT may slow down the virus and the effects it has on your body.

Many people who have HIV feel better while taking AZT. Sometimes AZT causes problems such as upset stomach, anemia (low blood), headache, or muscle soreness. These problems usually go away when AZT is stopped or the dose is lowered. Talk to your health care provider.

What We Have Learned about Babies and AZT

You may have heard about a research study by the National Institutes of Health called the 076 study. 076 is the number NIH gave to the study. The 076 study found that women with HIV who took AZT were much less likely to pass the virus to their babies.

Here Are the Facts:

• More than 500 pregnant women with HIV took part in the study.

• Half of the mothers and babies did not take AZT.

• The other half of the women took AZT, and their babies were given AZT for 6 weeks after they were born.

• Three of every 12 babies born to women who did not take AZT got HIV.

• One of every 12 babies born to mothers who took AZT got HIV.

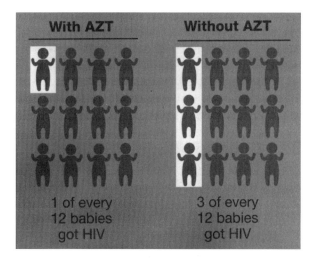

Figure 48.1. Results of the 076 AZT Study

About the Women in the AZT Study

The women in the AZT study:

- Began prenatal care early.

- Had HIV and began the study between 14 weeks (3½ months) and 34 weeks (8½ months) of pregnancy.

- Were 15 to 43 years old (average age 25).

- Were African-American (about 50 percent of the women), Hispanic (about 33 percent), and white (about 17 percent).

- Had not taken AZT for their own health before the study.

- Had T-cell counts over 200 at the start of the study. More than half had T-cell counts over 500.

What Are T Cells?

- T cells are white blood cells that protect the body from "germs" such as viruses and bacteria. T cells are also called T-helper cells and CD4 cells.

- When HIV enters the body, it infects the T cells. The virus kills these cells slowly. As more and more T cells die, the body loses its ability to fight infection.

- Counting the number of T cells in a person's blood is one way to find out how well the person's body can fight infection. A normal T-cell count is about 1,000.

Questions and Answers about the AZT Study

How was AZT given to the women and babies in the study?

The women and babies in the 076 study took AZT in three stages:

1. During pregnancy: The women took one AZT pill five times each day.

2. During labor and delivery: The women were given AZT through an IV.

3. Right after birth: The babies were given AZT syrup four times a day for 6 weeks.

426

Did AZT cause problems for the women?

Taking AZT did not seem to make the women in this study any sicker than the women who did not take AZT. Studies are being done to see if the women have any long-term problems.

Did AZT cause problems for the babies?

AZT did not cause any serious problems for the babies in the 076 study.

- AZT did not cause birth defects or cause babies to be born early.

- Babies born to women who did and did not take AZT were about the same size.

- Some of the AZT babies became anemic. The anemia went away soon after AZT was stopped.

- Babies born to women in both groups have been followed to at least 1 year of age. Growth and development are about the same for all babies.

- Studies are being done to see if AZT causes any long-term problems for the babies.

What do these results mean for me?

The results of the AZT study are very hopeful. But, we do not know if AZT will work the same for women and babies who are not like the women and babies in the study.

Is there anything else I can do?

- Do not breast feed your baby. HIV can pass to your baby through breast milk.

- Your baby should be given a medicine when he or she is 4 to 6 weeks old to help prevent pneumonia.

Thinking about AZT

Here are some important points to keep in mind as you make a decision about using AZT:

- HIV can be passed from mother to baby.

- Babies who are infected with HIV may become very sick. Some may die during their first year of life.

- With AZT you can lower the chance that you baby will get HIV.

- With AZT the chance that your baby will get HIV is lowered from about 3 out of 12 (25 percent) to 1 out of 12 (8 percent).

- Even if you take AZT, there is a small chance that your baby might get the virus.

- Taking AZT may cause anemia in your baby. The anemia will go away after the AZT is stopped.

- In the 076 study, AZT did not cause birth defects or problems in the growth or development of babies during the first year of life.

- Although AZT does not appear to cause any short-term problems for mothers or babies, no one knows if there will be any long-term problems.

Other Studies Are in Progress

- Studies are underway to see if other methods will lower the chances that HIV will pass from mothers to babies.

- It is too soon to know if these methods will work.

- To find out more about this research, call 1-800-TRIALS-A (1-800-874-2572).

Talking with Your Health Care Provider

Here are some questions to ask your health care provider about using AZT:

1. Could AZT help me and my baby?

2. Will AZT make me or my baby sick?

3. What if I am taking other medicines?

4. What if I use drugs or alcohol?

5. Will I need to keep taking AZT after I have my baby?

6. When will I know if my baby has HIV?

7. What if I need to take AZT later on for myself?

8. How will I pay for my care?

Write your own questions down so you won't forget them.

You Can Find Out More

Call the HIV/AIDS Treatment Information Service:

1-800-448-0440 (English and Spanish)
1-800-243-7012 (TTY/TDD)

You may qualify for Medicaid. Ask how you can find out more about Medicaid.

Or, you can write to:

Pregnancy and HIV
CDC National AIDS Clearinghouse
P.O. Box 6003
Rockville, MD 20849-6003

Chapter 49

Perinatal HIV Prevention

Over the past two years, researchers throughout the nation have documented dramatic declines in mother-to-infant (perinatal) transmission of HIV, indicating the success of recent perinatal prevention efforts. In 1994, clinical trials conducted by the National Institutes of Health (NIH) showed that HIV-infected women could reduce the risk of transmitting the virus to their babies by as much as two-thirds through administration of zidovudine (ZDV or AZT) during pregnancy, labor, and delivery, and by giving their babies AZT for the first 6 seeks after birth. In 1994, the Public Health Service (PHS) issued guidelines for using AZT during pregnancy, and in 1995, published guidelines for routinely counseling all pregnant women about HIV and offering them an HIV test.

As health care providers across the country have incorporated these guidelines into clinical practice, perinatal HIV transmission has dropped dramatically. On a national level, the number of children reported to CDC with perinatally acquired AIDS declined 27% between 1992 and 1995, with the most dramatic drop in cases occurring in 1994 and 1995. Additionally, research from numerous states has documented a declining rate of perinatal HIV transmission.

- Among women in CDC's Perinatal AIDS Collaborative Transmission Study (PACTS), AZT use increased following the publication of CDC guidelines, and the rate of perinatal transmission

CDC Update, National Center for HIV, STD, and TB Prevention, February 1997.

dropped from 21% to 11%. The PACTS study includes women from 4 cities: New York City, Newark, Atlanta, and Baltimore.

- Another multi-site study, the Women and Infants Transmission Study (WITS), tracks perinatal transmission in several groups of women from New York, Massachusetts, Illinois, Texas, and Puerto Rico. In the WITS study, the rate of perinatal transmission dropped to 8% in 1994, declining from a rate of 19% prior to the AZT guidelines.

- In North Carolina, perinatal HIV transmission dropped from 21% in 1993 to 6.2% in the first half of 1996.

Ongoing Research to Improve Perinatal HIV Prevention

Despite these encouraging findings, challenges remain for perinatal prevention. Perhaps greatest among these is the need to ensure pregnant women have access to quality prenatal care early in pregnancy and can sustain care throughout pregnancy and beyond. In order for HIV-infected women to benefit from treatment advances for themselves and their children, they must be reached early in pregnancy with the opportunity to learn their HIV status and to consider treatment for their health and for preventing transmission to their children. When women are provided appropriate information and counseling, studies show that acceptance of HIV testing and AZT treatment is extremely high.

Yet, some children are infected despite AZT use by their mothers. AZT is not 100% effective in preventing transmission, and a great deal remains unknown about the mechanisms by which AZT reduces transmission, as well as the potential for long-term side-effects for the exposed women and children. Moreover, new combination therapies offer promise for improved treatment for HIV-infected women. Researchers must explore the possibility that AZT treatment during pregnancy may reduce the effectiveness of these therapies for women later in life. CDC, NIH, and other researchers continue to study these questions to determine if there are more effective, simpler, or safer preventive therapies or practices available. Research is ongoing in a number of areas:

- PACTS and WITS are evaluating the impact of other factors on perinatal transmission, such as the mother's stage of HIV disease, and the time from rupture of membranes (water breaking) to delivery. These studies have found that when a mother's membranes have ruptured more than 4 hours before delivery, the risk of transmission is increased. These findings suggest that changes in obstetric practice may also help reduce HIV transmission. If physicians can reduce the duration of ruptured membranes, the chances of transmission can likely be reduced.

- If a shorter course of AZT during pregnancy were shown to be as effective as the treatment regimen now recommended, both the costs and potential risks from AZT use could be reduced. In developing countries where over 90% of new HIV infections occur, the extensive AZT course now recommended in the U.S. is generally not feasible. CDC and other researchers are now working with researchers in developing countries to determine if administering AZT or other antiretrovirals for a shorter time period during pregnancy and/or during delivery will be as effective in reducing perinatal HIV transmission.

- New combination therapies using protease inhibitors in combination with existing antiretroviral drugs such as AZT and 3TC have recently been shown to reduce the amount of HIV particles circulating in the blood of some infected individuals to non-detectable levels. While no one yet knows how long this effect will last or impact the disease progression, these results are promising for the quality of life of HIV-infected individuals. To determine if these or other therapies may be as, or ever more, effective than AZT alone in preventing perinatal transmission, NIH is beginning to study both the safety and efficacy of other options for perinatal prevention.

Efforts to Further Explore Potential Long-Term Side Effects

Neither the mothers nor the children studied have reported serious side effects immediately following the AZT regimen currently recommended. Effects have been limited largely to mild, reversible anemia in the infants. Researchers do not know if the mothers or the infants exposed to AZT will experience any side affects over time. Current recommendations stress that a woman should make a personal decision about taking AZT only after she discusses the benefits and potential risks for herself and her child with her health care provider. Researchers have long been aware that AZT could potentially cause rare long-term side effects, even though none have been reported to date in any of the exposed children. Since the discovery of AZT's effectiveness in perinatal HIV prevention occurred recently, the oldest children exposed to this regimen are now 5 years old. The guidelines recommend that they be followed until age 21 to ensure that any side effects are detected.

To further explore any theoretical or potential risks of long-term side effects of AZT, two laboratory studies have recently examined the question of whether AZT may cause cancer in the offspring or pregnant mice exposed to various doses of the drug. The relevance of these studies for human beings is not known, and the studies arrived at different conclusions. The first study was designed to determine if AZT, when given in extremely high doses to pregnant mice, could result in cancer in their offspring. Researchers found that when AZT is given in these high doses to pregnant mice, it can cause tumors in the liver, lung, and genital tract of their infants. The second study was designed to examine the long-term outcomes in the offspring of mice given much lower doses of AZT (designed to replicate the level of AZT in the blood of pregnant women following current treatment guidelines). This study found no increase in tumors.

The relationship between the doses of AZT used in these studies and those used in clinical practice in humans is not well understood. Since very few drugs have been studied in mice, scientists do not know if these studies can be used to reliably predict long-term effects in humans. Moreover, mice metabolize AZT very differently than humans. For example, AZT collects in high concentrations in the urine of mice, but does not do so in humans. Tumors seen in the vaginal tract of mice could be related to the direct contact with urine. But researchers do not know the mechanisms by which AZT caused the tumors in mice. Researchers are therefore uncertain if the outcomes of either of these mouse studies have any relevance to human beings. At this point, the long-term risks to humans remain theoretical. NIH and CDC, along with a "blue ribbon" panel of scientific experts, have concluded that the dramatic benefits of AZT in preventing perinatal transmission far outweigh the hypothetical concerns raised by these mouse studies, and that the current treatment guidelines should not be changed. However, both agencies continue to support additional research and the practice of informing women of any potential risks of AZT use.

Providing Women and Their Physicians the Best Possible Information

As the science continues to evolve in all of these areas, it continues to be critical that women and their health care providers have the information they need to make the best decisions for their health and the health of their babies. Community leaders and organizations should play a key role in reaching women at risk with complete information in terms they can understand. The agencies of the PHS regularly review research findings, and when necessary, the PHS perinatal task force reviews all relevant guidelines. The perinatal task force will soon be convened to review recent data on other risk factors, alternate therapies for HIV-infected individuals, and potential toxicity of AIDS drugs. The task force will outline areas requiring further study and ensure that current guidance reflects knowledge to date.

Chapter 50

Status of Perinatal HIV Prevention: Can Success Be Extended to the Developing World

During the early 1990s, before perinatal preventive treatments were available, an estimated 1,000-2,000 infants were born with HIV infection each year in the United States. Today, the U.S. has seen dramatic reductions in mother-to-child, or perinatal, HIV transmission rates. These declines reflect the widespread success of Public Health Service (PHS) recommendations made in 1994 and 1995 for routinely counseling and voluntarily testing pregnant women for HIV, and for offering zidovudine (AZT, also called ZDV) to infected women during pregnancy and delivery, and for the infant after birth.

Perinatal Prevention Saves Lives and Dollars

On a national level, and in numerous states, studies continue to demonstrate that perinatal HIV prevention is making a difference, both in terms of lives and resources saved:

- Between 1992 and 1996, perinatally acquired AIDS cases declined 43% in the U.S. In 1997, this trend continued with a 30% decline.

- A four-state study (Michigan, New Jersey, Louisiana, and South Carolina) found that the proportion of pregnant women voluntarily tested for HIV increased from 68% in 1993 to 79% in 1996. The percentage of women offered AZT increased from 27% in 1993 to 85% in 1996.

CDC Update, National Center for HIV, STD, and TB Prevention, June 1998.

437

- Among women in CDC's (Centers for Disease Control and Prevention) Perinatal AIDS Collaborative Transmission Study (PACTS), AZT use increased following the publication of PHS guidelines, and the rate of perinatal transmission dropped from 21% to 11%. The PACTS study includes women from four cities—New York City, Newark, Atlanta, and Baltimore.

- In North Carolina, perinatal HIV transmission dropped from 21% in 1993 to 6.2% in the first half of 1996.

- Prenatal care that includes HIV counseling and testing and AZT treatment for infected mothers and their children saves lives and resources. Without intervention, a 25% mother-to-infant transmission rate would result in the birth of an estimated 1,750 HIV-infected infants annually in the United States, with lifetime medical costs of $282 million.

- Researchers estimate that the annual cost of perinatal prevention is $67.6 million. This investment prevents 656 HIV infections and saves $105.6 million in medical care costs alone, for a net cost-savings of $38.1 million annually.

Despite these successes, challenges remain for further reducing HIV transmission to children in the United States, and for extending opportunities for perinatal prevention to nations in the developing world. Perhaps the greatest barriers in the U.S. are the continuing spread of HIV infection among minority women and the lack of early prenatal care for many of these women.

HIV Remains a Significant Problem for U.S. Women and Their Babies, Especially for Minority Women and Children

HIV infection in children is closely associated with the HIV epidemic in women. HIV transmission from mother to child during pregnancy, labor, and delivery or by breast-feeding has accounted for 91% of all AIDS cases reported among U.S. children. Obviously, the best way to prevent infection among children is to prevent infection in women.

Women of color and their children have always been disproportionately affected by the HIV epidemic. In 1997, of the 13,105 total AIDS cases reported among U.S. women, 10,458 (80%) were among African-American and Hispanic women. Of the 473 children reported with

AIDS last year, 402 (85%) were African-American and Hispanic. We must continue to improve HIV prevention efforts for women of color and ensure that interventions provide the information, skills, and support needed to reduce their HIV-related risks.

Moreover, perinatal HIV prevention efforts must work to ensure that all HIV-infected women are reached early in pregnancy with the opportunity to learn their HIV status and, if infected, to consider preventive therapy to improve the chances that their children will be born free of infection. Achieving this goal will require increased access to and utilization of prenatal care.

- A 1995 study analyzed data on approximately one-sixth of all HIV-exposed children born in the United States and found that only about half (53%) received the benefit of the full AZT treatment regimen (for the mother during pregnancy and delivery and for the infant following birth). The main reason for babies not having the advantage of therapy was that more than one-fourth of the mothers (26%) did not get prenatal care.

In addition to increasing access to preventive therapy in the United States, efforts must also focus on extending perinatal prevention to the developing world.

Critical Need to Extend Perinatal Prevention to the Developing World

Until recently, the only AZT regimen proven effective for perinatal HIV prevention was essentially out of reach for the countries where more than 90% of worldwide HIV infections occur. The AZT regimen used in the United States and other industrialized nations is costly and requires several months of treatment for the mother and the infant, and an intravenous dose during delivery that is not feasible in many developing countries. Additionally, HIV-infected mothers in these nations often have no practical alternative to breast-feeding, and this poses an additional risk of transmitting the virus to their newborns.

Earlier this year, researchers from CDC and the Ministry of Public Health in Thailand announced dramatic findings that offer real hope for extending perinatal prevention successes to many developing nations that previously had no realistic preventive options. Researchers found that a short course of AZT given late in pregnancy and during delivery reduced the rate of HIV transmission to infants of infected mothers by half and is safe for use in the developing world. However, the study did not address the efficacy of the regimen among women who breast-feed. Ongoing studies in Africa are expected to provide this critical information.

Policy makers believe that this regimen, using a much shorter course of AZT during pregnancy, an oral dose rather than an intravenous dose during delivery, and no infant dose, can more realistically be implemented in the developing world. The provision of safe alternatives to breast-feeding will still need to be addressed in every setting. The United Nations is now working with public health agencies around the globe to help make this short-course regimen available for as many women as possible and to continue to identify practical solutions for reducing the toll of the epidemic on women and children worldwide.

Chapter 51

Preventing Occupational Exposure to HIV

General Information on Occupational Exposures to Blood

Introduction

Health-care workers are at risk for occupational exposure to the human immunodeficiency virus (HIV). Exposures occur through needlesticks or cuts from other sharp instruments (percutaneous exposures) contaminated with an infected patient's blood or through contact of the eye, nose or mouth (mucous membrane) or skin with a patient's blood.

Most exposures do not result in infection. The risk of infection varies with the type of exposure and factors such as:

- The amount of blood involved in the exposure

- The amount of virus in the patient's blood at the time of exposure

- Whether postexposure treatment was taken

Your employer should have in place a system for reporting exposures in order to quickly evaluate the risk of infection from the exposure, counsel you about recommendations for treatments available to

Centers for Disease Control and Prevention (CDC) and U.S. Department of Health and Human Services (DHHS), June 1997.

441

prevent infection, and monitor you for side effects of treatments and determine if infection occurs. This may involve testing your blood and that of the source patient and offering appropriate postexposure treatment.

How can occupational exposures be prevented?

Many needlesticks and other cuts can be prevented by using medical devices with safety features designed to prevent injuries by using safer techniques (e.g. not recapping needles by hand), and by disposing of used needles in appropriate sharps disposal containers. Many exposures to the eyes, nose, mouth, or skin can be prevented by using appropriate barriers (e.g., gloves, eye and face protection, gowns) when contact with blood is expected.

If an Exposure Occurs

What should I do if I am exposed to the blood of a patient?

1. Immediately following an exposure to blood:

- Needlesticks and cuts should be washed with soap and water
- Splashes to the nose, mouth, or skin should be flushed with water
- Eyes should be irrigated with clean water, saline or sterile irrigants

No scientific evidence shows that the use of antiseptics for wound care or squeezing the wound will reduce the risk of transmission of HIV. The use of a caustic agent such as bleach is not recommended.

2. Following any blood exposure you should:

- Report the exposure to the department (e.g., occupational health infection control) responsible for managing exposures. Prompt reporting is essential because, in some cases, HIV postexposure treatment may be recommended and it should be started as soon as possible—preferably within 1-2 hours.

- In addition to HIV, discuss the possible risks of acquiring hepatitis B and hepatitis C with your health-care provider. You should have already received hepatitis B vaccine, which is extremely safe and effective in preventing hepatitis B.

Risk of Infection after Exposure

What is the risk of HIV infection after an occupational exposure?

While the risk is very low, it is not zero. HIV infection has been reported after occupational exposures to HIV-infected blood through needlesticks or cuts; splashes in the eyes, nose, or mouth; and skin contact.

- Exposure from needlesticks or cuts cause most infections. The average risk of HIV infection after a needlestick/cut exposure to HIV-infected blood is 0.3% (i.e., three-tenths of one percent, or about 1 in 300). Stated another way, 99.7% of needlestick/cut exposures do not lead to infection.

- The risk after exposure of the eye, nose, or mouth to HIV infected blood is estimated to be, on average, 0.1% (1 in 1,000).

- The risk after exposure of the skin to HIV-infected blood is estimated to be less than 0.1%. A small amount of blood on intact skin probably poses no risk at all. There have been no cases of HIV transmission documented due to an exposure involving a small amount of blood on intact skin. The risk may be higher if the skin is damaged (e.g., a recent cut) or if the contact involves a larger area or is prolonged.

Risk from all exposures is probably increased if the exposure involves a larger volume of blood or a higher amount of HIV in the patient's blood. (Source-patients near death with AIDS or patients with symptoms of acute HIV infection usually have higher amounts of HIV in their blood.)

How many health-care workers have been infected with HIV occupationally and under what circumstances?

As of December 1996, CDC had received reports of 52 documented cases and 111 possible cases of occupationally acquired HIV infection among health-care workers in the United States.

The 111 possible cases were in health-care workers who reported an occupational exposure to blood, body fluids, or HIV-infected laboratory material, and who did not have any other identifiable behavioral or transfusion risk for HIV infection. However, for these workers, infection specifically resulting from an occupational exposure was not documented.

443

Treatment for the Exposure

Is treatment available after an occupational exposure to HIV?

Yes. Results from a small number of studies suggest that the use of zidovudine (ZDV) and other antiviral drugs after certain occupational exposures may reduce the chance of HIV transmission. In one study, the use of ZDV after HIV exposure from a needlestick or cut reduced the risk of HIV transmission by almost 80%.

Will treatment after exposure prevent HIV infection?

These studies suggest that postexposure treatment may prevent infection with HIV. However, because there have been at least 12 reported cases of ZDV failing to prevent HIV infection in health-care workers, postexposure treatment will probably not prevent all cases of infection transmission.

Type of occupational exposure	Number
Needlestick or cuts	45
Eye, nose, mouth, and/or skin	5
Both injury & mucous membrane	1
Unknown	1
TOTAL	52

Type of fluid involved in exposure	Number
Blood	47
Concentrated virus in a laboratory	3
Visibly bloody fluid	1
Unspecified fluid	1
TOTAL	52

Table 51.1. Health-Care Workers with Documented Occupationally Acquired HIV Infection

Is postexposure treatment recommended for all types of occupational exposure to HIV?

No. Because most occupational exposures do not lead to HIV infection, the chance of possible serious side effects (toxicity) from the drugs used to prevent infection may be much greater than the chance of infection from such exposure. Both risk of infection and possible side effects of drugs should be carefully considered when deciding whether to take postexposure treatment. Exposures with a lower infection risk may not be worth the risk of the side effects associated with these drugs.

What about exposures to blood for which the HIV status of the source patient is unknown?

If the source individual cannot be identified or tested, decisions regarding follow-up should be based on the exposure risk and whether the source is likely to be a person who is HIV positive. Follow-up HIV testing should be available to all workers who are concerned about possible HIV infection through occupational exposure.

Treatments Available

What specific drugs are recommended for postexposure treatment?

In June 1996 the Public Health Service recommended that zidovudine (ZDV), lamivudine (3TC), and a protease inhibitor, preferably indinavir (IDV), be used as follows:

- ZDV should be considered for treatment of all exposures involving HIV-infected blood, fluid containing visible blood, or other potentially infectious fluid or tissue.

- 3TC should be added to ZDV for increased effectiveness and for use against ZDV-resistant types of virus. Used in combination, ZDV and 3TC are very effective in treating HIV infection, and considerable information shows that they are safe when used for a short time.

- IDV should be added for the highest risk exposures, such as those involving a larger volume of blood with a larger amount of HIV. IDV is a potent antiviral drug that appears to be safe when taken for a short period, although less information is available about the safety of this drug.

Since June 1996, several new antiviral drugs have been licensed for use in the United States. The Public Health Service recommendations will be reviewed and may be modified in 1997, taking into account the availability of additional drugs.

Can other antiviral drugs be used or substituted if these drugs are not available?

These recommendations are intended to provide guidance to clinicians and may be modified on a case-by-case basis. Whenever possible, consulting an expert with experience in the use of antiviral drugs is advised, especially if a recommended drug is not available, if the source patient's virus is likely to be resistant to one or more recommended drugs, or if the drugs are poorly tolerated.

Should zidovudine ever be used alone?

ZDV alone may be considered for some lower risk exposures when the virus is likely to be sensitive to the drug.

How soon after exposure to HIV should treatment start?

Treatment should be started promptly, preferably within 1-2 hours after the exposure. Although animal studies suggest that treatment is not effective when started more than 24-36 hours after exposure, it is not known if this time frame is the same for humans. Starting treatment after a longer period (e.g., 1-2 weeks) may be considered for the highest risk exposures; even if HIV infection is not prevented, early treatment of initial HIV infection may lessen the severity of symptoms and delay the onset of AIDS.

How long do the drugs need to be taken?

The optimal course of treatment is unknown; because 4 weeks of ZDV appears to provide protection against HIV infection, if tolerated, treatment should probably be taken for 4 weeks.

Has the FDA approved these drugs to prevent HIV following an occupational exposure?

No. The FDA has approved these drugs for the treatment of HIV infection, but not for preventing infection. However, physicians may prescribe any approved drug when, in their professional judgement, the use of the drug is warranted.

Safety and Side Effects

What is known about the safety and side effects of these drugs?

Most of the information known about the safety and side effects of these drugs is based on studies of their use in HIV-infected individuals. For these individuals, ZDV and 3TC have usually been well tolerated when taken in the doses recommended. There is less information about IDV, but it also may be well tolerated when used for a short period. IDV should not be used in combination with certain other drugs, including some prescription antihistamines (consult your health-care provider). Some of the more frequent side effects reported in HIV-infected patients include the following:

- Upset stomach (e.g., nausea, vomiting, diarrhea), tiredness, or headache for people taking ZDV

- Upset stomach and, in rare instances, pancreatitis for people taking 3TC

- Jaundice and kidney stones in people taking IDV, although these side effects are infrequent when IDV is taken less than one month. The risk of kidney stones may be reduced by drinking 48oz of fluid per 24-hour period.

There is some information about ZDV use by health-care workers as postexposure treatment. ZDV is usually tolerated, but reported side effects have included upset stomach, tiredness, and headache, all of which stopped when the drug was stopped. There is little information on the side effects of 3TC and IDV in uninfected individuals.

Should pregnant health-care workers take these drugs?

Based on limited information, ZDV taken in the second and third trimesters of pregnancy has not caused serious side effects in mothers or infants. There is very little information on the safety of ZDV when taken during the first trimester or on the safety of other antiviral drugs taken during pregnancy. If you are pregnant at the time you have an occupational exposure to HIV, you should consult a physician about the use of antiviral drugs for postexposure treatment.

447

Follow-up after the Exposure

What follow-up should be done after an exposure?

- You should be tested for HIV antibody as soon as possible after the exposure (baseline), and periodically for at least 6 months after the exposure (e.g., at 6 weeks, 12 weeks, and 6 months).

- If you take antiviral drugs for postexposure treatment, you should be checked for drug toxicity including a complete blood count and kidney and liver function test just before starting treatment and 2 weeks after starting treatment.

- You should report any sudden or severe flu-like illness that occurs during the follow-up period, especially if it involves fever, rash, muscle aches, tiredness, malaise, or swollen glands. Such an illness or symptoms may suggest HIV infection, drug reaction, or other medical condition.

- You should contact your health-care provider if you have any questions or problems during the follow-up period.

What precautions should be taken during the follow-up period?

During the follow-up period, especially the first 6-12 weeks when most infected persons are expected to show signs of infection, you should follow recommendations for preventing transmission of HIV. These include refraining from blood, semen, or organ donation and abstaining from sexual intercourse. If you choose to have sexual intercourse, using a latex condom consistently and correctly may reduce the risk of HIV transmission. In addition, women should not breast-feed infants during the follow-up period to prevent exposing their infants to HIV in breast milk.

HIV Occupational Exposure Registry

What is being done to learn more about the use of antiviral drugs for treatment after an occupational exposure to HIV?

Because information is limited about the side effects/toxicity of antiviral drugs in uninfected people like you, the Centers for Disease Control and Prevention, Glaxo Wellcome Inc., and Merck & Co., Inc., have begun the **HIV Postexposure Prophylaxis (PEP) Registry**, to collect information about the safety, tolerability, and outcome of taking antiviral drugs for postexposure treatment.

What kind of information will be collected by the Registry?

If you give permission, your health-care provider will provide information to the Registry about the exposure, the antiviral drugs taken, and abnormal laboratory findings and physical symptoms associated with the use of these drugs. Participation is voluntary and confidential. No information that would identify you will be collected.

How can I learn more about or enroll in the Registry?

Ask your health-care provider; he or she can obtain information about the Registry by calling toll-free 1-888-PEP4HIV (1-888-737-4448).

Other Sources of Information

How can I learn more about health-care workers and occupational exposures to HIV?

Information specialists who staff the CDC National AIDS Hotline (1-800-342-2437) can answer questions or provide information on HIV infection and AIDS and resources available in your area. The AIDS Treatment Information Service (1-800-933-4313) can also be contacted for information on the clinical treatment of HIV/AIDS. For free copies of printed material on HIV infection and AIDS, please call or write:

CDC National AIDS Clearinghouse
P.O. Box 6003
Rockville, MD 20849-6003
Telephone 1-800-458-5231.
Internet address http://www.cdcnac.aspensys.com:86

Chapter 52

Recent HIV/AIDS Treatment Advances and the Implications for Prevention

In recent years, medical science has made great progress in our ability to successfully treat HIV infection and associated opportunistic infections (OIs). Wider use of medications for preventing tuberculosis, *Pneumocystis carinii* pneumonia (PCP), toxoplasmosis, and *Mycobacterium avium* complex (MAC), for example, has helped reduce the number of people with HIV who develop serious illness and die from AIDS. Also, several new compounds in a new class of drugs, called protease inhibitors, have been federally approved to treat HIV infection. These drugs, when taken in combination with previously approved drugs such as zidovudine (ZDV, also called AZT), lamivudine (3TC) and dideoxyinosine (ddI), reduce the level of HIV particles circulating in the blood (viral load) to very low levels in many individuals. Treatment results using these drugs have been extremely encouraging, as these drug combinations are more effective than any previously available therapies. Researchers are hopeful that this type of combination therapy, with further study, will prove effective long-term and increase the healthy life span of more HIV-infected individuals.

Is It Time to Declare Victory Over HIV and AIDS?

Not yet, as there remain several areas of uncertainty and reasons for caution. Even though an estimated two-thirds of all HIV-infected people in the United States have been tested and know their serostatus, many remain unaware of their HIV infection until they

CDC Update, National Center for HIV, STD, and TB Prevention, June 1998.

are diagnosed with an AIDS-associated illness. People need to know they are infected so they can take steps to protect their health and prevent the transmission of HIV to others. People who learn their HIV serostatus early in the course of infection can benefit from taking medications specifically to prevent OIs, as well as other drugs to suppress HIV in their bodies.

Another significant concern is the effect that knowledge about success of the new combination therapies will have on prevention efforts. It is critical that individuals at risk do not relax their preventive behaviors because of the availability of more effective treatments. It is also important for prevention services to reach the increasing numbers of people living with HIV and help them maintain safer behaviors.

What Is the Long-Term Effectiveness and Safety of These New Combination Therapies?

Most patients have been studied for less than 2-3 years. Because these drugs are so new, their long-term effectiveness and safety are still unknown. What we do know is that:

- the new combination therapies reduce the concentration of HIV circulating in the blood of most individuals, but there is no evidence that the therapies completely eradicate the virus from all parts of the body. It is not known how long these drugs will be effective in maintaining reduced levels of HIV in the bloodstream. HIV may rebound from such areas as the lymph nodes, brain, or white blood cells.

- these drugs do not work for all people with HIV infection. In some individuals, substantial levels of circulating virus persist despite use of the newer drug combinations.

- many patients develop serious side effects which prevent them from continuing to take the drugs. Moreover, the long-term health consequences of taking these drugs for many years are unknown.

- these drugs are extremely expensive ($12,000 or more per year for the drugs alone), and paying for the drugs is a challenge for many people.

- because of the high costs, these therapies are not widely available in developing countries where over 90% of new HIV infections are occurring. Fighting the epidemic globally will require more cost-effective solutions.

- these drugs will be added to the long list of drugs taken by people with HIV infection, and they sometimes have adverse interactions with other medications. In particular, there are serious problems with taking protease inhibitors in conjunction with drugs commonly used to treat TB. Physicians prescribing these drugs must carefully consider all potential interactions.

Can HIV Develop Resistance to the New Drugs?

Yes. The new combination therapies require patients to follow complex treatment regimens, taking multiple medications several times each day. Some must be taken with food, and some must be taken on an empty stomach—and these drugs may have to be taken for the rest of the patient's life.

People who miss doses of their medication may be at increased risk for developing drug-resistant strains of HIV. If these strains are transmitted to others and spread widely, HIV infection could become much more difficult to treat.

Do These New Drug Therapies Block Transmission of HIV?

While studies are being conducted to investigate how new drug therapies relate to infectivity, conclusive findings are not yet available about their protection against HIV transmission. As we learn more about the impact of new combination therapies on infectiousness, it is possible that our treatment and prevention strategies will become more closely intertwined. In the meantime, it is critical that people adopt or maintain protective behaviors that are known to be effective in preventing the spread of HIV infection.

How Has Information about These New Drugs Affected Behavior in At-Risk Populations?

Research suggests that some individuals are less concerned about becoming infected than in the past and may be inclined to take more risks. Moreover, some may assume that HIV-positive individuals taking protease inhibitors are not infectious. As a result, some people may believe there is no longer a need to avoid high-risk sex and drug use. CDC is concerned that people may be placing themselves at unnecessary risk because of these assumptions. Another concern, as mentioned above, is the transmission of resistant strains, which could undermine the benefits of treatment advances.

Are the New Drug Therapies the Key to Controlling the HIV/AIDS Epidemic?

A wide range of behavioral and biomedical strategies are needed to control the epidemic. No medical advance, by itself, can succeed unless it is accompanied by appropriate behavior change. Even a vaccine does not stop a disease unless it is available and people have access to it. As researchers continue working to develop better treatment and prevention options, we must continue to focus on preventing HIV infection, which precludes the need for people to undergo complex, costly treatment regimens. A strong foundation of behavioral interventions must be maintained and, at the same time, there must be a focus on developing and strengthening biomedical prevention interventions such as vaccines, microbicides, and the treatment of other STDs.

How Can Care, Treatment, and Prevention Work Better Together?

Better integrating care and treatment services, including those for STD and substance abuse, would allow us to take advantage of multiple opportunities for prevention—first, to help the uninfected stay that way; second, to help infected people stay healthier; and third, to help those who are infected initiate and sustain behaviors that will keep themselves safe and prevent transmission to others.

In some cases, treatment is prevention. When pregnant women and their newborns are treated with ZDV, for example, the chances of mother-to-infant HIV transmission are greatly reduced. We also know that treating other STDs can greatly reduce the risk of transmitting or acquiring HIV infection. Substance abuse treatment that succeeds in getting a drug user to stop using drugs can prevent his or her own infection through sharing needles, as well as possible future HIV transmission to sex partners.

Reaching the HIV-Infected

Among those who are infected, using new drug combination therapies to suppress the virus and medications that we know are effective in preventing the development of opportunistic illnesses will keep people healthier longer. Also, prevention case management services have proven effective in helping people with HIV adopt and sustain safer behaviors. With HIV-infected persons living longer and healthier lives, prevention will be even more important. Ongoing services for people who are HIV positive must balance medical advances with the behavioral and social support needed to preserve their quality of life and prevent the spread of infection.

Chapter 53

HIV/AIDS Vaccine and
Prevention Strategies

Developing safe and effective prevention strategies to curb the human and economic costs of the HIV/AIDS pandemic has become an international health priority. Toward this end, NIAID, which spearheads federal funding for biomedical research on HIV/AIDS for the National Institutes of Health (NIH), supports a broad-based HIV vaccine and prevention research program.

NIAID's Division of AIDS (DAIDS) directs this program. Institute staff meet regularly with scientific, public health and community advisors to review the priorities and operation of the program.

The program has two main thrusts:

- to foster basic research on the structure and function of HIV, vaccine formulations, vaccine delivery systems, laboratory studies of vaccine performance and microbicides, and

- to promptly evaluate promising candidate vaccines, microbicides and other intervention strategies in animal models and, if warranted, in humans.

Traditional investigator-initiated research forms the foundation for HIV/AIDS vaccine research. NIAID supports several special collaborative and interdisciplinary initiatives to accomplish specific research objectives.

National Institute of Allergy and Infectious Diseases (NIAID) January 1997.

- *National Cooperative Vaccine Development Groups (NCVDGs)* constitute the core of preclinical HIV vaccine design and evaluation efforts sponsored by NIAID. Teams of scientists from industry, academia and government collaborate to develop and test novel experimental HIV vaccine concepts in the laboratory and in animal models.

- *The Cooperative Mucosal Immunology Group for Investigations on AIDS Vaccines* supports research on methods to stimulate and evaluate mucosal immune responses to HIV and its monkey counterpart, simian immunodeficiency virus (SIV). Investigators use this information to design new vaccines that will protect against mucosal exposure to HIV.

- *The Antibody Serologic Project* identifies and standardizes panels of monoclonal antibodies to characterize the antigenic components of HIV and SIV. This collaborative project involves investigators from around the world.

- *The HIV Variation Project* examines the rates and magnitudes of genetic and immunologic changes in HIV and related retroviruses and their consequences for vaccine design. The project includes a laboratory that determines the genetic sequences of large numbers of viral isolates (Genetic Variation Contract), a laboratory to assess the immunologic significance of genetic variation (Antigenic Variation Contract), and the **HIV Sequence Database and Analysis Unit** at the Los Alamos National Laboratory, which compiles and analyzes genomic sequences contributed by sequence laboratories. The HIV Variation Project is carried out in collaboration with the Centers for Disease Control and Prevention (CDC) and the World Health Organization (WHO).

- *Primate Research Laboratories* answer HIV-vaccine-related questions by testing HIV and HIV-like vaccines in chimpanzees and monkeys. The **Simian Vaccine Evaluation Units (S-VEUs)** evaluate vaccine concepts in the macaque model and compare immunologic and protection data, permitting standardized and directly comparable evaluations of various vaccine candidates. Substantial effort is being made to develop the chimeric SIV-HIV (SHIV) model for use in challenge studies. The **Chimpanzee Unit**, operated through an interagency agreement with the National Cancer Institute, has been used to prepare chimpanzee stocks and to evaluate candidate vaccine concepts and products in chimpanzees. The **Immunology Laboratory Support for Assessment of AIDS Vaccines in Primates** (which includes several contracts) develops, standardizes and performs cellular and serologic immune assays to assess responses to SIV and HIV vaccines in the S-VEUs, and is also available to NCVDG laboratories. This permits the direct comparison of candidate vaccines evaluated in independent laboratories and facilitates selection of the most promising vaccine designs.

* *The Reagent/Resource AIDS Vaccine Project* acquires or produces biological and chemical substances for comparative immunologic analyses, preclinical vaccine development, adjuvant development and standardized immunologic assessments of clinical samples from volunteers in vaccine trials.

* *The Master Agreement for Preclinical HIV Vaccine Development* provides flexible resources for the preclinical evaluation of the most promising HIV vaccine candidates. These resources include preclinical evaluation of vaccines in nonhuman primates, vaccine production and the development of reagents for preclinical and clinical vaccine studies.

* *The AIDS Vaccine Evaluation Group (A VEG)* conducts Phase I and Phase II trials in humans to evaluate the safety of and immune responses stimulated by experimental HIV vaccines. AVEG includes the following:

  — **A Vaccine Selection Group** independently evaluates the rationale and preclinical safety and immunogenicity data of candidate vaccines prior to their study in AVEG trials.

  — Six **AIDS Vaccine Evaluation Units (AVEUs),** located at research centers throughout the United States, conduct Phase I and II clinical trials of candidate HIV vaccines in volunteers who are not infected with HIV.

  — A **Central Immunology Laboratory** provides state-of-the-art evaluation of antibody and cellular immune responses of vaccinated volunteers in AVEG trials. Laboratory scientists evaluate samples from the AVEUs using standardized assays, permitting the comparison of responses in volunteers who receive different candidate vaccines at different AVEUs.

459

- A **Mucosal Immunology Laboratory** evaluates human mucosal immune responses to candidate vaccines in standardized assays, permitting the comparison of responses in volunteers who receive different candidate vaccines at different AVEUs.

- A **Data Coordinating and Analysis Center** provides a central facility for collecting and analyzing data from the trials conducted by the AVEUs.

- A **Data and Safety Monitoring Board** periodically reviews data from AVEG studies.

Planning for Efficacy Trials

NIAID is laying the groundwork for large-scale Phase III efficacy trials of candidate HIV vaccines and other prevention strategies to ensure that such trials begin promptly once suitable candidates are identified.

To assess the feasibility of conducting vaccine trials in the United States, NIAID initially provided supplemental funds to help support ongoing studies sponsored by the Centers for Disease Control and Prevention and the National Institute on Drug Abuse, and to other investigators working with populations at high risk of HIV infection.

To determine the feasibility of and develop the capability for conducting such trials abroad, NIAID in 1992 awarded eight two-year *Preparation for AIDS/HIV Vaccine Evaluations (PAVE)* grants to U.S. researchers and their international collaborators.

In 1993 the NIAID unified and extended these efforts by establishing the *HIV Network for Prevention Trials (HIVNET)*. HIVNET is charged with preparing for and conducting large-scale, randomized, controlled trials to evaluate the efficacy of vaccines and other strategies to prevent sexual, parenteral and perinatal transmission of HIV. In addition, HIVNET provides a unique opportunity to study the epidemiology of HIV transmission in different populations, and to examine the natural history and pathogenesis of early HIV infection and disease. HIVNET consists of five contracts:

- A domestic master contractor subcontracts with clinical sites to conduct activities in preparation for efficacy trials. These sites will evaluate the efficacy of HIV vaccines and other prevention strategies in U.S. populations once suitable candidates are identified.

460

- An international master contractor subcontracts with clinical sites to prepare for efficacy trials and to evaluate prevention strategies in international populations.

- A statistical and data coordinating center provides statistical and data management support for the domestic and international trials.

- A central laboratory provides quality assurance and specialized testing for the domestic and international trials, and preparatory research trials.

- A specimen repository collects, stores and distributes samples from the domestic and international clinical sites.

HIVNET investigators are collecting baseline data on virus strains being transmitted, rates of new HIV infections and the prevalence of other sexually transmitted diseases and other potential cofactors of HIV transmission from various populations at high risk for HIV infection. They also are collecting data on the willingness of high-risk individuals to enroll in vaccine trials.

Several of the HIVNET sites are conducting randomized controlled trials of various methods to prevent sexual and perinatal HIV infection. These interventions include microbicides to prevent sexual transmission, and antiretroviral drugs and HIV immune globulin to prevent perinatal transmission. Behavioral interventions also are being evaluated.

Institute staff assist public health and government officials, community members, scientists and others affiliated with potential trial sites to resolve legal, practical and ethical issues involved in planning for vaccine efficacy trials. These concerns include vaccine cost and delivery, liability issues, training of medical personnel and conduct of trials at potential overseas sites.

NIAID, a component of the National Institutes of Health (NIH), supports research on AIDS, tuberculosis and other infectious diseases, as well as allergies and immunology. NIH is an agency of the U.S. Department of Health and Human Services. NIAID press releases, fact sheets and other materials are available on the Internet via the NIAID home page at http://www.niaid.nih.gov.

Part Five

Where Do HIV/AIDS Drugs Come From?

Chapter 54

Where Do HIV/AIDS Drugs Come From?

Drug Discovery

Designing drugs to fight disease-causing viruses is a relatively young science that poses special challenges. Viruses live and multiply inside cells in the body that perform vital, day-to-day functions. Thus, to be safe for human use, an antiviral drug must kill its target without harming the cells it infects.

Until recently, the problems inherent to developing compounds to selectively kill viruses inside cells seemed insurmountable. The new tools of biotechnology, however, have enabled scientists to amass staggering amounts of information about the molecular biology and life cycles of viruses and how they cause diseases. This knowledge lets researchers zero in on a virus' most vulnerable features and design drugs to disarm it.

Bringing a new drug to market requires three principal steps. First, the candidate drug must either be discovered in the laboratory or the natural environment or be designed from scratch, based on information known about the microbe. This step involves evaluating the activity of the candidate drug in test-tube and tissue culture experiments and in animal models that mimic the human disease. Then the candidate drug must be purified and produced in large enough amounts so that its safety in animals can be assessed. Finally, its safety and effectiveness must be established in human clinical trials.

National Institute of Allergy and Infectious Diseases, (NIAID), August 1996.

465

As the number of people infected with the human immunodeficiency virus type 1 (HIV-1) continues to grow, efforts by government, university and private industry scientists to find treatments that inhibit HIV infection or slow the progress of HIV disease have expanded markedly. The National Institute of Allergy and Infectious Diseases (NIAID), through its Division of AIDS (DAIDS), plays a major role in fostering the discovery of promising anti-HIV agents and assuring their development into drugs for use in people infected with the virus. NIAID also has assumed this role for agents showing promise against microorganisms that cause opportunistic infections (OIs) associated with AIDS.

Drug Screening Versus Drug Design

Therapeutics for HIV disease and its associated OIs are discovered through a variety of approaches including high-volume screening of drug libraries, targeted drug screening, evaluation of natural products, and rational drug design.

Nearly all approved drugs used to fight infections were discovered through random screening of naturally occurring and synthetic compounds. Natural products or compounds synthesized in the laboratory can be submitted to the National Cancer Institute (NCI) to be initially screened for anti-HIV activity. Some 12,000 compounds are screened through this program yearly. About one out of every 50 compounds tested shows some measurable activity against HIV.

DAIDS staff use chemical databases, or drug libraries, to identify promising anti-HIV compounds that have not been synthesized or tested. An advantage of these databases is that they allow researchers to examine the potential effects of specific chemical changes on the activity and pharmacokinetics of the drug molecule without having to do tissue culture or animal model experiments.

Many compounds that inhibit HIV in screening tests, however, also seriously damage human cells. These compounds may be modified to reduce their toxicity and then be submitted for retesting. Only those that inhibit the virus while causing minimal damage to HIV-infected cells are candidates for development into drugs for human use. The compounds that meet these criteria amount to less than one percent of those screened each year.

A growing number of HIV researchers are pursuing a newer approach to drug discovery: rational, or targeted, drug design. The goal is to identify and learn as much as possible about vulnerable features of the disease-causing microbe and use these features as targets of drugs designed to thwart it.

DAIDS supports targeted drug discovery through the National Cooperative Drug Discovery Groups for HIV (NCDDG-HIV) and OIs (NCDDG-OI) programs and through a limited number of grants to individual investigators. In addition, the Strategic Program for Innovative Research on AIDS Treatments (SPIRAT) supports research on state-of-the-art therapeutic strategies from the advanced preclinical stage through pilot clinical studies in humans.

The NCDDG and SPIRAT programs provide major support for researchers pursuing targeted approaches to the discovery of anti-HIV as well as anti-OI drugs. But to design such drugs scientists first must gather extensive information about how HIV works.

The Biology of HIV

Since 1983 when HIV was discovered as the cause of AIDS, the virus has received an extraordinary amount of scientific attention. In that short time, researchers worldwide have learned more about the biology of HIV than of any other disease-causing virus. Information about the life cycle, reproduction and disease-causing mechanisms of HIV has come from studies of the genetics, biochemistry and molecular biology of HIV and its behavior once it infects and establishes itself within the cells.

HIV only multiplies inside cells. The virus gains access to the cell's interior through special attachment sites, or receptors, on the cell surface. Once inside, the virus uses its own enzyme, reverse transcriptase, to transcribe its genetic material, which is in the form of RNA, into DNA. HIV DNA then enters the cell nucleus and becomes inserted into the cell's DNA. From here, HIV genes govern the reproduction of new virus.

HIV's regulatory genes encode proteins that control virus replication. When the regulatory signals are turned on, the HIV DNA is copied back into RNA molecules, which then may become genetic material for a new virus or may be used to make structural proteins of HIV such as those of its outer coat or core.

Before leaving the cell, HIV particles assemble into whole viruses and are released through the cell membrane, picking up additional cellular proteins and other molecular components for their outer coats. Once the new viruses are outside the cell, they can infect new cells.

Targets for New Drugs

Because progression of HIV infection to AIDS depends greatly on the virus multiplying in and destroying immune system cells, many attempts to halt advancing disease are aimed at preventing HIV from replicating. Scientists designing anti-HIV drugs study each step in HIV's life cycle, looking for places where drugs may disrupt it. Candidate drugs might block receptors, inhibit essential enzymes, suppress replication signals or interfere with viral protein processing and assembly. Combinations of drugs may be aimed at two or more different steps in the virus' life cycle.

Examples of HIV drug targets include the following:

- reverse transcriptase—translates viral genetic information from RNA to DNA;
- protease—cleaves viral proteins into their mature, active forms;
- gp120—mediates entry of the virus into the host cell;
- integrase—inserts viral DNA into the host cell chromosome.

Other viral proteins may yet prove to be good targets for drug discovery and, through additional studies, their mechanisms of action will be understood.

To make copies of itself, HIV takes over the cell's normal machinery. Thus, researchers must be careful to target compounds to specific virus or cell components without disrupting the normal workings of the cell. Such accidental disruptions in cell function are a major cause of toxic side effects and a key obstacle to designing safe and effective drugs against HIV and other viruses.

Drug designers must understand the physical characteristics of anti-HIV drugs and how HIV interacts with various components of the human immune system. X-ray crystallography is invaluable for determining the three-dimensional shape of HIV proteins and cell proteins so that critical sites can be targeted or the shape of existing drugs can be improved to fit more precisely the target site. The three-dimensional structures of three viral proteins—CD4 (the cell surface binding site for HIV), protease, and reverse transcriptase—have been determined and have been used to design candidate anti-HIV drugs.

Drawing on the findings of basic research, NCDDG scientists develop laboratory procedures that allow candidate drugs to be tested for activity against HIV and its associated opportunistic infections. These researchers develop cell culture assays, biochemical screening tests and immunotherapies, or try to isolate and characterize active compounds from natural sources. The development of several new biochemical screens for agents blocking important HIV enzymes now enables investigators to screen more than 20,000 potential drugs annually without having to work directly with HIV.

So far, NCDDG scientists have helped advance several anti-HIV drugs into clinical testing. These include the following:

- stavudine (d4T), which like zidovudine (AZT), slows virus replication by inhibiting reverse transcriptase; approved for treatment of adults with advanced HIV infection who no longer respond to or who are intolerant of other antiviral drugs;

- oral and intravenous inhibitors of protease, the enzyme that cuts up the larger HIV proteins made first by an HIV-infected cell into smaller pieces that can reassemble into a new virus; in particular, early work on discovery of protease inhibitors at Abbott Laboratories; the company's drug, ritonavir, was recently approved by the U.S. Food and Drug Administration (FDA);

- genetically engineered CD4 and its derivatives, which act as decoys to bind free HIV and prevent its entry into cells;

- two novel BHAP compounds, which also inhibit reverse transcriptase activity but by a different mechanism.

The Drug Development Pipeline

Whether promising anti-HIV agents are discovered by scientists in government, academia or private industry, these compounds must be carefully evaluated before they can be licensed for use in people. Such an evaluation, consisting of test-tube, cell culture and animal model studies of a drug's safety and potential effectiveness, is called preclinical drug development.

To determine whether a drug is safe and effective enough to be tested in humans, results from certain preclinical studies are reviewed by the FDA. Turning promising agents into effective drugs depends upon strong, efficient partnerships between government agencies and private industry. NIAID facilitates this process by collaborating and consulting with drug sponsors to ensure that sufficient and appropriate preclinical data are generated for FDA review.

Drug development advances in steps, not all of which are required before a drug enters clinical testing. These steps include: cell culture tests to determine anti-HIV activity, safety studies in animals, efficacy evaluations in animals, investigations into mechanisms of drug action and chemical synthesis and formulation. Those studies required to obtain FDA permission to begin clinical studies are termed "critical path" steps. Other studies not required by the FDA also may be conducted to help determine a drug's appropriateness for clinical trials. Critical path steps fall into three general areas: efficacy, chemistry and safety. After a compound has shown activity against HIV in the test tube and in cultured cells, NIAID scientific staff and drug company representatives plan a drug development strategy that emphasizes critical path components. Initial studies are designed to confirm a drug's anti-HIV activity. The design of such studies is important because anti-HIV activity can be evaluated in many test systems, each of which provides different kinds of information. These confirmatory tests validate and sometimes duplicate the original observation.

Next, researchers must learn whether a drug's anti-HIV activity observed in laboratory studies can be duplicated in animal models of AIDS. Because HIV does not infect animals other than humans (except specifically designed experimental animal models), candidate drugs are tested in animals that are infected with viruses that cause AIDS-like disease symptoms, such as weight loss, abnormal blood cells and diarrhea. These model diseases are caused by viruses closely related to HIV.

Currently, DAIDS has available animal models of AIDS-like diseases in mice, cats and monkeys. Before carrying out studies in animal models, scientists conduct laboratory experiments to determine a drug's activity against the virus that produces the model disease. Results of such tests establish whether or not the virus is as susceptible as HIV to the new drug, and they also help in interpreting any negative study results.

Although the importance of animal model testing is widely accepted and recognized, it cannot be used alone in determining the drug's efficacy because it does not directly measure the drug's effect on HIV. Still, the FDA currently recommends animal model testing, if available, for drugs that will be used to treat people with HIV infection. Until a predictive model is established, however, the FDA does not require that the experimental drug cure the disease in the animal.

Even though the FDA does not require efficacy in an animal model before allowing clinical trials to begin, clinical researchers often use data from animal model tests as the basis for selecting which compounds will be given priority for entering clinical trials.

Drugs developed to combat OIs also take a critical path toward clinical trials. All people with AIDS are infected with HIV, but the virus is rarely the direct cause of death. The deterioration and eventual collapse of the immune system triggered by HIV infection enable common microbial organisms to flourish. These normally are present in the body but are held in check by a healthy immune system. In people infected with HIV, an OI can become life-threatening owing to the inability of the immune system to control the infection.

The second major critical path area of preclinical drug development is chemistry. The quantities of a newly synthesized drug required for initial test-tube studies are very small. Animal model testing, however, requires much larger quantities of drug, and early clinical safety trials require even more drug. Consequently, if test-tube studies show promising results, chemists begin producing quantities of drug that may be 1,000 times greater than the original amount made. Most academic chemical laboratories, which synthesize many potential anti-HIV drugs, do not have the capacity or expertise to make large quantities of drugs, and it can take six to 12 months to produce enough drug to supply all studies required by the FDA for approving a new agent. DAIDS currently has the resources to assist drug sponsors with producing large quantities of new drugs, particularly those drugs used to combat OIs.

After animal model testing is completed, candidate drugs may need to be refined with certain chemical changes in the original drug for better efficacy or stability into a form easily given to humans. Thus, at the same time that animal model studies proceed, and while larger quantities of drug are synthesized, other chemists search for ways to modify the drug to make it easily administered and of greater benefit to people. DAIDS also has the capacity to develop these formulations and to help manufacture them in quantities and purities that can be administered to patients.

The final step in the critical path development of a new drug is to establish the safety of the drug before giving it to people for the first time. These studies, carried out in animals, are carefully designed to answer critical questions about how the drug will be metabolized by humans, how long it will remain in the blood after administration, in which tissues will it be localized and what toxic side effects it may have. Based on the results of these studies, researchers can decide how best to administer the new drug and which doses to use. Because of the importance of these studies to the safety of patients, the FDA requires that these studies be conducted under stringent laboratory control and monitoring. DAIDS currently has the capacity to provide such safety studies to drug sponsors.

Although preclinical drug development obviously emphasizes the critical path steps, many ancillary studies take place simultaneously throughout the development and clinical testing of a new drug. These studies may identify the molecular target of the new drug; describe the mechanisms by which the drug inhibits HIV replication; evaluate the effects of the drug on healthy, non-HIV-infected cells or on viruses other than HIV; and determine how chemically related drugs affect HIV.

With its resources for chemistry, as well as its capacity to determine drug safety, DAIDS continues to exert a strong leadership role in seeing promising new chemicals through the preclinical drug development process into clinical trials.

Clinical Trials

If laboratory and animal studies show that a candidate drug is safe and likely to be effective, it is ready to be evaluated in humans in clinical trials. NIAID asks a committee of expert advisors to prioritize promising drugs for advance into clinical trials. Because a drug may act much differently in humans than it does in animals, evaluating the safety and effectiveness of a candidate drug in people must be done in discrete phases.

A drug's sponsor, which may be a drug company, a university or a government agency, must first file an investigational new drug (IND) application with the FDA. This application presents the results of test-tube, tissue culture and animal model studies for FDA review. If these studies indicate that the drug is safe enough to be given to people, the sponsor can then begin the first phase of clinical trials.

The largest network in the United States conducting human clinical trials of experimental AIDS therapies is the NIAID-supported AIDS Clinical Trials Group (ACTG). The ACTG coordinates studies involving drug companies, university hospitals and other government agencies to conduct trials to determine the dosage, safety and side effects of candidate drugs, as well as their effectiveness in fighting HIV infection or the immune deficiencies and opportunistic infections associated with AIDS.

In addition to the ACTG, NIAID supports clinical trials performed in community-based clinics under the Terry Beirn Community Programs for Clinical Research on AIDS (CPCRA). By involving community physicians in clinical trials, this program makes promising, experimental drugs available to patients who may not have access to clinical trials taking place at university-based medical centers.

A third mechanism for conducting clinical trials, the Division of AIDS Treatment Research Initiative (DATRI), was instituted by NIAID in October 1991. DATRI allows NIAID to rapidly address critical questions about new therapies and therapeutic approaches.

The Institute also sponsors AIDS clinical trials at the research hospital on the campus of the National Institutes of Health. Several important studies have been conducted and published by these researchers.

A Phase I clinical trial is the first setting in which an experimental drug is given to humans. These trials are thus designed to answer initial questions about a drug's safety. Researchers look for information about the drug's side effects, how much of the drug can be given to a patient and how the drug is handled by the body. Such information usually can be gathered in less than one year. Phase I trials are conducted on a small number of people, usually fewer than 20, and all participants receive the drug. Participants in Phase I trials for HIV and OI drugs usually have HIV infection.

If results from Phase I trials show that a drug is safe, it can enter the second phase of drug testing. Phase II trials enroll larger numbers of patients, as many as a few hundred. In these studies, researchers begin to ask questions about whether the drug is effective against HIV infection, AIDS-related immune deficiencies or opportunistic infections. Phase II clinical trials may take one to two years to complete.

To best answer questions about a drug's effectiveness, researchers try to avoid introducing psychological or intuitive biases into their studies. One way they can try to control conditions is by dividing study participants into two groups and giving the candidate drug to only one group. The other patients receive another drug already approved for their disorder or, if no such drug is available, they may get an inactive agent called a placebo. Doctors compare the outcomes in the two groups to see if the people who got the experimental drug have fewer symptoms, stay healthy longer or have fewer side effects. Currently, very few clinical trials of experimental AIDS drugs use placebos.

Another method of controlling bias in a clinical trial is to ensure that neither the health care providers nor the patients know who is getting which drugs. This is called "double blinding." Drugs are disguised and given code numbers so they cannot be recognized. The codes are kept secret, known only to a small number of people who oversee the progress of the clinical trial, until the study has ended.

Phase III clinical trials continue to answer questions about the drug's effectiveness and also look for long-term side effects that may not show up in earlier testing. For that reason, they may take up to four years to complete. Phase III trials often enroll several hundred to a few thousand patients and are controlled and blinded.

Traditionally, drug approval has been based on clinical efficacy, that is, an improvement in the patient's condition. With AIDS, however, the FDA is provisionally accepting efficacy based on improvements of the patient's laboratory tests, such as the number of certain immune system cells in the patient's blood. A drug approved under these guidelines is then re-evaluated when the final clinical data are submitted. This strategy is designed to speed the approval process.

The FDA has modified other regulations to speed the testing and approval processes for drugs aimed at life-threatening diseases. Under these guidelines, Phases II and III may be combined. This means that large Phase III trials to determine a drug's effectiveness may begin alongside Phase II trials that continue to evaluate an experimental drug's safety.

When Phase III clinical trials are complete, drug sponsors present results from all laboratory, animal and human studies to the FDA for review in the form of a new drug application (NDA) for approval to market the drug.

The magnitude and urgency of the AIDS epidemic have led researchers to look closely at the drug evaluation process to determine how it might be streamlined without compromising health and safety. One option is to conduct some controlled trials that measure fewer parameters and include more patients. Such studies are being conducted by the Terry Beirn CPCRA. The Public Health Service also has instituted a mechanism to make some promising drugs more available at the same time that they are being studied in clinical trials. Under this "parallel track" system, patients who do not qualify for or do not have access to clinical trials and who have no other therapeutic option can receive certain experimental drugs once these drugs have entered clinical trials.

Information on HIV/AIDS drug trials being conducted across the nation can be obtained by calling the AIDS Clinical Trials Information Service, a service of the U.S. Department of Health and Human Services, Public Health Service. The telephone number is 1-800-TRIALS-A (1-800-874-2572), and the service is open Monday through Friday from 9:00 a.m. through 7:00 p.m. Eastern Time. Spanish-speaking information specialists are available.

Chapter 55

CCR5 and Protection Against HIV-1 Infection

Recent findings from AIDS research suggest that a newly discovered variant gene may affect both susceptibility to HIV-1 infection and disease progression in persons who have become infected. The variant gene occurs primarily in persons of Western European heritage, but only about 1 % appear to have two copies of it (i.e., they are "homozygotes"). About 15%-20% have one copy (i.e., are "heterozygotes"). Persons with two copies of the gene appear to have some resistance to HIV-1 infection, while those with one copy can become infected but appear to have a slower rate of disease progression.

The gene determines the structure of a protein called chemokine receptor 5 ("CKR5," now called "CCR5") found on the surface of cells which can be infected by HIV-1. Scientists have recently discovered that CCR5 is one of the proteins to which HIV-1 attaches when it enters cells to infect them. In persons with two copies of the variant CCR5 gene, the protein is always defective and does not appear at the cell surface, apparently preventing most strains of HIV-1 from entering the cell.

While evidence indicates that persons with two copies of the variant CCR5 gene may be protected against HIV-1 transmission, it is not known whether the protection is partial or complete. There is at least one other protein (called "fusin") which some strains of HIV can use instead of CCR5 to enter $CD4^+$ T-lymphocytes, the cells targeted by HIV.

HIV/AIDS Prevention, Centers for Disease Control and Prevention (CDC), February 1997.

Persons with one copy of the variant CCR5 gene (heterozygotes) are not protected from becoming infected with HIV. However, studies conducted by the National Cancer Institute and other research groups indicate that among persons sexually infected with HIV, those who have one copy of the variant gene may not develop AIDS quite as quickly as those who have the normal gene only. Because persons with one copy of the variant gene have some of the defective protein and some normal CCR5 protein, their cells can be infected through the normal protein.

Further research is being conducted to learn more about CCR5 and the possible protective effect of the variant gene. This information may provide help in the development of effective therapies. However, because there is no evidence of complete genetic or other natural protection against HIV infection, all persons should continue to avoid behaviors that may place them at risk for infection, primarily unprotected sexual intercourse with an HIV-infected or at-risk partner and sharing of drug-injection equipment among persons who inject drugs.

Testing for the variant gene in order to predict whether an individual is susceptible to HIV is not recommended because protection associated with the variant gene may not be complete. Although some HIV-infected persons may request testing for the variant gene to help predict the course of their disease, it is not yet clear whether the test results would be truly predictive. In addition, the test for the variant gene is only performed in a few research laboratories at present. HIV-infected persons wishing to obtain more information about the test should contact their physicians. HIV-infected persons should be under the care of a physician to enable them to receive currently available antiretroviral therapy and prophylactic treatments to prevent the development of AIDS-related opportunistic illnesses.

Chapter 56

Challenges in Designing HIV Vaccines

Designing an effective vaccine to protect people from infection with the human immunodeficiency virus (HIV) or from becoming ill if already exposed to the virus is a high priority of worldwide efforts to control the epidemic.

The ideal HIV vaccine would be inexpensive, easy to store and administer and would elicit strong, appropriate immune responses that confer long-lasting protection against both bloodborne and mucosal (sexual) exposure to many HIV subtypes. The following describes why this ideal has not been easily achieved.

What Constitutes Immune Protection?

Researchers face unprecedented scientific challenges in trying to develop vaccines for HIV. The easiest way to design an effective vaccine is to know what immune responses protect against the specific infection and construct a vaccine that stimulates those responses. Although scientists have found clues about these so-called correlates of immunity or correlates of protection for HIV, these factors have not been precisely identified.

Unlike other viral diseases for which successful vaccines have been made, complete recovery from HIV infection has not been documented. Therefore, HIV vaccine researchers have no human model of protection to guide them. Indeed, whether a natural protective state against HIV can exist remains unknown.

National Institute of Allergy and Infectious Diseases (NIAID), January 1997.

However, now that the pandemic has matured, long-term survivors—those who remain clinically asymptomatic and maintain a CD4+ T cell count greater than 200 for at least 10 years following infection—provide ample evidence that some people appear better able than others to resist progression of HIV infection or the development of AIDS. Long-term survivors can be divided into two groups: (1) long-term nonprogressors, those who maintain healthy or steady levels of CD4+ T cells despite many years of infection, and (2) HIV-infected individuals who lose a significant proportion of CD4+ T cells but still remain healthy.

Recent attention also has been directed to those people who remain uninfected despite repeated exposure to HIV. If these multiply exposed but uninfected individuals can be proven to have resisted HIV by an active immune mechanism, they would represent the natural protective state upon which a vaccine could be modeled.

Another clue to why some people resist HIV infection has come from studies of recently identified co-receptors for HIV. Scientists have found that individuals who have inherited two copies of a mutated gene coding for one of these co-receptors, CCKR5, appear to be protected from HIV infection. This suggests that a single targeted intervention may be capable of preventing HIV infection.

To determine the factors that influence the body's response to HIV exposure and infection, investigators are comparing long-term HIV survivors with people who quickly became infected or sick. Leading areas of research include genetics, individual variations in the immune response and exposure to or infection by less deadly HIV variants. Such studies will help clarify what contributes to protective immunity against HIV.

Immune Responses

The ability to stimulate immune responses is called immunogenicity. Two main types of immunity exist: humoral immunity and cellular immunity. Humoral (antibody-mediated) immunity refers to protection provided by the secreted products of one type of white blood cell called a B lymphocyte. These products, custom-made proteins known as antibodies, circulate in body fluids, primarily blood and lymph. B lymphocytes (B cells) produce antibodies in response to a specific foreign invader like HIV or a vaccine.

Several different antibodies can be generated. So-called binding antibodies simply attach to part of HIV and may or may not have antiviral effects. Functional antibodies are binding antibodies that

478

actually do something more. For example—neutralizing antibodies—inactivate HIV or prevent it from infecting cells.

Scientists have identified the outer envelope of HIV as important for stimulating neutralizing antibodies. A major protein, gpl20 (glycoprotein 120), is found on the surface or envelope of HIV. Together with its parent protein gpl60, gpl20 forms the basis of many recombinant subunit vaccines, so-called because each is genetically engineered to contain only one small piece of the virus.

The second type of immunity, cellular (cell-mediated) immunity, refers to activities of T lymphocytes. Cytotoxic T lymphocytes (CTLs), nicknamed killer T cells, directly destroy HIV-infected cells. A subset called CD8+ CTLs (CD8+ T cells) bear CD8 receptors on their surfaces and kill cells that are producing HIV. Other CD8+ T cells can suppress HIV replication without necessarily killing the infected cell. CD8+ T cells may be critical to resisting HIV infection.

Regulatory T cells, another component of cellular immunity, direct antibody- and cell-mediated immune responses, like a conductor leading a symphony orchestra. The chief regulatory T cell, the helper T cell, also is HIV's main target. The virus attaches to the cell through a receptor on the cell's surface called CD4. Hence, helper T cells are called CD4+ T cells.

A subset of helper T cells, memory T cells, are evoked on first exposure to an invading organism. The name "memory" reflects their function, which is to create a criminal record file on that virus or microorganism. If the virus enters the body again, memory T cells will quickly stir the immune system into action. The most common way to measure memory T cells is by a test called the T lymphocyte proliferation assay, which indicates the strength of such cellular responses to HIV.

To be effective, an HIV vaccine may have to stimulate a third type of immunity, mucosal immunity. Immune cells lining the mucous membranes of the genital tract and other HIV portals into the body produce different responses that are not well understood.

HIV Strain Variation

HIV continually evolves as a result of genetic mutation and recombination. Thus, researchers must estimate the significance of strain variation within individuals and among populations when developing AIDS vaccines. Usually a person does not appear to be infected with more than one HIV variant. But once HIV infection becomes established, the virus continually undergoes changes, and many variants may arise within an infected person.

Whenever a drug or immune response destroys one variant, a distinct but related one can emerge. Also, certain variants may thrive in specific tissues or become dominant in an individual because they replicate faster than others. Any of these changes may yield a virus that can escape immune detection.

The envelope and core genes of many HIV isolates, the viruses taken from patients, have been analyzed and compared. On this basis, scientists have grouped HIV isolates worldwide into two groups, M and O. At least nine subtypes or clades have been identified in group M, and only a few in group O. Each subtype within a group is about 30 percent different from any of the others. In contrast, successful vaccines for other viruses have only had to protect against one or a limited number of virus strains.

The first AIDS vaccines made were based on the LAI strain (also known as IIIB and LAV). Subsequently, LAI has been shown to differ from most strains found in infected people. Newer vaccines have been based on the SF-2 and MN isolates, which belong to the same subtype as LAI but better represent HIV strains isolated from North Americans and Europeans.

A preventive vaccine will need to generate immune responses that protect uninfected individuals from all the different HIV subtypes to which they may be exposed.

Scientists are looking for conserved regions of HIV genes, those that produce proteins common to all or most subtypes. If such common proteins are not found, a cocktail vaccine comprising several proteins or peptides from different HIV strains may be necessary to invoke broad-based immunity.

HIV Transmission is Complex

Unlike some other viruses, HIV can be transmitted and can exist in the body not only as free virus but also within infected cells. Thus, a vaccine against HIV may be required to stimulate the two main types of immunity. Humoral immunity uses antibodies to defend against free virus. Cellular immunity directly or indirectly results in the killing of infected cells by immune cells. A major unanswered question is how important each type of immunity is for protection from HIV. Data from animal models and long-term HIV survivors, and human clinical trials of experimental HIV vaccines, may offer clues to the answer.

Another factor complicates the attempt to define HIV protection. According to WHO (World Health Organization), 80 percent of all HIV transmission worldwide occurs sexually. Thus, to be effective, an HIV vaccine also may need to stimulate mucosal immunity. Mucosal immune cells that line the respiratory, digestive and reproductive tracts and those found in nearby lymph nodes are the first line of defense against infectious organisms. Unfortunately, relatively little is known about how the mucosal immune system protects against viral infection.

Immune System Breakdown

Perhaps the most difficult challenge for vaccine researchers is that the major target of HIV is the immune system itself. HIV infects the key CD4+ T cells that regulate the immune response, modifying or destroying their ability to function.

After infection, HIV incorporates its genetic material into that of the host cell. If the cell reproduces itself, each new cell also contains the HIV genes. There the virus can hide its genetic material for prolonged periods of time until the cell is activated and makes new viruses. Other cells act as HIV reservoirs, harboring intact viruses that may remain undetected by the immune system.

Understanding how HIV disease evolves, especially during early infection, is a high priority for the Institute. Scientists at NIAID and elsewhere have shown that no true period of biological latency exists in HIV infection. After entering the body, the virus rapidly disseminates, homing to the lymph nodes and related organs where it replicates and accumulates in large quantities. Paradoxically, the filtering system in these lymphoid organs, so effective at trapping pathogens and initiating an immune response, may help destroy the immune system: HIV infects the steady stream of CD4+ T cells that travel to the lymph organs in response to HIV infection.

Basic research in immunology, epidemiology studies of long-term survivors, and vaccine trials in animal models and humans all contribute to a greater understanding of the immune system breakdown and ways vaccines may be designed to prevent or slow down the progress of HIV disease.

Adjuvants, Other Immune Enhancers

Because of safety concerns, most candidate HIV/AIDS vaccines use one or more proteins of HIV, not the whole infectious virus. These new generation vaccines contain no intact live virus and thus stimulate less potent immune responses than traditional vaccines made from whole viruses that have been inactivated or attenuated (weakened).

To augment the immune responses elicited by these and other vaccines, scientists use immunologic adjuvants, which can increase the type, strength and durability of immune responses evoked by a vaccine. Some vaccine antigen/adjuvant combinations can induce cell-mediated immune responses in animals, even if the vaccine antigen by itself does not. Some adjuvants also stimulate mucosal immunity.

Currently, only one adjuvant—alum, first discovered in 1926—is incorporated into vaccines licensed for human use by the U.S. Food and Drug Administration (FDA). An adjuvant may work well with one experimental vaccine but not another. Therefore, the FDA licenses the vaccine formulation, or the antigen-adjuvant combination, rather than the adjuvant alone. Alum primarily increases the strength of antibody responses generated by the vaccine antigen. Because of alum's limited activity, other adjuvants now being evaluated in animal models and human studies may be better suited for the newer candidate HIV vaccines.

A different way to enhance immune responses to HIV is the prime-boost vaccine strategy. Researchers first prepare or prime the immune systems of volunteers with a live vector vaccine, a bacterium or virus that has been genetically engineered to contain a gene for an HIV protein such as gp160 but that cannot infect the person with HIV or cause disease.

The best studied vector is vaccinia virus, formerly used to immunize against smallpox. Vaccinia carries the foreign HIV gene into the body. There, the vaccine directs cells to make the HIV protein that the body perceives as foreign, stimulating production of protective antibodies. Later, the volunteers receive booster shots of a different vaccine made from the same HIV protein.

By itself, a gp160-containing vaccinia virus vaccine stimulates production of memory T cells but few antibodies. The prime-boost combination, however, can stimulate a strong cellular immune response—including persistent killer CD8+ T cells—as well as antibodies that neutralize the virus or inhibit formation of syncytia, giant cells formed when HIV-infected cells fuse with cells that are not infected.

Because of concerns that a vaccinia-based vaccine might cause serious vaccinia infection in some people with compromised immune systems, such as people with HIV who have not been exposed to either smallpox or the vaccine, other vector vaccines are being developed and evaluated.

Several experimental vector vaccines made from a canarypox virus, which closely resembles vaccinia, are in clinical trials. Canarypox virus infects but does not reproduce in human cells and therefore should be much safer. Another example of a vector under development for HIV vaccines is *Salmonella*, bacteria that infect the human gut. Plasmid DNA vaccines, direct injections of genes coding for HIV proteins, are a recent innovation that have shown good ability to induce cellular immune responses. When the DNA is injected, the encoded viral proteins, e.g., HIV gp160, are produced, just as with live vectors. The potential of this vaccine concept is actively being pursued.

Animal Model Studies

Animal model studies can answer critical questions that cannot be answered either in humans, because of undue risk, or by using computer modeling or laboratory tests. For example, animals can be inoculated with an experimental vaccine and then challenged with virus to test the vaccine's effectiveness—a study that would be unethical to conduct in humans. However, AIDS researchers lack an ideal animal model.

Although chimpanzees can be infected with HIV, only one chimpanzee has been observed to develop disease, making it difficult to extrapolate findings to humans. Moreover, chimpanzees are an endangered species and both difficult and expensive to maintain.

Most non-human primate AIDS research is conducted with macaque monkeys. They can be infected with SIV, a retrovirus similar to HIV that causes an AIDS-like disease. The genetic and physical structures of SIV differ enough from those of HIV, however, that the results of SIV experiments may not wholly apply to humans.

Nonetheless, important information has been obtained from both monkeys and chimpanzees. Experiments in both species have demonstrated the feasibility of developing a protective vaccine. Moreover, a new animal model—infection of macaques with a chimeric virus (SHIV) based on SIV but including the HIV envelope, with subsequent development of disease—may become extremely valuable for evaluating candidate HIV vaccines.

In late 1992, NIAID-funded investigators first reported results from their experiments with a live-attenuated SIV vaccine made by deleting the SIV *nef* gene. The vaccine demonstrated durable protection against high intravenous doses of a lethal SIV strain different from that used in the vaccine. These findings provide hope that safe and effective human HIV vaccines can be developed. Optimism for the live-attenuated approach itself however, is tempered by concerns about its safety.

NIAID, a component of the National Institutes of Health (NIH), supports research on AIDS, tuberculosis and other infectious diseases, as well as allergies and immunology. NIH is an agency of the U.S. Department of Health and Human Services. NIAID press releases, fact sheets and other materials are available on the Internet via the NIAID home page at http://www.niaid.nih.gov.

Chapter 57

Clinical Research on HIV/AIDS Vaccines

The National Institute of Allergy and Infectious Diseases (NIAID) conducts clinical trials of candidate vaccines to discover which might most successfully protect people from human immunodeficiency virus (HIV) infection (preventive vaccine) or from becoming ill after they acquire the virus (therapeutic vaccine).

Scientists have identified important immunologic targets on HIV and on infected cells. For example, they know that the glycoprotein 120 (gp120) on the outer coat of the virus contains the region that attaches to cells of the host, the CD4 binding site. Scientists also know that most neutralizing antibodies (proteins that block a virus from infecting cells) in HIV-infected people are directed against gp120. For these reasons, vaccines based on genetically engineered HIV envelope proteins—gp160 and one of its cleavage products, gp120—have been the most well-studied to date.

More than 40 experimental HIV vaccines have been tested in humans worldwide. Vaccine approaches in development or in clinical trials include the following:

* *subunit vaccine*: a piece of the outer surface of HIV, such as gp160 or gp120, produced by genetic engineering.

* *recombinant vector vaccine*: a live bacterium or virus such as vaccinia (used in the smallpox vaccine) modified to transport into the body a gene that makes one or more HIV proteins.

National Institute of Allergy and Infectious Diseases (NIAID), May 1997.

- *vaccine combination*: for example, use of a recombinant vector vaccine to induce cellular immune responses followed by booster shots of a subunit vaccine to stimulate antibody production, referred to as a prime-boost strategy.

- *peptide vaccine*: chemically synthesized pieces of HIV proteins (peptides) known to stimulate HIV-specific immunity.

- *virus-like particle vaccine (pseudovirion vaccine)*: a non-infectious HIV look-alike that has one or more, but not all, HIV proteins.

- *anti-idiotype vaccine*: antibodies generated against antibodies to the virus.

- *plasmid DNA vaccine (nucleic acid vaccine)*: direct injection of genes coding for HIV proteins.

- *whole-inactivated virus vaccine*: HIV that has been inactivated by chemicals, irradiation or other means so it is not infectious.

- *live-attenuated virus vaccine*: live HIV from which one or more apparent disease-promoting genes of the virus have been deleted.

Clinical Trials Background

After an experimental vaccine performs well in preclinical safety and immunogenicity tests, it must successfully complete three stages of testing in people before development into a licensed product.

A Phase I trial is the first setting in which an experimental HIV vaccine is given to people. Such a trial enrolls about 20 to 80 non-HIV-infected volunteers at apparent low risk of HIV infection. A Phase I trial primarily seeks information on safety, usually assessing any vaccine-related side effects by comparing the vaccine with an inactive placebo or control that looks like the test product. A Phase I trial also can provide data on the vaccine's immunogenicity, including the dose and administration schedule required to achieve optimal immune responses. If the vaccine elicits neutralizing antibodies, scientists can study how these react against HIV strains from the same or other clades to determine the potential breadth of protection. A Phase I trial may last one to two years.

Once Phase I trials show that the experimental HIV vaccine is well-tolerated, it can advance into Phase II trials. These trials enroll more people, up to a few hundred, and often include some volunteers at higher risk for acquiring HIV. Researchers gather data about safety and immune responses, asking more sophisticated questions that such larger trials allow. Optimally, the trials are randomized and double-blind, meaning that volunteers are assigned at random to a study group and that neither the health care workers nor the patients know what preparations the patients receive. Phase II trials usually last one to two years.

The most promising candidate vaccines move into Phase III or efficacy trials, enrolling large numbers of non-HIV-infected people at high risk for exposure to the virus. A Phase III trial usually is designed to ensure the collection of enough data on safety and effectiveness to support a license application, if warranted. The vaccine may be tested against a placebo or a vaccine such as hepatitis B of known potential benefit to the study population. An efficacy trial can involve thousands of volunteers and therefore takes much longer, at least four years, to complete.

Clinical Trials of Preventive Vaccines

In August 1987, NIAID opened the first clinical trial of an experimental HIV vaccine at the NIH Clinical Center in Bethesda, Md. This safety trial eventually enrolled 138 non-infected healthy volunteers. The gp160 subunit candidate vaccine tested caused no serious adverse effects.

Since the first trial, more than 40 preventive HIV vaccine trials have been initiated worldwide. These Phase I/II trials examine the vaccine's safety and provide preliminary information on its ability to stimulate immune responses.

The *NIAID AIDS Vaccine Evaluation Group (AVEG)* is the largest U.S. cooperative HIV vaccine clinical trials group. The AVEG, which began enrolling volunteers in February 1988, includes the following:

- The *AIDS Vaccine Evaluation Units (AVEUs)*, located at six U.S. research centers, conduct phase I and II clinical trials of candidate HIV vaccines in low-risk and high-risk HIV-seronegative volunteers.

- The *Central Immunology Laboratory* provides state-of-the-art evaluation of humoral and cellular immune responses of vaccinees in AVEG trials. The evaluations use standardized tests, permitting comparison of responses in different individuals and to different candidate vaccines.

- The *Data Coordinating and Analysis Center* provides a central facility for collecting and analyzing data from the trials conducted by the AVEUs.

- The *Immunology Laboratory Support for Assessment of Mucosal Immune Responses Induced by AIDS Vaccines* evaluates human mucosal immune responses to candidate vaccines in standardized tests, permitting the comparison of responses in volunteers at different AVEUs and in volunteers who receive different candidate vaccines.

- The *Specimen Repository* collects and maintains blood samples and other specimens from volunteers in AVEG trials for use in current and future studies.

- A *Data and Safety Monitoring Board* periodically reviews data from AVEG studies.

As of January 1997, more than 2,000 men and women have participated in preventive HIV vaccine trials conducted at six medical center AVEU sites located in Baltimore, Nashville, Seattle, St. Louis, Birmingham and Rochester, N.Y.

To date, all the vaccine candidates tested have been well-tolerated, generally producing only mild side effects typical of most vaccines. The first candidates tested stimulated production of antibodies, although levels decreased within a relatively short period of time. Initial formulations and dosages of these vaccines produced few or low levels of neutralizing antibodies and rarely elicited cytotoxic T cells, which are invoked through cell-mediated immunity to kill HIV-infected cells.

With newer protocols, using increased vaccine dosages, different immunization schedules, experimental adjuvants and new recombinant proteins, more promising data regarding the induction of neutralizing antibodies and cytotoxic T cells have emerged.

In December 1992, NIAID launched the first Phase II HIV vaccine clinical trial. Earlier trials enrolled noninfected people at low risk of HIV infection and primarily sought data on safety. This trial includes noninfected volunteers with a history of high-risk behavior—injection drug use, multiple sex partners or sexually transmitted diseases. Participants are counseled repeatedly to avoid any behavior that puts them at risk of HIV infection. Follow-up for this trial has been extended to four years.

The trial will help determine if these distinct populations, representative of people likely to be enrolled in large-scale efficacy trials, respond differently to vaccines. The trial also will provide more detailed data on the safety and ability of vaccines to stimulate immune responses.

A second Phase II HIV vaccine clinical trial is now under way at AVEU sites and in the HIV Network for Prevention Trials (HIVNET).

Experimental HIV vaccines are growing in number and kind. Clinical trials will yield valuable information about the relative effects on immune response of different formulations and delivery methods.

Future Directions

Although the challenges are daunting, scientists remain optimistic that safe and effective HIV vaccines can be developed. Novel ways to present HIV proteins to the immune system continue to be designed and tested, as do new antigen/adjuvant vaccine formulations. A growing number and variety of experimental vaccines are entering clinical tests in primates and humans, and more trials are exploring whether changing immunization schedules, increasing booster doses or using a combination vaccine strategy can stimulate stronger, more durable immune responses. Together, progress in basic and clinical research is moving scientists closer toward identifying products suitable for large-scale HIV vaccine efficacy trials.

NIAID, a component of the National Institutes of Health (NIH), supports research on AIDS, tuberculosis and other infectious diseases, as well as allergies and immunology. NIH is an agency of the U.S. Department of Health and Human Services. NIAID press releases, fact sheets and other materials are available on the Internet via the NIAID home page at http://www.niaid.nih.gov.

Chapter 58

Clinical Trials for AIDS Therapies

The National Institute of Allergy and Infectious Diseases (NIAID) has the lead responsibility within the National Institutes of Health for the discovery and development of interventions to treat or prevent HIV infection and its complications in adults and children. In keeping with this mission, the Institute's research effort encompasses primary HIV disease, opportunistic infections, oncology and neurology. There is also a comprehensive HIV research program that focuses on identifying and improving interventions for the prevention of HIV infection and its sequelae in infants.

NIAID's extensive portfolio of clinical research on new HIV therapeutics includes studies conducted through several multicenter clinical trials networks and within its intramural facilities in the Clinical Center in Bethesda. Although each network has distinct capabilities, the research is very much intertwined and, taken together, represents the largest AIDS therapy research initiative in the world. These networks serve a large patient base and provide extensive clinical expertise and sophisticated laboratory capabilities, thereby giving NIAID an extraordinary ability to assess state-of-the-art therapies and further our understanding of HIV pathogenesis.

The extramural clinical trials networks supported by NIAID's Division of AIDS include: the Adult AIDS Clinical Trials Group (AACTG), the Pediatric AIDS Clinical Trials Group (PACTG), the Terry Beirn Community Programs for Clinical Research on AIDS (CPCRA) and the Strategic Program for Innovative Research on AIDS (SPIRAT).

National Institute of Allergy and Infectious Diseases (NIAID), February 1997.

The Adult and Pediatric ACTGs are multicenter cooperative clinical trials groups involved in all phases of clinical research, from early safety studies to large-scale efficacy trials; they evaluate new drugs and drug combinations for the treatment of HIV infection in adults and children, respectively. The PACTG also evaluates regimens for the prevention of maternal-fetal HIV transmission. The CPCRA is based mainly in primary care settings and principally conducts large (clinical endpoint) studies. The SPIRAT integrates both clinical and preclinical research focused on innovative therapeutic approaches, such as immune system restoration, DNA-based therapeutic vaccines and gene therapy.

Scientists in NIAID's Division of Intramural Research focus primarily on intensive clinical/laboratory investigations involving novel agents or modalities.

The clinical research conducted by investigators in these networks has yielded valuable information that has provided the basis for much of the current state-of-the-art treatment for HIV disease. For example, NIAID-supported clinical trials have:

- demonstrated and defined the efficacy of zidovudine (AZT), zalcitibine (ddC), didanosine (ddI) and stavudine (d4T) as monotherapies and in combination regimens for a wide variety of clinical conditions.

- demonstrated that combination regimens employing two or more antiretroviral agents are more effective than AZT monotherapy, particularly early in disease.

- defined the standard of care for acute treatment and prophylaxis of *Pneumocystis carinii* pneumonia, treatment and maintenance for cryptococcal meningitis (fluconazole), treatment and maintenance therapy for disseminated histoplasmosis (itraconazole), treatment of disseminated *Mycobacterium avium* complex (clarithromycin), management of cytomegalovirus retinitis and acyclovir-resistant herpes simplex (foscarnet).

- assessed and validated assays for use as surrogate markers of drug effectiveness including p24 antigen, quantitative peripheral blood mononuclear cells (PBMC), microculture and DNA/ RNA (PCR).

- developed state-of-the-art study design methodology for HIV disease (e.g., endpoints) to permit rapid clinical and laboratory evaluation of antiretroviral compounds.

NIAID's pediatric clinical research effort has significantly advanced the treatment and prevention of HIV infection in infants and children. Through clinical trials, NIAID has:

- demonstrated that AZT therapy reduced dramatically the likelihood of childhood HIV infection resulting from transmission from infected mothers during pregnancy or delivery.

- demonstrated that ddI or ddI plus AZT are superior to AZT monotherapy for children with symptomatic HIV infection or AIDS.

- demonstrated the effectiveness of IVIG for preventing serious bacterial infections in children with HIV.

- developed guidelines for the prevention of PCP in HIV-infected children.

Over the next several years, NIAID research will continue to define the standard of care for HIV-infected people of all ages. Particular emphasis will be placed on the use of combination regimens with protease inhibitors.

For More Information about Clinical Trials

For further information about any NIAID-supported clinical trials, call 1-800-TRIALS-A (1-800-243-7012 TTY/TDD) weekdays from 9 a.m. to 7 p.m. Eastern Time, or visit the web site at http://www.actis.org or http://www.hivatis.org. For further information about clinical trials conducted by the NIAID DIR AIDS program, call 1-800-243-7644 weekdays from 9 a.m. to 5 p.m. Eastern Time.

NIAID, a component of the National Institutes of Health (NIH), supports research on AIDS, tuberculosis and other infectious diseases, as well as allergies and immunology. NIH is an agency of the U.S. Department of Health and Human Services. NIAID press releases, fact sheets and other materials are available on the Internet via the NIAID home page at http://www.niaid.nih.gov.

Chapter 59

HIV/AIDS Clinical Trials: Knowing Your Options

HIV/AIDS Clinical Trials

HIV/AIDS clinical trials are research studies that involve people and are designed to answer specific questions about the safety and effectiveness of treatments for HIV/AIDS and related conditions.

Clinical trials are vitally important because there are no other direct ways to learn how different people respond to medications, treatments, or therapeutic approaches. Clinical trials are also called experimental programs, research studies, and protocols.

All approved treatments for HIV/AIDS must be tested through clinical trials before they can be marketed to treat HIV infection or related conditions.

HIV/AIDS clinical trials may provide critical information that can help people to live longer, healthier, and more comfortable lives.

People join clinical trials for many reasons. Some want to try the newest medications and others want to receive HIV/AIDS health services related to the clinical trial. Other people seek clinical trials because they offer hope.

Should You Participate?

Your decision is an important one, both for yourself and others living with HIV/AIDS. You can follow these steps to become informed about clinical trials:

An undated brochure produced by the AIDS Clinical Trials Information Service (ACTIS); included in current list of publications available from the Centers for Disease Control and Prevention (CDC), inventory no. D845.

495

- Learn
- Consider
- Choose

Learn

You owe it to yourself to learn everything that is involved in a clinical trial. Depending on the type of research, you may be one of only a small group of people, or one of many people involved in a particular study. The clinical trial may take place in a hospital, medical center, university, doctor's office, or a community clinic. You will need to commit the time required for the study and travel to your appointments.

To ensure reliable results, clinical trials follow precise medical guidelines called protocols. If you choose to participate, you accept the responsibility to observe these guidelines. So before you decide, make sure you know the number and length of appointments, medical tests required, and other medications allowed. Although you can leave a clinical trial at any time, do not start one if you think you may drop out.

Each trial is part of one of three possible steps, or phases, in development of a medication or treatment.

Phase I Trials: A study medication is given to a small group of people for the first time, to measure its safety.

Phase II Trials: In Phase II, the study medication is given to larger groups of people to see if it works and to further evaluate its safety.

Phase III Trials: In this phase, the study medication is given to very large groups of people to develop information that will allow the drug to be marketed and used safely.

Are Clinical Trials Safe?

There are some risks to participants in clinical trials, but the federal government has imposed mandatory safeguards to protect them. Each clinical trial is reviewed by an Institutional Review Board (IRB), a diverse group of people that must approve the trial. The IRB periodically reviews the clinical trial operations to ensure that the risks are as low as possible, and worth the potential benefits. Some trials also have community advisory boards. In addition, all study participants must read and sign informed consent documents. These documents ensure that participants understand the risks and potential benefits as well as their rights and responsibilities should they decide to participate in the study.

Consider

Considering whether to get involved in a clinical trial means understanding both the benefits and risks related to clinical trials.

Benefits

- You may be among the first people helped by a new study medication.
- You will get HIV/AIDS health care related to the research study.
- You can help others by adding to the medical information about HIV/AIDS.
- Medications and appointments related to the research will usually be free of charge.
- Medical information obtained during the clinical trial can be shared with your own health care provider.

Risks

- A study medication may not be helpful; in fact it may be harmful to you, or have side effects.
- While in the study, you can use only treatments approved by the researchers—some you are taking now may not be allowed.
- After your part of the trial ends, you may not be able to continue receiving the tested drug—even if it worked for you.
- The study medications are usually free, but you may have some other expenses related to the clinical trial.

Choose

You may choose to join a clinical trial, but the researchers must decide whether you are eligible. Each clinical trial includes people who have the same or very similar health profiles. When selecting participants, researchers may consider these or other factors:

- Age
- Your CD4 or T-cell count
- Past medical history
- Current medical status
- Your willingness and ability to follow all of the trial's instructions and schedules

Informed Consent

Before you agree to join a clinical trial, researchers must be sure that you understand everything about the study—risks, benefits, obligations, etc. The staff will explain the study in detail. Then they will ask you to read and sign an informed consent document that is printed in a language you understand.

Questions to Ask

- What is the purpose of the clinical trial?
- What will I need to do to join the clinical trial?
- Are there standard treatments for my current medical condition? How does this study compare with any standard treatments?
- Will I know what drug I am taking?
- How often will I need to come to appointments, use study medications, and have medical tests?
- Will I need to be hospitalized during the clinical trial? If so, how often and for how long?
- What side effects can I expect from participating in this clinical trial?
- What should I do if I get any side effects or feel uncomfortable during the clinical trial?
- How will my confidentiality be protected during the clinical trial?
- What kind of long-term followup care will be provided as part of the clinical trial?
- Will my insurance cover any of the expenses related to the clinical trial?

- Will the study medications be free? Will there be any costs involved in participating in the study?
- Can I get help with child care or transportation related to the study?

Learn More about Clinical Trials

- Talk with your health care provider
- Call the AIDS Clinical Trials Information Service (ACTIS) at 1-800-TRIALS-A (1-800-874-2572)
- Contact clinical trial programs in your area

Part Six

Additional Help and Information

Chapter 60

Glossary of
HIV/AIDS-Related Terms

Terms in **bold** type indicate other entries in the glossary.

A

ABT-538: *See* **ritonavir.**

acquired immunodeficiency syndrome (AIDS): The most severe manifestation of infection with the **human immunodeficiency virus (HIV)**. The **Centers for Disease Control and Prevention (CDC)** lists numerous **opportunistic infections** and **neoplasms** (cancers) that, in the presence of HIV infection, constitute an AIDS diagnosis. There are also instances of presumptive diagnoses when a person's HIV status is unknown or not sought. This was especially true before 1985 when there was no HIV-antibody test. In 1993, CDC expanded the criteria for an AIDS diagnosis to include **CD4+ T cell** count at or below 200 cells per microliter in the presence of HIV infection. In persons (age 5 and older) with normally functioning immune systems, CD4+ T cell counts usually range from 500 to 1,500 cells per microliter. Persons living with AIDS often have infections of

Compiled from *Glossary of HIV/AIDS-Related Terms*, HIV/AIDS Treatment Information Service, U.S. Department of Health and Human Services (DHHS), March 1997, (800) HIV-0440; and *HIV Vaccine Glossary*, AIDS Clinical Trials Information Service, National Institute of Allergy and Infectious Diseases National Institutes of Health (NIAID), June 1997, (800) TRIALS-A. The use of brand names is for identification purposes only; it does not constitute an endorsement.

the lungs, brain, eyes, and other organs, and frequently suffer debilitating weight loss (**wasting syndrome**), **diarrhea**, and a type of cancer called **Kaposi's sarcoma**. (*See also* **HIV disease**.)

ACTG: *See* **AIDS Clinical Trials Group**.

acupuncture: A Chinese medical treatment involving the insertion of very fine sterile needles into the body at specific points according to a mapping of "energy pathways." Historically, acupuncture is one component of an overall program of Chinese medicine that includes theory, practice, diagnosis, physiology, and the use of herbal preparations. Acupuncture is used to control pain and to treat other conditions such as allergies or addiction withdrawal. (*See also* **alternative medicine**.)

acute HIV infection: The 4-to-7-week period of rapid viral replication immediately following exposure. The number of **virions** produced during primary infection is similar to that produced during several subsequent years of established, asymptomatic infection. An estimated 30 to 60 percent of individuals with primary HIV infection develop an acute syndrome characterized by fever, **malaise**, lymphadenopathy, pharyngitis, headache, myalgia, and sometimes rash. Following primary infection, **seroconversion** and a broad HIV-1 specific **immune response** occur, usually within 30 to 50 days. It was previously thought that HIV was relatively dormant during this phase. However, it is now known that during the time of primary infection, high levels of **plasma** HIV **RNA** can be documented.

acyclovir (acycloguanosine): A **nucleoside analog** antiviral drug used to treat the symptoms of **herpes simplex virus** infection, **herpes zoster** (**shingles**), and sometimes acute **varicella zoster virus** (chicken pox). Also known as Zovirax.

ADAP: *See* **AIDS Drugs Assistance Programs**.

ADCC: *See* **antibody-dependent cellular cytotoxicity**.

adenopathy: Any disease involving or causing enlargement of glandular tissues, especially one involving the **lymph nodes**.

adjuvant: An ingredient—as in a prescription or solution—that facilitates or modifies the action of the principal ingredient; may be used in HIV therapies or for HIV vaccines.

administration (route of administration): How a drug or therapy is introduced into the body. Systemic administration means that the drug goes throughout the body (usually carried in the bloodstream), and includes oral (by mouth), intravenous (injection into the vein, IV), intramuscular (injection into a muscle, IM), intrathecal (into the spinal canal), subcutaneous (beneath the skin, SQ), and rectal administrations. Local administration means that the drug is applied or introduced into the specific area affected by the disease, such as application directly onto the affected skin surface (topical administration). The effects of most therapies depend upon the ability of the drug to reach the affected area, thus the route of administration and consequent distribution of a drug in the body are important determinants of its effectiveness.

adverse reaction (adverse event): An unwanted effect detected in clinical trial in participants. The term is used whether or not the effect can be attributed to the intervention under study. (*See* **side effects.**)

aerosolized: A form of administration in which a drug, such as **pentamidine**, is turned into a fine spray or mist by a nebulizer and inhaled.

AETC: *See* **AIDS Education and Training Centers.**

affected community: Persons living with HIV and AIDS, and other related individuals including their families, friends, and advocates whose lives are directly influenced by HIV infection and its physical, psychological, and sociological ramifications.

agammaglobulinemia: A nearly total absence of immunoglobulins. (*See* **antibodies.**)

Agency for Health Care Policy and Research (AHCPR): An agency of the **Department of Health and Human Services** supporting activities to enhance health care services and improve access to them.

AHCPR: *See* **Agency for Health Care Policy and Research.**

AIDS: *See* **Acquired Immunodeficiency Syndrome.**

AIDS Clinical Trials Group (ACTG): Composed of a number of U.S. medical centers that evaluate treatment for HIV and HIV-associated infections. ACTG studies—both adult and pediatric—are sponsored by the **National Institute of Allergy and Infectious Diseases** and the **National Institute of Child Health and Human Development** (for many of the pediatric studies) of the **National Institutes of Health.**

AIDS Dementia Complex (ADC): A degenerative neurological condition attributed to HIV infection, characterized by a group of clinical presentations including loss of coordination, mood swings and loss of inhibitions, and widespread cognitive dysfunctions. It is the most common central nervous system complication of HIV infection. Characteristically, it manifests itself after the patient develops major **opportunistic infections** or **AIDS-related cancers**. However, patients can also have this syndrome before these major systemic complications occur. The cause of ADC has not been determined exactly, but it may result from HIV infection of cells or inflammatory reactions to such infections.

AIDSDRUGS: An online database service of the **National Library of Medicine**, with information about drugs undergoing testing against **AIDS, AIDS-related complex**, and related opportunistic diseases. For information about access call the National Library of Medicine, 1-800-638-8480.

AIDS Drugs Assistance Programs (ADAP): State-based programs funded in part by Title II of the **Ryan White CARE Act** that provide therapeutics (including devices necessary to administer pharmaceuticals) to treat HIV disease or prevent the serious deterioration of health, including treatment of **opportunistic infections**. ADAP formularies and eligibility criteria are determined state-by-state with a focus on serving low-income individuals.

AIDS Education and Training Centers (AETC): The Health Resources and Services Administration (HRSA) supports a network of 15 regional centers that serve as resources for educating health professionals in prevention, diagnosis, and care of HIV-infected patients. The centers train primary caregivers to incorporate HIV prevention strategies into their clinical priorities, along with diagnosis, counseling, and care of HIV-infected persons and their families.

AIDSLINE: An online database service of the **National Library of Medicine**, with citations and abstracts covering the published scientific and medical literature on AIDS and related topics. For information about access call the National Library of Medicine, 1-800-638-8480.

AIDS-related cancers: Several cancers are more common or more aggressive in persons living with HIV. These malignancies include certain types of immune system cancers known as **lymphomas**, **Kaposi's sarcoma**, and anogenital cancers that primarily affect the anus and the cervix. HIV, or the immune suppression it induces, appears to play a role in the development of these cancers.

AIDS-Related Complex (ARC): 1. A term that has been used by some clinicians to describe a variety of symptoms and signs found in some persons living with HIV. These may include recurrent fevers, unexplained weight loss, swollen **lymph nodes, diarrhea, herpes, hairy leukoplakia,** and/or fungus infection of the mouth and throat. Also more accurately described as symptomatic HIV infection. 2. Symptoms that appear to be related to infection by HIV. They include an unexplained, chronic deficiency of white blood cells (**leukopenia**) or a poorly functioning lymphatic system with swelling of the lymph nodes (**lymphadenopathy**) lasting for more than 3 months without the **opportunistic infections** required for a diagnosis of AIDS. (*See* **wasting syndrome.**)

AIDS Research Advisory Committee (ARAC): A board that advises and makes recommendations to the Director, **National Institute of Allergy and Infectious Diseases,** on all aspects of HIV-related research, **vaccine** development, **pathogenesis,** and **epidemiology.**

AIDS Service Organization (ASO): A health association, support agency, or other service actively involved in the prevention and treatment of AIDS.

AIDSTRIALS: An online database service of the **National Library of Medicine,** with information about **clinical trials** of agents (e.g., drugs) under evaluation against HIV infection, AIDS, and related opportunistic diseases. For information about access, call the National Library of Medicine, 1-800-638-8480.

AIDS wasting syndrome: Involves involuntary weight loss of 10 percent of baseline body weight plus either chronic diarrhea (two loose stools per day for more than 30 days) or chronic weakness and documented fever (for 30 days or more, intermittent or constant) in the absence of a concurrent illness or condition other than HIV infection that would explain the findings.

alpha interferon: A protein—one of three major classes of **interferons**—that the body produces in response to infections. In persons who are HIV positive, elevated interferon levels are regarded as an indication of disease progression. Genetically engineered alpha interferon has been approved by the FDA as a treatment for **Kaposi's sarcoma.**

alkaline phosphatase: An enzyme normally present in certain cells within the liver, bone, kidney, intestine, and placenta. When the cells are destroyed in those tissues, more of the enzyme leaks into the blood, and levels rise in proportion to the severity of the condition. Measurement of this enzyme is used as an indication of the health of the liver.

alopecia: Loss of hair that frequently occurs in patients undergoing chemotherapy for cancer or suffering from other diseases, such as AIDS, where cell-killing, or **cytotoxic**, drugs are used.

alternative medicine: A broad category of treatment systems (e.g., chiropractic, herbal medicine, **acupuncture**, homeopathy, naturopathy, and spiritual devotions) or culturally based healing traditions such as Chinese, Ayurvedic, and Christian Science. Alternative medicines share the common characteristic of nonacceptance by the biomedical (i.e., mainstream Western) establishment. Alternative medicine is also referred to as **complementary medicine**. The designation alternative medicine is not equivalent to **holistic medicine**, a narrower term.

alum: Potassium aluminum sulfate, or ammonium aluminum sulfate, used especially as an emetic (i.e., an agent that induces vomiting), an astringent (i.e., a substance that contracts tissues), and a styptic (i.e., a substance that tends to check bleeding by contracting the tissues or blood vessels).

ALVAC-HIV™: A genetically engineered HIV vaccine composed of a live, weakened **canarypox** virus (ALVAC™) into which parts of genes for non-infectious components of HIV have been inserted. When ALVAC™ infects a human cell, the inserted HIV genes direct the cell to make HIV proteins. These proteins are packaged into HIV-like particles that bud from the cell membrane. These particles are not infectious but fool the immune system into mounting an immune response to HIV. ALVAC™ can infect but not grow in human cells, an important safety feature. (*See also* **canarypox**.)

alveolar: Pertaining to the alveoli sac, the site of gas exchange in the lungs.

amebiasis: An inflammation of the intestines caused by infestation with *Entameba histolytica* (a type of ameba) and characterized by frequent, loose stools flecked with blood and mucus.

amino acids: Any of a class of nitrogen-containing acids. Some 22 amino acids are commonly found in animals and humans. Chains of amino acids synthesized by living systems are called polypeptides (up to about 50 amino acids) and proteins (more than 50 amino acids). (*See* **peptide**; **proteins**.)

analog: In chemistry, a compound with a structure similar to that of another compound but differing from it in respect to certain components or structural makeup, which may have a similar or opposite action metabolically.

anamnestic response: The heightened immunologic reaction elicited by a second or subsequent exposure to a particular antigen such as a pathogenic microorganism (e.g., bacterium, fungus) or **antigen**.

anaphylactic shock: A life-threatening allergic reaction characterized by a swelling of body tissues (including the throat) and a sudden decline in blood pressure.

anemia: A lower than normal number of red blood cells.

anergy: 1. The loss or weakening of the body's immunity to an irritating agent, or **antigen**. Anergy can be thought of as the opposite of allergy, which is an overreaction to a substance. The strength of the body's immune response is often quantitatively measured by means of a skin test where a solution containing an antigen known to cause a response, such as mumps or **candida**, is injected immediately under the skin. Patients may be so immunologically suppressed that they are unable to produce cutaneous (skin) delayed-type hypersensitivity reaction (DTH). Such patients will usually not test positive for **tuberculosis** on a tuberculin skin test (or Mantoux test). The lack of a reaction to these common antigens indicates anergy. 2. Researchers, in cell culture, have shown that **CD4+ T cells** can be turned off by a signal from HIV that leaves them unable to respond to further immune system stimulation.

angiogenesis: The process of forming new blood vessels. Angiogenesis is essential for the growth of tumors, especially **Kaposi's sarcoma**.

anorexia: The lack or loss of appetite that leads to significant decline in weight.

antibiotic: A substance, especially one similar to those produced by certain fungi, that kills or inhibits the growth of microorganisms such as bacteria or fungi. Some antibiotics are used to treat infectious diseases.

antibodies: Molecules in the blood or secretory fluids that tag, destroy, or neutralize bacteria, viruses, or other harmful toxins (**antigens**). They are members of a class of proteins known as immunoglobulins, which are produced and secreted by **B lymphocytes** in response to stimulation by antigens. An antibody is specific to an antigen.

antibody-dependent cell-mediated cytotocicity (ADCC): An immune response in which **antibodies** bind to target cells, identifying them for attack by the immune system.

antibody-mediated immunity: *See* **humoral immunity**.

antifolate: An agent that inhibits intracellular (i.e., inside cells) production of **folinic acid**.

antigen: Any substance that antagonizes or stimulates the immune system to produce **antibodies** (i.e., proteins that fight antigens). Antigens are often foreign substances such as bacteria or viruses that invade the body.

antigen-presenting cell (APC): B cell, **macrophage**, **dendritic cell**, or other cell that ingests and processes foreign bodies such as viruses and displays the resulting antigen fragments on its surface to attract and activate the **CD4+ T cells** that respond specifically to that antigen.

antiidiotype: An antibody that recognizes and binds to another antibody (idiotype).

antineoplastic: Inhibiting or preventing the proliferation of tumor cells.

antiretroviral agents: Substances used against **retroviruses** such as HIV.

antisense drugs: An antisense, nucleic acid-related compound is the mirror image of the genetic sequence that it is supposed to inactivate. It is a synthetic segment of **DNA** or **RNA** that locks onto a strand of natural DNA or RNA with a complementary sequence of **nucleotide** (*see* **ribonucleic acid**) bases. Antisense drugs are designed to block viral genetic instructions, marking them for destruction by cellular enzymes, in order to prevent the building of new virus or the infection of new cells.

antitoxins: Antibodies that recognize and inactivate toxins produced by certain bacteria, plants, or animals.

antiviral: A substance or process that destroys a virus or suppresses its replication (i.e., reproduction).

aphasia: Loss of ability to speak or understand speech.

aphthous ulcer: A painful oral or esophageal sore of unknown cause that has a deep eroded base. Aphthous ulcers are common in persons living with HIV and are treated with corticosteroids. Thalidomide—a drug used in Europe as a sedative before it was discovered that it caused birth defects—is an experimental, alternate therapy.

apoptosis: "Cellular suicide" also known as programmed cell death. HIV may induce apoptosis in both infected and uninfected immune system cells. Normally when **CD4+ T cells** mature in the **thymus gland**, a small proportion of these cells are unable to distinguish self from nonself. Because these cells would otherwise attack the body's own tissues, they receive a biochemical signal from other cells that results in apoptosis. (*See* **tumor necrosis factor**.)

ARC: *See* **AIDS-related complex**.

arm: One group of participants in a comparative **clinical trial**, all of whom receive the same treatment. The other arm(s) receive(s) a different treatment regimen.

arthralgia: A pain in a joint.

ASO: *See* **AIDS service organization**.

aspergillosis: A fungal infection—resulting from the **fungus** *Aspergillus*—of the lungs that can spread through the blood to other organs. Symptoms include fever, chills, difficulty in breathing, and coughing up blood. If the infection reaches the brain, it may cause **dementia**. Amphotericin B is a recommended treatment. Itraconazole may be considered for less serious disease or for those who cannot tolerate amphotericin B.

assembly and budding: Names for a portion of the processes by which new HIV is formed in infected host cells. Viral core proteins, **enzymes**, and **RNA** (**ribonucleic acid** gather just inside the cell's membrane, while the viral **envelope** proteins aggregate within the membrane. An immature viral particle is formed and then pinches off from the cell, acquiring an envelope and the cellular and HIV proteins from the cell membrane. The immature viral particle then undergoes processing by an HIV enzyme called protease to become an infectious virus.

asymptomatic: Without symptoms. Usually used in the HIV/AIDS literature to describe a person who has a positive reaction to one of several tests for HIV antibodies but who shows no clinical symptoms of the disease.

ataxia: Lack of muscular coordination.

attenuated: Weakened or decreased. For example, an attenuated virus can no longer produce disease but might be used to produce a **vaccine**.

autoantibody: 1. An **antibody** that is active against some of the tissues of the organism that produced it. 2. An antibody directed against the body's own tissue.

autoimmunization: The induction in an individual of an **immune response** to its own cells (tissue).

autoinoculation: Inoculation of a microorganism obtained by contact with a lesion on one's own body, producing a secondary infection.

autologous: Pertaining to the same organism or one of its parts; originating within an organism itself. For instance, donating your own blood for your future surgery is known as an autologous transfusion.

AZT: Azidothymidine, also called Retrovir™, zidovudine, or ZDV. The first **antiretroviral** drug against HIV infection to be approved by the FDA (1987). A thymidine (RNA constituent) analog that suppresses replication of HIV. AZT is increasingly administered in combination with other antiviral drugs. Possible side effects include bone marrow suppression leading to **anemia, leukopenia,** or **neutropenia**; nausea; muscle weakness; and headaches. (*See also* **nucleoside analog**; **ribonucleic acid**.)

B

bactericidal (bacteriocidal): Capable of killing bacteria.

bacteriostatic: Capable of inhibiting reproduction of bacteria.

bacterium: A microscopic organism composed of a single cell. Many bacteria can cause disease in humans.

Bactrim: *See* **TMP/SMX**.

baculovirus: A virus of insects used in the production of some HIV vaccines. (*See* **vaccine.**)

baseline: 1. Information gathered at the beginning of a study from which variations found in the study are measured. 2. A known value or quantity with which an unknown is compared when measured or assessed. 3. The initial time point in a **clinical trial**, just before a volunteer starts to receive the experimental treatment undergoing testing. At this reference point, measurable values such as **CD4** count are recorded. Safety and efficacy of a drug are often determined by monitoring changes from the baseline values.

basophil: A type of white blood cell, also called a granular leukocyte, filled with granules of toxic chemicals that can digest microorganisms. Basophils, as well as other types of white blood cells, are responsible for the symptoms of allergy.

B cell lymphoma: *See* **lymphoma.**

B cells: *See* **B lymphocytes.**

bDNA test: *See* **branched DNA assay.**

beta 2 microglobulin (B2M): Protein tightly bound to the surface of many nucleated cells, particularly those of the immune system. Elevated B2M levels occur in a variety of diseases. While elevated B2M is not specific to HIV, there is a correlation between this marker and the progression of HIV disease. (*See* **immune system.**)

bilirubin: A red pigment occurring in liver bile, blood, and urine. Its measurement can be used as an indication of the health of the liver. Bilirubin is the product of the breakdown of hemoglobin in red blood cells. It is removed from the blood and processed by the liver, which secretes it into the digestive tract. The normal value is 0.1 to 1.5 milligrams per liter of blood. An elevated level of bilirubin in blood serum is an indication of liver disease or drug-induced liver impairment.

binding antibody: As related to HIV infection: An **antibody** that attaches to some part of HIV. Binding antibodies may or may not adversely affect the virus.

bioavailability: The extent to which an oral medication is absorbed in the digestive tract and reaches the bloodstream.

biological response modifiers (BRM): Substances, either natural or synthesized, that boost, direct, or restore normal immune defenses.

BRMs include **interferons, interleukins, thymus**, hormones, and **monoclonal antibodies**.

biopsy: Surgical removal of a piece of tissue from a living subject for microscopic examination to make a diagnosis (e.g., to determine whether abnormal cells such as cancer cells are present).

biotechnology: 1. Use of living organisms or their products to make or modify a substance. These include recombinant **DNA** techniques (**genetic engineering**) and hybridoma technology. 2. Industrial application of the results of biological research, particularly in fields such as recombinant DNA or gene splicing, which permits the production of synthetic hormones or enzymes by combining genetic material from different species.

blinded study: A **clinical trial** in which participants are unaware as to whether they are in the experimental or control **arm** of the study. (*See* **double blind study**.)

blood-brain barrier: A selective barrier (obstacle) between brain blood vessels and brain tissues whose effect is to restrict what may pass from the blood into the brain. Certain compounds readily cross the blood-brain barrier; others are completely blocked.

B lymphocytes (B cells): One of the two major classes of **lymphocytes**, B lymphocytes are blood cells of the **immune system**, derived from the bone marrow and spleen, and involved in the production of **antibodies**. During infections, these cells are transformed into plasma cells that produce large quantities of antibody directed at specific pathogens. When antibodies bind to foreign proteins, such as those that occur naturally on the surfaces of bacteria, they mark the foreign cells for consumption by other cells of the immune system. This transformation occurs through interactions with various types of **T cells** and other components of the immune system. In persons living with AIDS, the functional ability of both the B and the T lymphocytes is damaged, with the T lymphocytes being the principal site of infection by HIV.

body fluids: Any fluid in the human body, such as blood, urine, saliva (spit), sputum, tears, semen, mother's milk, or vaginal secretions. Only blood, semen, mother's milk, and vaginal secretions have been linked directly to the transmission of HIV.

bone marrow: Soft tissue located in the cavities of the bones where blood cells such as **erythrocytes, leukocytes,** and **platelets** are formed.

bone marrow suppression: A side effect of many anticancer and antiviral drugs, including **AZT**. Leads to a decrease in white blood cells, red blood cells, and platelets. Such reductions, in turn, result in anemia, bacterial infections, and spontaneous or excess bleeding.

booster: A second or later dose of a **vaccine** given to increase the immune response to the original dose.

branched DNA assay (bDNA test): A test developed by the Chiron Corporation for measuring the amount of HIV (as well as other viruses) in blood plasma. The test uses a method that creates a luminescent signal whose brightness depends on the amount of viral **RNA** present. Test results are calibrated in numbers of virus particle equivalents per milliliter of plasma. The bDNA test is similar in results but not in technique to the **PCR test**. bDNA testing is currently being used to evaluate the effectiveness of drug treatment regimens and to gauge HIV disease progression. Newer versions, or generations, of these assays are being developed; they will be able to detect smaller numbers of copies of HIV in a blood sample. (*See* **viral burden**.)

breakthrough infection: An infection, caused by the infectious agent the **vaccine** is designed to protect against, that occurs during the course of a vaccine trial. These infections may be caused by exposure to the infectious agent before the vaccine has taken effect, or before all doses of the vaccine have been given.

bronchoscopy: Visual examination of the bronchial passages of the lungs through the tube of an endoscope (usually a curved flexible tube containing fibers that carry light down the tube and project an enlarged image up the tube to the viewer) that is inserted into the upper lungs. Can be used for extraction of material from the lungs.

budding: *See* **assembly and budding**.

Burkitt's lymphoma: *See* **lymphoma**.)

C

cachexia: General ill health and malnutrition, marked by weakness and emaciation, usually associated with serious disease. (*See* **wasting syndrome**.)

canarypox: a virus that infects birds and is used as a **live vector** for HIV vaccines. It can carry a large quantity of foreign genes.

515

Canarypox virus cannot grow in human cells, an important safety feature. (*See also* **ALVAC- HIV™**; **vector**.)

Candida: Yeast-like fungi commonly found in the normal flora of the mouth, skin, intestinal tract, and vagina, which can become clinically infectious in immune-compromised persons. (*See* **fungus**; **thrush**.)

candidiasis: An infection with a yeast-like **fungus** of the *Candida* family, generally *Candida albicans*. It most commonly involves the skin (dermatocandidiasis), oral mucosa (**thrush**), respiratory tract (bronchocandidiasis), and vagina (vaginal candidiasis, formerly called monilia). Candidiasis of the esophagus, trachea, bronchi, or lungs is an indicator disease for AIDS. Oral or recurrent vaginal candida infection is an early sign of immune system deterioration. (*See* **opportunistic infection**.)

carcinogen: Any cancer-producing substance.

catheter: A tubular medical device for insertion into canals, vessels, passageways, or body cavities, usually to permit injection (e.g., through an intravenous catheter into a vein), withdrawal of fluids, or to keep a passage open.

CBCT: *See* **community-based clinical trial**.

CBO: *See* **community-based organization**.

CC CKR5: Cell surface **molecule**, which is needed along with the primary receptor, the **CD4** molecule, in order to fuse with the membranes of the immune system cells. Researchers have found that the strains of HIV most often transmitted from person to person require the CC CKR5 molecule and CD4 molecule in order for HIV to enter the cell. In addition to its role in fusion, CC CKR5 is a receptor for certain immune-signaling molecules called **chemokines** that are known to suppress HIV infection of cells. (*See also* **CXCR4**.)

CD: abbreviation for "cluster of differentiation," referring to cell surface molecules that are used to identify stages of maturity of immune cells, for example, **CD4+ T cells**.

CD4 (T4) or CD4+ cells: 1. A type of T cell involved in protecting against viral, fungal, and protozoal infections. These cells normally orchestrate the **immune response**, signaling other cells in the immune system to perform their special functions. Also known as T helper cells. 2. HIV's preferred targets are cells that have a docking molecule called "cluster designation 4" (CD4) on their surfaces. Cells with this molecule are known as CD4-positive (or CD4+) cells. Destruction of CD4+ lymphocytes is the major cause of the immunodeficiency observed in AIDS, and decreasing CD4+ lymphocyte levels appear to be the best indicator for developing **opportunistic infections**. Although CD4 counts fall, the total T cell level remains fairly constant through the course of HIV disease, due to a concomitant increase in the **CD8+ cells**. The ratio of CD4+ to CD8+ cells is therefore an important measure of disease progression. (*See also* **immunodeficiency**.)

CD8 (T8) Cells: A protein embedded in the cell surface of suppressor **T lymphocytes**. 1. Also called **cytotoxic T cells**. Some CD8 cells recognize and kill cancerous cells and those infected by intracellular pathogens (some bacteria, viruses, and mycoplasma). These cells are called **cytotoxic T lymphocytes**. 2. Also called T-suppressor cells. Immune cells that shut down the immune response after it has effectively wiped out invading organisms. Sensitive to high concentrations of circulating **lymphokines**, T8 cells release their own lymphokines when an **immune response** has achieved its goal, signaling all other participants to cease their coordinated attack. A number of **B lymphocytes** remain in circulation in order to fend off a possible repeat attack by the invading organism. With HIV, however, the immune system's response system does not work. **T4 cells** are dysfunctional, lymphokines proliferate in the bloodstream, and T8 cells compound the problem by misreading the oversupply of lymphokines as meaning that the immune system has effectively eliminated the invader. So while HIV is multiplying, T8 cells are simultaneously attempting to further shut down the immune system. The stage is set for normally repressed infectious agents, such as **PCP** or **CMV**, to proliferate unhindered and to cause disease.

CDC: *See* **Centers for Disease Control and Prevention**.

CDC National AIDS Clearinghouse: CDC's (**Centers for Disease Control and Prevention**) comprehensive reference, referral, and publication distribution service for HIV and AIDS information. The Clearinghouse works in partnership with national, regional, state, and local organizations that develop and deliver HIV prevention and treatment programs and services.

CDC National AIDS Hotline: Provides education, information, and referrals for persons living with HIV, their families and friends, health professionals, and the general public on HIV/AIDS issues, including transmission, prevention, and testing. The Hotline number is 1-800-342-AIDS.

cell lines: Specific cell types artificially maintained in the laboratory (i.e., *in vitro*) for scientific purposes.

cell-mediated immunity (CMI): This branch of the **immune system** exists primarily to deal with viruses that are more insidious than bacteria because they invade the host (e.g., human) cells where they can hide from the antibody-making cells of the immune system. With this system, the reaction to foreign material is performed by specific defense cells, such as **killer T cells**, **macrophages**, and other **white blood cells** rather than by **antibodies**.

cellular immunity: *See* **cell-mediated immunity**.

Centers for Disease Control and Prevention (CDC): The **Department of Health and Human Services** agency with the mission to promote health and quality of life by preventing and controlling disease, injury, and disability. CDC operates 11 Centers including the National Center for **HIV**, **STD**, and **TB** prevention. CDC assesses the status and characteristics of the HIV epidemic and conducts epidemiologic, laboratory, and surveillance investigations. CDC supports the design, implementation, and evaluation of prevention activities for HIV/AIDS, and maintains various HIV/AIDS information services, such as the **CDC National AIDS Clearinghouse** and the **CDC National AIDS Hotline**.

central nervous system (CNS) damage: By HIV infection: The central nervous system is composed of the brain, spinal cord, and the **meninges** (protective membranes surrounding them). Although **monocytes** and **macrophages** can be infected by HIV, they appear to be relatively resistant to killing. However, these cells travel throughout the body and carry HIV to various organs, especially the lungs and the brain. Persons living with HIV often experience abnormalities in the central nervous system. Investigators have hypothesized that an accumulation of HIV in brain and nerve cells or the inappropriate release of **cytokines** or toxic byproducts of these cells may be to blame for the neurological manifestations of HIV disease.

cerebral: Pertaining to the cerebrum, the main portion of the brain.

cerebrospinal fluid (CSF): Fluid that bathes the brain and the spinal cord. A sample of this fluid is often removed from the body for diagnostic purposes by a **lumbar puncture** (spinal tap).

cervical cancer: A neoplasm of the uterine cervix that can be detected in the early curable stage by the Papanicolaou (Pap) test. (*See* **cervical dysplasia**; **cervix**; **Pap smear**.)

cervical dysplasia: Abnormality in the size, shape, and organization of adult cells of the **cervix**. Often a precursor lesion for cervical cancer. Studies indicate an increase in prevalence of **cervical dysplasia** among women living with HIV. Additional studies have documented that a higher prevalence is associated with greater immune suppression. HIV infection also may adversely affect the clinical course and treatment of cervical dysplasia and cancer.

cervical intraepithelial neoplasia (CIN1, CIN2, CIN3): Dysplasia of the **cervix epithelium**, often premalignant (i.e., precancerous), characterized by various degrees of **hyperplasia**, abnormal keratinization (forming horny epidermal tissue), and condylomata. Considerable evidence implicates **human papilloma virus (HPV)** in the development of CIN. Immunosuppression may also play an important role in facilitating infection or persistence of HPV in the genital tract and progression of HPV-induced neoplasia. (*See* **condyloma**; **neoplasm**.)

cervix: The lower, cylindrical terminus of the uterus that juts into the vagina and contains a narrow canal connecting the upper and lower parts of a woman's reproductive tract.

challenge: In vaccine experiments, the exposure of an immunized animal to the infectious agent.

chancroid: A highly contagious **sexually transmitted disease** caused by the *Hemophilus ducreyi* **bacterium**. It appears as a pimple, chancre, sore, or ulcer on the skin of the genitals. The lesion appears after an incubation period of 3 to 5 days and may help the transmission of HIV.

chemokines: Also called beta chemokines. Studies of the relationship between HIV and these **immune system** chemicals have shown the complex exchanges that take place when HIV and white blood cells meet. Chemokines are intracellular messenger molecules secreted by **CD8+ cells** whose major function is to attract immune cells to sites of infection. Recent research has shown that HIV-1 needs access to chemokine receptors on the cell surface to infect the cell. Several chemokines—called RANTES, MIP-1A and MIP-1B—interfere with HIV replication by occupying these receptors. Findings suggest that one mechanism these **molecules** use to suppress HIV infectivity is to block the process of **fusion** used by the virus to enter cells.

chemotherapy: The treatment, mostly of cancer, using a series of **cytotoxic** drugs that attack cancerous cells. This treatment commonly has adverse **side effects** that may include the temporary loss of the body's natural immunity to infections, loss of hair, digestive upset, and a general feeling of illness. Although unpleasant, the adverse effects of treatment are tolerated considering the life-threatening nature of the cancers.

chlamydia: A **sexually transmitted disease (STD).** The most common sexually transmitted **bacterium** (*Chlamydia trachomatis*) that infects the reproductive system. In fact, in 1995, chlamydia was the most common STD in the United States. The infection is frequently asymptomatic (i.e., shows no symptoms), but if left untreated, can cause sterility in women.

CHO (Chinese hamster ovary) cell: A cell used as a "factory" in genetic engineering to make certain **subunit** vaccines. CHO cells are derived from mammals and are advantageous because they add carbohydrates (a sugar coat) to the protein, much like naturally infected human cells do.

chronic idiopathic demyelinating polyneuropathy (CIPD): Chronic, spontaneous loss or destruction of **myelin**. Myelin is a soft, white, somewhat fatty material that forms a thick sheath around the core of myelinated nerve fiber. Patients show progressive, usually symmetric weakness in the upper and lower extremities. Patients with clinical progression of the **syndrome** after 4 to 6 weeks by definition have CIPD. Treatment in most centers consists of giving IV-immune globulin for 4 to 5 days or **plasmapheresis** (5 to 6 exchanges over 2 weeks).

CIPD: *See* **chronic idiopathic demyelinatingpolyneuropathy**.

circulating immune complexes: *See* **immune complex**.

circumoral paresthesia: An abnormal touch sensation, such as burning or prickling around the mouth, often in the absence of an external stimulus. (*See* **paresthesia**.)

clade: Also called a **subtype**. A group of related HIV isolates classified according to their degree of genetic similarity (such as of their envelope proteins). There are currently two groups of HIV-1 **isolates**,

M and O. M consists of at least nine clades, A through I. Group O may consist of a similar number of clades.

clinical: Pertaining to or founded on observation and treatment of patients, as distinguished from theoretical or basic science.

Clinical Alert: The **National Institutes of Health** in conjunction with the editors of several biomedical journals publish those bulletins on urgent cases in which timely and broad dissemination of results of clinical trials could prevent morbidity (sickness) and mortality (death). The Clinical Alert does not become a barrier to subsequent publication of the full research paper. Clinical Alerts are widely distributed electronically through the **National Library of Medicine** and through standard mailings.

clinical endpoint: *See* **endpoint**.

clinical latency: The state or period of an infectious agent, such as a virus or bacterium, living or developing in a host without producing clinical symptoms. Pertaining to HIV infection, infected individuals usually exhibit a period of clinical latency with little evidence of disease, but **viral load** studies show that the virus is never truly latent (dormant). Even early in the disease, HIV is active within **lymphoid organs** where large amounts of virus become trapped in the FDC (**follicular dendritic cells**) network. Surrounding tissues are areas rich in **CD4+ T cells**. These cells increasingly become infected and viral particles accumulate both in infected cells and as free virus.

clinical practice guidelines: Standards for physicians to adhere to in prescribing care for a given condition or illness.

clinical trial: A scientifically designed and executed investigation of the effects of a drug (or vaccine) administered to human subjects. The goal is to define the safety, clinical efficacy, and pharmacological effects (including toxicity, side effects, incompatibilities, or interactions) of the drug. The U.S. government, through the **Food and Drug Administration (FDA)**, requires strict testing of all new drugs and vaccines prior to their approval for use as therapeutic agents. (*See also* entries for **Phase I, II, III,** and **IV Trials**.)

clone: 1. A group of genetically identical cells or organisms descended from a common ancestor. 2. To produce genetically identical copies. 3. A genetically identical replication of a living cell that is valuable for the investigation and reproduction of test cultures.

521

CMV: *See* **cytomegalovirus**.

CNS: *See* **central nervous system**.

coccidioidomycosis: An infectious fungal disease caused by the inhalation of spores of *Coccidioides immitis*, which are carried on windblown dust particles. The disease is endemic in hot, dry regions of the Southwestern United States and Central and South America, and is an opportunistic disease associated with AIDS. Also called desert fever, San Joaquin fever, or **Valley fever**. (*See* **fungus**; **opportunistic infection**.)

codon: A sequence of three **nucleotides** of **messenger RNA** that specifies addition of a particular **amino acid** to, or termination of, a polypeptide chain during protein synthesis. (*See* **ribonucleic acid**.)

cofactors: 1. Substances, microorganisms, or characteristics of individuals that may influence the progression of a disease or the likelihood of becoming ill. 2. A substance, such as a metallic ion or coenzyme, that must be associated with an enzyme for the enzyme to function. 3. A situation or activity that may increase a person's susceptibility to AIDS. Examples of cofactors are: other infections, drug and alcohol use, poor nutrition, genetic factors, and stress. In HIV immunology, the concept of cofactors is being expanded and new cofactors have been identified. A recent example is the discovery of the interaction of **CXCR4** (fusin) and **CD4** to facilitate entry of HIV into cells.

cognitive impairment: Loss of the ability to process, learn, and remember information.

cohort: In epidemiology, a group of individuals with some characteristics in common.

colitis: Inflammation of the colon.

combination therapy: For HIV infection or AIDS: Two or more drugs or treatments used together to achieve optimum results against HIV infection and/or AIDS. Combination therapy may offer advantages over single-drug therapies by being more effective in decreasing **viral load**. An example of combination therapy would be the use of two **nucleoside analog** drugs (such as **3TC** and **AZT**) plus either a **protease inhibitor** or a **non-nucleoside reverse transcription inhibitor**. (*See* **synergism**.)

community-based clinical trial (CBCT): A **clinical trial** conducted primarily through primary-care physicians rather than academic research facilities.

community-based organization (CBO): A service organization that provides social services at the local level.

community planning: Community planning groups are responsible for developing comprehensive HIV prevention plans that are directly responsive to the epidemics in their jurisdictions. The goal of HIV Prevention Community Planning is to improve the effectiveness of HIV prevention programs. Together in partnership, representatives of affected populations, epidemiologists, behavioral scientists, HIV/ AIDS prevention service providers, health department staff, and others analyze the course of the epidemic in their jurisdiction, determine their priority intervention needs, and identify interventions to meet those needs. **CDC** supports implementation of an effective planning process.

Community Programs for Clinical Research on AIDS (CPCRA): An initiative of NIAID (**National Institute of Allergy and Infectious Diseases**) to broaden the base of clinical investigations by involving community physicians in AIDS research and trials. NIAID started CPCRA in 1989. It is one of four HIV **clinical trials** programs supported by NIAID. In 1992, the name of the program was officially changed to the Terry Beirn Community Programs for Clinical Research on AIDS.

compassionate use: A method of providing experimental therapeutics (including experimental drugs) prior to final **Food and Drug Administration (FDA)** approval for use in humans. This procedure is used with very sick individuals who have no other treatment options. Often, case-by-case approval must be obtained from the FDA for "compassionate use" of a drug or therapy.

complement: A group of proteins in normal blood serum and plasma that, in combination with **antibodies**, causes the destruction of **antigens**, particularly bacteria and foreign blood cells.

complement cascade: A precise sequence of events, usually triggered by an antigen-antibody complex, in which each component of the complement system is activated in turn. (*See* **antibodies**; **antigen**.)

complementary therapy: A whole range of services designed to complement traditional medical practice as part of a practitioner's primary care plan for an individual.

concomitant drugs: Drugs that are taken together. Certain concomitant medications may have adverse interactions.

concorde study: Joint French/British clinical trial of **AZT** in asymptomatic HIV-infected individuals.

condyloma (*Condyloma acuminatum*): A **papilloma** with a central core of connective tissue in a treelike structure covered with **epithelium**, usually occurring on the **mucous membrane** or skin of the external genitals or in the perianal (tissue surrounding the anus) region. Although the lesions are usually few in number, they may aggregate to form large cauliflower-like masses. Caused by the **human papilloma virus (HPV)**, it is infectious and autoinoculable (i.e., capable of being transmitted by inoculation from one part of the body to another). Also called genital warts, venereal warts, or *verruca acuminata*.

contagious: In the context of HIV, has come to be more popularly known as any infectious disease capable of being transmitted by casual contact from person to another. Casual contact can be defined as normal day-to-day contact among people at home, school, work, or in the community. A contagious pathogen (e.g., chicken pox) can be transmitted by casual contact. An infectious pathogen, on the other hand, is transmitted by direct or intimate contact (e.g., sex). HIV is infectious, not contagious.

contraindication: A specific circumstance when the use of certain treatments could be harmful.

controlled trials: Control is a standard against which experimental observations may be evaluated. In **clinical trials**, one group of patients is given an experimental drug, while another group (i.e., the control group) is given either a standard treatment for the disease or a **placebo**.

co-receptors: A group of proteins that have been found to block the entry of HIV into immune cells.

core: the protein capsule surrounding a virus' **DNA** or **RNA**. In HIV, p55, the precursor molecule to the core, is broken down into the smaller molecules p24, p17, p7 and p6. HIV's core is primarily composed of **p24**.

core protein: As related to HIV: An integral core protein.

correlates of immunity/correlates of protection: The immune responses that protect an individual from a certain disease. The precise identities of the correlates of immunity in HIV are unknown.

CPCRA: *See* **Community Programs for Clinical Research on AIDS.**

creatinine: A protein found in muscles and blood, and excreted by the kidneys in the urine. The level of creatinine in the blood or urine provides a measure of kidney function.

Crixivan: *See* **indinavir.**

cross-resistance: The phenomenon in which a microbe that has acquired resistance to one drug through direct exposure, also turns out to have resistance to one or more other drugs to which it has not been exposed. Cross-resistance arises because the biological mechanism of resistance to several drugs is the same and arises through the identical genetic mutations.

cryotherapy: The use of liquid nitrogen to freeze and destroy a lesion or growth, sometimes used to induce scar formation and healing to prevent further spread of a condition (e.g., warts or molluscum contagiosum).

cryptococcal meningitis: A life-threatening infection of the membranes (**meninges**) that line the brain and the spinal cord. Cryptococcal disease is caused by a **fungus** (*Cryptococcus neoformans*). Most people have been exposed to this organism, which is found in soil contaminated by bird droppings, but it usually does not cause disease in healthy people. The majority of persons with cryptococcal meningitis have immune systems that are damaged by disease, such as AIDS, or suppressed by drugs. The organism can infect almost all organs of the body, although it most commonly causes disease of the meninges, skin, or lungs. (*See* **cryptococcosis.**)

cryptococcosis: An infectious disease seen in HIV-infected patients due to the **fungus** *Cryptococcus neoformans*, which is acquired via the respiratory tract. It can spread from the lungs to the brain, the central nervous system, the skin, the skeletal system, and the urinary tract. (*See* **cryptococcal meningitis.**)

cryptosporidiosis: A gastrointestinal disease caused by the microscopic protozoan parasite *Cryptosporidium parvum*. It is recognized as one of the three most common diarrhea-causing intestinal pathogens in the world. Transmission occurs by the oral-fecal route. Persons with **CD4+** counts greater than 300/mm^3 are more likely to have self-limiting disease, while those with fewer than 200 CD4+ cells/mm^3 almost always have persistent disease.

CT scan (CT or **computed tomography):** Radiography (using x-ray) in which a three-dimensional image of a body structure is constructed by computer from a series of cross-sectional images made along an axis. Also referred to as CAT scan. (*See also* **magnetic resonance imaging (MRI).**)

CTL: *See* **cytotoxic T lymphocyte.**

cutaneous: Of, pertaining to, or affecting the skin.

CXCR4 (also known as **fusin**): A cell molecule that acts as a **cofactor** or co-receptor for the entry of HIV into **immune system** cells. Early in the epidemic, **CD4** molecules were found to be the primary receptor for HIV on immune system cells. Recent data indicate that a second molecule, CXCR4, is also required for fusion and entry of certain strains of HIV into cells. New studies indicate a multistage interplay between HIV and two receptors on white blood cells. After binding to the receptor CD4, the virus fuses with a second receptor, CXCR4, which normally binds to **chemokines**. This double clasp may then signal the receptors to move the virus into the cell.

cytokines: Cytokines are among the proteins produced by white blood cells that act as chemical messengers between cells and can stimulate or inhibit the growth and activity of various immune cells. HIV replication is regulated by a delicate balance among the body's own cytokines. By altering that balance one can influence the replication of the virus in the test tube and potentially even in the body. (*See also* **interleukins**; **tumor necrosis factor.**)

cytomegalovirus (CMV): A **herpes virus** that is a common cause of opportunistic diseases in persons with AIDS and other persons with immune suppression. While CMV can infect most organs of the body, persons with AIDS are most susceptible to **CMV retinitis** (disease of the eye) and **colitis** (disease of the colon).

cytomegalovirus (CMV) retinitis: Most adults in the United States have been infected by cytomegalovirus, although the virus usually does not cause disease in healthy people. Because the virus remains in the body for life, it can cause disease if the **immune system** becomes severely damaged by disease or suppressed by drugs. CMV retinitis is an eye disease common among persons who are living with HIV. Without treatment, persons with CMV retinitis can lose their vision. CMV infection can affect both eyes and is the most common cause of blindness among persons with AIDS.

cytopenia: Deficiency in the cellular elements of the blood.

cytoplasm: All of the substance of a cell other than the nucleus.

cytotoxic: An agent or process that is toxic to cells (i.e., it causes suppression of function or cell death).

cytotoxic T lymphocyte (CTL): A **lymphocyte** that is able to kill foreign cells marked for destruction by the cellular immune system. (*See* **CD8 (T8) cells.**)

D

dapsone: An approved oral **antibiotic** of the sulfone class used for the treatment and **prophylaxis** of **PCP** and **toxoplasmosis**.

Data Safety and Monitoring Board (DSMB): An independent committee, composed of community representatives and clinical research experts, that reviews data while a **clinical trial** is in progress to ensure that participants are not exposed to undue risk. A DSMB may recommend that a trial be stopped if there are safety concerns or if the trial objectives have been achieved.

ddC: Dideoxycytidine, a **nucleoside analog** drug that inhibits the replication of HIV. FDA-approved treatment for selected patients with advanced HIV disease. Also called Zalcitabine, HIVID.

ddI: Dideoxyinosine, a **nucleoside analog** drug that inhibits the replication of HIV. It is an FDA-approved treatment for patients with advanced HIV disease. Also called didanosine or Videx.

delavirdine: A **non-nucleoside reverse transcription inhibitor** drug that noncompetitively inhibits the enzyme, HIV-1 **reverse transcriptase**, through direct binding.

deletion: Elimination of a **gene** (i.e., from a chromosome) either in nature or in the laboratory.

dementia: Chronic intellectual impairment (i.e., loss of mental capacity) with organic origins that affects a person's ability to function in a social or occupational setting. (*See* **AIDS dementia complex.**)

demyelination: Destruction, removal, or loss of the **myelin** sheath of a nerve or nerves.

dendrite: Any of the usual branching protoplasmic processes that conduct impulses toward the body of a nerve cell. (*See* **protoplasm.**)

dendritic cells: Patrolling **immune system** cells that may begin the HIV disease process by carrying the virus from the site of the infection to the **lymph nodes**, where other immune cells become infected. Dendritic cells travel through the body and bind to foreign invaders—such as HIV—especially in external tissues, such as the skin and the membranes of the gut, lungs, and reproductive tract. They then ferry the foreign substance to the lymph nodes to stimulate **T cells** and initiate an **immune response**. In laboratory experiments, the dendritic cells that carry HIV also bind to **CD4+ T cells**, thereby allowing HIV to infect the CD4+ T cells. CD4+ T cells are the primary immune system cells targeted by HIV and depleted during HIV infection.

deoxyribonucleic acid (DNA): The molecular chain found in genes within the nucleus of each cell, which carries the genetic information that enables cells to reproduce. DNA is the principal constituent of chromosomes, the structures that transmit hereditary characteristics.

Department of Health and Human Services (DHHS): The U.S. government's principal agency for protecting the health of all Americans and providing essential human services, especially for those who are least able to help themselves. DHHS includes some 250 programs, administered by 10 principal operating divisions such as **CDC**, **FDA**, and **NIH**. DHHS works closely with state and local governments, and many DHHS-funded services are provided at the local level by state or county agencies, or through private sector grantees.

desensitization: Gradually increasing the dose of a medicine in order to overcome severe reactions. Desensitization procedures have become popular when administering Bactrim to persons with a history of adverse reactions to the drug. Bactrim (**TMP/SMX**) is an important drug against **PCP** infection.

DHHS: *See* **Department of Health and Human Services**.

d4T: A dideoxynucleoside pyrimidine analog. Like other **nucleoside analogs**, d4T inhibits HIV replication by inducing premature viral **DNA** chain termination. d4T has been **FDA** approved for patients with advanced HIV infection intolerant to, or failing on, other antiretroviral drugs. Also known as stavudine or Zerit.

diagnosis: The determination of the presence of a specific disease or infection, usually accomplished by evaluating clinical symptoms and laboratory tests.

diarrhea: Uncontrolled, loose, and frequent bowel movements. In the United States, almost all persons living with AIDS develop diarrhea at some time in the course of their disease. Severe or prolonged diarrhea can lead to weight loss and malnutrition. The excessive loss of fluid that may occur with AIDS-related diarrhea can be life threatening. There are many possible causes of diarrhea in persons who have AIDS. The most common infectious organisms causing AIDS-related diarrhea include **cytomegalovirus (CMV)** the parasites *Cryptosporidium, Microsporidia,* and *Giardia lamblia*; and the bacteria *Mycobacterium avium* and *Mycobacterium intracellulare*. Other bacteria and parasites that cause diarrheal symptoms in otherwise healthy people may cause more severe, prolonged, or recurrent diarrhea in persons with HIV or AIDS. (*See also* **giardiasis**; **microsporidiosis**; **mycobacterium avium complex (MAC)**.)

didanosine: *See* **ddI**.

diplopia: Double vision.

disseminated: Spread (of a disease) throughout the body.

DNA: *See* **deoxyribonucleic acid**.

DNA vaccine (nucleic acid vaccine): direct injection of a **gene**(s) coding for a specific antigenic protein(s), resulting in direct production of such **antigen**(s) within the vaccine recipient in order to trigger an appropriate **immune response**.

domain: A region of a **gene** or gene product.

dormancy: *See* **latency**.

dose-ranging study: A **clinical trial** in which two or more doses of an agent (such as a drug) are tested against each other to determine which dose works best and is least harmful.

dose-response relationship: The relationship between the dose of some agent (such as a drug), or the extent of exposure, and a physiological response. A dose-response effect means that as the dose increases, so does the effect.

double-blind study: A **clinical trial** design in which neither the participating individuals nor the study staff know which patients are receiving the experimental drug and which are receiving a **placebo** or another therapy. Double-blind trials are thought to produce objective results, since the doctor's and patient's expectations about the experimental drug do not affect the outcome. (*See also* **blinded study**.)

drug-drug interaction: A modification of the effect of a drug when administered with another drug. The effect may be an increase or a decrease in the action of either substance, or it may be an adverse effect that is not normally associated with either drug.

drug resistance: The ability of some disease-causing microorganisms, such as bacteria, viruses, and mycoplasma, to adapt themselves, to grow, and to multiply even in the presence of drugs that usually kill them. (*See* **cross-resistance**.)

DSMB: *See* **Data Safety and Monitoring Board**.

dysplasia: Any abnormal development of tissues or organs. In pathology, alteration in size, shape, and organization of adult cells.

dyspnea: Difficult or labored breathing.

E

edema: An abnormal swelling resulting from the accumulation of fluid in the spaces between tissues.

efficacy: Of a drug or treatment: The maximum ability of a drug or treatment to produce a result regardless of dosage. A drug passes efficacy trials if it is effective at the dose tested and against the illness for which it is prescribed. In the procedure mandated by the **FDA**, **Phase II clinical trials** gauge efficacy, and **Phase III trials** confirm it.

ELISA (enzyme-linked immunosorbent assay): A type of enzyme immunoassay (EIA) to determine the presence of **antibodies** to HIV in the blood or oral fluids. Repeatedly reactive (i.e., two or more) ELISA test results should be validated with an independent supplemental test of high specificity. In the United States the validation test used most often is the **Western Blot** test.

empirical: Based on experimental data, not on a theory.

emulsion: a suspension of droplets of one liquid in another liquid (such as oil and water). The two liquids do not actually combine but are instead suspended within one another.

encephalitis: A brain inflammation of viral or other microbial origin. Symptoms include headaches, neck pain, fever, nausea, vomiting, and nervous system problems. Several types of **opportunistic infections** can cause encephalitis.

endemic: Pertaining to diseases associated with particular locales or population groups.

endogenous: Relating to or produced by the body.

endoscopy: Viewing the inside of a body cavity (e.g., colon) with an endoscope, a device using flexible fiber optics.

endotoxin: A toxin present inside a bacterial cell.

endpoint: A category of data used to compare the outcome in different **arms** of a **clinical trial**. Common endpoints are severe toxicity, disease progression, or—especially in HIV disease—surrogate markers, such as **CD4** count; sometimes death is used as an endpoint. The term is confusing because it often incorrectly implies that patients in a study are no longer followed after they experience an endpoint. This is obviously true where the event is death, but need not be so for nonfatal events. In fact, the design of the trial may require continued treatment and followup of patients over the entire course of the trial, regardless of the number of nonfatal "endpoints" observed.

end-stage disease: Final period or phase in the course of a disease leading to a person's death.

enhancing antibody: a type of **binding antibody**, detected in the test tube and formed in response to HIV infection, that may enhance the ability of HIV to produce disease. Theoretically, enhancing antibodies could attach to HIV virions and enable **macrophages** to engulf the viruses. However, instead of being destroyed, the engulfed virus may remain alive within the macrophage, which then can carry the virus to other parts of the body. It is currently unknown whether enhancing antibodies have any effect on the course of HIV infection. Enhancing antibodies can be thought of as the opposite of **neutralizing antibodies**.

enteric: Pertaining to the intestines.

enteritis: Inflammation of the intestine.

env: A **gene** of HIV that codes for the protein **gp160**, the precursor of the envelope proteins **gp120** and **gp41**.

envelope: In virology, a protein covering that packages the virus's genetic information. The outer coat, or envelope, of HIV is composed

531

of two layers of fat-like molecules called **lipids** taken from the membranes of human cells. Embedded in the envelope are numerous cellular proteins, as well as mushroom-shaped HIV proteins that protrude from the surface. Each mushroom is thought to consist of a cap made of four **glycoprotein** molecules called **gp120**, and a stem consisting of four **gp41** molecules embedded in the envelope. The virus uses these proteins to attach to and infect cells.

enzyme: A cellular protein whose shape allows it to hold together several other **molecules** in close proximity to each other. In this way, enzymes are able to induce chemical reactions in other substances with little expenditure of energy and without being changed themselves. Basically, an enzyme acts as a catalyst.

eosinophil: A type of white blood cell, called **granulocyte**, that can digest microorganisms. The granules can be stained by the acid dye, eosin, for microscopic examination.

eosinophillic folliculitis: An inflammatory reaction around hair follicles, characterized by very itchy papules (small elevation or bump on the skin) that may grow together to form plaques. The cause of this condition in persons with AIDS has yet to be established; it involves invasion of the follicles by **eosinophils**. Partially successful treatment has been reported with ultraviolet light, steroids, antihistamines, and itraconazole.

epidemic: A disease that spreads rapidly through a demographic segment of the human population, such as everyone in a given geographic area; a military base, or similar population unit; or everyone of a certain age or sex, such as the children or women of a region. Epidemic diseases can be spread from person to person or from a contaminated source such as food or water.

epidemiological surveillance: The ongoing and systematic collection, analysis, and interpretation of data about a disease or health condition. As part of a surveillance system to monitor the HIV epidemic in the United States, the **Centers for Disease Control and Prevention (CDC)**, in collaboration with state and local health departments, other federal agencies, blood collection agencies, and medical research institutions, conducts standardized HIV **seroprevalence** surveys in designated subgroups of the U.S. population. Collecting blood samples for the purpose of surveillance is called serosurveillance.

epidemiology: The branch of medical science that deals with the study of incidence and distribution and control of a disease in a population.

epithelium: The covering of the internal and external organs of the body. Also the lining of vessels, body cavities, glands, and organs. It consists of cells bound together by connective material and varies in the number of layers and the kinds of cells.

epitope: A unique shape or marker carried on an antigen's surface that triggers a corresponding antibody response. (*See* **antibodies**; **antigen.**)

Epivir: *See* **3TC**.

Epstein-Barr virus (EBV): A herpes-like virus that causes one of the two kinds of mononucleosis (the other is caused by **CMV**). It infects the nose and throat and is contagious. EBV lies dormant in the **lymph glands** and has been associated with **Burkitt's lymphoma** and **hairy leukoplakia**.

erythema: Redness or inflammation of the skin or mucous membranes.

erythema multiforme: A skin disease characterized by papular (small, solid, usually conic elevation of the skin) or vesicular lesions (blisters), and reddening or discoloration of the skin often in concentric zones about the **lesion**. Associated with many infections, collagen disease, drug sensitivities, allergies, and pregnancy. A severe form of this condition is **Stevens-Johnson syndrome**.

erythrocytes: Red blood cells whose major function is to carry oxygen to cells.

etiology: The study or theory of the factors that cause disease.

exclusion/inclusion criteria: The medical or social standards determining whether a person may or may not be allowed to enter a **clinical trial**. For example, some trials may not include persons with chronic liver disease, or may exclude persons with certain drug allergies; others may exclude men or women or only include persons with a lowered **T cell** count.

exogenous: Developed or originating outside the body.

exotoxin: A toxic substance, made by bacteria released outside the bacterial cell.

expanded access: Refers to any of the **FDA** procedures, such as compassionate use, parallel track, and **treatment IND**, that distribute experimental drugs to patients who are failing on currently available treatments for their condition and also are unable to participate in ongoing **clinical trials**.

expression system: In HIV **vaccine** production, cells into which an HIV gene has been inserted to produce desired HIV proteins.

F

fallopian tubes: Part of the female reproductive system. A pair of ducts opening at one end into the uterus and at the other end into the peritoneal cavity, over the ovary. Each tube serves as a passage through which the ovum (egg) is carried to the uterus and through which spermatozoa (sperm) move out toward the ovary.

FDA: *See* **Food and Drug Administration**.

FDC: *See* **follicular dendritic cells**.

floaters: Drifting dark spots within the field of vision. Floaters can be caused by infection with **cytomegalovirus (CMV) retinitis**, but also can appear in persons as a normal part of the aging process.

folic acid: A crystalline vitamin of the B complex that is used especially in the treatment of nutritional **anemias**. It occurs in green plants, fresh fruit, liver, and yeast. Also called folacin, folate, and vitamin B9.

folinic acid: Also called citrovorum factor. A metabolically active form of **folic acid** that has been used in cancer therapy to protect normal cells against methotrexate—a cancer chemotherapy agent. Also used to treat megaloblastic **anemias**.

follicle: A small anatomical sac, cavity, or deep narrow-mouthed depression (e.g., a hair follicle).

follicular dendritic cells (FDC): Cells found in the germinal centers of lymphoid organs. FDCs have thread-like tentacles that form a weblike network to trap invaders and present them to other cells of the **immune system** for destruction. (*See* **lymphoid organs**.)

fomite: An inanimate object that can harbor pathogenic microorganisms and thus serve as an agent of transmission of an infection.

Food and Drug Administration (FDA): The **Department of Health and Human Services** agency responsible for ensuring the safety and effectiveness of drugs, biologics, **vaccines**, and medical devices used (among others) in the diagnosis, treatment, and prevention of HIV infection, **AIDS**, and AIDS-related **opportunistic infections**. The FDA also works with the blood banking industry to safeguard the nation's blood supply.

functional antibody: An **antibody** that binds to an **antigen** and has an effect. For example, **neutralizing antibodies** inactivate HIV or prevent it from infecting other cells.

fungus: 1. One of a group of primitive, nonvascular organisms including mushrooms, yeasts, rusts, and molds. 2. Fungi, which were once classified as plants, have since been reclassified as unmoving organisms that lack chlorophyll. Some fungi are single-celled but differ from bacteria in that they have a distinct nucleus and other cellular structures. Reproduction is accomplished by spores. Mycologists (scientists working with fungi) estimate that there are 100,000 species of fungi, ranging from baker's yeast to dermatophytes (fungi that cause ringworm and athlete's foot) to potentially invasive species such as *Candida albicans* and *Aspergillus*. As many as 150 of these organisms have now been linked to animal or human diseases.

fusin: *See* **CXCR4.**

fusion mechanism: Fusion is an integral step in the process whereby HIV enters cells. Researchers have found that in addition to the primary receptor, the **CD4** molecule, other cofactors, such as **CC CKR5** and **CXCR4**, are needed in order for HIV to fuse with the membranes of the **immune system** cells.

G

gag: a gene of HIV that codes for p55, the **core protein**. p55 is the precursor of HIV proteins p17, **p24**, p7 and p6 that form HIV's capsid or core, the inner protein shell surrounding HIV's strands of **RNA**.

gamma globulin: One of the proteins in blood serum that contains **antibodies**. Passive immunizing agents obtained from pooled human plasma. (*See* **globulins, immunoglobulins.**)

gamma interferon: A T cell-derived stimulating substance that suppresses virus reproduction, stimulates other **T cells**, and activates **macrophage** cells.

ganglion: A mass of nervous tissue, composed principally of nerve-cell bodies, usually lying outside the **central nervous system**.

gastrointestinal (GI): Relating to the stomach and intestines.

gene: 1. A unit of **DNA** that carries information for the biosynthesis of a specific product in the cell. 2. Ultimate unit by which inheritable characteristics are transmitted to succeeding generations in all living organisms. Genes are contained by, and arranged along the length of, the chromosome. The gene is composed of deoxyribonucleic acid (DNA). Each chromosome of each species has a definite number and arrangement of genes, which govern both the structure and metabolic functions of the cells and thus of the entire organism. They provide information for the synthesis of enzymes and other proteins and specify when these substances are to be made. Alteration of either gene number or arrangement can result in mutation (a change in the inheritable traits).

gene therapy: Any of a number of experimental treatments in which cell **genes** are altered. Some gene therapies attempt to provoke new immune activity; some try to render cells resistant to infection; some involve the development of **enzymes** that destroy viral or cancerous genetic material within cells.

genetic engineering: New research techniques that manipulate the **DNA** (genetic material) of cells. The gene-splicing technique, which produces recombinant DNA, is a method of transporting selected genes from one species to another. For example, in this technique, the genes, which are actually portions of **molecules** of DNA, are removed from the donor (insect, plant, mammal, or other organism) and spliced into the genetic material of a virus; the virus is then allowed to infect recipient bacteria. In this way the bacteria become recipients of both viral and foreign genetic material. When the virus replicates within the bacteria, large quantities of the foreign as well as viral material are made.

genital ulcer disease: Ulcerative lesions on the genitals usually caused by a **sexually transmitted disease** such as herpes, **syphilis**, or **chancroid**. The presence of genital ulcers may increase the risk of transmitting HIV.

genitourinary tract: The organs concerned with the production and excretion of urine and those concerned with reproduction. Also called genitourinary system, urogenital system, or urogenital tract.

genital warts: *See* **condyloma**.

genome: The complete set of **genes** in the chromosomes of each cell of a particular organism.

germinal centers: One of a series of **follicles** or cavities around the periphery of **lymph nodes**. Germinal centers are the site of antibody production and are populated mostly by **B cells** but include a few **T cells** and **macrophages**. As HIV infection progresses, the germinal centers gradually decay.

giardiasis: A common protozoal infection of the small intestine, spread via contaminated food and water and direct person-to-person contact. (*See also* **diarrhea**.)

globulins: Simple proteins found in the blood serum, which contain various **molecules** central to the **immune system** function. (*See* **immunoglobulin**.)

glycoprotein: A conjugated protein in which the nonprotein group is a carbohydrate (i.e., a sugar molecule); also called glucoprotein.

gp: Abbreviation for **glycoprotein**. A protein **molecule** that is glycosylated, that is, coated with a carbohydrate, or sugar. The outer coat proteins of HIV are glycoproteins. The number after the gp (e.g., **gp 160, gp 120, gp41**) is the molecular weight of the glycoprotein.

gp41: Glycoprotein 41, a protein embedded in the outer **envelope** of HIV. Plays a key role in HIV's infection of **CD4+ T cells** by facilitating the fusion of the viral and the cell membranes. (*See also* **gp120**.)

gp120: Glycoprotein 120, a protein that protrudes from the surface of HIV and binds to **CD4+ T cells**. In a two-step process that allows HIV to breach the membrane of **T cells**, gp120-CD4 complex refolds to reveal a second structure that binds to **CC CKR5**, one of several **chemokine** co-receptors used by the virus to gain entry into T cells.

gp160: Glycoprotein 160, a precursor of HIV **envelope** proteins **gp41** and **gp120**.

granulocyte: A type of white blood cell filled with granules of compounds that digest microorganisms. Granulocytes are part of the innate **immune system** and have broad-based activity. They do not respond only to specific **antigens** as do **B cells** and **T cells**. **Basophils, eosinophils**, and **neutrophils** are all granulocytes.

granulocytopenia: A lack or low level of **granulocytes** in the blood. Often used interchangeably with **neutropenia**.

H

hairy leukoplakia: *See* **oral hairy leukoplakia**.

half-life: The time required for half the amount of a drug to be eliminated from the body.

Health Resources and Services Administration (HRSA): An agency in the **Department of Health and Human Services** that puts primary health care providers and services in the places they are needed most. HRSA administers the **Ryan White CARE Act** Titles I, II, III(b), IV, SPNS, and AETCs (see explanations for these terms under Ryan White CARE Act) to provide treatment and services for those affected by HIV/AIDS. HRSA administers programs to demonstrate how communities can organize their health care resources to develop an integrated, comprehensive, culturally competent system to care for those with AIDS and HIV infection. HRSA also administers education and training programs for health care providers and community service workers who care for persons living with HIV or AIDS.

helper/suppressor ratio (of T cells): T cells are **lymphocytes** (white blood cells) that are formed in the **thymus** and are part of the **immune system**. They have been found to be abnormal in persons with AIDS. The normal ratio of helper T cells (**CD4+ cells**) to suppressor T cells (**CD8+ cells**) is approximately 2:1. This ratio becomes inverted in persons with AIDS but also may be abnormal for a host of other temporary reasons.

helper T cells: Lymphocytes bearing the **CD4** marker that are responsible for many **immune system** functions, including turning **antibody** production on and off.

hematocrit: A laboratory measurement that determines the percentage of packed red blood cells in a given volume of blood. In women, red blood cells are normally 37 to 47 percent of their blood, and in men, red blood cells are normally 40 to 54 percent of their blood.

hematotoxic: Poisonous to the blood or bone marrow.

hemoglobin: The component of red blood cells that carries oxygen.

hemolysis: The rupture of red blood cells.

hemophilia: An inherited disease that affects mostly males and prevents normal blood clotting. It is treated by lifelong injections of a synthetic version of the clotting factor lacking in persons with the disease. The new recombinant clotting factor replaces the natural product, which was extracted from people's blood and, when not heat treated, could carry HIV.

hepatic: Pertaining to the liver.

hepatitis: An inflammation of the liver. May be caused by bacterial or viral infection, parasitic infestation, alcohol, drugs, toxins, or transfusion of incompatible blood. Although many cases of hepatitis are not a serious threat to health, the disease can become chronic and can sometimes lead to liver failure and death. There are four major types of viral hepatitis: (a) hepatitis A, caused by infection with the hepatitis A virus, which is spread by fecal-oral contact; (b) hepatitis B, caused by infection with the hepatitis B virus (HBV), which is most commonly passed on to a partner during intercourse, especially during anal sex, as well as through sharing of drug needles; (c) non-A, non-B hepatitis, caused by the hepatitis C virus, which appears to be spread through sexual contact as well as through sharing of drug needles (another type of non-A, non-B hepatitis is caused by the hepatitis E virus, principally spread through contaminated water); (d) delta hepatitis, which occurs only in persons who are already infected with HBV and is caused by the HDV virus; most cases of delta hepatitis occur among people who are frequently exposed to blood and blood products such as persons with **hemophilia.**

hepatomegaly: Enlargement of the liver.

herpes viruses: A group of viruses that includes **herpes simplex type 1 (HSV-1), herpes simplex type 2 (HSV-2), cytomegalovirus (CMV), Epstein-Barr virus (EBV), varicella zoster virus (VZV),** human herpes virus type 6 (HHV-6), and HHV-8, a herpes virus associated with **Kaposi's sarcoma.**

herpes simplex virus I (HSV-I): A virus that causes cold sores or fever blisters on the mouth or around the eyes, and can be transmitted to the genital region. Stress, trauma, other infections, or suppression of the **immune system** can reactivate the latent virus.

herpes simplex virus II (HSV-II): A virus causing painful sores of the anus or genitals that may lie dormant in nerve tissue. It can be reactivated to produce the symptoms. HSV-II may be transmitted to a neonate (newborn child) during birth from an infected mother, causing retardation and/or other serious complications. HSV-II is a precursor of **cervical cancer**.

herpes varicella zoster virus (VZV): The varicella virus causes chicken pox in children and may reappear in adults as herpes zoster. Also called shingles, herpes zoster consists of very painful blisters on the skin that follow nerve pathways.

histocompatibility testing: A method of matching the self-antigens on the tissues of a transplant donor with those of a recipient. The closer the match, the better the chance that the transplant will not be rejected. (*See also* **human leukocyte antigens (HLA)**.)

histoplasmosis: A fungal infection, commonly of the lungs, caused by the **fungus** *Histoplasma capsulatum*. This fungus is commonly found in bird and/or bat droppings in the Ohio and Mississippi Valley region, the Caribbean Islands, and in Central and South America. It is spread by breathing in the spores of the fungus. The most definitive test for the fungus has been from fungal stains and bone marrow cultures. Blood testing has proved to be less reliable. In areas where *H. capsulatum* is prevalent, 80 percent or more of the population has been exposed to infection through breathing in airborne spores produced by the fungus. Persons with severely damaged **immune systems**, such as those with AIDS, are vulnerable to a very serious disease known as progressive disseminated histoplasmosis. Nationwide, about 5 percent of persons with AIDS have histoplasmosis, but in geographic areas where the fungus is common, persons with AIDS are at high risk for disseminated histoplasmosis.

HIV-1: *See* **human immunodeficiency virus type 1**.

HIV-2: *See* **human immunodeficiency virus type 2**.

HIV disease: During the initial infection with HIV, when the virus comes in contact with the mucosal surface, and finds susceptible T cells (**T lymphocytes**), the first site at which there is truly massive production of the virus in lymphoid tissue. This leads to a burst of massive **viremia** with wide dissemination of the virus to **lymphoid organs**. The resulting **immune response** to suppress the virus is only partially successful and some virus escapes. Eventually, this results

540

in high viral turnover that leads to destruction of the **immune system**. HIV disease is, therefore, characterized by a gradual deterioration of immune functions. During the course of infection, crucial immune cells, called **CD4+ T cells**, are disabled and killed, and their numbers progressively decline. (*See* **acquired immunodeficiency syndrome**; **human immunodeficiency virus type 1.**)

HIV-related tuberculosis: *See* **tuberculosis**.

HIV set point: The rate of virus replication that stabilizes and remains at a particular level in each individual after the period of primary infection.

HIV viral load: *See* **viral load**.

HIVID: *See* **ddC**.

HLA: *See* **human leukocyte antigens**.

HLA class I: Molecules that exist on all nucleated cells and identify the cell as "self." In addition, if the cell is infected by a virus or other microbe, the cell displays the invader's **antigens** in combination with the cell's HLA class I molecules. The presence of the foreign **peptide** antigen with the HLA class I molecule activates **CD8+ cytotoxic T lymphocytes** specific for that antigen.

HLA class II: Molecules that are found on antigen-presenting cells such as **macrophages**. These cells process soluble **antigens** such as toxins or other proteins made by microbes and then display them on their surface as **peptide** antigens in combination with HLA Class II molecules. **Helper T cells** specific for these antigens are then able to be activated and respond to the presence of the invading microbe.

Hodgkin's disease: A progressive malignant cancer of the lymphatic system. Symptoms include lymphadenopathy, wasting, weakness, fever, itching, night sweats, and anemia. Treatment includes radiation and chemotherapy. (*See* **lymphoma.**)

holistic medicine: Healing traditions that promote the protection and restoration of health through theories reputedly based on the body's natural ability to heal itself and through manipulation of various ways body components affect each other and are influenced by the external environment.

homologous: Similar in appearance or structure, but not necessarily in function.

hormone: An active chemical substance formed in one part of the body and carried in the blood to other parts of the body where it stimulates or suppresses cell and tissue activity. (*See also* **pituitary gland.**)

host: A plant or animal harboring another organism.

host factors: The body's potent mechanisms for containing HIV, including immune system cells called **CD8+ T cells**, which may prove more effective than any **antiretroviral** drug in controlling HIV infection.

HPV: *See* **human papilloma virus.**

HRSA: *See* **Health Resources and Services Administration.**

HTLV-I: *See* **human T cell lymphotropic virus type I.**

HTLV-II: *See* **human T cell lymphotropic virus type II.**

human growth hormone (HGH): A **peptide hormone** secreted by the anterior **pituitary gland** in the brain. HGH enhances tissue growth by stimulating protein formation. A recombinant (genetically engineered) HGH, called serostim, has been FDA approved as a treatment for **AIDS wasting syndrome.**

human immunodeficiency virus type 1 (HIV-1): 1. The **retrovirus** isolated and recognized as the etiologic (i.e., causing or contributing to the cause of a disease) agent of **AIDS**. HIV-1 is classified as a **lentivirus** in a subgroup of retroviruses. 2. Most viruses and all bacteria, plants, and animals have genetic codes made up of **DNA**, which uses **RNA** to build specific **proteins**. The genetic material of a retrovirus such as HIV is the RNA itself. HIV inserts its own RNA into the host cell's DNA, preventing the host cell from carrying out its natural functions and turning it into an HIV factory.

human immunodeficiency virus type 2 (HIV-2): A virus closely related to **HIV-1** that has also been found to cause **AIDS**. It was first isolated in West Africa. Although HIV-1 and HIV-2 are similar in their viral structure, modes of transmission, and resulting **opportunistic infections**, they have differed in their geographic patterns of infection.

human leukocyte antigens (HLA): Markers that identify cells as "self" and prevent the immune system from attacking them.

human papilloma virus (HPV): The virus that causes genital warts and is linked to **cervical dysplasia** and **cervical cancer**. HPV affects more than 24 million Americans, and **CDC** estimates that there are at least 500,000 new cases each year. There is no specific cure for an HPV infection, but the warts can be removed or controlled by podophyllo-toxin, the active ingredient in podophyllin. **Cryotherapy**, laser treat-ment, or conventional surgery can remove the warts. **Interferon** is used in the treatment of refractory or recurrent genital warts. The virus can be transmitted through sexual contact. HPV is a frequently seen infection in women with HIV/AIDS.

human T cell lymphotropic virus type I (HTLV-I): HTLV-I and **HTLV-II,** like all **retroviruses**, are single-stranded **RNA** viruses containing a **genome** that replicates through a **DNA** intermediate. This unique life cycle is made possible by the presence of a virally encoded **enzyme**, **reverse transcriptase**, which converts a single-stranded viral RNA into a double-stranded DNA **provirus** that can then be integrated into the **host** genome. HTLV-I has an affinity for **T lymphocytes**; it appears to be the causative agent of certain T cell leukemias, **T cell lymphomas**, and HTLV-I-associated myelopathy/tropical spastic paraparesis (HAM/TSP).

human T cell lymphotropic virus type II (HTLV-II): A virus closely related to **HTLV-I**, shares 60 percent genomic homology (struc-tural similarity) with HTLV-I. Found predominantly in injection drug users and Native Americans, as well as Caribbean and South Ameri-can Indian groups. HTLV-II has not been clearly linked to any dis-ease, but has been associated with several cases of myelopathy/tropical spastic paraparesis (HAM/TSP)-like neurological disease.

humoral immunity: The branch of the **immune system** that relies primarily on **antibodies**. (*See* **cell-mediated immunity**.)

hybrid: An offspring produced from mating plants or animals from different species, varieties, or genotypes.

hybridoma: A **hybrid** cell produced by the fusion of an antibody-producing **lymphocyte** with a tumor cell. Hybridomas are used in the production of **monoclonal antibodies**.

hypergammaglobulinemia: Abnormally high levels of **immunoglo-bulins** in the blood. Common in persons with HIV.

hyperplasia: Abnormal increase in the elements composing a part (as tissue cells).

hyperthermia: An unproven and dangerous experimental procedure that involves temporarily heating a patient's body core to temperatures of up to 108° F on the theory that this temperature kills free HIV and

HIV-containing cells. One method for accomplishing this is by passing patients' blood through an external heater. This is called extracorporeal whole body hyperthermia.

hypogammaglobulinemia: Abnormally low levels of **immunoglobulins**. (*See* **antibodies**.)

hypothesis: A specific statement or proposition, stated in a testable (researchable) form, predicting a particular relationship among multiple variables.

hypoxia: Reduction of oxygen supply to tissue.

I

idiopathic: Without a known cause.

idiopathic thrombocytopenia purpura (ITP): *See* **immune thrombocytopenic purpura**.

idiotypes: The unique and characteristic parts of an **antibody**'s variable region, which can themselves serve as **antigens**.

IHS: *See* **Indian Health Service**.

immune complex: Clusters formed when **antigens** and **antibodies** bind together.

immune deficiency: A breakdown or inability of certain parts of the **immune system** to function, thus making a person susceptible to certain diseases that they would not ordinarily develop.

immune response: The activity of the **immune system** against foreign substances.

immune system: The body's complicated natural defense against disruption caused by invading foreign agents (e.g., microbes, viruses). There are two aspects of the immune system's response to disease: innate and acquired. The innate part of the response is mobilized very quickly in response to infection and does not depend on recognizing specific proteins or **antigens** foreign to an individual's normal tissue. It includes **complement, macrophages, dendritic cells**, and **granulocytes**. The acquired, or learned, **immune response** arises when dendritic cells and macrophages present pieces of **antigen** to **lymphocytes**, which are genetically programmed to recognize very specific **amino acid** sequences. The ultimate result is the creation of **cloned** populations of antibody-producing **B cells** and **cytotoxic T lymphocytes** primed to respond to a unique **pathogen**.

immune thrombocytopenic purpura (ITP): Also idiopathic immune thrombocytopenic purpura. A condition in which the body produces **antibodies** against the **platelets** in the blood, which are cells responsible for blood clotting. ITP is very common in persons infected with HIV.

immunity: A natural or acquired resistance to a specific disease. Immunity may be partial or complete, long lasting or temporary.

immunization: The process of inducing immunity by administering an **antigen** (**vaccine**) to allow the **immune system** to prevent infection or illness when it subsequently encounters the infectious agent.

immunocompetent: 1. Capable of developing an **immune response**. 2. Possessing a normal **immune system**.

immunocompromised: Refers to an **immune system** in which the ability to resist or fight off infections and tumors is subnormal.

immunodeficiency: Breakdown in **immunocompetence** when certain parts of the **immune system** no longer function. This condition makes a person more susceptible to certain diseases.

immunogen: A substance, also called an **antigen**, capable of provoking an **immune response**.

immunogenicity: The ability of an **antigen** or **vaccine** to stimulate an **immune response**.

immunoglobulin (IG): A general term for **antibodies**, which bind onto invading organisms, leading to their destruction. There are five classes: **IgA**, IgD, IgE, **IgG**, and IgM.

immunoglobulin A (IgA): An immunoglobulin found in body fluids such as tears and saliva and in the respiratory, reproductive, urinary, and gastrointestinal tracts. IgA protects the body's mucosal surfaces from infection.

immunoglobulin G (IgG): The prominent type of immunoglobulin existing in the blood. Also called gamma globulin.

immunomodulator: Any substance that influences the **immune system**. (*See* **interleukin-2**; **immunostimulant**; **immunosuppression**.)

immunostimulant: Any agent or substance that triggers or enhances the body's defense; also called immunopotentiator.

immunosuppression: A state of the body in which the **immune system** is damaged and does not perform its normal functions. Immunosuppression may be induced by drugs (e.g., in **chemotherapy**) or result from certain disease processes, such as HIV infection.

immunotherapy: Treatment aimed at reconstituting an impaired **immune system**.

immunotoxin: A plant or animal toxin (i.e., poison) that is attached to a **monoclonal antibody** and used to destroy a specific target cell.

incidence: The number of new cases (e.g., of a disease) occurring in a given population over a certain period of time.

inclusion/exclusion criteria: The medical or social standards determining whether a person may or may not be allowed to enter a **clinical trial**. For example, some trials may not allow persons with chronic liver disease or with certain drug allergies; others may exclude men or women, or only include persons with a lowered **T cell** count.

incubation period: The time interval between the initial infection with a **pathogen** (e.g., HIV) and the appearance of the first symptom or sign of disease.

IND: *See* **investigational new drug**.

Indian Health Service (IHS): The federal agency charged with administering the health programs for American Indians and Alaska Natives (AI/AN), who are enrolled members of federally recognized Indian tribes.

indinavir: A peptide-based **protease inhibitor**. Approved by the **FDA** for use as monotherapy or in combination with approved **nucleoside inhibitors** in persons living with HIV. Indinavir, in combination with the **nucleoside analog** drugs 3TC and **AZT**, has been shown to decrease **viral load** and increase **CD4** counts in patients. Patients taking indinavir must drink plenty of fluids to prevent the development of kidney stones. Also known as Crixivan, MK-639, and L735,524.

infection: The state or condition in which the body (or part of the body) is invaded by an infectious agent (e.g., a **bacterium**, **fungus**, or **virus**), which multiplies and produces an injurious effect (active infection). As related to HIV: Infection typically begins when HIV encounters a **CD4+ cell**. The HIV surface protein **gp120** binds tightly to the CD4 molecule on the cell's surface. The membranes of the virus and the cell fuse, a process governed by **gp41**, another surface protein. The **viral core**, containing HIV's **RNA**, **proteins**, and **enzymes**, is released into the cell.

infectious: An infection capable of being transmitted by direct or intimate contact (e.g., sex).

informed consent: The permission granted by a participant in a research study (including medical research) after he/she has received comprehensive information about the study. This is a statement of trust between the institution performing the research procedure and the person (e.g., a patient) on whom the research procedures are to be performed. This includes, for example, the type of protection available to people considering entering a drug trial. Before entering the trial, participants must sign a consent form that contains an explanation of: (a) why the research is being done, (b) what the researchers want to accomplish, (c) what will be done during the trial and for how long, (d) what the risks associated with the trial are, (e) what benefits can be expected from the trial, (f) what other treatments are available, and (g) the participant's right to leave the trial at any time. Informed consent also pertains to situations where certain tests need to be performed. (*See* **clinical trial**.)

infusion: The process of administering therapeutic fluid, other than blood, to an individual by slowly injecting a dilute solution of the compound into a vein. Infusions are often used when the digestive system does not absorb appreciable quantities of a drug or when the drug is too toxic or the volume is too large to be given by quick injection.

inoculation: The introduction of a substance (inoculum; e.g., a **vaccine**, **serum**, or **virus**) into the body to produce or to increase immunity to the disease or condition associated with the substance.

Institutional Review Board (IRB): 1. A committee of physicians, statisticians, researchers, community advocates, and others that ensures that a **clinical trial** is ethical and that the rights of study participants are protected. All clinical trials in the United States must be approved by an IRB before they begin. 2. Every institution that conducts or supports biomedical or behavioral research involving human subjects must, by federal regulation, have an IRB that initially approves and periodically reviews the research so as to protect the rights of human subjects.

integrase: A little-understood **enzyme** that plays a vital role in the HIV-infection process. Integrase inserts HIV's genes into a cell's normal **DNA**. It operates after **reverse transcriptase** has created a DNA version of the **RNA** form of HIV genes present in virus particles. Substances that inhibit integrase are being studied in HIV-infected patients.

integration: The process by which the different parts of an organism are made a functional and structural whole, especially through the activity of the nervous system and of hormones. As related to HIV: The process by which the viral **DNA** migrates to the cell's nucleus, where it is spliced into the host's DNA with the help of viral **integrase**. Once incorporated, HIV DNA is called the **provirus** and is duplicated together with the cell's genes every time the cell divides. Recent reports suggest that HIV's DNA also can integrate into the DNA of non-dividing cells such as **macrophages** and brain and nerve cells.

intent to treat: Analysis of **clinical trial** results that includes all data from patients in the groups to which they were randomized (i.e., assigned through random distribution) even if they never received the treatment.

interferon: One of a number of **antiviral** proteins that modulate the **immune response**. Interferon alpha (IFNa) is secreted by a virally infected cell and strengthens the defenses of nearby uninfected cells. A manufactured version of IFNa (trade names: Roferon, Intron A) is an FDA-approved treatment for **Kaposi's sarcoma**, **hepatitis** B virus, and hepatitis C virus. Interferon gamma (IFNy) is synthesized by **immune system** cells (**natural killer [NK] cells** and **CD4** cells). It activates **macrophages** and helps orient the immune system to a mode that promotes **cellular immunity**. (*See* **Th1 response**).

interleukins: One of a large group of **glycoproteins** that act as **cytokines**. The interleukins are secreted by and affect many different cells in the **immune system**. (*See also* **biotechnology**; **B lymphocytes**; **genetic engineering**; **killer T cells**; **natural killer cells (NK)**; **lymphocyte**; **T cells**.)

interleukin-1 (IL-1): A **cytokine** that is released early in an immune system response by **monocytes** and **macrophages**. It stimulates T cell proliferation and protein synthesis. Another effect of IL-1 is that it causes fever.

interleukin-2 (IL-2): A **cytokine** secreted by **Th1 CD4** cells to stimulate **CD8 cytotoxic T lymphocytes**. IL-2 also increases the proliferation and maturation of the CD4 cells themselves. During HIV infection, IL-2 production gradually declines. Commercially, IL-2 is produced by recombinant DNA technology and is approved by the **FDA** for the treatment of metastatic renal (i.e., kidney) cell cancer. Recent data suggests that therapy with subcutaneous IL-2, in combination with **antiretroviral agents**, has the potential to halt the usual progression of HIV disease by maintaining an individual's CD4+ T cell count in the normal range for prolonged periods of time.

interleukin-4 (IL-4): A **cytokine** secreted by **Th2 CD4** cells that promotes **antibody** production by stimulating **B cells** to proliferate and mature.

interleukin-12 (IL-12): A **cytokine** released by **macrophage** in response to infection that promotes the activation of **cell-mediated immunity**. Specifically, IL-12 triggers the maturation of **Th1 CD4** cells, specific **cytotoxic T lymphocyte responses**, and an increase in the activity of **NK cells**. IL-12 is under study as an **immunotherapy** in HIV infection.

interstitial: Relating to or situated in the small, narrow spaces between tissues or parts of an organ.

intramuscular (IM): Injected directly into a muscle.

intrathecal: Injected into the fluid surrounding the spinal cord.

intravenous (IV): Of or pertaining to the inside of a vein, as of a thrombus. Injection directly into a vein.

intravenous immunoglobulin (IVIG): A sterile solution of concentrated **antibodies** extracted from healthy people. IVIG is used to prevent bacterial infections in persons with low or abnormal antibody production. Injected into a vein.

intravitreal: Within the eye.

investigational new drug (IND): The status of an experimental drug after the **FDA** agrees that it can be tested in people.

Invirase: *See* **saquinavir**.

in vitro **("in glass"):** An artificial environment created outside a living organism (e.g., a test tube or culture plate) used in experimental research to study a disease or process.

549

in vivo (**"in life"**): Studies conducted within living organisms (e.g., animal or human studies).

IRB: *See* **Institutional Review Board.**

isolate: An individual (as a spore or a single organism), viable part of an organism (as a cell), or a strain that has been separated (as from diseased tissue, contaminated water or the air) from the whole. Also, a pure culture produced from such an isolate. A particular strain of HIV taken from a patient.

ITP: *See* **immune thrombocytopenic purpura.**

IVIG: *See* **intravenous immune globulin.**

J

jaundice: Yellow pigmentation of the skin and whites of the eyes caused by elevated blood levels of **bilirubin**. The condition is associated with either liver or gallbladder disease or excessive destruction of red blood cells.

JC virus: *See* **PML**; **papilloma.**

K

Kaposi's sarcoma (KS): An AIDS-defining illness consisting of individual cancerous lesions caused by an overgrowth of blood vessels. KS typically appears as pink or purple painless spots or nodules on the surface of the skin or oral cavity. KS also can occur internally, especially in the intestines, **lymph nodes**, and lungs, and in this case is life threatening. The cancer may spread and also attack the eyes. There has been considerable speculation that KS is not a spontaneous cancer but is sparked by a virus. A species of **herpes virus** also referred to as Kaposi's sarcoma herpes virus (KSHV) or HHV-8—similar to the **Epstein-Barr virus** is currently under extensive investigation. Up to now, KS has been treated with **alpha interferon**, radiation therapy (outside the oral cavity), and various systemic and intralesional cancer chemotherapies.

Karnofsky score: A score between 0 and 100 assigned by a clinician based on observations of a patient's ability to perform common tasks. Thus, 100 signifies normal physical abilities with no evidence of disease.

Decreasing numbers indicate a reduced ability to perform activities of daily living.

killer T cells: Because viruses lurk inside **host** (e.g., human) cells where **antibodies** cannot reach them, the only way they can be eliminated is by killing the infected host cell. To do this, the **immune system** uses a kind of white blood cell, called killer T cells. These cells act only when they encounter another cell that carries a "marker" (i.e., a **protein**) that links it to a foreign protein—that of the invading virus. Killer T cells can themselves become infected by HIV or other viruses, or transformed by cancer. Also known as cytotoxic T cells (or cytotoxic T lymphocytes). (*See* **NK (natural killer) cells; null cell; T cells.**)

KSHV: Kaposi's sarcoma herpes virus. (*See* **Kaposi's sarcoma.**)

Kupffer cells: Specialized **macrophages** in the liver.

L

LAI: A group of closely related HIV **isolates** that includes the LAV, IIIB, and BRU strains of HIV. Used in HIV **vaccine** development.

LAK cells: Lymphocytes transformed in the laboratory into **lymphokine** activated killer cells, which attack tumor cells.

lamivudine: *See* **3TC.**

Langerhans cells: Dendritic cells in the skin that pick up an **antigen** and transport it to the **lymph nodes.**

LAS: *See* **lymphadenopathy syndrome.**

latency: An inactive or resting period during a disease process. Clinical latency is an asymptomatic period in the early years of HIV infection. The period of latency is characterized in the peripheral blood by near normal **CD4** counts. Recent research indicates that HIV remains quite active in the **lymph nodes** during this period. Cellular latency is the period after HIV has integrated its **genome** into a cell's **DNA** but has not yet begun to replicate.

LAV (lymphadenopathy associated virus): *See* **human immunodeficiency virus type I.**

LD50 (short for "Lethal Dose 50"): In toxicology, the amount of a substance sufficient to kill one half of the population of test subjects (e.g., mice or rats).

lentivirus: "Slow" virus characterized by a long interval between infection and the onset of symptoms. HIV is a lentivirus as is the **simian immunodeficiency virus (SIV)** that infects nonhuman primates.

lesion: A general term to describe an area of altered tissue (e.g., the infected patch or sore in a skin disease).

leukocytes: Any of the various white blood cells that together make up the **immune system. Neutrophils, lymphocytes,** and **monocytes** are all leukocytes.

leukocytosis: An abnormally high number of **leukocytes** in the blood. This condition can occur during many types of infection and inflammation.

leukopenia: A decrease in the number of white blood cells. The threshold value for leukopenia is usually taken as less than 5,000 white blood cells per cubic millimeter of blood.

leukoplakia: *See* **oral hairy leukoplakia**.

LIP: *See* **lymphoid interstitial pneumonitis**.

lipid: Any of a group of fats and fatlike compounds, including sterols, fatty acids, and many other substances.

liposomes: A spherical particle in an aqueous (watery) medium (e.g., inside a cell) formed by a **lipid** bilayer enclosing an aqueous compartment. Microscopic globules of lipids are manufactured to enclose medications. The liposome's fatty layer is supposed to protect and confine the enclosed drug until the liposome binds with the outer membrane of target cells. By delivering treatments directly to the cells needing them, drug **efficacy** may be increased while overall toxicity is reduced.

live vector vaccine: As pertaining to HIV, a **vaccine** that uses an attenuated (i.e., weakened) **virus** or **bacterium** to carry pieces of HIV into the body to directly stimulate a **cell-mediated immune response**.

liver function test: A test that measures the blood serum level of any of several enzymes (e.g., **SGOT** and **SGPT**) produced by the liver. An elevated liver function test is a sign of possible liver damage.

log: Changes in **viral load** are often reported as logarithmic or "log changes." This mathematical term denotes a change in value of what is being measured by a factor of 10. For example, if the baseline viral load by **PCR** were 20,000 copies/ml plasma, then a 1-log increase equals a 10-fold (10 times) increase or 200,000 copies/ml plasma. A 2-log increase equals 2,000,000 copies/ml plasma, or a 100-fold increase. Using the same starting point of 20,000 copies/ml plasma, a 1-log decrease means that the viral load has dropped to 2,000 copies/ml. A 2-log decrease equals a viral load of 200 copies/ml plasma. An easy way to figure out log changes is to either drop the last "0" or add "0" to the original number.

long terminal repeat sequence (LTR): The genetic material at each end of the HIV **genome**. When the HIV genome is integrated into a cell's own genome, the LTR interacts with cellular and viral factors to trigger the **transcription** of the HIV-integrated HIV **DNA** genes into an **RNA** form that is packaged in new virus particles. Activation of LTR is a major step in triggering HIV replication.

long-term nonprogressors: Individuals who have been living with HIV for at least 7 to 12 years (different authors use different time spans) and have stable **CD4+ T cell** counts of 600 or more cells per cubic millimeter of blood, no HIV-related diseases, and no previous antiretroviral therapy. Data suggest that this phenomenon is associated with the maintenance of the integrity of the lymphoid tissues and with less virus trapping in the **lymph nodes** than is seen in other individuals living with HIV.

LTR: *See* **long terminal repeat sequence**.

lumbar: Lower back region. Of, relating to, or constituting the vertebrae between the thoracic vertebrae and the sacrum region. The sacrum is the triangular bone made up of five fused vertebrae and forming the posterior section of the pelvis. The thorax is the part of the human body between the neck and the diaphragm, partially encased by the ribs and containing the heart and lungs (i.e., the chest).

lumbar puncture: A procedure in which sero-spinal fluid from the **subarachnoid space** in the **lumbar** region is tapped for examination. Also known as spinal tap.

lymph: A transparent, slightly yellow fluid that carries **lymphocytes**. Lymph is derived from tissue fluids collected from all parts of the body and is returned to the blood via **lymphatic vessels**.

lymph nodes: Small, bean-sized organs of the **immune system**, distributed widely throughout the body. Lymph fluid is filtered through the lymph nodes in which all types of **lymphocytes** take up temporary residence. **Antigens** that enter the body find their way into lymph or blood and are filtered out by the lymph nodes or spleen respectively, for attack by the immune system.

lymphadenopathy syndrome (LAS): Swollen, firm, and possibly tender **lymph nodes**. The cause may range from an infection such as HIV, the flu, or mononucleosis to **lymphoma** (cancer of the lymph nodes).

lymphatic vessels: A body-wide network of channels, similar to the blood vessels, that transport **lymph** to the immune organs and into the bloodstream.

lymphocyte: A white blood cell. Present in the blood, **lymph**, and lymphoid tissue. (*See* **B Lymphocytes**; **T Cells**.)

lymphoid interstitial pneumonitis (LIP): A type of pneumonia that affects 35 to 40 percent of children with AIDS, which causes hardening of the lung membranes involved in absorbing oxygen. LIP is an AIDS-defining illness in children. The etiology (cause) of LIP is not clear. There is no established therapy for LIP, but the use of corticosteroids for progressive LIP has been advocated.

lymphoid organs: Include tonsils, adenoids, **lymph nodes**, **spleen**, **thymus**, and other tissues. These organs act as the body's filtering system, trapping invaders (i.e., foreign particles, e.g., bacteria and viruses) and presenting them to squadrons of immune cells that congregate there. Within these lymphoid tissues, immune activity is concentrated in regions called **germinal centers**, where the thread-like tentacles of **follicular dendritic cells (FDCs)** form networks that trap invaders.

lymphokines: 1. Products of the lymphatic cells that stimulate the production of disease-fighting agents and the activities of other lymphatic cells. Among the lymphokines are **gamma interferon** and **interleukin-2**. 2. Non-antibody mediators of **immune responses**, released by activated **lymphocytes**.

lymphoma: Cancer of the lymphoid tissues. Lymphomas are often described as being "large cell" or "small cell" types, cleaved or noncleaved, or diffuse or nodular. The different types often have different prognoses (i.e., prospect of survival or recovery). Some of these lymphomas are named after the physicians who first described them (e.g., **Burkitt's lymphoma, Hodgkin's disease**). Lymphomas can also be referred to by the organs where they are active such as CNS lymphomas, which are in the **central nervous system**, and GI lymphomas, which are in the **gastrointestinal** tract. The types of lymphomas most commonly associated with HIV infection are called **non-Hodgkin's lymphomas** or B cell lymphomas. In these types of cancers, certain cells of the lymphatic system grow abnormally. They divide rapidly, growing into tumors.

lymphoproliferative response: A specific **immune response** that entails rapid **T cell** replication. Standard **antigens**, such as tetanus toxoid, that elicit this response, are used in lab tests of **immunocompetency**.

lysis: Rupture and destruction of a cell.

M

MAC: *See* **mycobacterium avium complex**.

macrophage: A large immune cell that devours invading **pathogens** and other intruders. Stimulates other immune cells by presenting them with small pieces of the invader. Macrophages can harbor large quantities of HIV without being killed, acting as reservoirs of the virus.

macrophage-tropic virus: HIV strains that preferentially infect **macrophages** in cell culture experiments. They readily fuse with cells that have both **CD4** and **CC CKR5** molecules on their surfaces, whereas the same viral **isolates** fail to fuse with cells expressing only **CD4**. These isolates are the main strains found in patients during the symptom-free stage of HIV disease.

magnetic resonance imaging (MRI): A noninvasive, non-x-ray diagnostic technique—also called nuclear magnetic resonance or NMR—based on the magnetic fields of hydrogen atoms in the body. MRI provides computer-generated images of the body's internal tissues and organs.

MAI: *See* **mycobacterium avium complex**.

major histocompatibility complex (MHC): Two classes of molecules on cell surfaces. MHC class I molecules exist on all cells, and hold and present foreign **antigens** to CD8 **cytotoxic T lymphocytes** if the cell is infected by a virus or other microbe. MHC class II molecules are the billboards of the **immune system**. **Peptides** derived from foreign proteins are inserted into MHC's binding groove and displayed on the surface of antigen-presenting cells. These peptides are then recognized by T lymphocytes so that the immune system is alerted to the presence of foreign material. (*See also* **histocompatibility testing**).

malabsorption syndrome: Decreased intestinal absorption resulting in loss of appetite, muscle pain, and weight loss. (*See* **wasting syndrome**).

malaise: A generalized, nonspecific feeling of discomfort.

malignant: Refers to cells or tumors growing in an uncontrolled fashion. Such growths may spread to and disrupt nearby normal tissue, or reach distant sites via the bloodstream. By definition, cancers are always malignant, and the term "malignancy" implies cancer. (*See* **metastasis**.)

mast cell: A **granulocyte** found in tissue. The contents of the mast cells, along with those of **basophils**, are responsible for the symptoms of allergy.

mean: The arithmetic average, or the sum of all the values divided by the number of values.

median: The midpoint value obtained by ranking all values from highest to lowest and choosing the value in the middle. The median divides a population into two equal halves.

memory T cells: A subset of **T lymphocytes** that have been exposed to specific **antigens** and can then proliferate (i.e., reproduce) on subsequent **immune system** encounters with the same antigen.

meninges: Membranes surrounding the brain or spinal cord. Part of the so-called **blood-brain barrier**. (*See also* **meningitis**.)

meningitis: An inflammation of the **meninges** (membranes surrounding the brain or spinal cord), which may be caused by a **bacterium**, **fungus**, or **virus**. (*See also* **cryptococcal meningitis**; **central nervous system**.)

messenger RNA: Also referred to as mRNA. An RNA (**ribonucleic acid**) that carries the genetic code for a particular protein from the **DNA** in the cell's nucleus to a **ribosome** in the **cytoplasm** and acts as a template, or pattern, for the formation of that **protein**.

metabolism: The sum of the processes by which a particular substance is handled (as by assimilation and incorporation, or by detoxification and excretion) in the living body.

metabolite: Any substance produced by **metabolism** or by a metabolic process.

metastasis: Transfer of a disease-producing agent (e.g., cancer cells or bacteria) from an original site of disease to another part of the body, with development of a similar **lesion** in the new location (e.g., spread of cancer from an original site to other sites in the body).

MHC: *See* **major histocompatibility complex**.

microbes: Microscopic living organisms, including bacteria, protozoa, viruses, and fungi.

microbicide: An agent (e.g., a chemical or **antibiotic**) that destroys **microbes**. New research is being carried out to evaluate the use of rectal and vaginal microbicides to inhibit the transmission of **sexually transmitted diseases**, including HIV.

microencapsulated: Surrounded by a thin layer of protection. A means of protecting a drug or vaccine from rapid breakdown.

microsporidiosis: An intestinal infection that causes **diarrhea** and wasting in persons with HIV. It results from two different species of microsporidia, a protozoal parasite. (*See* **pathogen**; **protozoa**; **wasting syndrome**.)

mitochondria: Organelles (particles of a living substance) within the **cytoplasm** of the cells, mitochondria have their own independent **DNA**, and serve as a source of energy for the cell.

MN: A strain of HIV used in **vaccine** development.

molecule: The smallest particle of a compound that has all the chemical properties of that compound. Molecules are made up of two or more atoms, either of the same element or of two or more different elements. Ionic compounds, such as common salt, are made up not of molecules, but of ions arranged in a crystalline structure. Unlike ions, molecules carry no electrical charge. Molecules differ in size and molecular weight as well as in structure.

molluscum contagiosum: A disease of the skin and **mucous membranes** caused by a poxvirus (molluscum contagiosum virus, MCV) infection. It is characterized by small dome-shaped papules (bumps) on the face, upper trunk, or extremities. The disease most frequently occurs in children and adults with impaired **immune response**. It is transmitted from person to person by direct contact. It is also autoinocuable (i.e., a secondary infection produced by contact with a

lesion on one's own body). In persons living with HIV, molluscum contagiosum is often a progressive disease, resistant to treatment. When **CD4+** cells fall below 200, the lesions tend to proliferate and spread.

monoclonal antibodies: Antibodies produced in the laboratory by a **hybridoma** or antibody-producing cell source for a specific **antigen**. Monoclonal antibodies are useful as tools for identifying specific protein molecules.

monocyte: A large white blood cell that ingests microbes or other cells and foreign particles. When a monocyte enters tissues, it develops into a **macrophage**.

mononeuritis multiplex (MM): A rare type of **neuropathy** that has been described with HIV infection. It may fall into two different settings. One type occurs during the early period of the infection and has a more benign outcome. The second form occurs later and is more aggressive, leading to progressive paralysis and death in some patients. It has been suggested that MM is related to multifocal **cytomegalovirus (CMV)** infection.

monovalent vaccine: A vaccine that is specific for only one **antigen**.

MRI: *See* **magnetic resonance imaging**.

mucocutaneous: Anything that concerns or pertains to **mucous membranes** and the skin (e.g., mouth, eyes, vagina, lips, or anal area).

mucosa: *See* **mucous membrane**.

mucosal immunity: Resistance to infection across the **mucous membranes**. Dependent on immune cells and **antibodies** present in the lining of the urogenital tract, **gastrointestinal** tract, and other parts of the body exposed to the outside world.

mucous membrane: Moist layer of tissue lining the digestive, respiratory, urinary, and reproductive tracts—all the body cavities with openings to the outside world except the ears.

multiple drug resistant tuberculosis (MDR-TB): A strain of **tuberculosis (TB)** that does not respond to two or more standard anti-TB drugs. MDR-TB usually occurs when treatment is interrupted, thus allowing organisms, in which mutations for drug resistance have occurred, to proliferate.

mutation: In biology, a sudden change in a **gene** or unit of hereditary material that results in a new inheritable characteristic. In higher animals and many higher plants, a mutation may be transmitted to future generations only if it occurs in germ—or sex cell—tissue; body cell mutations cannot be inherited. Changes within the chemical structure of single genes may be induced by exposure to radiation, temperature extremes, and certain chemicals. The term mutation may also be used to include losses or rearrangements of segments of chromosomes, the long strands of genes. Mutation, which can establish new traits in a population, is important in evolution. As related to HIV: During the course of HIV disease, HIV strains may emerge in an infected individual that differ widely in their ability to infect and kill different cell types, as well as in their rate of replication. Of course, HIV does not mutate into another type of virus.

myalgia: Diffuse muscle pain, usually accompanied by **malaise** (vague feeling of discomfort or weakness).

mycobacterium: Any **bacterium** of the genus *Mycobacterium* or a closely related genus.

mycobacterium avium complex (MAC): 1. A common **opportunistic infection** caused by two very similar mycobacterial organisms, *Mycobacterium avium* and *Mycobacterium intracellulare* (MAI), found in soil and dust particles. 2. A bacterial infection that can be localized (limited to a specific organ or area of the body) or disseminated throughout the body. It is a life-threatening disease, although new therapies offer promise for both prevention and treatment. MAC disease is extremely rare in persons who are not infected with HIV.

mycoplasma: 1. Smallest free-living organisms known to infect humans. Mycoplasma cause a variety of illnesses, especially of the lungs and sexual organs. 2. Any microorganism of the genus *Mycoplasma*, also called pleuropneumonia-like organism.

mycosis: Any disease caused by a **fungus**.

myelin: A substance that sheathes nerve cells, acting as an electric insulator that facilitates the conduction of nerve impulses. (*See also* **chronic idiopathic demyelinating polyneuropathy**.)

myelopathy: Any disease of the spinal cord.

myelosuppression: Suppression of bone marrow activity, causing decreased production of red blood cells (**anemia**), white blood cells (**leukopenia**), or **platelets** (**thrombocytopenia**). Myelosuppression is an effect of some drugs, such as **AZT**.

myelotoxic: Destructive to bone marrow.

myocardial: Refers to the heart's muscle mass.

myopathy: Progressive muscle weakness. Myopathy may arise as a toxic reaction to **AZT** or as a consequence of the HIV infection itself.

N

National AIDS Clearinghouse: *See* **CDC National AIDS Clearinghouse**.

National AIDS Hotline: *See* **CDC National AIDS Hotline**.

National Cancer Institute (NCI): An institute of the **National Institutes of Health (NIH)** with the overall mission of conducting and supporting research, training, and disseminating health information with respect to the causes, diagnosis, and treatment of cancer. NCI also performs these functions for HIV-related cancers.

National Institute of Allergy and Infectious Diseases (NIAID): An **NIH** institute that conducts and supports research to study the causes of allergic, immunologic, and infectious diseases, and to develop better means of preventing, diagnosing, and treating illnesses. NIAID is responsible for the federally funded, national basic research program in AIDS. It supports basic research, **epidemiology**, and natural history studies; blood screening tests; drug discovery and development; **vaccine** development and testing; and treatment studies, some directly and some through contracts and cooperative agreements with other institutions. It administers the Adult and Pediatric **AIDS Clinical Trial Group (ACTG)** network of testing units at hospitals around the country and the **Community Programs for Clinical Research on AIDS (CPCRA)**, a community-based network of AIDS treatment research centers.

National Institute of Child Health and Human Development (NICHD): An **NIH** institute that conducts and supports research on the reproductive, developmental, and behavioral processes that determine the health of children, adults, families, and populations. Thus, NICHD supports clinical research related to the transmission of HIV from infected mothers to their offspring, the progression of disease in HIV-infected infants and children, and the testing of potential therapies and preventatives for this population.

National Institutes of Health (NIH): A multi-institute agency of the **Department of Health and Human Services,** NIH is the federal focal point for health research. It conducts research in its own laboratories and supports research in universities, medical schools, hospitals, and research institutions throughout this country and abroad.

National Library of Medicine (NLM): An **NIH** institute, NLM is one of three U.S. national libraries. It is the world's largest research library in a single scientific and professional field (i.e., medicine). In the HIV/AIDS area, NLM provides electronic and print information services including the online services **AIDSLINE, AIDSTRIALS,** and **AIDSDRUGS.**

natural history study: Study of the natural development of something (such as an organism or a disease) over a period of time.

natural killer cells (NK cells): A type of **lymphocyte.** Like **cytotoxic T cells,** NK cells attack and kill tumor cells and protect against a wide variety of infectious microbes. They are "natural" killers because they do not need additional stimulation or need to recognize a specific **antigen** in order to attack and kill. Persons with **immunodeficiencies** such as those caused by HIV infection have a decrease in "natural" killer cell activity. (*See also* **B Lymphocytes; T Cells; Null Cell.**)

NCI: *See* **National Cancer Institute.**

NDA: *See* **new drug application.**

nebulized: *See* **aerosolized.**

necrolysis: Shedding of surface components of tissue, such as cells from internal body surfaces, due to death of a portion of tissue.

nef: One of the regulatory **genes** of HIV. Three HIV regulatory genes—*tat, rev,* and *nef*—and three so-called auxiliary genes—*vif, vpr,* and *vpu*—contain information necessary for the production of proteins that control the virus' ability to infect a cell, produce new copies of itself, or cause disease. (*See* **rev; tat.**)

neonatal: Concerning the first 4 weeks of life after birth.

neoplasm: An abnormal and uncontrolled growth of tissue; a tumor.

nephrotoxic: Poisonous to the kidneys.

neuralgia: A sharp, shooting pain along a nerve pathway.

neurological complications of AIDS: *See* **central nervous system (CNS) damage**.

neuropathy: The name given to a group of disorders involving nerves. Symptoms range from a tingling sensation or numbness in the toes and fingers to paralysis. It is estimated that 35 percent of persons with HIV disease have some form of neuropathy. (*See* **peripheral neuropathy**.)

neutralization: The process by which an **antibody** binds to specific **antigens**, thereby "neutralizing" the microorganism.

neutralizing antibody: An **antibody** that keeps a **virus** from infecting a cell, usually by blocking **receptors** on the cell or the virus.

neutralizing domain: The section of the HIV **envelope** protein, **gp120**, that elicits **antibodies** with neutralizing activities.

neutropenia: An abnormal decrease in the number of **neutrophils** (the most common type of white blood cells) in the blood. The decrease may be relative or absolute. Neutropenia may also be associated with HIV infection or may be drug induced.

neutrophil: Also called polymorphonuclear neutrophil (PMN) leukocyte. A white blood cell that plays a central role in defense of a **host** against infection. Neutrophils engulf and kill foreign microorganisms.

nevirapine: The first **non-nucleoside reverse transcriptase inhibitor (NNRTI)** to be approved by the **FDA** (6/24/96). It is used in combination with **nucleoside analogs** for the treatment of HIV-infected adults experiencing clinical and/or immunologic deterioration. Also known as Viramune.

new drug application (NDA): An application submitted by the manufacturer of a drug to the FDA—after clinical trials have been completed—for a license to market the drug for a specified indication.

NIAID: *See* **National Institute of Allergy and Infectious Diseases**.

NICHD: *See* **National Institute of Child Health and Human Development**.

night sweats: Extreme sweating during sleep. Although they can occur with other conditions, night sweats are also a symptom of HIV disease.

NIH: *See* **National Institutes of Health.**

NK cell: *See* **natural killer cells.**

NLM: *See* **National Library of Medicine.**

NNRTI: *See* **non-nucleoside reverse transcriptase inhibitors.**

non-Hodgkin's lymphoma (NHL): A **lymphoma** made up of **B cells** and characterized by nodular or diffuse tumors that may appear in the stomach, liver, brain, and bone marrow of persons with HIV. After **Kaposi's sarcoma**, NHL is the most common opportunistic cancer in persons with AIDS.

non-nucleoside reverse transcriptase inhibitors (NNRTIs): A new, third class of anti-HIV drugs, including **delavirdine**, loviride, and **nevirapine**, that act to directly combine with and block the action of HIV's **reverse transcriptase** enzyme. In contrast, **nucleoside analogs** block reverse transcriptase by capping the unfinished **DNA** chain that the enzyme is constructing.

Norvir: *See* **ritonavir.**

NSAID: Nonsteroidal anti-inflammatory (reduces inflammation) drug.

nucleic acid: Organic substance, found in all living cells, in which the hereditary information is stored and from which it can be transferred. Nucleic acid molecules are long chains that generally occur in combination with **proteins.** The two chief types are **DNA (deoxyribonucleic acid)**, found mainly in cell nuclei, and **RNA (ribonucleic acid)**, found mostly in **cytoplasm.** (*See also* **gene**; **genetic engineering**; **mutation.**)

nucleoli: Bodies in the nucleus that become enlarged during protein synthesis and contain the **DNA** template for ribosomal RNA. (*See* **ribonucleic acid**; **ribosome.**)

nucleoside: A building block of **DNA** or **RNA**, the genetic material found in living organisms. (*See* **nucleic acid.**)

nucleoside analog: A type of synthetic antiviral drug, such as **AZT**, **ddI, ddC, d4T**, or **3TC**, whose makeup constitutes a defective version of a natural **nucleoside**. Nucleoside analogs may take the place of the natural nucleosides, blocking the completion of a viral DNA chain during infection of a new cell by HIV. The HIV enzyme **reverse transcriptase** is more likely to incorporate the nucleoside analogs into the DNA it is constructing than is the DNA polymerase normally used for DNA creation in cell nuclei. (*See also* **nucleic acid**.)

nucleus: 1. The central controlling body within a living cell, usually a spherical unit enclosed in a membrane and containing genetic codes for maintaining the life systems of the organism and for issuing commands for growth and reproduction. 2. The nucleus of a cell is essential to such cell functions as reproduction and protein synthesis. It is composed of nuclear sap and a nucleoprotein-rich network from which chromosomes and **nucleoli** arise, and is enclosed in a definite membrane.

nucleotide: Nucleic acid chains are composed of subunits called nucleotides. **Nucleosides** are related to nucleotides, the subunits of nucleic acids; however, nucleosides do not carry the phosphate groups of the nucleotides.

nucleotide analogs: Chemically related to **nucleoside analogs**, nucleotide analogs are beginning to draw attention as agents that could fight AIDS-related infections as well as HIV. Cidofovir (also known as HPMPC), the first of this new class of antiviral drugs, is under investigation for the treatment of **cytomegalovirus retinitis**. (*See* **nucleotide**.)

null cell: A **lymphocyte** that develops in the bone marrow and lacks the characteristic surface markers of the B and T lymphocytes. Null cells represent a small proportion of the lymphocyte population. Stimulated by the presence of **antibody**, null cells can attack certain cellular targets directly and are known as "natural killer" or **NK cells**.

O

ocular: Pertaining to the eye.

Office of AIDS Research (OAR): An office within the **National Institutes of Health (NIH)** that coordinates AIDS research in all of the participating NIH institutes.

off-label use: Use of a drug for a disease or condition other than the specific disease or condition for which the **FDA** approved it.

oncology: Study of cancers or other tumors.

open-label trial: A **clinical trial** in which doctors and participants know which drug or vaccine is being administered.

opportunistic infections: Illnesses caused by various organisms, some of which usually do not cause disease in persons with normal immune systems. Persons living with advanced HIV infection suffer opportunistic infections of the lungs, brain, eyes, and other organs. Opportunistic infections common in persons diagnosed with AIDS include ***Pneumocystis carinii* pneumonia (PCP)**; **Kaposi's sarcoma**; **cryptosporidiosis**; **histoplasmosis**; other parasitic, viral, and fungal infections; and some types of cancers.

oral hairy leukoplakia (OHL): A whitish **lesion** that appears on the side of the tongue and inside cheeks. The lesion appears raised, with a ribbed or "hairy" surface. OHL occurs mainly in persons with declining immunity and may be caused by **Epstein-Barr virus** infection. OHL was not observed before the HIV epidemic.

organelle: Any one of various particles of living substance bound within most cells, such as the **mitochondria**, the Golgi complex, the endoplastic reticulum, the lysosomes, and the centrioles.

oropharyngeal: Relating to that division of the pharynx between the soft palate and the epiglottis. Pharynx is a tube that connects the mouth and nasal passages with the esophagus, the connection to the stomach. Epiglottis is a thin, valvelike structure that covers the glottis, the opening of the upper part of the larynx (the part of the throat containing the vocal cords), during swallowing.

orphan drugs: An **FDA** category that refers to medications used to treat diseases and conditions that occur rarely. Therefore, there is little financial incentive for the pharmaceutical industry to develop such medications. Orphan drug status gives a manufacturer specific financial incentives to develop and provide such medications.

P

p24: A bullet-shaped core made of another protein that surrounds the viral **RNA** within the **envelope** of HIV. The p24 antigen test looks for the presence of this protein in a patient's blood. A positive result for the p24 antigen suggests active HIV replication. P24 found in the peripheral blood is also thought to correlate with the amount of virus in the peripheral blood. Measurement of p24 levels in the blood have been used to monitor viral activity, although this is not considered a very accurate method due to the existence of the p24 antibody that binds with the antigen and makes it undetectable. (*See* **branched DNA assay**.)

package insert: A document, approved by the **FDA** and furnished by the manufacturer of a drug, for use when dispensing the drug (i.e., inserted into the package). The document indicates approved uses, contraindications, and potential side effects.

palliative: A treatment that provides symptomatic relief but not a cure.

palliative care: Palliative care is an approach to life-threatening chronic illnesses, especially at the end of life. Palliative care combines active and compassionate therapies to comfort and support patients and their families who are living with life-ending illness. Palliative care strives to meet physical needs through pain relief and maintaining quality of life while emphasizing the patient's and family's rights to participate in informed discussion and to make choices. This patient- and family-centered approach uses the skills of interdisciplinary team members to provide a comprehensive continuum of care including spiritual and emotional needs.

pancreas: A gland situated near the stomach that secretes a digestive fluid into the intestine through one or more ducts and also secretes the hormone insulin.

pancreatitis: Inflammation of the **pancreas** that can produce severe pain and debilitating illness. An occasional side effect of treatment with **ddI**, can result in severe abdominal pain and death. Its onset can be predicted by rises in blood levels of the pancreatic enzyme, amylase.

pancytopenia: Deficiency of all cell elements of the blood.

pandemic: A disease prevalent throughout an entire country, continent, or the whole world. (*See also* **epidemic**.)

Pap smear: A method for the early detection of cancer and other abnormalities of the female genital tract, especially of the **cervix**, employing scraped as well as exfoliated cells (cells that have been shed into the vaginal fluid) and a special staining technique for microscopic examination that differentiates diseased tissue. Also known as Papanicolaou Smear after George Papanicolaou, the American cytologist who developed this method.

papilloma: 1. A benign tumor (as a wart or **condyloma**) resulting from an overgrowth of epithelial tissue on papillae of vascularized connective tissue (as of the skin). 2. An epithelial tumor caused by a virus. (*See also* **epithelium**).

parallel track: A system of distributing experimental drugs to patients who are unable to participate in ongoing clinical efficacy trials and have no other treatment options. (*See* **clinical trial**.)

parasite: A plant or animal that lives and feeds on or within another living organism (**host**), causing some degree of harm to the host organism.

parenchyma: The tissue of an organ (as distinguished from supporting or connective tissue).

parenteral: Not in or through the digestive system. For example, parenteral can pertain to blood being drawn from a vein in the arm or introduced into that vein via a transfusion (intravenous), or to injection of medications or vaccines through the skin (subcutaneous) or into the muscle (intramuscular).

paresthesia: Abnormal sensations such as burning, tingling, or a "pins-and-needles" feeling. Paresthesia may constitute the first group of symptoms of **peripheral neuropathy**, or it may be a limited drug side effect that does not worsen with time. Circumoral paresthesia affects the area around the mouth.

passive immunotherapy: Process in which individuals with advanced disease (who have low levels of HIV antibody production) are infused with plasma rich in HIV **antibodies** or an **immunoglobulin** concentrate (HIVIG) from such plasma. The plasma is obtained from asymptomatic HIV-positive individuals with high levels of HIV antibodies.

pathogen: Any disease-producing microorganism or material.

pathogenesis: The origin and development of a disease.

PBMC: *See* **peripheral blood mononuclear cell**.

PCP: *See* ***Pneumocystis carinii* pneumonia (PCP)**.

PCR: *See* **polymerase chain reaction**.

567

pelvic inflammatory disease (PID): Gynecological condition caused by an infection (usually sexually transmitted) that spreads from the vagina to the upper parts of a women's reproductive tract in the pelvic cavity. PID takes different courses in different women, but can cause abscesses and constant pain almost anywhere in the genital tract. If left untreated, it can cause infertility or more frequent periods. Severe cases may even spread to the liver and kidneys causing dangerous internal bleeding and death.

pentamidine: An approved antiprotozoal drug used for the treatment and prevention of ***Pneumocystis carinii* pneumonia (PCP)** infection. It can be delivered intravenously or intramuscularly or inhaled as an aerosol. Aerosolized pentamidine is approved for the **prophylaxis** of PCP in persons living with HIV with **CD4+** counts below 200 per cubic millimeter, or for those with prior episodes of PCP. Intravenous (IV) and intramuscular (IM) pentamidine are used for acute PCP. The drug is also known under the name Pentam 300 (IV and IM form) and NebuPent (aerosolized form). (*See also* **TMP/SMX.**)

peptide (also polypeptide): Biochemical formed by the linkage of up to about 50 **amino acids** to form a chain. Longer chains are called **proteins**. The amino acids are coupled by a peptide bond, a special linkage in which the nitrogen atom of one amino acid binds to the carboxyl carbon atom of another. Many peptides, such as the hormones vasopressin and ACTH, have physiological or antibacterial activity.

perianal: Around the anus.

perinatal: Events that occur at or around the time of birth.

perinatal transmission: Transmission of a pathogen, such as HIV, from mother to baby before, during, or after the birth process. Ninety percent of children reported with AIDS acquired HIV infection from their HIV-infected mothers.

peripheral blood mononuclear cell (PBMC): Cells in the bloodstream with one **nucleus**. Generally refers to **lymphocytes** and **macrophages**.

peripheral neuropathy: Condition characterized by sensory loss, pain, muscle weakness, and wasting of muscle in the hands or legs and feet. It may start with burning or tingling sensations or numbness in the toes and fingers. In severe cases, paralysis may result. Peripheral neuropathy may arise from an HIV-related condition or be the side effect of certain drugs, some of the **nucleoside analogs** in particular.

persistent generalized lymphadenopathy (PGL): Chronic, diffuse, noncancerous **lymph node** enlargement. Typically it has been found in persons with persistent bacterial, viral, or fungal infections. PGL in HIV infection is a condition in which lymph nodes are chronically swollen in at least two areas of the body for 3 months or more with no obvious cause other than the HIV infection.

PGL: *See* **persistent generalized lymphadenopathy**.

PHA (phytohemagglutinin): A plant chemical used to stimulate the multiplication (proliferation) of **T lymphocytes** in laboratory tests.

phagocyte: A cell that is able to ingest and destroy foreign matter, including bacteria.

phagocytosis: The process of ingesting and destroying a virus or other foreign matter by phagocytes. (*See* **macrophage**; **monocyte**.)

pharmacokinetics: The processes (in a living organism) of absorption, distribution, metabolism, and excretion of a drug or vaccine.

Phase I Trials: Involves the initial introduction of an investigational new drug into humans. Phase I trials are closely monitored and may be conducted in patients or healthy volunteers. The studies are designed to determine the metabolism and pharmacologic actions of the drug in humans, safety, side effects associated with increasing doses, and if possible, early evidence of effectiveness. The trials also can include studies of structure-activity relationships, mechanisms of action in humans, use of the investigational drug as research tools to explore biological phenomena, or disease processes. The total number of patients included in Phase I studies varies but is generally in the range of 20 to 80. Sufficient information should be obtained in the trial to permit design of well-controlled, scientifically valid Phase II studies. (*See* **clinical trials**.)

Phase II Trials: Includes controlled clinical studies of effectiveness of the drug for a particular indication or indications in patients with the disease or condition under study, and determination of common, short-term side effects and risks associated with the drug. Phase II studies are typically well controlled, closely monitored, and usually involve no more than several hundred patients. (*See* **clinical trials**.)

Phase III Trials: Expanded controlled and uncontrolled studies. They are performed after preliminary evidence of drug effectiveness has been obtained. They are intended to gather additional information about effectiveness and safety that is needed to evaluate the overall benefit-risk relationship of the drug and to provide adequate basis for physician labeling. These studies usually include anywhere from several hundred to several thousand subjects. (*See* **clinical trials.**)

Phase IV Trials: Postmarketing studies, carried out after licensure of the drug. Generally, a Phase IV trial is a randomized, controlled trial that is designed to evaluate the long-term safety and efficacy of a drug for a given indication. Phase IV trials are important in evaluating AIDS drugs because many drugs for HIV infection have been given accelerated approval with small amounts of clinical data about the drugs' effectiveness. (*See* **clinical trials.**)

photosensitivity: Heightened skin response to sunlight or ultraviolet light (rapid burning when exposed to the sun).

PHS: *See Public Health Service.*

pituitary gland: Small, oval endocrine gland that lies at the base of the brain. It is called the master gland because the other endocrine glands depend on its secretions for stimulation. The pituitary has two distinct lobes, anterior and posterior. The anterior lobe secretes at least six **hormones**: human growth hormone, which stimulates overall body growth; ACTH (adrenocorticotropic hormone), which controls steroid hormone secretion by the adrenal cortex; thyrotropic hormone, which stimulates the activity of the thyroid gland; and three gonadotropic hormones, which control growth and reproductive activity of the gonads (ovaries and testes). The posterior lobe secretes an antidiuretic hormone, which causes water retention by the kidneys, and oxytocin, which stimulates the mammary glands to release milk and also causes uterine contractions. An overactive pituitary during childhood can cause gigantism. Dwarfism results from pituitary deficiency in childhood.

placebo: An inactive substance (may look like the real medication) against which investigational treatments are compared for efficacy and safety. (*See* **placebo controlled study.**)

placebo controlled study: A method of investigation of drugs in which an inactive substance (the **placebo**) is given to one group of patients, while the drug being tested is given to another group. The results obtained in the two groups are then compared to see if the investigational treatment is more effective in treating the condition.

placebo effect: A physical or emotional change, occurring after a substance is taken or administered, that is not the result of any special property of the substance. The change may be beneficial, reflecting the expectations of the patient and, often, the expectations of the person giving the substance.

plasma: That 10 percent of the blood that contains nutrients, electrolytes (dissolved salts), gases, albumin, clotting factors, wastes, and hormones.

plasma cells: Large antibody-producing cells that develop from B cells. (*See* **antibodies**; **B lymphocytes**.)

plasmapheresis: The selective removal of certain **proteins** or **antibodies** from the blood (followed by reinjection of the blood). This process is sometimes used in the treatment of some **peripheral neuropathies** and is an integral part of passive **immunotherapies** for HIV.

plasmid: an extrachromosomal ring of **DNA**, especially of bacterial origin, that replicates autonomously.

platelets: Active agents of inflammation when damage occurs to a blood vessel. They are not actually cells, but fragments released by megakaryocyte cells. Megakaryocyte is a large cell in the bone marrow whose function it is to produce platelets. When vascular damage (i.e., damage to blood vessels) occurs, the platelets stick to the vascular walls, forming clots to prevent the loss of blood. Thus, it is important to have adequate numbers of normally functioning platelets to maintain effective coagulation (clotting) of the blood. There are drugs that can potentially alter the platelet count, making it necessary to monitor the count. Also, some persons living with HIV develop **thrombocytopenia**—a condition characterized by a platelet count of less than 100,000 platelets per cubic millimeter of blood. The normal value for men is 154,000 to 354,000 platelets per cubic millimeter of blood. For women, it is 162,000 to 380,000 platelets per cubic millimeter of blood.

PML: *See* **progressive multifocal leukoencephalopathy**.

***Pneumocystis carinii* pneumonia (PCP):** An infection of the lungs caused by *Pneumocystis carinii*, which is thought to be a **protozoa**

but may be more closely related to a **fungus**. *P. carinii* grows rapidly in the lungs of persons with AIDS and is a frequent AIDS-related cause of death. *P. carinii* infection sometimes may occur elsewhere in the body (skin, eye, spleen, liver, or heart). The standard treatment for persons with PCP is either a combination of trimethoprim and sulfamethoxazole (**TMP/SMX**, also called Bactrim or Septra), **dapsone**, or **pentamidine**.

pol: A **gene** of HIV that codes for the enzymes **protease, reverse transcriptase**, and **integrase**.

polymerase: Any of several **enzymes** that catalyze the formation of **DNA** or **RNA** from precursor substances in the presence of preexisting DNA or RNA acting as templates (i.e., patterns).

polymerase chain reaction (PCR): 1. A laboratory process that selects a **DNA** segment from a mixture of DNA chains and rapidly replicates it; used to create a large, readily analyzed sample of a piece of DNA. It is used in DNA fingerprinting and in medical tests to identify diseases from the infectious agent's DNA. See DNA. 2. As related to HIV—also called RT-PCR—a sensitive laboratory technique that can detect and quantify HIV in a person's blood or **lymph nodes**. PCR works by repeatedly copying genetic material using heat cycling and enzymes similar to those used by cells. It is an **FDA**-approved test to measure **viral load**.

polyneuritis: Inflammation of many nerves at once.

polypeptide: *See* **peptide**.

polyvalent vaccine: A vaccine that is active against multiple viral strains.

PPD test: *See* **purified protein derivative**.

preclinical: Refers to the testing of experimental drug in the test tube or in animals—the testing that occurs before trials in humans may be carried out.

precursor cells: Cells from which natural processes form other cells.

prevalence: A measure of the proportion of people in a population affected with a particular disease at a given time.

preventive HIV vaccine: A vaccine designed to prevent HIV infection.

primary HIV infection: *See* **acute HIV infection**.

prime-boost: In HIV vaccine research, administration of one type of vaccine, such as a **live-vector vaccine**, followed by or together with a second type of vaccine, such as a **recombinant** subunit vaccine. The intent of this combination regimen is to induce different types of **immune responses** and enhance the overall immune response, a result that may not occur if only one type of vaccine were to be given for all doses.

priming: Giving one **vaccine** dose(s) first to induce certain **immune responses**, followed by or together with a second type of vaccine. The intent of priming is to induce certain immune responses that will be enhanced by the booster dose(s).

proctitis: Inflammation of the rectum.

prodrome: A symptom that indicates the onset of a disease.

progenitor: Parent or ancestor.

progressive multifocal leukoencephalopathy (PML): A rapidly debilitating **opportunistic infection** caused by the **JC virus** that infects brain tissue and causes damage to the brain and the spinal cord. Symptoms vary from patient to patient but include loss of muscle control, paralysis, blindness, problems with speech, and an altered mental state. PML can lead to coma and death. There are no standard treatments for this disease.

prophylaxis: Treatment to prevent the onset of a particular disease ("primary" prophylaxis), or the recurrence of symptoms in an existing infection that has been brought under control ("secondary" prophylaxis, maintenance therapy).

protease: An **enzyme** that breaks down **proteins** into their component **peptides**. HIV's protease enzyme breaks apart long strands of viral protein into the separate proteins making up the **viral core**. The enzyme acts as new virus particles are budding off a cell membrane. Protease is the first HIV protein whose three-dimensional structure has been characterized.

protease inhibitors: HIV protease is an enzyme essential to the replicative life cycle of HIV. The three-dimensional molecular structure of the HIV protease has been fully determined. Pharmaceutical developers therefore are able to rationally design drugs to inhibit the enzyme and thus interfere with replication of the virus. These drugs act by preventing cleavage of HIV viral polyproteins into active proteins;

this occurs during the process by which HIV normally replicates. The drugs bind to the enzyme's active site, blocking cleavage of the polyprotein. The FDA has approved the following protease inhibitors as drugs to treat HIV disease: **saquinavir** (Invirase™), **indinavir** (Crixivan™), and **ritonavir** (Norvir™).

proteins: Highly complex organic compounds found in all living cells. Protein is the most abundant class of all biological molecules, comprising about 50 percent of cellular dry weight. Structurally, proteins are large molecules composed of one or more chains of varying amounts of the same 22 **amino acids** that are linked by **peptide** bonds. Each protein is characterized by a unique and invariant amino acid sequence. The information for the synthesis of the specific amino acid sequence in a protein, from free amino acids, is carried by the cell's **nucleic acid.**

protocol: The detailed plan for conducting a **clinical trial.** It states the trial's rationale, purpose, drug or vaccine dosages, length of study, routes of administration, who may participate, and other aspects of trial design. (*See also* **inclusion/exclusion criteria.**)

protozoa: Large group of one-celled (unicellular) animals, including amoebas. Some protozoa cause parasitic diseases in persons with AIDS, notably **toxoplasmosis** and **cryptosporidiosis.** (*See also Pneumocystis carinii* **pneumonia.**)

provirus: Viral genetic material, in the form of **DNA** that has been integrated into the **host genome.** HIV, when it is dormant in human cells, is in a proviral form.

pruritis: Itching.

pseudovirion: A virus-like particle.

pulmonary: Pertaining to the lungs.

purified protein derivative (PPD): Material used in the **tuberculin skin test (TST)**; the most common test for exposure to *Mycobacterium tuberculosis,* the **bacterium** that causes **tuberculosis (TB).** PPD is sometimes used synonymously with TST. In the PPD test, a small amount of protein from TB is injected under the skin. If patients have been previously infected, they will mount a delayed-type hypersensitivity reaction, characterized by a hard red bump called an induration.

R

radiology: The science of diagnosis and/or treatment using radiant energy. Includes x-rays, **CT scan**, and destruction of tumors by radiation.

randomized trial: A study in which participants are randomly (i.e., by chance) assigned to one of two or more treatment **arms** or regimen of a **clinical trial**. Occasionally **placebos** are utilized. Randomization minimizes the differences among groups by equally distributing people with particular characteristics among all the trial arms.

reactogenicity: The capacity to produce adverse reactions.

reagent: any chemical used in a laboratory test or experiment.

receptor: A molecule on the surface of a cell that serves as a recognition or binding site for **antigens**, **antibodies**, or other cellular or immunological components.

recombinant: An organism whose **genome** contains integrated genetic material from a different organism. Also used in relation to compounds produced by laboratory or industrial cultures of genetically engineered living cells. The cells' genes have been altered to give the capability of producing large quantities of the desired compound for use as a medical treatment. Recombinant compounds often are altered versions of naturally occurring substances.

recombinant DNA: *See* **biotechnology**; **genetic engineering**.

regulatory genes: As related to HIV: Three regulatory HIV genes — *tat*, *rev*, and *nef* — and three so-called auxiliary genes — *vif, vpr*, and *vpu* — contain information for the production of proteins that regulate the virus's ability to infect a cell, produce new copies of the virus, or cause disease.

regulatory T cells: T cells that direct other immune cells to perform special functions. The chief regulatory cell, the **CD4+ T cell** or T helper cell, is HIV's chief target.

remissions: The lessening of the severity or duration of outbreaks of a disease, or the abatement (diminution in degree or intensity) of symptoms altogether over a period of time.

renal: Pertaining to the kidneys.

resistance: Reduction in a pathogen's sensitivity to a particular drug. Resistance is thought to result usually from a genetic **mutation**. In HIV, such mutations can change the structure of viral **enzymes** and **proteins** so that an antiviral drug can no longer bind with them as well as it used to. Resistance detected by searching a pathogen's genetic makeup for mutations thought to confer lower susceptibility is called "genotypic resistance." Resistance found by successfully growing laboratory cultures of the **pathogen** in the presence of a drug is called "phenotype resistance."

reticuloendothelial cells: A system of **interstitial** cells that includes all the phagocytic cells, which trap and consume foreign agents, except the **leukocytes** circulating in the bloodstream. This system forms a network throughout the body and is another of the body's defense systems against invading organisms in the connective tissues of the body. (*See* **phagocyte**.)

retina: Light-sensitive tissue at the back of the eye that transmits visual impulses via the optic nerve to the brain. (*See* **retinitis**.)

retinal detachment: Condition in which a portion of the **retina** becomes separated from the inner wall of the eye. In AIDS patients, it can result from retinal disease such as **CMV retinitis**. The condition can rapidly lead to vision loss but is treatable by adding silicone to the eye's vitreous humor to increase the pressure on the retina.

retinitis: Inflammation of the **retina**, linked in AIDS to **cytomegalovirus (CMV)** infection. Untreated, it can lead to blindness.

Retrovir: *See* **AZT**.

retrovirus: A type of virus that, when not infecting a cell, stores its genetic information on a single-stranded **RNA** molecule instead of the more usual double-stranded **DNA**. HIV is an example of a retrovirus. After a retrovirus penetrates a cell, it constructs a DNA version of its genes using a special enzyme called **reverse transcriptase**. This DNA then becomes part of the cell's genetic material.

rev: One of the regulatory genes of HIV. Three HIV regulatory genes— *stat*, *rev*, and *nef*—and three so-called auxiliary genes—*vif*, *vpr*, and *vpu*—contain information necessary for the production of proteins that control the virus's ability to infect a cell, produce new copies of the virus, or cause disease.

reverse transcriptase: This **enzyme** of HIV—and other **retroviruses**—converts the single-stranded viral **RNA** into **DNA**, the form in which the cell carries its genes. Some antiviral drugs approved by the FDA for the treatment of HIV infection (e.g., **AZT, ddC, ddI, 3TC,** and **D4T**) work by interfering with this stage of the viral life cycle. They are also referred to as reverse transcriptase inhibitors (RTIs).

ribonucleic acid (RNA): 1. A **nucleic acid,** found mostly in the **cytoplasm**—rather than the nucleus—of cells, that is important in the synthesis of **proteins.** The amount of RNA varies from cell to cell. RNA, like the structurally similar **DNA,** is a chain made up of subunits called **nucleotides.** In protein synthesis, **messenger RNA (mRNA)** replicates the DNA code for a protein and moves to sites in the cell called **ribosomes.** There, transfer RNA (tRNA) assembles amino acids to form the protein specified by the messenger RNA. Most forms of RNA (including messenger and transfer RNA) consist of a single nucleotide strand, but a few forms of viral RNA that function as carriers of genetic information (instead of DNA) are double-stranded. Some viruses, such as HIV, carry RNA instead of the more usual genetic material DNA. (*See also* **retrovirus.**)

ribosome: A cytoplasmic **organelle,** composed of **ribonucleic acid** and **protein,** that functions in the synthesis of protein. Ribosomes interact with **messenger RNA (mRNA)** and transfer RNA to join together amino acid units into a polypeptide chain according to the sequence determined by the genetic code. (*See* **peptide.**)

ritonavir: A peptide-based **protease inhibitor** drug. **FDA** approved for use alone or in combination with **nucleoside analogs** for treatment of HIV infection. It has been reported that ritonavir can cause extreme nausea and can interact adversely with many drugs. Gradual dose escalation when initiating therapy may provide relief from some of the side effects. Also known as Norvir, ABT-538.

RNA: *See* **ribonucleic acid.**

RO 31-8959: *See* **saquinavir.**

route of administration: *See* **administration.**

RTI (reverse transcriptase inhibitors): *see* **reverse transcriptase.**

RT-PCR (reverse transcriptase polymerase chain reaction): An FDA-approved test to measure **viral load.** The test is also known as **polymerase chain reaction (PCR).**

Ryan White CARE Act: Through the Ryan White Comprehensive AIDS Resources Emergency (CARE) Act, health care and support services are provided for persons living with HIV/AIDS. **HRSA** administers this Act, which was reauthorized by the Congress in 1996 for 5 years. The metropolitan areas most affected by the HIV epidemic are awarded Title I grants to improve and expand health care. Title II grants to states and territories support essential health care and support services for persons living with HIV/AIDS, including health insurance and **AIDS Drug Assistance Programs**. Title III(b) supports early intervention in clinical settings such as community and migrant health centers, health care for the homeless programs, and Native Hawaiian health programs. Title IV supports services for women, children, adolescents, and families affected by the HIV epidemic. Part F of the Act supports **Special Projects of National Significance (SPNS)** and **AIDS Education and Training Centers (AETCs)**.

S

SAMHSA: *See* **Substance Abuse and Mental Health Services Administration**.

sarcoma: A malignant (cancerous) tumor of the skin and soft tissue.

saquinavir: A peptide-based, **protease inhibitor**. FDA-approved for combination use with **nucleoside analogs** for treatment of advanced HIV infection in selected patients. Also known as Invirase. Saquinavir has been shown to have less bioavailability than the other approved protease inhibitors.

seborrheic dermatitis: A chronic inflammatory disease of the skin of unknown cause or origin, characterized by moderate **erythema**; dry, moist, or greasy scaling; and yellow crusted patches on various areas, including the mid-parts of the face, ears, supraorbital regions (above the orbit of the eye), umbilicus (the navel), genitalia, and especially the scalp. Seborrheic dermatitis in patients infected with HIV responds to a variety of therapies but tends to reoccur. Topic antifungal agents and corticosteroids suppress the process, but therapy must be applied repeatedly.

sepsis: The presence of harmful microorganisms or associated toxins in the blood.

seroconversion: The development of **antibodies** to a particular **antigen**. When people develop antibodies to HIV, they "seroconvert" from antibody negative to antibody positive. It may take from as little as 1 week to several months or more after infection with HIV for antibodies to the virus to develop. After antibodies to HIV appear in the blood, a person should test positive on antibody tests. (*See* **incubation period**; **window period**.)

serologic test: Any of a number of tests that are performed on the clear portion of blood (**serum**). Often refers to a test that determines the presence of **antibodies** to **antigens** such as viruses.

seroprevalence: As related to HIV infection, the proportion of persons who have serologic (i.e., pertaining to **serum**) evidence of HIV infection at any given time.

serostatus: Results of a blood test for specific **antibodies**.

serum: The clear, thin, and sticky fluid portion of the blood that remains after coagulation (clotting). Serum contains no blood cells, platelets, or fibrinogen.

sexually transmitted disease (STD): Also called venereal disease or VD (an older public health term). Sexually transmitted diseases are infections spread by the transfer of organisms from person to person during sexual contact. In addition to the "traditional" STDs (syphilis and gonorrhea), the spectrum of STDs now includes HIV infection, which causes AIDS; *Chlamydia trachomatis* infections; **human papilloma virus (HPV)** infection; genital herpes; **chancroid;** genital **mycoplasmas**; **hepatitis** B; trichomoniasis; **enteric** infections; and ectoparasitic diseases (i.e., diseases caused by organisms that live on the outside of the host's body). The complexity and scope of STDs have increased dramatically since the 1980's; more than 20 organisms and syndromes are now recognized as belonging in this category.

SF-2: A strain of HIV used in **vaccine** development.

SGOT (serum glutamic oxaloacetic transaminase): Also known as AST (aspartate aminotransaminase), a liver enzyme that plays a role in **protein metabolism**, such as **SGPT**. Elevated **serum** levels of SGOT are a sign of liver damage from disease or drugs.

SGPT (serum glutamic pyruvate transaminase): Also known as ALT (alanine aminotransaminase), a liver enzyme that plays a role in **protein metabolism** like **SGOT**. Elevated **serum** levels of SGPT are a sign of liver damage from disease or drugs.

shingles: *See* **herpes varicella zoster virus.**

SHIV: Genetically engineered **hybrid** virus having an HIV **envelope** and an SIV core. (*See also* **genetic engineering**; **simian immunodeficiency virus (SIV)**.)

side effects: The actions or effects of a drug (or vaccine) other than those desired. The term usually refers to undesired or negative effects, such as headache, skin irritation, or liver damage. Experimental drugs must be evaluated for both immediate and long-term side effects.

simian immunodeficiency virus (SIV): An HIV-like virus that infects monkeys, chimpanzees, and other nonhuman primates.

sinusitis: Inflammation of the nasal cavity and sinuses.

SIV: *See* **simian immunodeficiency virus**.

Special Projects of National Significance (SPNS): The SPNS Program is the research and demonstration program of the **Ryan White CARE Act**. The program's mission is to advance knowledge and skills in health and support services for persons with HIV/AIDS. The authorizing legislation specifies three objectives for this program: (1) to assess the effectiveness of particular models of care, (2) to support innovative program design, and (3) to promote replication of effective models.

spinal tap: *See* **lumbar puncture**.

spleen: Large lymphatic organ in the upper left of the abdominal cavity with several functions: (1) trapping of foreign matter in the blood, (2) destruction of degraded red blood cells and foreign matter by **macrophages**, (3) formation of new **lymphocytes** and **antibody** production, and (4) storage of excess red blood cells.

splenomegaly: An enlarged spleen.

sputum analysis: Method of detecting certain infections (especially **tuberculosis**) by culturing of sputum—the mucus matter that collects in the respiratory and upper digestive passages and is expelled by coughing.

standards of care: Treatment regimen or medical management based on state-of-the-art patient care.

staphylococcus: Type of bacteria that may cause various types of infections.

statistical significance: In **vaccine** research, the probability that an event or difference occurred as the result of the intervention (vaccine) rather than by chance alone. This probability is determined by using statistical tests to evaluate collected data. Guidelines for defining significance are chosen before data collection begins.

stavudine: *See* **d4T**.

STD: *See* **sexually transmitted disease**.

stem cells: Cells from which all blood cells derive. Bone marrow is rich in stem cells. **Clones** of stem cells may become any one of the repertoires of immune cells depending upon what **cytokines** and **hormones** they are exposed to.

sterilizing immunity: An **immune response** that completely eliminates an infection.

steroid: Member of a large family of structurally similar **lipid** substances. Steroid molecules have a basic skeleton consisting of four interconnected carbon rings. Different classes of steroids have different functions. All the natural sex hormones are steroids. Anabolic steroids increase muscle mass. Antiinflammatory steroids (or corticosteroids) can reduce swelling, pain, and other manifestations of inflammation.

Stevens-Johnson syndrome: A severe and sometimes fatal form of **erythema multiforme** that is characterized by severe skin manifestations; conjunctivitis (eye inflammation), which often results in blindness; Vincent's angina (trench mouth); and ulceration of the genitals and anus.

stomatitis: Any of numerous inflammatory diseases of the mouth having various causes, such as mechanical trauma, irritants, allergy, vitamin deficiency, or infection.

strain: Subgroup of a species (also called taxon).

stratification: A layered configuration.

subarachnoid space: The space through which the spinal fluid circulates.

subclinical infection: An infection, or phase of infection, without readily apparent symptoms or signs of disease.

subcutaneous (SQ): Beneath the skin or introduced beneath the skin (e.g., subcutaneous injections).

Substance Abuse and Mental Health Services Administration (SAMHSA): An agency of the **Department of Health and Human Services**, with the mission to assure that quality substance abuse and mental health services are available to the people who need them, and to ensure that prevention and treatment knowledge is used more efficiently in the general health care system.

subtype (also called a clade): With respect to HIV **isolates**, a classification scheme based on genetic differences.

subunit HIV vaccine: A genetically engineered **vaccine** that is based on only part of the HIV molecule. (*See* **genetic engineering**.)

sulfa drug: A **sulfonamide** drug used to treat bacterial infections. These drugs inhibit the action of p-aminobenzoic acid, a substance bacteria needed in order to reproduce. Sulfa drugs are now used primarily in the treatment of urinary tract infections and ulcerative colitis. In the HIV area, the sulfa drug, sulfadiazine, is used in combination with pyrimethamine as standard therapy for **toxoplasmosis**. Trimethoprim is used in combination with another sulfa drug, sulfamethoxazole (**TMP/SMX), against PCP**.

sulfonamides: Synthetic derivatives of paminobenzenesulfonamide. (*See* **sulfa drug**.)

superantigen: Investigators have proposed that a molecule known as a superantigen, either made by HIV or an unrelated agent, may stimulate massive quantities of **CD4+ T cells** at once, rendering them highly susceptible to HIV infection and subsequent cell death. (*See* **antigen**.)

suppressor phenomenon: Process where **CD8+ cells** not only kill HIV-infected cells directly by a process called cytolysis, but also secrete soluble factors that suppress HIV replication in both blood and **lymph nodes**. It appears that CD8+ cells secrete signaling molecules, called beta-chemokines, which normally recruit inflammatory cells to the site of an infection. Three of these beta-chemokines, RANTES, MIP-1a, and MIP-1b, appear to block HIV replication by occupying receptors necessary for the entry of some strains of HIV into their target cells. (*See* **chemokines**.)

suppressor T cells (T8, CD8): Subset of **T cells** that halts **antibody** production and other **immune responses**.

surrogate marker: Laboratory tests that may predict a patient's clinical outcome or indicate whether a drug is effective without having to rely on the traditional clinical **endpoints** of death or development of a major **opportunistic infection**. Surrogate markers under study in HIV disease include **CD4** counts, CD4/CD8 cell ratios, **p24**

antigen, **beta-2 microglobulin**, heparin, neopterin, and assays of levels of HIV such as plasma **viremia**, quantitative **polymerase chain reaction**, or **viral load**.

surveillance: *See* **epidemiologic surveillance**.

susceptible: Vulnerable or predisposed to a disease.

symptoms: Any perceptible, subjective change in the body or its functions that indicates disease or phases of disease, as reported by the patient.

syncytia ("giant cells"): Dysfunctional multicellular clumps formed by cell-to-cell fusion. Cells infected with HIV may also fuse with nearby uninfected cells, forming balloonlike giant cells called syncytia. In test tube experiments, these giant cells have been associated with the death of uninfected cells. The presence of so-called syncytia-inducing variants of HIV has been correlated with rapid disease progression in HIV-infected individuals.

syndrome: A group of symptoms as reported by the patient and signs as detected in an examination that together are characteristic of a specific condition.

synergism, synergistic: An interaction between two or more treatments (e.g., drugs) that produces or enhances an effect that is greater than the sum of the effects produced by the individual treatments.

synthesis: 1. In chemistry, the formation of a compound from simpler compounds or elements. 2. The production of a substance (e.g., as in protein synthesis) by the union of chemical elements, groups, or simpler compounds, or by the degradation (i.e., breaking down) of a complex compound.

syphilis: A disease—primarily sexually transmitted—resulting from infection with the spirochete (a **bacterium**), *Treponema pallidum*. Syphilis can also be acquired in the uterus during pregnancy.

systemic: Concerning or affecting the body as a whole. A systemic therapy is one that the entire body is exposed to, rather than just the target tissues affected by a disease.

T

tat: One of the regulatory genes of HIV. Three HIV regulatory genes—*tat*, *rev*, and *nef*—and three so-called auxiliary genes—*vif*, *vpr*, and *vpu*—contain information necessary for the production of proteins that control the virus' ability to infect a cell, produce new copies of the virus, or cause disease. The tat gene is thought to enhance virus replication.

TB: *See* **tuberculosis**.

T cells (T lymphocytes): T cells are white blood cells, derived from the **thymus gland**, that participate in a variety of **cell-mediated immune reactions**. Three fundamentally different types of T cells are recognized: **helper, killer,** and **suppressor**. They are the immune system's "border police," responsible for finding infected or cancerous cells. The killer T cell receptors (TCR) bind to an infected cell's distress signal—a combination of one of the cell's own proteins and a tiny fragment of the invader's protein. The bits of foreign **protein** are made with the help of **enzymes** inside the invaded cell that chew up the **pathogens** into protein fragments (**peptides**), which are then scooped up by the **major histocompatibility complex (MHC)** and carted through the cell membrane.

T4 cell: *See* **CD4 (T4) or CD4+ cells**.

T8 cell: *See* **CD8 (T8 cells)**.

template: A gauge, pattern, or mold used as a guide to the form of the piece being made. In biology, a **molecule**—such as **DNA**—that serves as a pattern for the generation of another macromolecule (e.g., **messenger RNA**). (*See also* **ribonucleic acid**.)

teratogenicity: The production of physical defects in offspring *in utero* (i.e., causing birth defects). Teratogenicity is a potential side effect of some drugs, such as thalidomide.

Terry Beirn Community Programs for Clinical Research on AIDS: *See* **CPCRA**.

testosterone: Naturally occurring male hormone. When administered as a drug it can cause gain in lean body mass, increased sex drive, and possibly aggressive behavior. Many men with HIV have low testosterone levels.

therapeutic HIV vaccine: Also called treatment vaccine. A **vaccine** designed to boost the immune response to HIV in persons already infected with the virus. A therapeutic vaccine is different from a preventive vaccine, which is designed to prevent a disease from becoming established in a person.

3TC: Similar to other **nucleoside analog** drugs, 3TC inhibits HIV replication through viral **DNA** chain termination. **FDA** approved for combination use with **AZT** as a treatment option for HIV infection in adults and pediatric patients (3 months old or older). Also known as lamivudine, Epivir.

Th1 response: An acquired **immune response** whose most prominent feature is high **cytotoxic T lymphocyte** activity relative to the amount of **antibody** production. The Th1 response is promoted by **CD4+** "Th1" T-helper cells. (*See also* **Th2 response**.)

Th2 response: An acquired **immune response** whose most prominent feature is high **antibody** production relative to the amount of **cytotoxic T lymphocyte** activity. The Th2 response is promoted by **CD4+** "Th2" T-helper cells. (*See also* **Th1 response**.)

thrombocytopenia: A decreased number of blood **platelets** (cells important for blood clotting). (*See* **immune thrombocytopenia purpura**.)

thrush: Sore patches in the mouth caused by the **fungus** *Candida albicans*. Thrush is one of the most frequent early symptoms or signs of an immune disorder. The fungus commonly lives in the mouth, but only causes problems when the body's resistance is reduced either by antibiotics that have reduced the number of competitive organisms in the mouth, or by an immune deficiency such as HIV disease. (*See* **candidiasis**.)

thymosin: A polypeptide **hormone** of the **thymus** gland that influences the maturation of **T cells** destined for an active role in **cell-mediated immunity**.

thymus: A mass of glandular tissue (**lymphoid organ**) found in the upper chest under the breastbone in humans. The thymus is essential to the development of the body's system of immunity beginning in fetal life (i.e., before birth). The thymus processes white blood cells (**lymphocytes**), which kill foreign cells and stimulate other immune cells to produce **antibodies**. An important function of the thymus is to weed out lymphocytes that react to **proteins** produced by the body (self-antigens), thus preventing autoimmune disease. The gland grows throughout childhood until puberty and then gradually decreases in size. (*See* **thymosin**.)

tissue: A collection of similar cells acting together to perform a particular function. There are four basic tissues in the body: epithelial, connective, muscle, and nerve.

titer (also "titre"): A laboratory measurement of the amount—or concentration—of a given compound in solution.

T lymphocyte proliferation assay: Measures the strength of response of **T memory cells**—a subgroup of **T lymphocytes**—to HIV.

T lymphocytes: *See* **T cells**.

TMP/SMX (Trimethoprim/sulfamethoxazole; also called **Bactrim, Septra, or Trimoxazole):** A combination antibiotic drug effective at preventing and treating **PCP**. May also be effective against **toxoplasmosis** and some bacterial infections. Possible side effects include skin rash (which on rare occasions spreads to other body surfaces and becomes the life-threatening **Stevens-Johnson syndrome**), digestive disturbances, bone marrow suppression, and liver impairment. **Desensitization** procedures have become popular when administering TMP/SMX to persons with a history of adverse reactions to the drug.

toxicity: The extent, quality, or degree of being poisonous or harmful to the body.

toxoplasmic encephalitis: *See* **toxoplasmosis**.

toxoplasmosis: Toxoplasmosis is an infection that is caused by the protozoan (see **protozoa**) parasite, *Toxoplasma gondii*. The parasite is carried by cats, birds, and other animals, and is found in soil contaminated by cat feces and in meat, particularly pork. The parasite can infect the lungs, retina of the eye, heart, pancreas, liver, colon, and testes. Once *T. gondii* invades the body, it remains there, but the **immune system** in a healthy person usually prevents the parasite from causing disease. If the immune system becomes severely damaged, as in HIV-infected persons, or is suppressed by drugs, *T. gondii* can begin to multiply and cause severe disease. In HIV-infected persons, the most common site of toxoplasmosis is the brain. When *T. gondii* invades the brain, causing inflammation, the condition is called toxoplasmic encephalitis. While the disease in HIV-infected persons can generally be treated with some success, lifelong therapy is required to prevent its reoccurrence.

transaminase: A liver enzyme. A laboratory test that measures transaminase levels is used to assess the health of the liver.

transcription: The process of constructing a **messenger RNA** molecule, using a **DNA** molecule as a **template**, with the resulting transfer of genetic information to the messenger RNA. As related to HIV:

The process by which the **provirus** produces new viruses. RNA copies, called messenger RNA, must be made that can be read by the **host** cell's protein-making machinery. Cellular enzymes, including RNA polymerase II, facilitate transcription. The viral genes may partly control this process. For example, *tat* encodes a **protein** that accelerates the transcription process by binding to a section of the newly made viral RNA. (*See also* **integration; ribonucleic acid**.)

transfer factor: A fraction of white blood cells that apparently "transfers" capability to mount an **immune response** to a specific **antigen**.

transfusion: 1. The process of transfusing fluid (such as blood) into a vein. 2. The transfer of whole blood or blood products from one individual to another.

translation: As related to HIV: The process by which HIV **messenger RNA** is processed in a cell's **nucleus** and transported to the **cytoplasm**, the cellular material outside the nucleus. In the cytoplasm, the cell's protein-making machinery translates the messenger RNA into viral **protein** and **enzymes**.

transmission: In the context of HIV disease: HIV is spread most commonly by sexual contact with an infected partner. The virus can enter the body through the mucosal lining of the vagina, vulva, penis, rectum or, rarely, the mouth during sex. The likelihood of transmission is increased by factors that may damage these linings, especially other **sexually transmitted diseases** that cause ulcers or inflammation. HIV also is spread through contact with infected blood, most often by the sharing of drug needles or syringes contaminated with minute quantities of blood containing the virus. Children can contract HIV from their infected mothers either during pregnancy or birth, or postnatally, through breast-feeding. In developed countries, HIV is now only rarely transmitted by transfusion of blood or blood products because of screening measures.

treatment IND: A program to provide experimental treatments to a class of patients who lack satisfactory alternative treatments. IND stands for **investigational new drug** application, which is part of the process to get approval from the **FDA** for marketing a new prescription drug in the United States.

tuberculin skin test (TST): A **purified protein derivative (PPD)** of the tubercle bacilli, called tuberculin, is introduced into the skin by scratch, puncture, or intradermal injection. If a raised, red, or hard

587

zone forms surrounding the test site, the person is said to be sensitive to tuberculin, and the test is read as positive.

tuberculosis (TB): A bacterial infection caused by *Mycobacterium tuberculosis*. TB bacteria are spread by airborne droplets expelled from the lungs when a person with active TB coughs, sneezes, or speaks. Exposure to these droplets can lead to infection in the air sacs of the lungs. The immune defenses of healthy people usually prevent TB infection from spreading beyond a very small area of the lungs. If the body's immune system is impaired because of infection with HIV, aging, malnutrition, or other factors, the TB bacterium may begin to spread more widely in the lungs or to other tissues. TB is seen with increasing frequency among persons infected with HIV. Most cases of TB occur in the lungs (pulmonary TB). However, the disease may also occur in the larynx, lymph nodes, brain, kidneys, or bones (extrapulmonary TB). Extrapulmonary TB infections are more common among persons living with HIV. (*See* **multidrug resistant TB**.)

tumor necrosis factor (TNF): A **cytokine**, produced by **macrophages**, which helps activate **T cells**. It also may stimulate HIV activity. TNF levels are very high in persons with HIV, and the **molecule** is suspected to play a part in HIV-related **wasting syndrome, neuropathy**, and **dementia**. TNF triggers a biochemical pathway that leads to the programmed form of cell suicide known as **apoptosis**. It also activates a key molecule that can block this very pathway, and so set up a delicate life-death balance within the cell.

V

V3 loop: Section of the **gp120** protein on the surface of HIV. Appears to be important in stimulating **neutralizing antibodies**.

vaccination: Inoculation of a substance (i.e., the **vaccine**) into the body for the purpose of producing active **immunity** against a disease.

vaccine: A substance that contains antigenic components from an infectious organism. By stimulating an **immune response**—but not the disease—it protects against subsequent infection by that organism. There can be **preventive vaccines** (e.g., measles or mumps) as well as **therapeutic (treatment) vaccines**. (*See also* **antigen**.)

vaccinia: A cowpox virus, formerly used in human smallpox vaccines. Employed as a vector in HIV vaccine research to transport HIV genes into the body. (*See* **vaccination**; **vector**.)

Valley fever: *See* **coccidioidomycosis**.

variable region: The part of an antibody's structure that differs from one **antibody** to another.

varicella zoster virus (VZV): A virus in the herpes family that causes chicken pox during childhood and may reactivate later in life to cause **herpes zoster (shingles)** in **immunosuppressed** individuals.

vector: A nonpathogenic bacterium or virus used to transport an **antigen** into the body to stimulate protective **immunity** (e.g., in vaccine; see).

vertical transmission: Transmission of a **pathogen** such as HIV from mother to fetus or baby during pregnancy or birth. (*See* **perinatal transmission**.)

Videx: *See* **ddI**.

viral burden: The amount of HIV in the circulating blood. Monitoring a person's viral burden is important because of the apparent correlation between the amount of virus in the blood and the severity of the disease: sicker patients generally have more virus than those with less advanced disease. A new, sensitive, rapid test—called the viral load assay for HIV-1 infection—can be used to monitor the HIV viral burden. This procedure may help clinicians to decide when to give anti-HIV therapy. It may also help investigators determine more quickly if experimental HIV therapies are effective. (*See* **viral load test**; **polymerase chain reaction**.)

viral core: 1. Typically a virus contains an RNA (**ribonucleic acid**) or DNA (**deoxyribonucleic acid**) core of genetic material surrounded by a protein coat. 2. As related to HIV: Within HIV's **envelope** is a bullet-shaped core made of another protein, **p24**, that surrounds the viral RNA. Each strand of HIV RNA contains the virus' nine genes. Three of these—*gag*, *pol*, and *env*—are structural genes that contain information needed to make structural proteins. The *env* gene, for example, codes for **gp160**, a **protein** that is later broken down to **gp120** and **gp41**. (*See* **surrogate marker**.)

viral culture: A laboratory method for growing viruses.

viral envelope: As related to HIV: HIV is spherical in shape with a diameter of 1/10,000 of a millimeter. The outer coat, or **envelope**, is composed of two layers of fat-like molecules called **lipids**, taken from the membranes of human cells. Embedded in the envelope are numerous cellular proteins, as well as mushroom-shaped HIV proteins that protrude from the surface. Each mushroom is thought to consist of four **gp41** molecules embedded in the envelope. The virus uses these proteins to attach to and infect cells.

viral load test: As related to HIV: Test that measures the quantity of HIV **RNA** in the blood. Results are expressed as the number of copies per milliliter of blood plasma. Research indicates that viral load is a better predictor of the risk of HIV disease progression than the **CD4** count. The lower the viral load the longer the time to AIDS diagnosis and the longer the survival time. Viral load testing for HIV infection is being used to determine when to initiate and/or change therapy. (*See* **viral burden.**)

Viramune: *See* **nevirapine**.

viremia: The presence of virus in the bloodstream. (*See* **sepsis.**)

virion: A virus particle existing freely outside a **host** cell. A mature virus.

virology: The study of viruses and viral disease.

viricide: Any agent that destroys or inactivates a virus.

virus: Organism composed mainly of **nucleic acid** within a **protein** coat, ranging in size from 100 to 2,000 angstroms (unit of length; 1 angstrom is equal to 10^{-10} meters). When viruses enter a living plant, animal, or bacterial cell, they make use of the **host** cell's chemical energy and **protein**—and nucleic acid—synthesizing ability to replicate themselves. **Nucleic acids** in viruses are single stranded or double stranded, and may be DNA (**deoxyribonucleic acid**) or RNA (**ribonucleic acid**). After the infected host cell makes viral components and virus particles are released, the host cell is often dissolved. Some viruses do not kill cells but transform them into a cancerous state; some cause illness and then seem to disappear, while remaining latent and later causing another, sometimes much more severe, form of disease. In humans, viruses cause—among others—measles, mumps, yellow fever, poliomyelitis, influenza, and the common cold. Some viral infections can be treated with drugs.

visceral: Pertaining to the major internal organs.

W

wasting syndrome: *See* **AIDS wasting syndrome**.

Western Blot: A laboratory test for specific **antibodies** to confirm repeatedly reactive results on the HIV **ELISA** or EIA tests. In the United States, Western Blot is the validation test used most often for confirmation of these other tests.

white blood cells: *See* **leukocytes**.

window period: Time from infection with HIV until detectable **seroconversion**.

Y

yeast infection: *See* **candidiasis**.

Z

Zalcitabine: *See* **ddC**.

Zerit: *See* **d4T**.

zidovudine: *See* **AZT**.

Chapter 61

HIV/AIDS-Related Internet Resources

Introduction

The main text in this chapter has been prepared by the CDC National AIDS Clearinghouse (CDC NAC) as an introduction to the Internet and HIV/AIDS information. The first section provides information about what the Internet is, software packages and services available to access the Internet, and how to read an Internet address. The second section covers the various Internet tools and how they can be used. It covers the World Wide Web, FTP, gopherspace, electronic mail, listservs, telnet, Usenet newsgroups, and freenets. The third section discusses how to navigate the World Wide Web, FTP, and gopherspace to find and organize the information you need. In the fourth section, a selection of World Wide Web sites on a variety of HIV/AIDS-related topic areas helps you begin your search for information. This section also lists Usenet newsgroups and listservs that may be of interest. The fifth section presents a list of books and journals for further information. Fact sheets on the CDC National AIDS Clearinghouse's and the National Library of Medicine's Internet services are included at the end of the chapter.

"Guide to Selected HIV/AIDS-Related Internet Resources," CDC National AIDS Clearinghouse, Centers for Disease Control and Prevention (CDC), June 1996; and "National Library of Medicine (NLM) Internet-Accessible Resources," National Institutes of Health (NIH), March 1995; URLs updated and verified in October 1998.

About the Internet

What Is the Internet?

The Internet is a "global network" of networks. The Internet requires a "Local Network" computer to connect the various users and route the various requests to the Internet destinations. Local network computers are run by Internet Service Providers. No single company or group "owns" or runs the Internet; every computer connected to the Internet is responsible only for its own part of the Internet.

Computers connected to the Internet can contain anything that can be put into digital form. This includes databases, library catalogs, government archives, messages on every conceivable topic, photographs, movies, and sound recordings.

To access the Internet, you need a computer with communications software, a modem, and an Internet account. An Internet account can be acquired in several ways. One way is to find out if your organization/company provides Internet accounts. Ask your computer/information systems staff if they can provide you with access to the Internet. You can also get an Internet account through a number of Internet service providers which allow you to use their connections to the Internet (for a fee). To get a list of Internet service providers, check magazines such as *Internet World, PCWorld, Online, MacWorld,* and *Byte,* which are available at most newsstands and local libraries.

To become familiar with using the Internet, the publishing industry has produced several books on getting access to and using the Internet. See the sampling of Internet-related books and magazines which may be helpful listed near the end of this chapter; you can also look in the computer section of your local library or bookstore.

Software Packages and Services

In this chapter, we describe the various Internet services and how to use them in a manner general enough so that you can apply this information to the type of software and service you are using to access the Internet. However, this means that we cannot provide you with step-by-step instructions for accessing the Internet for each type of software or service. We recommend that you read any and all materials (both paper and electronic) that you received when you set up your Internet access. We also recommend speaking with your service's Help Desk or System Administrator if you encounter problems along the way. They are familiar with the software you are using, and can most efficiently guide you through the steps to carry out a particular function. There are also several books available at your local public library and bookstores to assist you in accessing the Internet. The bibliography near the end of this chapter lists some of the currently published books. Spend some time browsing the shelves and select the book that is right for you based on the type of computer and access software you are using.

How to Read an Internet Address

The addresses in this chapter are given as URLs. URL stands for Uniform Resource Locator, and is the format an Internet address takes when used by the World Wide Web. URLs are a fairly standard, widely recognized way to present addresses, and can be broken down into three basic parts: the type of tool or resource, the address of the site, and the location of the file on the site. URLs look like this:

http://www.cdc.gov/diseases/hivqa.html

URLs are read from left to right. The first section, the part which ends with ://, tells the Web browser (and you) what type of tool you will be looking at. The tool type in this example is http:// which tells us that it is a World Wide Web site.

These are the other major tool types:

gopher:// = Gopher
telnet:// = Telnet connection
ftp:// = FTP site
file:// = file on an FTP site

The section between the tool type and the first single slash (/) is the address of the site. In our examples, this is the address: www.cdc.gov.

Anything after the first single slash is the path to the file. In our example, "/diseases/" is the directory path and "hivqa. html" is the file name.

Internet Tools and Technology

World Wide Web

The recent explosion in Internet popularity and use is attributable in large part to the World Wide Web and the browsers which make using the Web so easy. The Web allows users to follow a trail of their

595

interests by linking pages of information together using hypertext. Hypertext is a non-linear method of joining information and uses highlighted words or phrases as "live" links to other parts of the document or other documents. As the user, all you need to do is click with your mouse on the link (or press return if you're using the text browser, Lynx) and you go to the document that the link represents.

A "browser," or special software, is used to navigate the World Wide Web. Some examples of Web browsers are Netscape, Mosaic, and Lynx. Lynx is a text-based Web browser. Web browsers are also capable of linking to non-Web Internet sites such as gophers, FTP archives, and telnet sites. This pulling together of a variety of Internet tools makes the World Wide Web valuable.

The browser you use will have an option such as "Open URL" which will allow you to type in the URL and go directly to that site. You will probably develop a list of Web sites which you find useful. These sites can be saved and organized using a "hotlist" or list of "bookmarks."

Helper Applications: Helpers are applications that assist in accessing, downloading, and decompressing data from other networks. They can also enable you to view multimedia displays like video, animation, and sound recordings. These applications can run independently of a Web browser or can work with the browser to provide access to a variety of information formats. There are many helper applications to choose from and most are dependent on the type of computer being used (PC or Macintosh). A "plug-in" is a helper application that works seamlessly within the browser. Some examples of helper applications are the Adobe® Acrobat® Reader, L-View©, and Apple QuickTime© movie player.

Anonymous FTP

Many files, especially larger ones, are stored on the Internet in sites called FTP archives. FTP stands for File Transfer Protocol, the "language" computers use to transfer a copy of the files from where they are stored to where you want them. (FTP is based on Unix, the computer platform and language on which many Internet sites are based.)

To retrieve a file from an FTP archive, you need to know three things: the name of the archive, the name of the file, and where the file is located (directory path) in the archive. If you've been given a URL, it should tell you all you need to know. If you know only the address and path, you may need to look at some files until you find the right one.

Most often, the files you would like to access are on remote computers—computers for which you do not have a user account. To access these files, you must use "Anonymous FTP." This means that when asked for a user name (or login name), you enter the name: anonymous. You will next be asked to provide a password. While not required, it is considered good Internet manners (netiquette) to provide your E-mail address.

At this point, you will either type in the directory path or click with the mouse on the directory, depending on how your service works. You may need to issue some commands to retrieve the file, or simply click on the file and drag it to where you want it stored on your computer.

To help you find files on FTP sites, a tool called Archie was developed. For more information about using Archie, see the section titled "Navigating the Internet."

Gopher

Gopher is a means of navigating through parts of the Internet using a menu-based interface. It's an improvement over FTP and telnet because you don't need to know the address of a resource to use it. To use a gopher, follow the instructions given to you by your account administrator. You may have to type the word "gopher" at your account prompt, or use a gopher software package.

Once you've gotten into gopher, you can follow the menu choices to other gophers all over the world. A good place to start is the "mother gopher," (gopher://gopher.micro.umn.edu:70/1) maintained by the creators of Internet gopher at the University of Minnesota. One of the menu items is "All the Gophers in the World" which is then further broken down by geographic region. Many universities maintain gophers.

Files can be read while online or mailed to your E-mail account. Some gopher software clients also allow you to save a file directly to your account or your computer. If you find a gopher you visit frequently, you can create a list of "bookmarks" which becomes a personal menu of your favorite sites.

To help you find information on gopher, a tool called Veronica was developed. For more information about using Veronica, see the section titled "Navigating the Internet."

Usenet Newsgroups

One of the most popular methods for communicating with other people, Usenet newsgroups are subject-oriented and cover a wide range of topics, from sports to medicine to lifestyles to cooking. To access the thousands of available newsgroups, your system must have a newsreader (check with your administrator to see if you have one). Some World Wide Web browsers include newsreaders.

Some newsgroups are very busy, with as many as 100 postings in one day; others receive only a few postings each week. Newsgroups are organized in hierarchies; the major categories are listed below and will give you a good idea of where you might find different topics:

- alt = alternative

- bit = gatewayed BITNET mailing lists

- biz = business

- comp = computers

- rec = recreation

- sci = science

- soc = society

- talk = discussion

The newsgroup's name indicates its level of specificity; reading the name sci.med.aids from left to right tells you that the newsgroup is broadly related to science, in the field of medicine, and most specifically, deals with AIDS.

The first step you need to take is to subscribe to the newsgroups which interest you. How you do this will depend on your newsreader (again, ask your administrator for assistance). Once you have subscribed, you will receive all the messages posted (sent) to that newsgroup. You will also be able to post your own messages.

Some advantages to newsgroups are that you can obtain quick answers to tough questions and receive prompt notification of important news related to specific topics. For a list of HIV/AIDS-related newsgroups, see "Usenet Newsgroups" near the end of this chapter.

E-mail

The most frequently used tool on the Internet is electronic mail (E-mail), a very effective medium for communicating with other people. Any user with an Internet address can send electronic mail messages to any other user with an address. This includes users of the commercial services such as America Online and CompuServe.

Popular uses of E-mail are mailing lists, known as listservs, and electronic journals.

Listservs

Listservs cover a specific topic, e.g., AIDS. Once you have subscribed, you may send (post) a message to be read by all other people who subscribe to the listserv.

There are two parts to a listserv address. Addresses take the form listservname@hostname. The listservname is the name used when posting messages to the listserv. The hostname is the machine on which the listserv's software and other files are located.

To subscribe to a listserv, send the following command in the text of the message (leave the subject line blank): subscribe <listservname> <yourfirstname> <yourlastname> to the address: listserv@hostname. Some listservs use other subscribing language, however, this is the most common.

The listserv@hostname address is the address you should use when subscribing, unsubscribing, or executing other commands to the listserv (to find out what other commands you can use, send the command "help" to the listserv@hostname address). Send your discussion contributions to the listservname@hostname address; do not send subscribe or unsubscribe messages to this address. See "Listservs" near the end of this chapter for a list of some of the HIV/AIDS-related listservs.

Telnet

Telnet allows you to log in to other computers which are connected to the Internet, called remote computers. To use telnet, you'll need to know the address of the machine and the login name/password required to gain access. Special software is also required to use telnet. Most World Wide Web browsers can be configured to call up telnet software so that you can telnet directly through your Web browser.

A popular telnet site for government information is the FedWorld bulletin board system. To access it, at your system prompt, type: telnet://fedworld.gov.

When connected, you will see a login: prompt. At that point, type: new. (These commands are for the FedWorld site and may vary for other sites.)

You will then see a menu of many options available to you. When you are done, type quit, bye, exit, logoff, or logout. If the system tells

599

you which command to use, use that one; otherwise, try any of them until you are disconnected.

Freenets

Freenets are open-access, free, community computer systems. One such system is the Cleveland Freenet sponsored by Case Western Reserve University (CWRU). There's no charge for the registration process and no charge to use the system. To register, telnet to any one of the following addresses: telnet://freenet-in-a.cwru.edu, telnet://freenet-in-b.cwru.edu, or telnet://f reenet-in-c.cwru.edu.

Freenets are community-based systems that provide Internet access, electronic mail, bulletin boards, and other types of information access to members of the community at no charge. The Freenet concept originated with Dr. Tom Grundner, Department of Family Medicine at Case Western Reserve University.

The National Public Telecomputing Network is the organization which oversees development of freenets. For more information about freenets in your area, contact: National Public Telecomputing Network, P.O. Box 1987, Cleveland, Ohio 44106; (216) 247-5800 voice; (216) 247-3328 fax; E-mail: info@nptn.org; http://www.nptn.org. You can also contact your local public library for information about freenets in your area.

Navigating the Internet

The Internet provides access to a wealth of information, however, users often find it difficult to locate the specific information they need. Fortunately, there are tools to help you navigate the World Wide Web, FTP sites, and gopherspace.

Searching on the World Wide Web: Search Engines and Directories

There are a couple of ways to find information on the World Wide Web: directories of Internet sites and search engines which search for terms you specify.

Yahoo is the most commonly used and comprehensive directory listing of sites on the Internet. Yahoo is an extensive subject tree of Internet sites, broken down by subject category and subcategory. You can also use a search engine to search the sites listed in Yahoo. The URL for Yahoo is http://www. yahoo. com/.

To search Web pages by subject using a search engine, type the search term or terms you are looking for in the space provided and the search engine will generate a list of Web sites that include that subject. Some popular search engines are Alta Vista (http://altavista.digital.com/), InfoSeek (http://www2.infoseek. com/), Lycos (http://www.lycos. com), and Open Text (http://www.opentext.com/omw/f -omw.html). Some search engines allow you to search gopher or FTP sites as well as the World Wide Web and will even search links within a page. The Internet does not have a standard language or thesaurus to use for searching; all search engines use a different mechanism for searching. Therefore, search results will differ depending on the search engine you choose. To find the information you are looking for, you may need to try a couple of search engines.

Hotlists: Hotlists are a convenient way to organize Internet sites of interest or sites you plan to visit often. Hotlists are collections of Web addresses that you can store in a file on your Web browser. Sometimes called "bookmarks," these lists are compiled by the user and allow you to directly access saved Internet addresses. You can create a hotlist (done differently in different browsers) of sites which you can then use each time you visit the Web without having to remember the URL.

Searching FTP Sites: Archie

Finding files on FTP archives can be a bit tricky and difficult. To help, there is a search tool called Archie. To use it, you must access an Archie server using telnet. There are several Archie servers; here are some addresses:

- telnet://archie.au
- telnet://archie.funet.fi
- telnet://archie.sogang.ac.kr
- telnet://archie.nz
- telnet://archie.luth.se
- telnet://archie.hensa.ac.uk
- telnet://archie.rutgers.edu

Once connected, log in as Archie unless the system tells you differently. To search, the command is: prog <search term>

You can change how Archie searches by setting the search type. Searches are either exact or substring. Exact means that the file name must match your search string exactly. Substring means that the file must contain your search string somewhere in its name. To change the search type, the command is: set search sub or set search exact.

When your search results are several screens long or you don't want to read them immediately, you can have Archie searches mailed to your E-mail account. The command is: set mailto <e-mail address>.

Once a search has been run, issue the command to mail the results to yourself. The command is: mail.

To leave Archie, the command is: quit. This will exit you out of the Archie server and return you to your account.

Searching Gopher Sites: Veronica

Information found on gophers is searchable using a tool called Veronica. Veronica searches directory titles on all registered gopher servers and looks for words that match a search term. Veronica works well because compared to the World Wide Web, gopherspace is relatively small and better organized.

The "Search Gopherspace Using Veronica" option can be found on many gopher menus. Select any of the search options (usually between 14 and 20 menu items) and enter your search term(s) in the space provided. Veronica will then look through gopher menus for the term, and build a menu of items meeting your search requirements. You may then use that menu as you would any other gopher menu.

Selected Internet Resources on HIV/AIDS

World Wide Web Sites

This section includes a selection of World Wide Web sites on a variety of HIV/AIDS-related topic areas to help you begin your search for information. It also lists Usenet newsgroups that may be of interest. Due to the continuously changing nature of the Internet, you might find that some of the resources listed may no longer be available. Listings contain the following information: the resource's name, the access address(es), and a brief description of its contents and scope. Inclusion of a service does not imply endorsement by the Centers for Disease Control and Prevention, CDC NAC, or any other organization. A description of Internet services provided by the CDC National AIDS Clearinghouse and the National Library of Medicine is included near the end of this chapter.

Adolescents

The Center for AIDS Prevention Studies (CAPS)

URL: http://chanane.ucsf.edu/capsweb/index.html
Among the many valuable resources at the CAPS site at the University of California, San Francisco, are Teens *Teach Kids About HIV* (http://www.epibiostat.ucsf.edu/capsweb/hotindex.html), a curricula for educating peer educators, and *What are Adolescent's Prevention Needs* (http://chanane.ucsf.edu/capsweb/adoltext.html), a fact sheet which includes links to references and other sources of information.

Funding

Community of Science

URL: http://cos.com
The Community of Science is a global registry designed to provide accurate, timely, easy-to-access information about what new funding opportunities exist, who is working on what subject, and where. The Funding Opportunities database (http://cos.fundingopps2.cos.com/) includes information on funding opportunities announced by federal agencies, state/provincial and commercial organizations, non-profit foundations and professional associations. The NIH Grants database (http://fundedresearch.cos.com/hih/index.html) offers information on federally funded research in the U.S.

The Foundation Center's Home Page

URL: http://fdncenter.org/2index.html
This site offers a wealth of information about Foundation Center services in particular and fundraising in general. Use the site's search engine to locate all HIV/AIDS related information on the page. Browse the links to private and corporate foundations. The Publications section provides access to information about ordering AIDS fundraising guides and catalogs.

Harm Reduction / Syringe Exchange

North American Syringe Exchange Network (NASEN)

URL: http://www.nasen.org/
NASEN is dedicated to the creation, expansion, and continued existence of syringe exchange programs as a proven method of stopping the transmission of bloodborne pathogens, especially HIV, in the injecting drug using community. The NASEN site includes information

on syringe exchange programs, syringe exchange reports and literature, national drug policy and drug treatment, a syringe exchange mailing list, and upcoming events.

Does Needle Exchange Work?
URL: http://www.epibiostat.ucsf.edu/capsweb/needletext.html
This fact sheet at the Center for AIDS Prevention Studies Web site (http://www.epibiostat.ucsf.edu/capsweb/index.html) answers many questions about the strategy of harm reduction and needle exchange, and provides links to bibliographies of research literature on the topic.

International

Joint United Nations Programme on HIV/AIDS
URL: http://undcp.or.at/undcp/activ/intecoop/unaids.htm
This site includes graphs and statistics on the global AIDS epidemic as well as information on conferences, human rights, and other organizations concerned with world health.

Pan American Health Organization
URL: http://lwww. paho.org/default.htm
The technical information area of this site includes the full text of AIDS Surveillance in the Americas which reports statistics on the AIDS epidemic in the region of the Americas.

U.S. Census Bureau International Program Center
URL: http://www.census.gov/ftp/pub/ipc/www/
This site offers access to the HIV/AIDS Surveillance Database, a compilation of information from studies appearing in the medical and scientific literature, presented at international conferences, and appearing in the press.

Race / Ethnicity

The Center for AIDS Prevention Studies (CAPS)
URL: http://www.caps.ucsf.edu/capsweb/index.html
This site contains the fact sheets, *What Are African-Americans' HIV Prevention Needs?* (http://www.caps.ucsf.edu/capsweb/afamtext.html) and *What Are Latinos' HIV Prevention Needs?* (http://www.caps.ucsf. edu/capsweb/latinotext.html). It also provides access to bibliographies of CAPS publications on African Americans and HIV/AIDS and multiethnic minorities.

National Institute of Allergy and Infectious Disease (NIAID) Publications

URL: http://www.niaid.nih.gov/facts/facts.htm
The fact sheet area of this site provides access to the NIAID fact sheet, *Minorities and HIV Infection* (http://www.niaid.nih.gov/facts/mwhhp0.htm).

AIDS & the Latino Community

URL: http://latino.sscnet.ucla.edu/research/aids/aidscomm.html
This site is a comprehensive collection of HIV/AIDS resources for the Latino community. It is one of the many useful areas on the Chicano/Latino Network (http://latino.sscnet.ucla.edu/).

Religion

The Body: A Multimedia AIDS and HIV Information Resource

URL: http://www.thebody.com/index.html
The Body is a multimedia AIDS and HIV education resource produced by The Body Health Resources Corporation. Its Web site houses the AIDS National Interfaith Network site (http://www.thebody.com/anin/aninpage. html) which provides information on HIV and AIDS activities of more than 2,000 religious organizations, and Religion and AIDS (http://www.thebody.com/religion.html), which contains full text of articles on Christianity, Judaism, and interfaith aspects of HIV/AIDS.

Religion and AIDS/HIV

URL: http://web.bu.edu/COHIS/aids/new/religion.htm
This resource guide, produced by the CDC National AIDS Clearinghouse, is available in the HIV/AIDS section of the Boston University Medical Center, Community Outreach Health Information System (http://web.bu.edu/COHIS/). It covers issues relevant to HIV/AIDS and the religious community and includes information about national religious organizations involved in AIDS work.

Safer Sex & Condoms

New York Online Access to Health (NOAH)

URL: http://www.noah.cuny.edu/
NOAH contains useful information about condoms and safe sex, including the Sexuality Information and Education Council of the U.S. (SIECUS) fact sheet, *The Truth About Latex Condoms* (http://www.noah.cuny.edu/sexuality/siecus/fact1.html), the Gay Men's Health

Crisis brochure *Loving, Sharing, Caring* (http://www.noah.cuny.edu/ illness/aids/gmhc/brochure6.html), STD Prevention: Condoms section of the site (http://www.noah.cuny.edu/illness/stds/stds.html#Prevention), and more.

The Safer Sex Page
URL: http://www.safersex.org/
This site is full of useful information on condoms in particular and safe sex/HIV transmission prevention in general. The site includes a media gallery with a how to put on a condom video and cartoons, as well as text of brochures, articles, handouts, and more. It includes a section of information for counselors and links to other resources.

Stop AIDS Project
URL: http://www.stopaids.org/AIDSpre.html#Pleasure
This site includes *Condoms: What's Your Pleasure?* a review of condom brands (Avanti, Maxx, Lifestyles, Pleasure Plus and Rough Rider, and Glyde's Lollyes dental dams) and *How to Use Condoms*, a step-by-step explanation of the proper use of condoms.

Coalition for Positive Sexuality
URL: http://www.positive.org/cps/
The Coalition for Positive Sexuality Web site is full of useful information on safe sex in general and condoms in particular. The Just Say Yes (http://www.positive.org/cps/JustSayYes/index.html) page contains detailed information about how to use condoms to practice safer sex.

Sexually Transmitted Diseases (STDS)

CDC National Center for HIV, STD and TB Prevention
Division of Sexually Transmitted Disease Prevention
URL: http://www.cdc.gov/nchstp/dstd/dstdp.html
This site offers access to general information and publications on sexually transmitted diseases and information on the work of CDC's Division of Sexually Transmitted Disease Prevention.

Ask NOAH About: Sexually Transmitted Diseases
URL: http://www.noah.cuny.edu/stds/stds.html
The STD section of NOAH: New York Online Access to Health (http://www.noah.cuny.edu) provides comprehensive information on preventing, identifying, and treating sexually transmitted diseases and links to other sources of information.

Statistics

CDC National Center for HIV, STD, and TB Prevention, Division of HIV/AIDS Prevention
URL: http://www.cdcnac.org/
The Basic Statistics section of this site (http://www.cdc.gov/nchstp/hiv-aids/statisti.htm) provides information on cumulative cases, exposure categories, the HIV/AIDS Surveillance Report, international projections statistics, and the 10 states/territories and cities reporting the highest number of AIDS cases.

Testing

Center for AIDS Prevention Studies (CAPS)
URL: http://www.caps.ucsf.edu/capsweb/index.html
The Center for AIDS Prevention Studies, at the University of California–San Francisco, produces a series of fact sheets, including *What Is Testing's Role in HIV Prevention?* (http://www.caps.ucsf.edu/capsweb/testtext.html) and *What Is the Role of HIV Testing at Home?* (http://www.caps.ucsf.edu/capsweb/hometext.html) which are available at the CAPS Web site.

A Guide to HIV Antibody Testing
URL: http://www.noah.cuny.edu/aids/gmhc/brochure4.html
This brochure, produced by Gay Men's Health Crisis (http://www.gmhc.org), explains what test results mean and examines the possible advantages and disadvantages of being tested.

Treatment and Clinical Trials

HIV/AIDS Treatment Information Service (ATIS)
URL: http://www.hivatis.org
ATIS provides information about federally approved HIV/AIDS treatment options, as well as treatment-related government press releases and links to related sites.

AIDS Clinical Trials Information Service (ACTIS)
URL: http://www.actis.org
ACTIS provides information on HIV/AIDS clinical trials open to enrollment and trial results.

National Institute of Allergy and Infectious Diseases (NIAID) Publications
URL: http://www.niaid.nih.gov/publications/publications.htm

The fact sheet area of this site (http://www. niaid.nih.gov/facts/facts.htm) provides access to 10 NIAID fact sheets on various opportunistic infections.

Project Inform (PI)
URL: http://www.projinf.org/
Project Inform prepares printed material on a variety of treatment and public policy issues related to HIV disease. This Web site makes PI's materials, which are continually revised and updated, available in an indexed and searchable format.

Seattle Treatment Education Project (STEP)
URL: http://www.thebody.com/step/steppage.html
STEP provides information on many treatment options and protocols. The STEP Web site includes the full text of selected publications.

HIV/AIDS Information Outreach Project
URL: http://www.aidsnyc.org/index.html
This site, developed by The New York Academy of Medicine, is a resource for community-based organizations working with people affected by HIV/AIDS. Its contents include the National AIDS Treatment Advocacy Project (http://www.natap.org) and the AIDS Treatment Data Network (http://www.aidsnyc.org/network/index.html).

Treatment Overview
URL: http://www.thebody.com/treat/treatovr.html
The Treatment Overview page, part of The Body Web site (http://www.thebody.com/treatment.html), contains text and links to useful treatment resources.

Tuberculosis

Tuberculosis
URL: http://www.cpmc.columbia.edu/tbcpp/index.html
This site provides information on tuberculosis for health care consumers and providers as well as links to other sources of information. It is part of the collaborative Web site maintained by Department of Medical Informatics, Columbia University, and the Clinical Information Services, Presbyterian Hospital (http://www.cpmc.columbia.edu).

World Health Organization (WHO) Global Tuberculosis Programme
URL: http://www.who.int/dsa/

This site provides the text of WHO reports on the TB epidemic, fact sheets on TB, and links to other sources of information.

The American Lung Association
URL: http://www.pbs.org/ppol/ala.html
The Tuberculosis Resources section of this site includes health information resources, educational resources, the text of *Facts and Figures*, and other information on TB.

Treatment Issues Fact Sheet: Tuberculosis
URL: http://www.gmhc.org/living/medcare/tb.html
This fact sheet provides information about TB infection and disease, signs and symptoms, multi-drug resistant strains, and treatment. It is located on the Gay Men's Health Crisis site on the Web (http://www.gmhc.org/).

Women

What Are Women's HIV Prevention Needs?
URL: http://chanane.ucsf.edu/capsweb/womentext.html
This is one of many useful fact sheets available at the Center for AIDS Prevention Studies, UCSF (http://www.caps.ucsf.edu/capsweb/index.html).

Women and Safer Sex
URL: http://www.safersex.org/women/
This site provides access to the CDC Fact Sheet *Women and AIDS* and articles on Women and HIV published in the Virginia AIDS Information Newsletter.

Workplace Issues

The Mid-Atlantic Americans with Disabilities Act (ADA) Information Center
URL: http://www.thebody.com/ada/adapage.html
This site explains the mission of the Mid-Atlantic ADA Information Center, one of 10 regional centers set up to provide training, information, and technical assistance, as well as the full text of articles produced by the Center.

Lambda Legal Defense and Education Fund, Inc.
URL: http://www.thebody.com/lambda/lambda.html
This site includes the full text of articles available from the Lambda Legal Defense and Education Fund, a national organization committed

to achieving full recognition of the civil rights of lesbians, gay men, and people with HIV/AIDS through impact litigation, education, and public policy work. The site is available at The Body (http://www.the body.com/index. html).

Usenet Newsgroups

This section includes a selection of Usenet newsgroups maintaining discussions on various aspects of the HIV/AIDS epidemic.

Bionet.molbio.hiv
This newsgroup focuses its discussion on the molecular biology of HIV.

Clari.tw.health.aids
This newsgroup discusses AIDS-related health issues, but is only available if your service provider provides access to the CLARI hierarchy (CLARI is a for-fee hierarchy, so a subscription must be purchased to gain access).

Misc.health.aids
This newsgroup is the only worldwide forum dedicated to a free and open exchange of ideas about AIDS. There are more than 42,000 readers of misc.health.aids worldwide.

Sci.med.aids
This is one of the oldest and most active AIDS-related discussion groups. The CDC's AIDS Daily Summary is posted here, and many current topics are discussed.

Listservs

Following are a few the listservs available on HIV/AIDS-related topics. To find out about other listservs available, visit the LISTZ Directory of E-mail Discussion Groups on the World Wide Web (http://www.liszt.com/). When subscribing to the listservs below, substitute your real first name and last name where the instructions say "firstname lastname."

aids
This is the AIDS mailing-list, which is the same as the sci.med.aids USENET newsgroup. It is a moderated mailing-list/newsgroup.

Questions about the mailing-list may be sent to "owner-aids@wubios. wustl. edu". For information about the list, mail the command "info aids" to Majordomo@wubios.wustl.edu.

AIDS
For information about the AIDS Educators Discussion List, mail the command "info AIDS" to LISTSERV%SIUCVMB.BITNET@UBVM. CC.BUFFALO.EDU.

AIDSBKRV
This listserv disseminates updates to the *AIDS Book Review Journal* on a monthly basis. You can join this group by sending the message "sub AIDSBKRV firstname lastname" to listserv@uicvm.uic. edu.

AIDSNEWS
The CDC National AIDS Clearinghouse maintains this list for individuals who wish to receive AIDS-related documents, including the *AIDS Daily Summary*, a daily news clipping service, and selected *Morbidity and Mortality Weekly Report* articles. The listserv also distributes press releases from other Public Health Service agencies. To subscribe, Internet users should send the message "subscribe aidsnews firstname lastname" to listserv@cdcnac.org.

aidspat
This listserv distributes information about AIDS patents. For information, mail the command "information aidspat" to listserv@vinca. cnidr.org.

aids-stat
This list is a moderated list for the posting of official statistics about the rates of HIV infection and associated conditions such as AIDS. For information, mail the command "info aids-stat" to Majordomo@ wubios.wustl.edu.

aids-treatment-news
This listserv distributes *AIDS Treatment News* twice each month. *AIDS Treatment News* reports on experimental and standard treatments, especially those available now. It includes interviews with physicians, scientists, other health professionals, and persons with HIV/AIDS. It also collects information from meetings and conferences,

medical journals, and computer databases. *AIDS Treatment News* does not recommend particular therapies, but seeks to increase the options available. For information, mail the command "info aids-treatment-news" to Majordomo@igc.apc.org.

ca-aids
This is the discussion list of the AIDS and Anthropology Group. For information, mail the command "info ca-aids" to Majordomo@uva.nl.

caregivers
The purpose of this list is to help caregivers of people with HIV/AIDS support one another in the pressures and problems they encounter. It also includes discussions about death, and the cumulative grief that may build up after more than one death. For more information, mail the command "info caregivers" to Majordomo@QueerNet.ORG.

GAP
GAP is a listserv on HIV prevention and awareness. You can join this group by sending the message "sub GAP firstname lastname" to listserv@listserv.syr.edu.

HEALTH-PR
HEALTH-PR is a listserv for health promotion and disease prevention researchers. The listserv is based in Stockholm, Sweden. You can join this group by sending the message "sub HEALTH-PROMOTION firstname lastname" to listserv@sokrates.mip.ki.se.

HIVPSYCH
This listserv addresses HIV/AIDS psycho-social issues. You can join this group by sending the message "sub HIVPSYCH firstname lastname" to listserv@sjuvm.stjohns.edu.

PANET-L
You can join this medical education and health information discussion group by sending the message "sub PANET-L firstname lastname" to listserv@yalevm.cis.yale.edu.

4ACURE-L
This listserv focuses on possible cures for AIDS. For information about the listserv, mail the command "info 4ACURE-L" to listserv@health. state.ny.us.

Selected Resources for Additional Information

The following is a sampling of the many available publications about the Internet. Resources listed may be found in your local public library or bookstore.

Books

Benson, Allen C. *The Complete Internet Companion for Librarians.* New York: Neal-Schuman, 1994.

Dern, Daniel P. *The Internet Guide for New Users.* New York: McGraw-Hill, 1994.

Falk, Bennett. *The Internet Roadmap.* 2nd edition. Alameda: Sybex, 1994.

Gilster, Paul. *Finding It on the Internet: the Essential Guide to Archie, Veronica, Gopher, WAIS, WWW (including Mosaic), and Other Search and Browsing Tools.* New York: Wiley, 1994.

Hahn, Harley, and Rick Stout. *The Internet Complete Reference.* 3rd edition. Berkeley: Osborne McGraw-Hill, 1994.

Krol, Ed. *The Whole Internet: User's Guide & Catalog.* 2nd edition. Sebastopol, CA: O'Reilly & Associates, 1994.

LaQuey, Tracy L. *The Internet Companion: A Beginner's Guide to Global Networking.* 2nd edition. Reading, MA: Addison-Wesley, 1994.

Pomeroy, Brian. *BeginnerNet: A Beginner's Guide to the Internet and World Wide Web.* Thorofare: Slack, 1996.

Rosenfeld, Louis B., Joseph Janes, and Martha Vander Kolk. *The Internet Compendium: Subject Guides to Health Sciences Resources.* New York: Neal-Schuman, 1994.

Tittel, Ed, and Margaret Robbins. *Internet Access Essentials.* Boston: AP Professional, 1995.

Wiggins, Richard W. *The Internet for Everyone: A Guide for Users and Providers.* New York: McGraw Hill, 1995.

Journals

Computers in Libraries. Westport, CT: Mecklermedia.

Directory of Electronic Journals, Newsletters, and academic Discussion Lists. Washington, DC: Association of Research Libraries, Office of Scientific and Academic Publishing.

The Federal Internet Source: A Directory of Nearly 300 Sources of Government Information on the Internet and How to Find and Use Them. Washington, DC: National Journal, Inc. and NetWeek, Inc.

Gale Guide to Internet Databases. Detroit, MI: Gale Research, Inc.

HealthLink: Global Internet Resources and Databases. Marco Island, FL: M.P. Zillman.

The Internet Directory. New York: Fawcett Columbine.

The Internet Letter. Cabin John, MD: Net Week Inc.

Internet World. Westport, CT: Mecklermedia. (http://www.internet world.com)

NetGuide: The Guide to Online Services and the Internet. Manhasset, NY: CMP Media.

On Internet. Westport CT: Mecklermedia.

Wired. San Francisco, CA: Wired. (http://www.wired. com)

CDC National AIDS Clearinghouse

Internet Services

The CDC National AIDS Clearinghouse (CDC NAC) makes available a variety of Internet services to share HIV/AIDS related information and publications with people and organizations working in prevention, health care, research, and support services. To correspond with the Clearinghouse, send E-mail to aidsinfoecdenac.org

World Wide Web Sites

CDC National AIDS Clearinghouse
http://www.cdcnac.org
The CDC NAC Web site includes the following features:

- The **Internet Order Form** provides an easy-to-use way to order free HIV/AIDS-related materials online. It includes materials for professionals in the field and persons living with HIV/ AIDS, *HIV/AIDS Surveillance Reports*, and general information. Orders will be received by mail within 2-3 weeks.

614

- **QuickTime Movies of the CDC "Respect Yourself, Protect Yourself" Public Service Announcements** make use of the rapidly expanding multimedia capabilities of the Web. The movies and related materials allow quick access to information on the recent CDC campaign targeting youth.

- The *AIDS Daily Summary* provides summaries of AIDS-related articles from major newspapers and journals. It helps people keep up-to-date on HIV/AIDS prevention, treatment, and care issues. The *AIDS Daily Summary* can be obtained in a couple of ways: visit the Web site daily to read the new summary, or sign up to receive the *AIDS Daily Summary* directly via E-mail through the AIDSNEWS listserv.

HIV/AIDS Treatment Information Service (ATIS)
http://www.hivatis.org
The HIV/AIDS Treatment Information Service Web site provides information on federally approved treatments for HIV infection, treatment-related publications, and links to other treatment-related sites. ATIS is a Public Health Service coordinated project.

AIDS Clinical Trials Information Service (ACTIS)
http://www.actis.org
The AIDS Clinical Trials Information Service Web site provides information on HIV/AIDS clinical trials, including new trials open to enrollment, trial results, and links to other related sites. ACTIS is a Public Health Service coordinated project.

AIDSNEWS Listserv
listserv@cdcnac.org
CDC NAC maintains a list for individuals who wish to receive AIDS-related documents, including the *AIDS Daily Summary*, selected *Morbidity and Mortality Weekly Report* articles, and fact sheets. The listserv also distributes press releases from other Public Health Service agencies such as NIH and the Food and Drug Administration. To subscribe, Internet users should send the message

    subscribe aidsnews firstname lastname

to the address above, where your real first and last names are substituted for firstname and lastname. Anyone with E-mail access to the Internet, including members of networks such as America Online and CompuServe, can subscribe to the AIDSNEWS Listserv.

615

Anonymous File Transfer Protocol (FTP) Site

ftp://ftp.cdcnac.org

The Clearinghouse's anonymous FTP site contains files of documents such as the current *HIV/AIDS Surveillance Report*, Agency for Health Care Policy and Research's (AHCPR) clinical practice guidelines, Clearinghouse guides to AIDS information, and the Clearinghouse's Standard Search Series.

Questions?

Call 1-800-458-5231 or send E-mail to aidsinfo@cdcnac.org

National Library of Medicine (NLM) Internet-Accessible Resources

Introduction

NLM provides many services to the biomedical library community using the capabilities of the Internet. Internet users can reach these services through basic Internet processes, such as telnet and ftp (file transfer protocol), or through software clients such as Gopher for Gopher servers and Mosaic, Netscape, or other browsers for World Wide Web servers. This fact section describes the services that NLM makes available over the Internet.

World Wide Web (WWW) Servers

NLM provides documents and access to many services through its World Wide Web servers. Users must have a Web client, such as Mosaic (available for Unix, Macintosh, and MS Windows), Netscape, or MacWeb. The WWW allows NLM to distribute information in a publication-look format and to include hypertext links to documents, photographs, sound files, video clips, and online telnet sessions. There is no charge for most services.

NLM's Home Page, called HyperDOC, (http://www.nlm.nih.gov) provides information about Library programs, connections to NLM online services, and links to specialized NLM Web servers such as the Educational Technology Branch (ETB) World Wide Web server (http://wwwetb.nlm.nih.gov/). The ETB Web server has information about computer and multimedia technologies related to health professions education. The National Center for Biotechnology Information (NCBI) also has a Web server (http://www.ncbi.nlm.nih.gov/) that provides information about the GenBank® DNA sequence database. It also provides

GenBank searching, and information about other DNA and protein databases. Scientists can submit sequences directly to GenBank on the Web with a submission tool called BankIt.

Anonymous FTP Servers

NLM distributes many publications and software programs via anonymous ftp (ftp://nlmpubs.nlm.nih.gov/). NLM publications including fact sheets, bibliographies, AIDS information, and newsletters are available. The publications server provides many documents in both ASCII text and PostScript formats. These two formats allow users to select either plain text files that contain all the textual information or a PostScript file that allows printing the publication in its original format. Some files are also available in WordPerfect format. Users with only e-mail access to the Internet may obtain publications from the anonymous ftp server. Sending a message to mailserv@ nlm.nih.gov with only the word help in the message body will return basic instructions on this process. NCBI also has an anonymous ftp site (ftp://ncbi.nlm.nih.gov/). Through this service, NCBI makes available GenBank and other sequence databases, submission software, Entrez software, and documentation.

HSTAT

HSTAT (Health Services/Technology Assessment Texts) is a free, electronic resource that provides access to the full text of clinical practice guidelines and other documents useful in health care decision making. HSTAT is available via the NLM Full-Text Retrieval System (FTRS) which provides a menu-driven interface to the text. The FTRS can be accessed through telnet to text.nlm.nih.gov and login as hstat or HSTAT. The HSTAT resource is available via anonymous ftp (nlmpubs.nim.nih.gov in the /hstat directory) and on the NLM Gopher (gopher:// gopher.nim.nih.gov/) and the NLM HyperDOC Home Page (http://www.nlm.nih.gov/ and select NLM Online Information Services, then HSTAT).

Locator

NLM Locator is a client-server interface that allows menu-driven Internet access to NLM's CATLINE® (cataloged records of monographs and serials), AVLINE® (audiovisuals), and SERLINE® (serials owned by NLM and other libraries). NLM designed Locator for novice or infrequent users to access the files representing the NLM collection. The interface requires no training and allows searching these files without learning NLM's interactive command-driven search interface. To access Locator, use VTI00 emulation and telnet to locator.nlm.nih.gov, login as locator.

Services Available Via Telnet

Many of NLM's established services are available over the Internet through telnet. These services include MEDLARS, TOXNET, and DOCLINE. The MEDLARS system includes MEDLINE® and other biomedical databases covering AIDS, bioethics, cancer, chemicals, organizations, health planning and administration, history of medicine, population information, and toxicology. Individuals with accounts may telnet to medlars.nlm.nih.gov. The TOXNET system and its various databases are part of the MEDLARS system. Individuals with MEDLARS accounts may telnet to medlars.nim.nih.gov. A FILE TOXNET command will take users via the gateway into TOXNET databases. DOCLINE is NLM's automated interlibrary loan request and referral system for biomedical libraries. Registered libraries may telnet to DOCLINE at medlars.nlm.nih.gov.

Summary

NLM provides many services via the Internet. The easiest way for new Internet users to learn more about NLM and its Internet services is to use a tool such a World Wide Web browser. Using this software, users may explore the various documents and services which are available. For further information, contact NLM program areas by e-mail.

NLM E-mail addresses (Internet)
Office of Public Information
publicinfo@occshost.nlm.nih.gov

Anonymous ftp service
ftpadmin@nlmpubs.nlm.nih.gov

Grateful Med assistance
gmhelp@gmedserv.nlm.nih.gov

Gopher services
admin@gopher.nlm.nih.gov

History of Medicine Division
hmdref@nlm.nih.gov

Interlibrary Loan/DOCLINE
ill@nlm.nih.gov

International Programs Office
hsieh@nlm.nih.gov

Mailserv service
admin@mailserv.nim.nih.gov

MEDLARS Management Section
mms@nlm.nih.gov

MeSH® vocabulary suggestions
meshsugg@nlm.nih.gov

National Center for Biotechnology Information (NCBI)
info@ncbi.nlm.nih.gov

National Information Center on Health Services Research and Health
Care Technology
nichsr@nlm.nih.gov

Online Images from the History of Medicine
oli@nlm.nih.gov

Planning and Evaluation Office
siegel@nlm.nih.gov

Preservation information
pres@nlm.nih.gov

Reference assistance
ref@nlm.nih.gov

Technical services assistance
tsd@nlm.nih.gov

Toxicology and Environmental Health Information Program
tehip@teh.nlm.nih.gov

Chapter 62

National Organizations Providing HIV/AIDS Services

Introduction

National Organizations Providing HIV/AIDS Services: A Directory For Community-Based Organizations provides quick access to information on selected national HIV/AIDS service organizations located in the United States and Puerto Rico. This revised 1997 edition includes the most up-to-date information from the CDC National AIDS Clearinghouse Resources and Services Database on many of the organizations that were listed in the previous editions, as well as additional organizations.

Organizations are grouped alphabetically within seven categories: Epidemiology, Housing, Policy and Legal Issues, Prevention, Services for the Incarcerated, Support Services, Technical Assistance, and Treatment.

The Clearinghouse constantly adds new entries and updates the existing information in its databases. To obtain the most current information, to order a free Clearinghouse catalog of publications, or to ask specific questions about HIV/AIDS, please contact the CDC NAC Reference Service:

- 1-800-458-5231 (Voice)
- 1-800-243-7012 (TTY)
- 1-888-282-7681 (Fax)
- e-mail: info@cdcpin.org

Excerpted from *National Organizations Providing HIV/AIDS Services: A Directory For Community-Based Organizations*, CDC National AIDS Clearinghouse, September 1997; verified and updated in October 1998.

Other Reference Services

All of the HIV/AIDS reference services operate Monday–Friday from 9:00 a.m. to 7:00 p.m., EST. All calls are completely confidential. Spanish- and English-speaking reference specialists are available for the following specialized services operated by CDC NAC:

AIDS Clinical Trials Information Service (ACTIS) 1-800-874-2572

Provides up-to-date information on clinical trials that evaluate experimental drugs and other therapies for adults and children at all stages of HIV infection. ACTIS is sponsored by the Centers for Disease Control and Prevention, the Food and Drug Administration, the National Institute of Allergy and Infectious Diseases, and the National Library of Medicine.

HIV/AIDS Treatment Information Service (ATIS) 1-800-448-0440

Provides information about federally approved treatment guidelines for HIV and AIDS to healthcare providers and people living with HIV infection. ATIS is sponsored by Agency for Health Care Policy and Research, Centers for Disease Control and Prevention, Health Resources and Services Administration, Indian Health Service, National Institutes of Health, and Substance Abuse and Mental Health Services Administration.

CDC Business and Labor Resource Service (BLRS) 1-800-458-5231

Is a centralized information and referral service that links the business and labor communities with resources for developing HIV/AIDS in the workplace programs.

Electronic Information Dissemination

NAC FAX. NAC FAX is a service of the CDC National AIDS Clearinghouse through which you can obtain information directly via your fax machine. Selected documents, including CDC fact sheets, HIV/AIDS Surveillance Reports, and information on Clearinghouse services are available free through the service. NAC FAX is available 24 hours a day, 7 days a week at 1-800-458-5231.

Internet Services. The Clearinghouse has a World Wide Web site located at www.cdcnac.org.

Epidemiology

Rockefeller Archive Center
15 Dayton Ave.
Pocantico Hills
Sleepy Hollow, NY 10591
(914) 631-4505
(914) 631-6017 (Fax)
Website: http://www.rockefeller.edu/archive.ctr/
E-mail: archive@rockvax.rockefeller.edu

The Rockefeller Archive Center was created in 1974 to assemble, process, and make available for scholarly research the archival collections of members of the Rockefeller family and of various educational institutions. Major subjects researched at the Center include education, international relations, medicine, population, and women's history. The Center sponsors seminars and conferences on research topics and issues two annual publications containing information about medical research and public health, including epidemiological information on public health and models of diseases such as HIV/AIDS. A newsletter is produced annually.

U.S. Department of Health and Human Services
Public Health Service
Centers for Disease Control and Prevention (CDC)
Division of HIV/AIDS Prevention
Technical Information Activity (TIA)
1600 Clifton Rd., NE, #E-49
Atlanta, GA 30333
(404) 639-3311
(404) 332-4559 (Travel requirements—recorded message)
(404) 639-2007 (Fax)
Website: http://www.cdc.gov

The Centers for Disease Control and Prevention (CDC), Division of HIV/AIDS Prevention, Technical Information Activity (TIA) provides scientific, statistical, and programmatic information to other centers, institutes, and organizations of the CDC; staff of other federal agencies; health care professionals; public health officials; and, through contractual services provided by outside agencies, to the general public. It also produces recommendations and guidelines on the, prevention of transmission of HIV.

U.S. Department of Health and Human Services

Public Health Service
Centers for Disease Control and Prevention (CDC)
National Center for Health Statistics (NCHS)
6525 Belcrest Rd.
Hyattsville, MD 20782
(301) 436-8500
Website: http://www.cdc.gov/nchs
E-mail: nchsquery@cec.gov

The Centers for Disease Control and Prevention (CDC), National Center for Health Statistics (NCHS) is the federal government's principal vital and health statistics agency. It produces data on morbidity and mortality, utilization of health services, behaviors and practices related to HIV transmission, and the public's knowledge and attitudes on HIV/AIDS. From its many data systems, NCHS has produced an estimate of the prevalence of HIV infection in the general, household-based population; estimates of the hospital, ambulatory, and long-term care associated with AIDS; statistics on knowledge and attitudes about AIDS, including HIV transmission; and measures of changes in behavior in response to AIDS. Deaths from AIDS are tracked through the NCHS vital statistics system and reported on a monthly and annual basis. NCHS data are presented in publications and are also available on data tape, CD-ROM, and diskette. NCHS also offers catalogs of publications and electronic products, information on data availability, and assistance in locating and using NCHS data. A library is available and referrals are provided.

U.S. Department of Justice

Office of Justice Programs, Bureau of Justice Statistics
Corrections Unit
Quinquennial Prison Census
810 Seventh St., NW
Washington, DC 20531
(202) 307-0703
Website: http://www.ojp.usdoj.gov
E-mail: askocpa@ojp.usdoj.gov

The U.S. Department of Justice, Corrections Unit, Quinquennial Prison Census collects information relating to the number of deaths among inmates that are attributed to AIDS or AIDS-related diseases. The data collection consists of the Quinquennial Prison Census and

Quinquennial Census of State and Federal Adult Correctional Facilities and Census of Jails. The 1991 Census of Probation and Parole Agencies collected information on AIDS-related agency policies and on the number of AIDS cases among adult and juvenile clients. The annual National Prisoner Statistics' Summary of Sentenced Population Movement provides information on state and federal agency policies and on the number of inmates with confirmed AIDS or who were HIV-positive at year end. Quinquennial surveys of inmates provide information on HIV testing and prevalence through inmate self-reports. Brochures are produced and disseminated.

Housing

AIDS Housing of Washington (AHW)
2025 1ˢᵗ Ave., Suite 420
Seattle, WA 98121
(206) 448-5242
(206) 441-9485 (Fax)
Website: http://www.aidshousing.org

AIDS Housing of Washington (AHW), founded in 1988, addresses the housing needs of persons living with HIV/AIDS (PLWAs). AHW's National Technical Assistance Program was initiated in 1991 in response to the numerous requests for information and assistance from providers and developers across the country. AHW offers technical assistance in the areas of HIV/AIDS housing planning, development, operations, and policy. AHW staff provide technical assistance to individuals and agencies around the country to develop long-range plans for HIV/AIDS housing and the coordination of Ryan White CARE Act and Housing Opportunities for People with AIDS (HOPWA) funds. In support of the Technical Assistance Program and the benefit of sharing information among AIDS housing professionals, AHW maintains a comprehensive database of HIV/AIDS housing providers in the country. AHW also hosts the National HIV/AIDS Housing Conference. Manuals on developing HIV/AIDS care residences are also available.

National Alliance to End Homelessness
1518 K St., NW, Suite 206
Washington, DC 20005
(202) 638-1526
(202) 638-4664 (Fax)
Website: http:/www.endhomelessness.org

The National Alliance to End Homelessness works to increase the capacity of programs that provide housing for persons living with AIDS (PLWAs). It also disseminates information related to successful housing programs and how others may improve. Workshops and a database of resources are provided. Financial aid and housing referrals are available. Brochures and a speakers' bureau are also provided.

Policy and Legal Issues

AIDS Action Council (AAC)

1875 Connecticut Ave., NW, Suite 700
Washington, DC 20009
(202) 986-1300
(202) 986-1345 (Fax)

The AIDS Action Council (AAC) was established in 1984 by AIDS service providers nationwide to address AIDS public policy issues. The Council represents community-based service organizations serving persons living with HIV/AIDS (PLWAs) and is a nationally recognized organization whose role is to work with the federal government to develop a comprehensive response on AIDS research and policy issues. The organization encourages biomedical research on AIDS; expedites treatment therapies; implements medical, legal, and social policies; ensures access to care for the ill; develops reimbursement programs to share the expenses caused by HIV infection; and informs community service agencies of the federal government response to AIDS. AAC provides financial assistance to organizations working with AIDS policy issues. AAC also administers the Pedro Zamora Fund which is dedicated to educating the public about HIV prevention

AIDS Coalition To Unleash Power (ACT-UP)

332 Bleeker St., Suite G5
New York, NY 10014
(212) 966-4873 (Fax)
Website: http://www.actupny.org/
E-mail: actupny@panix.com

The AIDS Coalition to Unleash Power (ACT-UP) is a diverse, nonpartisan group of individuals committed to direct action to end the HIV epidemic. It focuses on the politics and public policy issues of the HIV epidemic. The Pediatric Committee focuses on self-empowerment of parents and HIV-positive children. The Women's Committee concentrates on services specifically for women. Real Treatments for Real People, a working group of ACT-UP, aims to jump start research on promising HIV/AIDS treatments currently in use and suggests that NIH fund studies for drugs approved for non-AIDS conditions, including drugs whose patents have expired, drugs developed outside the U.S., and alternative therapies.

Alan Guttmacher Institute (AGI)
1120 Connecticut Ave., NW, Suite 460
Washington, DC 20036-3902
(202) 296-4012
(202) 223-5756 (Fax)
Website: http://www.agi-usa.org
E-mail: policyinfo2agi-usa.org

The Alan Guttmacher Institute (AGI) is an independent, non-profit corporation for research, policy analysis, and public education in the field of women's reproductive health. AGI assists in the development of sound public policy in HIV prevention and is particularly interested in the role that family planning organizations play in HIV prevention and service strategies. All policy issues are handled out of this office; research activities are conducted out of the New York office.

American Association of Naturopathic Physicians (AANP)
601 Valley St., Suite 105
Seattle, WA 98109
(206) 298-0126
(206) 298-0125 (Reference line)
(206) 298-0129 (Fax)
Website: http://www.aanp.com

The American Association of Naturopathic Physicians (AANP) is an association of general physicians who are trained as specialists in natural medicine. They treat disease and restore health using botanical medicine, Oriental medicine, herbal medicine, homeopathy, physical medicine, exercise therapy, counseling, and acupuncture. AANP lobbies to increase the place of naturopathic medicine on the national health care agenda, supports constituent associations in their efforts to obtain licensing, and promotes research agendas among federally recognized colleges. It acts as a national referral service, provides assistance in obtaining reimbursement for treatment, and publishes education and resource materials.

American Bar Association (ABA)
AIDS Coordination Project
740 15th St., NW
Washington, DC 20005-1009
(202) 662-1025
(202) 662-1032 (Fax)
E-mail: aidsproject@attmaii.com

The American Bar Association (ABA), AIDS Coordination Project, provides technical support to attorneys and judges. It has developed a training course, manual, and video titled Creating a Pro-Bono Project for People with AIDS. Another resource available to judges is the AIDS Bench Book, which summarizes cases relating to HIV/AIDS. Legal assistance services are available for attorneys. A legal referral directory is also available.

American Civil Liberties Union (ACLU)
National Prison Project (NPP)
1875 Connecticut Ave., NW, Suite 410
Washington, DC 20009
(202) 234-4830
(202) 234-4890 (Fax)
Website: http://www.npp.org

The American Civil Liberties Union (ACLU), Aids Project is dedicated to the preservation of the particular liberties guaranteed inmates by the Constitution and is primarily concerned with the Constitution's ban on cruel and unusual punishment. The National Prison Project's primary work is in litigation and supporting others to negotiate and litigate civil rights cases on behalf of offenders. The AIDS in Prison Project serves as a resource center to provide educational and advocacy assistance regarding HIV/AIDS in correctional facilities. The project maintains a wide range of articles, including studies done on prisoners with HIV/AIDS, statistics, problems within correctional facilities, and policies. The project assists HIV/AIDS correctional support groups and peer education programs, and maintains a list of referrals for inmates, their families and friends, and HIV/AIDS service organizations.

American Counseling Association (ACA)
5999 Stevenson Ave.
Alexandria, VA 22304
P.O. Box 531
Annapolis Junction, MD 20701-0531
(703) 823-9800
(800) 347-6647 (Hotline, National)
(703) 604-0158 (Fax)
Website: http: //www. counseling. org

The American Counseling Association (ACA) is a private, nonprofit organization for the counseling and human development professions. Founded in 1952, the Association has more than 58,000 members in the U.S. and in 50 foreign countries. The organization helps to set professional and ethical standards for the counseling profession. Its Office on Government Relations lobbies on legislation at the federal level and addresses the health and mental health care needs of persons living with HIV/AIDS (PLWAs), their families, friends, and significant others. ACA also provides ongoing continuing educational programs and publications, including a newsletter, that may include information on AIDS and AIDS-related issues for its members.

American Foundation for AIDS Research (AmFAR)
Public Policy Office
120 Wall Street, 13th Floor
New York, NY 10005
(212) 806-1600
(212) 806-1601 (Fax)

The American Foundation for AIDS Research (AmFAR), Public Policy Office is a national nonprofit public foundation fighting AIDS through grant-making programs in biomedical and clinical research, education for HIV prevention, and public policy development. The Washington, DC, office of AMFAR concentrates on public policy development and makes policy recommendations. The AMFAR Public Policy office monitors government activities regarding the HIV/AIDS epidemic, not only in terms of government funding, but also through laws that affect persons living with HIV/AIDS (PLWAs) or the work of caregivers and researchers. AMFAR encourages Congress to boost funding for AIDS research, education, and care; defends the rights and dignity of all PLWAs; helps draft and pass legislation; and fights discrimination and inappropriate AIDS policies. AMFAR publications include a directory, information software, bilingual handbooks, and a newsletter.

American Immigration Lawyers Association (AILA)
1400 I St., NW, Suite 1200
Washington, DC 20005
(202) 216-2400
(202) 371-9449 (Fax)

American Immigration Lawyers Association (AILA) provides legal assistance and referrals to persons living with HIV/AIDS (PLWAs), especially recent immigrants and undocumented aliens. A newsletter and educational materials are also distributed.

American Nurses Association (ANA)
600 Maryland Ave., SW, Suite 100
West Washington, DC 20024-2571
(202) 651-7000
(800) 242-4ANA
(202) 651-7001 (Fax)
Website: http://www.ana.org

The American Nurses Association (ANA) is a member association representing registered nurses. It has issued a nondiscriminatory position statement regarding the treatment of persons living with HIV/AIDS (PLWAs), and also supports early testing of experimental medications. ANA supports legislation on increased funding for AIDS education and research, offers speakers' bureaus and educational services for nurses, and provides educational materials. A National Action Agenda focuses on practice, research, education, and policy.

American Psychological Association (APA)
Public Interest Directorate, Office on AIDS
750 1st St., NE
Washington, DC 20002-4242
(202) 336-5500
Website: http://www.apa.org
E-mail: publicinterest@apa.org

The American Psychological Association (APA), Public Interest Directorate, Office on AIDS, provides training on the social and psychosocial aspects of AIDS through multimedia interactive workshops (HOPE Program) to health and mental health care professionals.

These workshops are intended for professionals within community-based organizations, including hospices and clinics, who are involved in counseling persons living with HIV/AIDS (PLWAs). The APA Committee on Psychology and AIDS (COPA) offers a mental health AIDS training resource directory, a directory of educational materials on the neuropsychiatric complications of AIDS, and a training film. COPA develops AIDS-related policies, fosters the development of potential AIDS mental health services, and encourages seroprevalence studies in psychiatric hospitals. It also disseminates information regarding psychology and AIDS and provides leadership in survey methodology and evaluation research. A speakers' bureau and referrals to physicians and mental health services are available.

American Society of Law, Medicine, and Ethics (ASLME)
765 Commonwealth Ave., Suite 1634
Boston, MA 02215
(617) 262-4990
(617) 437-7596 (Fax)
Website: http://www.aslme.org

The American Society of Law, Medicine, and Ethics (ASLME) is concerned with health policy, law, and ethics in the AIDS epidemic. Educational conferences are scheduled on a regular basis on such topics as ethics and health law in relation to nursing homes, the elderly, and women's reproductive health and AIDS.

Asian and Pacific Islander American Health Forum (APIAHF)
Empowerment through Training and Technical Assistance Program
942 Market St., Suite 200
San Francisco, CA 94102
(415) 954-9959
(415) 954-9999 (Fax)

The Asian and Pacific Islander American Health Forum (APIAHF) is a national advocacy organization that lobbies government agencies' and collaborates with other organizations for improvement in the health status of Asian and Pacific Islander (API) Americans. The Empowerment Through Training and Technical Assistance Program (ETTA) provides technical assistance to API organizations in responding to HIV/AIDS and STDs. ETTA works with other API community organizations in the areas of program development, fundraising, administration, and

631

improvement of available technologies. APIAHF also produces a news-letter and educational materials targeting Asian and Pacific Islander populations.

Center for Women Policy Studies (CWPS)
National Resource Center on Women and AIDS Policy
1211 Connecticut Ave., NW, Suite 312
Washington, DC 20036
(202) 872-1770
(202) 296-8962 (Fax)

The Center for Women Policy Studies (CWPS) established the National Resource Center on Women and AIDS in 1987 to serve as a centralized resource for researchers, policymakers, advocates, and caregivers. The Center has taken leadership on a range of AIDS policy issues affecting women, working closely with members of Congress and community leaders. It is the principal national, nongovernmental policy and advocacy organization addressing AIDS issues from women's perspectives, with attention to the self-defined needs of women of color.

Children's Defense Fund (CDF)
25 E St., NW
Washington, DC 20001
(202) 628-8787
(202) 662-3560 (Fax)
http://www.childrensdefense.org
E-mail: cdinfo@childrensdefense.org

The Children's Defense Fund (CDF) is an advocacy and research group that lobbies for children's health issues. CDF publishes an annual report on maternal and child health titled Health of America's Children, which includes data on pediatric AIDS. A newsletter is produced quarterly.

Gay Men's Health Crisis (GMHC)
119 W 24th St.
New York, NY 10011
(212) 807-6664
Website: http://www.gmhc.org

Gay Men's Health Crisis (GMHC), founded in 1981, is a community-based, volunteer-supported, AIDS service organization. It has a three-fold mission: to provide support services to persons living with HIV/

AIDS (PLWAs), and their caregivers; to educate the general public, individuals at risk for HIV infection, and health care professionals about AIDS; and to advocate for fair and effective AIDS public policy. GMHC offers pediatric referrals, legal services, financial services, support groups, buddies, crisis intervention counseling, housing referrals, and recreational programs. It maintains an ombudsman unit. Financial services consist of grants to individuals, tokens for transportation, and referrals for further assistance. The nutrition counseling program offers a free monthly public nutrition forum that focuses on the nutritional needs of PLWAs. The forums emphasize food and water safety, the role of exercise, and vitamin and mineral supplementation. GMHC publishes a variety of educational materials on HIV/AIDS, developments in the field, and safer sex practices. It manages a speakers' bureau and sponsors meetings and forums, which include seminars and discussion groups to reinforce the safer sex practices of gay and bisexual men. GMHC's AIDS Treatment Library gives clients access to Medline.

Harvard AIDS Institute

651 Huntington Ave.
Boston, MA 02115
(617) 432-4400
(617) 432-4545 (Fax)
Website: http://www.hsph.harvard.edu/hai.html
E-mail: hai@hsph.harvard.edu

The Harvard AIDS Institute is a university-wide organization whose mission is fourfold: to promote research that enhances understanding of HIV prevention, transmission, diagnosis, and treatment; to advance AIDS education on local, national, and international levels; to provide multidisciplinary AIDS training to scientists and clinicians throughout the world; and to stimulate the development of policies and solutions that benefit those affected by the HIV epidemic. The Institute works to advance AIDS education through speakers' bureaus, conferences, publications, and programs. The Program for AIDS Clinical Research Training provides physician investigators with broad training in quantitative research methodologies. The Fogarty International Training Program in AIDS-Related Epidemiology prepares biomedical researchers and health care workers from developing countries to promote AIDS research in their own countries. The U.S. Medical Students' AIDS Training Program enables interested minority graduate professional school students to pursue careers in research.

Hemlock Society USA
P.O. Box 101810
Denver, CO 80250-1810
(303) 639-1202
(800) 247-7421
(303) 639-1224 (Fax)
Website: http://www.hemlock.org/hemlock

The Hemlock Society USA, founded in 1980, is a nonprofit educational and research organization that believes terminally ill people should have the right to self-determination for all end-of-life decisions. The Hemlock Society U.S.A. reveres life and believes dying people must be able to retain their dignity, integrity, and self-respect. The Society does not encourage suicide for emotional, traumatic, or financial reasons in the absence of terminal illnesses. It supports the work of those involved in suicide prevention programs and encourages, through a program of education and research, public acceptance of voluntary physician aid-in-dying for people with terminal illnesses. It offers a clearinghouse of information regarding legislation, court cases, and other legal activity relative to physician aid-in-dying. Members are encouraged to initiate and participate in local political processes to further the mission of Hemlock. It publishes a newsletter, brochures, and books to help persons decide the manner and means of their deaths. National conferences and speakers are dedicated to right-to-die and death-with-dignity issues each year.

Human Rights Campaign (HRC)
919 18th St., NW
Washington, DC 20006
(202) 628-4160
(202) 347-5323 (Fax)
Website: http://www.hrc.org
E-mail: hrc@hrc.org

The Human Rights Campaign (HRC) is a lesbian and gay political organization that works to end discrimination, secure equal rights, and protect the health and safety of all Americans. With a staff of volunteers, and members throughout the country, HRC lobbies the federal government on lesbian, gay, and health issues, including AIDS-related issues; educates the general public; participates in election campaigns; organizes volunteers; and provides expertise and training at the state and local levels. Through political contributions, lobbying, and grassroots activities, HRC works to ensure that the federal government is committed to HIV/AIDS research, prevention treatment, and care. HRC operates outreach and education programs and posts action alerts, congressional voting, and other information on the Internet. A newsletter is produced quarterly.

International Association of Physicians in AIDS Care (IAPAC)
225 W. Washington St., Suite 2200
Chicago, IL 60606
(312) 419-7074
(312) 419-7160 (Fax)
Website: http://www.iapac.org
E-mail: iapac@iapac.org

The International Association of Physicians in AIDS Care (IAPAC) is a nonprofit organization of 7,000 physicians in 41 countries concerned with the impact of HIV infection on medical practice, society, and the resources necessary to care for patients, their families, and friends. IAPAC is interdisciplinary, providing opportunities to formulate policy for various affiliated health care professionals, patient groups, insurers, and others concerned about the HIV epidemic. IAPAC also publishes a monthly news journal, which addresses the clinical, social, ethical, and financial dimensions of the HIV epidemic.

International Center for Research on Women (ICRW)
1717 Massachusetts Ave., NW, Suite 302
Washington, DC 20036
(202) 797-0007
(202) 797-0020 (Fax)
Website: http://www.icrw.org
E-mail: icrw@igc.apc.org

The International Center for Research on Women (ICRW), established in 1976, is dedicated to promoting women's full participation in social and economic development. ICRW works in collaboration with policy makers, practitioners, and researchers throughout Africa, Asia, and Latin America in formulating policy and actions concerning the economic, social, and health status of women in developing countries, women's critical contributions to development, and policy and program features that can improve the situation of poor women. The first phase of the Women and AIDS Research Program was initiated in 1990 with support from the Offices of Health and Women in Development of the U.S. Agency for International Development (USAID). Its objective is to support research in developing countries and to identify the behavioral, sociocultural, and economic factors that influence women's vulnerability to HIV infection. It also seeks to identify opportunities for intervention to reduce women's risk of HIV infection. It focuses on rural and urban communities, school-based and nonschool-based adolescents, and traditional women's associations. The second phase of the program, started in 1993, includes design, implementation, and evaluation of interventions. Research findings are available.

National Alliance of State and Territorial AIDS Directors (NASTAD)
444 N. Capitol St., NW, Suite 339
Washington, DC 20009
(202) 434-8090
(202) 434-8092 (Fax)
Website: http://www.nastad.org

The National Alliance of State and Territorial AIDS Directors (NASTAD) was formed in 1992 to promote a more effective national, state, and local response to the AIDS epidemic; to prevent the occurrence of HIV infection; and to ensure access to comprehensive care to persons living with HIV/AIDS (PLWAs). NASTAD represents HIV/AIDS program managers in each U.S. state and territory. NASTAD members are responsible for administering AIDS health care, prevention, education, and supportive service programs, including those funded under Title II of the Ryan White CARE Act. As one of the national partners funded by the Centers for Disease Control and Prevention (CDC), NASTAD began the Technical Assistance (TA) Project to identify and provide technical assistance and information exchange to increase the capacity of state health departments and HIV community planning groups to carry out social marketing activities related to HIV prevention. A newsletter is produced monthly.

National Association of Community Health Centers (NACHC)
1330 New Hampshire Ave., Suite 122 NW
Washington, DC 20036
(202) 659-8008
(202) 659-8519 (Fax)
Website: http://www.nachc.com
E-mail: nachc@erols.com

The National Association of Community Health Centers (NACHC) is the trade association for the nation's community health centers, migrant health centers, and health care for the homeless projects. These clinics receive Federal Health Center funding to provide comprehensive primary care in medically underserved rural and urban communities nationwide. NACHC provides training to centers on funding and program development. It also educates health policymakers on the effectiveness of the Community Health Center model and works for increased attention to resources for meeting the health care needs of underserved communities.

National Association of Protection and Advocacy Systems (NAPAS)

900 2nd St. NE, Suite 211
Washington, DC 20002
(202) 408-9514
(202) 489-9521 (TTY)
(202) 408-9520 (Fax)
Website: http://www. protectionandadvocacy.com
E-mail: napas@earthlink.net

The National Association of Protection and Advocacy Systems (NAPAS), established in 1989, aims to further the human, civil, and legal rights of persons with disabilities; advance the interests of member organizations and enhance their capacity to provide optimal advocacy services; and facilitate coordination and mutual support among member organizations. Since 1989, NAPAS has served as a clearinghouse on AIDS for its 80 member agencies representing the physically and mentally disabled nationwide. The project strives to develop links and information exchanges between state protection and advocacy systems and community-based AIDS organizations, as well as to produce a community training manual. In addition, publications, such as technical report updates on pertinent legal, service, and policy issues, are available.

National Center for Lesbian Rights (NCLR)

870 Market St., Suite 570
San Francisco, CA 94102
(415) 392-6257
(800) 528-6257
(415) 392-8442 (Fax)
Website: http://www.nclrights.org

The National Center for Lesbian Rights (NCLR), a public interest law firm, advocates on behalf of the rights of lesbians, gay men, and their families. It also provides legal assistance and litigation services, makes referrals, and undertakes community education and information dissemination. Other services include workshops and forums across the country and technical assistance to lawyers. Referrals to HIV-antibody testing are available.

National Conference of State Legislatures (NCSL)
1560 Broadway, Suite 700
Denver, CO 80202-5140
(303) 830-2200
(303) 863-8003 (Fax)
Website: http://www.ncsl.org

The National Conference of State Legislatures (NCSL) serves the legislators of the nation's 50 states, commonwealths, and territories, and was created to improve the quality and effectiveness of legislatures to assure a strong voice in the federal system. All state legislators become members of the NCSL upon election. The NCSL has an ongoing project to provide information services on HIV prevention and adolescent health issues to state legislatures through an information clearinghouse, publications, conferences, and presentations at NCSL meetings. This initiative derives from the perception that legislators play a key role in the appropriation of funds and the development of state programs for HIV risk reduction, education, and other services. In September 1996, the Intergovernmental Health Policy Project (IHPP) was transferred from the George Washington University to NCSL. (See below)

National Conference of State Legislatures
Intergovernmental Health Policy Project (IHPP)
444 N. Capitol St., NW
Washington, DC 20001
(202) 624-5400
(202) 737-1069 (Fax)
Website: http://www.ncsl.org

The National Conference of State Legislatures, Intergovernmental Health Policy Project (IHPP), researches the health laws and programs of individual states and provides information on recent laws and changes to state and local officials who formulate public policy on health care reform and health insurance issues. The IHPP also provides information on innovative state programs to federal officials, and maintains a legislative clearinghouse with files on proposed and recently enacted health legislation. In addition to its regular publications, IHPP also publishes research monographs, maintains files on health reports that are produced by the individual states, and conducts conferences on selected health topics. It also produces materials that can be used in workplace programs. In September 1996, IHPP joined with the National Conference of State Legislatures (NCSL) (see above) to greatly expand the capacity for state health policy research. IHPP is no longer affiliated with the George Washington University, and IHPP's Legislative Tracking Service has been renamed the Health Policy Tracking Service.

National Council of La Raza (NCLR)
1111 19th St., NW, Suite 1000
Washington, DC 20036
(202) 785-1670
(202) 776-1792 (Fax)
Website: http://www.nclr.org

The National Council of La Raza (NCLR) exists to improve life opportunities for Americans of Hispanic descent. It was incorporated in 1968 in Arizona as a nonprofit, tax-exempt organization, and serves as a national umbrella organization for more than 180 affiliates. It undertakes applied research, policy analysis, and advocacy on behalf of the needs of the entire Hispanic community. Policy analysis is provided for education, language issues, poverty, immigration, employment and training, civil rights enforcement, the elderly, housing and community development, and health. NCLR Center for Health Promotion houses the HIV/STD/TB Prevention Project and the Hispanic Immigration Program. The HIV/STD/TB Prevention Project serves as an information clearinghouse and source of training for NCLR affiliates and other groups committed to HIV/STD and TB Prevention and education. Its work has become the catalyst for broader NCLR involvement in health education, prevention., and promotion efforts.

National Gay and Lesbian Task Force (NGLTF)
2320 17th St., NW
Washington, DC 20009-2702
(202) 332-6483
(202) 332-6219 (TTY)
(202) 332-0207 (Fax)
Website: http://www.ngltf.org

The National Gay and Lesbian Task Force (NGLTF) is divided into four components: lobbying, organizing, education, and action. NGLTF works with Congress, the executive branch, and the full range of nongovernmental professional, religious, and advocacy groups in lobbying for general gay and lesbian rights issues and AIDS rights issues. Issues include increased federal funding for AIDS, protection against discrimination for persons living with AIDS (PLWAs), and increased AIDS education. The other three components of the NGLTF program-grass roots organizing, education, and action-involve, respectively, working on issue-oriented projects, publications and media work, and organizing and supporting demonstrations and direct action. Referrals to HIV-antibody testing, physicians, and mental health counseling services are available.

National Hemophilia Foundation (NHF)

Hemophilia and AIDS Network for the Dissemination of Information (HANDI)
116 West 32nd St., 11th Floor
New York, NY 10001
(212) 328-3700
(800) 42-HANDI
(212) 328-3799 (Fax)
Website: http://www.infonhf.org

The National Hemophilia Foundation (NHF), Hemophilia and AIDS Network for the Dissemination of Information (HANDI) is a nonprofit, voluntary health organization founded in 1948 and dedicated to the treatment and cure of hemophilia, related bleeding disorders, and complications, including HIV infection. NHF also promotes and supports research programs; patient, family, and community services; education; publications; and information services. NHF Chapters provide advocacy, patient and public education on hemophilia and HIV, AIDS risk and stress reduction programs, and support groups for persons with hemophilia and their families. NHF cooperates with the hemophilia treatment centers established by the Health Resources and Services Administration (HRSA), Maternal and Child Health Bureau (MCHB). The Chapter Outreach Demonstration Project (CODP) also provides AIDS-related services to culturally diverse people with hemophilia. NHF operates a Women's Outreach Network (WONN), a workshop for women who are spouses and sexual partners of persons with hemophilia, and the Men's Advocacy Network (MANN).

National Institutes of Health (NIH)

Office of Research on Women's Health (ORWH)
9000 Rockville Pike, Bldg. 1, Rm. 201
Bethesda, MD 20892-0161
(301) 402-1770
(301) 402-1798 (Fax)
Website: http://www4.od.nih.gov/orwh/index.html

The Office of Research on Women's Health (ORWH) was established in September 1990 to serve as a focal point for women's health research at the National Institutes of Health (NIH) in setting and monitoring policy, promoting and doing research, and enhancing scientific development. ORWH works to strengthen and enhance research related to diseases and conditions that affect women; to ensure that biomedical and behavioral research conducted and supported by NIH adequately addresses issues regarding women's health; to appropriately represent women in research studies; and to develop opportunities and support for recruitment, retention, re-entry, and advancement of women in biomedical careers. ORWH provides funding through NIH to support basic and clinical research, career development programs, conferences, and workshops. Current research priorities include immune diseases; STDs; risk factors for disease in women of different racial, ethnic, and socioeconomic groups; and behavioral and cultural factors associated with women and disease prevention and intervention. ORWH sponsors an annual Women's Health Seminar Series.

National Lesbian and Gay Health Association (NLGHA)

1407 S St., NW
Washington, DC 20009
(202) 797-3500
(202) 797-3504 (Fax)
Website: http://www. nlgha.org

The National Lesbian and Gay Health Association (NLGHA) disseminates information regarding health care issues in the gay and lesbian community. Topics include racial and ethnic diversity, transgender sexuality, and development of non-HIV services for lesbian and gay youth as well as poor and uninsured persons. NLGHA operates a research institute and develops resources for lesbian and gay health. It also provides technical assistance and policy analysis to emerging lesbian and gay health centers, community-based services related to HIV/AIDS, mental health services, and substance abuse services.

Referrals to HIV-antibody testing, physicians, housing, and financial aid services are available. Brochures and a quarterly newsletter are distributed.

National Minority AIDS Council (NMAC)
1931 13th St., NW
Washington, DC 20009-4432
(202) 483-6622
(202) 483-1135 (Fax)
Website: http://www.nmac.org

The National Minority AIDS Council (NMAC) was formed in 1987 to develop leadership within communities of color to address issues regarding HIV infection. These communities include African American, Latino, Asian, Pacific Islander, and Native American communities. NMAC also conducts policy analysis and makes recommendations to government leaders on the challenges of HIV infection. NMAC provides direct technical assistance to community-based organizations (CBOS) on management, fundraising, and strategic planning. The AIDS Treatment and Research Network assists people of color in gaining access to treatment information.

National Women's Health Network
514 10th St., NW, 4th Fl.
Washington, DC 20004
(202) 347-1140
(202) 347-1168 (Fax)

The National Women's Health Network is a public interest organization devoted solely to women and health issues. It provides safer sex counseling by phone, training, education, a library, and many information resources. It offers brochures on AIDS statistics, as well as information on living with AIDS. The Network publishes a newsletter and maintains a bibliography of current AIDS materials in print for women. It is involved in policy recommendations concerning women and HIV/AIDS.

National Victim Center, Arlington Office
2111 Wilson Blvd., Suite 300
Arlington, VA 22201
(703) 276-2880
(703) 276-2889 (Fax)
Website: http://www.nvc.org

The National Victim Center, Arlington Office, established in 1985, is an advocacy organization for the rights of victims of crime. It links victims of violent crimes and their advocates to services in their own communities; undertakes public opinion surveys to assess public reaction to crime; maintains a library collection on victimology; provides training for victim assistance workers, law enforcement and corrections officers, emergency room personnel, and prosecutors; educates the public on crime and victimization; and advocates for public policy programs to enact legislation to protect and enforce the rights of all individuals when a crime is committed. Information and training on HIV/AIDS and its impact on victim services is available. The Arlington office focuses on public policy, legislation, communications, education, training, program development, library services, a speakers' bureau, legal referrals, and distribution of brochures and a quarterly newsletter.

North American Task Force on Prostitution (NTFP), New York Office
2785 Broadway, Apt. 4L
New York, NY 10025-2834
(212) 866-8854
E-mail: prisalex@interport.net

The North American Task Force on Prostitution (NTFP), New York Office, was founded in 1979 to act as an umbrella organization for prostitutes' rights organizations in the U.S. In 1994, its mission was expanded to include sex workers' rights organizations and individuals who support the rights of prostitutes and other sex workers in the U.S. and Canada. The NTFP's goals include the repeal of existing prostitution laws and the use of occupational safety and health and other workplace regulations to ensure safe working conditions. It supports the rights of prostitutes and other sex workers to organize on their own behalf, work safely and without legal repression, travel without restrictions, have families and raise children, and enjoy the same rights and responsibilities as other people. It works to inform the public about a wide range of issues related to prostitution and other forms of sex work and to promote the development of support services for sex workers, including HIV/AIDS, STD, and violence prevention projects, rape and domestic violence services, legal assistance, health and social support services, and job retraining and other programs to assist prostitutes who wish to change their occupation. To this end, the NTFP engages in public education, producing and distributing position papers, bibliographies, program development materials, and other publications.

Panos Institute
1701 K St. NW, 11th Floor
Washington, DC 20006
(202) 223-7949
(202) 223-7947 (Fax)
Website: http://www.fundforpeace.org

The Panos Institute is an independent information institute working to provide sustainable international development. The Panos Institute combines research with dissemination, providing information that can be readily understood and used. To meet the growing demand for reliable, up-to-date information on AIDS, the agency has established an AIDS information unit. Working in collaboration with other groups, the unit produces information in a variety of formats, for different audiences, in both English and Spanish. A speakers' bureau is available.

Parents Families and Friends of Lesbians and Gays (PFLAG), National Office
1101 14th St., NW, Suite 1030
Washington, DC 20005
(202) 638-4200
(202) 638-0243 (Fax)
Website: http://www.pflag.org
E-mail: info@pflag.org

Parents Families and Friends of Lesbians and Gays (PFLAG), National Office, was founded in 1981 to help end the alienation that often results when gay men and lesbians disclose their homosexuality to their families and friends. PFLAG works through the national media and lobbies Congress to increase government funding and eliminate hate crimes and discrimination against gay men and lesbians. PFLAG also offers an information hotline and training to teachers and school administrators about the special needs of gay and lesbian youth. PFLAG provides information and referrals to persons living with HIV/AIDS (PLWAs), their families, and friends.

Public Health Foundation (PHF)
1220 L St., NW, Suite 350
Washington, DC 20005
(202) 898-5600
(202) 898-5609 (Fax)
Website: http://www.phf.org

The Public Health Foundation (PHF), in cooperation with the Association of State and Territorial Health Officials, the National Association of County Health Officials, the U.S. Conference of Local Health Officers, and other national organizations, has undertaken a series of AIDS-related consensus development projects. Since 1981, PHF has promoted consensus by convening a national meeting of AIDS experts representing a wide range of organizations and viewpoints and working with the other sponsoring organizations to develop and publish recommendations to assist health departments in implementing their AIDS programs. It illuminates national public policy discussions, improves public health practice by fostering the application of advances in science and technology, increases professional development in public health, promotes understanding and consensus about public health issues, and facilitates access to information and retrieval technologies. Publications include the Guides to Public Health Practice and comprehensive reviews of state health agencies' AIDS services and expenditures. Policy analysis of state legislative and regulatory barriers and studies of the utilization of hospice services by persons living with HIV/AIDS (PLWAs) are also provided.

San Francisco AIDS Foundation (SFAF), Client Services
995 Market St., #200
San Francisco, CA 94103
(415) 487-8000
(415) 487-8009 (Fax)
Website: http://www.sfaf.org

The San Francisco AIDS Foundation (SFAF), Client Services, was established in 1982. The Foundation networks with state and national policymakers to help them make informed public policy decisions. It also offers client services, education, and advocacy to at-risk persons in the community and, specifically, to persons living with HIV/AIDS (PLWAs). SFAF publishes and distributes a wide range of educational materials on HIV/AIDS.

University of California San Francisco
Institute for Health Policy Studies (IHPS)
1388 Sutter St., 11th Fl.
San Francisco, CA 94019
(415) 476-4921
(415) 476-0705 (Fax)

The University of California San Francisco, Institute for Health Policy Studies (IHPS), established in 1972, is a health research organization

645

that provides information and assistance to federal, state, and local policymakers. The purposes of the Institute are to conduct policy-oriented research and analysis on a wide range of health issues; to apply research findings to health policy issues; and to provide education and training opportunities in health policy and health services research. Areas of emphasis include health economics, the organization and financing of health care, effectiveness and appropriateness of care, the delivery of specialized clinical services, cost and policy issues related to the HIV epidemic and substance abuse, physician payment issues, peer review and dissemination of biomedical publications, medication use by the elderly, child health issues, and reproductive health services and policies.

U.S. Conference of Mayors (USCM), Health Programs
1620 I St., NW
Washington, DC 20006
(202) 293-7330
(202) 293-9445
(TTY) (202) 293-2352 (Fax)
Website: http://www.usmayors.org/uscm

The U.S. Conference of Mayors (USCM), Health Programs is concerned with the public health problems of people who live in cities. Its health programs address the delivery of health services in the inner city that treat minorities, people of low income, residents of public housing, and those who speak little or no English. With funding from the Centers for Disease Control and Prevention (CDC), the Conference provides grants to local health departments, and community-based organizations working collaboratively to implement prevention programs among populations at risk. The Conference is working with the CDC in the area of prevention community planning; has an intensive program of information exchange and technical assistance to local governments, health departments, and community-based organizations; publishes a wide variety of newsletters, profiles, and capsule reports on innovative and effective AIDS-related policies and programs; and maintains a comprehensive directory and database on local AIDS services. A permanent Mayors Task Force on AIDS meets regularly to discuss and guide Conference policy on HIV/AIDS issues.

Prevention

Advocates for Youth
1025 Vermont Ave., NW, Suite 200
Washington, DC 20005
(202) 347-5700; (202) 347-2263 (Fax)
Website: http://www.advocatesforyouth.org

Advocates for Youth aims to increase the opportunities for, and abilities of, youth to make healthy decisions about sexuality. The National Adolescent AIDS and HIV Prevention Initiative assists organizations that educate adolescents in developing HIV/AIDS education programs. Advocates for Youth also develops educational materials for professionals serving youth. A model peer education program, Teens for AIDS Prevention (TAP), trains a core group of youth in sexuality issues and then assists these young people in designing activities to educate their peers. The National School Condom Availability Clearinghouse maintains information about school condom availability programs that are in development, in existence, or have been considered but rejected. Staff are available to provide technical assistance to individuals and school districts that are trying to move programs forward or that need assistance in program design and evaluation.

American Lung Association (ALA)
Lung Disease Care and Education Program
1740 Broadway
New York, NY 10019-4374
(212) 315-8700; (800) 586-4872; (212) 315-8872 (Fax)
Website: http://www.lungusa.org

The American Lung Association (ALA), Lung Disease Care and Education Program, is dedicated to fighting lung disease. Because the lung is a major target of attack for persons living with HIV/AIDS (PLWAs), ALA produces and distributes pamphlets and videos on HIV/AIDS as well as TB and other opportunistic lung diseases. Pamphlets and a quarterly newsletter are distributed.

American Red Cross
Hispanic HIV/AIDS Program
8111 Gatehouse Rd., 6th Fl.
Falls Church, VA 22042-1203
(703) 206-7090; (703) 206-7754 (Fax)
Website: http://www.redcross.org/

647

The American Red Cross, Hispanic HIV/AIDS Program, provides HIV/AIDS information to Hispanics in a culturally relevant manner, taking into consideration the psychosocial issues that surround this disease. Instructors involve audience members in a dialogue, or "platica," by exchanging knowledge and encouraging them to share their interests, concerns, and everyday experiences. The program staff collaborate with other organizations to deliver the program wherever there is a need, including communities throughout the U.S., Central and South America, and the Caribbean. Videos, posters, teaching guides, comic books, and a newsletter are available.

American Red Cross, National Headquarters
Health and Safety Services, HIV/AIDS Education Program
8111 Gatehouse Rd.
Falls Church, VA 22042-1203
(800) HELP-NOW
(703) 206-7090; (703) 206-7754 (Fax)
Website: http://www.redcross.org

The American Red Cross, National Headquarters, Health and Safety Services, HIV/AIDS Education Program, provides HIV/AIDS-related products and services through the HIV/AIDS coordinators at local Red Cross chapters and statewide HIV/AIDS Networks nationwide. These chapters and their phone numbers are listed in local telephone directories. Many chapters have an HIV/AIDS coordinator and an HIV/AIDS education program, and each distributes HIV/AIDS-related brochures. Other HIV/AIDS-related services at selected chapters include youth, workplace, and minority programs; counseling; home care; and training. The American Red Cross also offers training and certification of HIV educators.

American Social Health Association
CDC National AIDS Hotline (CDC NAH)
P.O. Box 13827
Research Triangle Park, NC 27709-3827
(919) 361-8430; (800) 342-2437 (Hotline)
(800) 243-7889 (TTY, Hotline, Mon.-Fri., 10am-10pm)
(800) 344-7432 (Spanish, Hotline, Mon.-Sun., 8am-2am)
(919) 361-4855 (Fax)
Website: http://sunsite.unc.edu/ASHA

The CDC National AIDS Hotline (CDC NAH) is a toll-free service available to the general public 24 hours a day, 7 days a week throughout the U.S. and its territories. The Hotline provides callers with confidential information, education, and referrals related to AIDS and HIV infection. Trained information specialists are available to answer calls in English and Spanish or through a TTY machine for the deaf and hearing impaired. The specialists can answer questions about HIV transmission, HIV prevention, risk reduction behaviors, HIV-antibody testing, symptoms, treatment, resources, and other topics. Callers can be given referrals specific to their needs, including public health clinics and hospitals, alternative HIV-antibody test site locations, counseling and support groups, AIDS educational organizations, local hotlines, financial and legal services, and many others.

Americans for the Arts
1000 Vermont Ave., NW
Washington, DC 20005
(202) 371-2830
(202) 371-0424 (Fax)
Website: http://www.artsusa.org

Americans for the Arts provides various resources to its members in response to the AIDS epidemic. Information provided includes model health care, insurance, and staff policies to protect persons living with AIDS (PLWAs). It also produces and disseminates resource directories on the AIDS epidemic and related workplace issues. A focus group of members on AIDS interest areas meets at the national convention and networks through the rest of the year. A speakers' bureau is also available.

Athletes and Entertainers for Kids
1845 Camino Dos Rios, 2nd Fl.
Newbury Park, CA 91320
(805) 376-6067
(800) 933-KIDS
(805) 376-6070 (Fax)

Athletes and Entertainers for Kids is a national, nonprofit youth service educational organization comprised of athletes and members of the arts community. Its mission is prevention through education. The members are committed to brightening the lives of all youth, including children and teens who have serious illnesses such as AIDS. They teach youth decision-making skills with programs that showcase athletes and entertainers who provide basic educational information.

The organization administers the Ryan White HIV/AIDS Education Program for Youth, an education information presentation performed by athletes and entertainers at individual schools. Brochures are distributed.

Boys and Girls Club of America (B&GCA), National Headquarters
1230 W. Peachtree St., NW
Atlanta, GA 30309-3447
(404) 815-5700
(404) 815-5789 (Fax)
Website: http://www.bgca.org

Boys and Girls Clubs of America (B&GCA), National Headquarters is a private, nonprofit, national youth organization. It provides Boys and Girls Clubs across the country with the resources, consultation, and support services necessary for them to become the most effective youth development organizations in their communities. Since 1860, the Boys and Girls Clubs of America have offered guidance and youth development programs that build self-esteem, character, and positive relationships for boys and girls. B&GCA programs serve at-risk and disadvantaged youth and provide opportunities for young people to contribute, learn, grow, and advance on merit to their full potential. SMART Moves is a national prevention effort focusing on alcohol, tobacco, and other drug use, as well as early sexual involvement and pregnancy. The Act SMART program is an HIV/AIDS education curriculum produced in cooperation with the American Red Cross.

Concern for Health Options, Information, Care, and Education (CHOICE)
1233 Locust St., 3rd Fl.
Philadelphia, PA 19107-5414
(215) 985-3355
(215) 985-3309 (TTY)
(215) 985-3369 (Fax)

Concern for Health Options, Information, Care, and Education (CHOICE) is a nonprofit social service organization providing advocacy for reproductive health care, health care for persons living with HIV/AIDS (PLWAs), and children's health. With special concern for low-income individuals and teenagers, CHOICE and its Community AIDS Hotline link people with needed services, from maternity and infertility care to treatment for STDs and AIDS. Workshops and seminars for health care professionals, community groups, and school and youth-oriented agencies are available. A variety of brochures are available, and referrals to HIV-antibody testing and physicians are provided.

Coyote Radio
622 Andamar Way
Goleta, CA 93117
(805) 967-0274
(805) 967-0274 (Fax)
E-mail: coyoteradio@igc.org.apc

Coyote Radio produces noncommercial radio segments on HIV/AIDS in the form of interviews, features, and documentaries. Segments have also been produced on underserved populations.

Do It Now (DIN) Foundation
2750 S. Hardy Dr., Suite 2
Tempe, AZ 85282
P.O. Box 27568
Tempe, AZ 85285
(602) 736-0599
(602) 736-0771 (Fax)
Website: http://www.doitnow.org

The Do It Now (DIN) Foundation is a national, independent educational organization established in 1968 to provide alternative approaches to substance abuse prevention and recovery. It distributes publications on chemical dependency and recovery, AIDS, safer sex, eating disorders, suicide, and emotional health topics. It maintains a specialized library of drug abuse and alcoholism information, with a particular emphasis on human development, health promotion, and alternative resources.

Gay Men's Health Crisis (GMHC)
(See listing under Policy and Legal Issues)

General Federation of Women's Clubs (GFWC)
1734 N St., NW
Washington, DC 20036
(202) 347-3168
(202) 347-3168 (Fax)
Website: http://www.gfwc.org
E-mail: gfwc@gfwc.org

The General Federation of Women's Clubs (GFWC) is a member service organization of nearly 300,000 members that is dedicated to community improvement through volunteer service. It supports the goals and objectives of "Healthy People 2000" and the "Campaign for Women's Health." Members are encouraged to organize and support awareness of a range of topics such as literacy, environmental conservation, and HIV/AIDS.

Girls, Incorporated, Keeping Healthy, Keeping Safe AIDS/HIV Project
3959 N Central
Indianapolis, IN 46205
(317) 283-0086
(317) 283-0301 (Fax)
Website: http://www.girlsinc.org

Girls, Incorporated, Keeping Healthy, Keeping Safe AIDS/HIV Project has developed age-appropriate educational materials centered around the needs of girls 6-18 years old for use by youth-serving organizations. The materials incorporate information about HIV transmission, AIDS risks, and human sexuality programs. All organizations receive training at regional meetings. A survey and a project guide are available. The staff include a human sexuality expert and an evaluation specialist. The Project also advocates for girls issues and provides technical assistance, library services, and behavioral research.

Hispanic Designers Incorporated (HDI)
National Hispanic Education and Communications Projects
1000 Thomas Jefferson St., NW, Suite 310
Washington, DC 20007
(202) 337-9636
(202) 337-9635 (Fax)

Hispanic Designers, Incorporated (HDI), National Hispanic Education and Communications Projects, is a nonprofit educational organization specializing in Spanish and English-language education and information programs targeting the Hispanic community. HDI provides AIDS education and public service announcements (PSAs) and broadcasts culturally appropriate messages on two major Spanish networks, Univision and Telemundo, as well as other commercial stations. HDI is particularly concerned with reaching Hispanic youth and women of all ages. It created the Educational Leadership Council Latinas: Partners for Health, a national network of Hispanic women leaders involved in public health that aims to facilitate HIV prevention services in communities nationally. Meetings and information production services are provided. As one of the national partners funded by the Centers for Disease Control and Prevention (CDC), HDI operates the Teatro AIDS Prevention Project for Latinas (TAPP for Latinas) at the national and local levels to address the need for HIV prevention among Latinas under the age of 25. Training sessions, technical assistance workshops, and focus groups will adapt the standard curriculum to community needs, provide quality control for cultural and linguistic competency, and mobilize new groups of community leaders to join in the fight against HIV/AIDS. Referrals to HIV-antibody testing, counseling, housing, and physician services are available.

Jackson State University
National Alumni AIDS Prevention Project (NAAPP)
P.O. Box 18890
Jackson, MS 39217-0154
1400 J.R. Lynch St.
Jackson, MS 39217
(601) 968-2519
(601) 974-5951 (Fax)

The Jackson State University, National Alumni AIDS Prevention Project (NAAPP) is a collaborative effort among Jackson State alumni chapter affiliates in 27 states to develop and implement HIV intervention and prevention strategies aimed at decreasing the transmission of HIV within the African American community. Technical assistance is provided to minority community-based organizations (CBOS) and other agencies that serve racial and ethnic minorities at high risk for HIV and STDs. NAAPP provides technical assistance and training in the following specific topic areas: needs assessment, board training and development, program planning and development, grant writing, fiscal/grant management, resource development, information dissemination, marketing, staff and volunteer recruitment and retention, networking and collaboration, and program evaluation.

Kaleidoscope (KTV)
1777 NE, Loop 410, Suite 300
San Antonio, TX 78217
(210) 824-7446
(210) 824-1666 (TTY)
(210) 829-1388 (Fax)
Website: http://www.ktv-i.com

653

Kaleidoscope (KTV) is a national cable programming service by and for Americans with disabilities, their families, and the organizations, corporations, government agencies, departments, and professionals who work with them. Kaleidoscope has produced HIV/AIDS-related television shows and several public service announcements (PSAs) for the Centers for Disease Control and Prevention (CDC). Services are available in open captioning, audio descriptive narration, and full sound.

Kids on the Block, Incorporated (KOB)
9385-C Gerwig Lane
Columbia, MD 21046-1583
(410) 290-9095
(800) 368-5437
(410) 290-9358 (Fax)
Website: http://www.kotb.com

Kids on the Block, Incorporated (KOB) is an educational puppet company that develops curricula for children to teach them about disabilities, differences, and social concerns. The Kids on the Block program on HIV prevention teaches later elementary school and early middle school children about HIV/AIDS, abstinence, safer sex, and the dangers associated with alcohol and other drugs, while dispelling myths and misconceptions about transmission. One script for younger children focuses on basic hygiene and the differences between viruses that are easy to catch (like colds and flu) and viruses that are hard to catch (like HIV). A newsletter is produced biannually.

Metro TeenAIDS, Teen AIDS Youth Coalition
651 Pennsylvania Ave., SE
Washington, DC 20003-5577
P.O. Box 15577
Washington, DC 20003-5577
(202) 543-9355
(202) 543-3963 (Youth line)
(202) 543-3343 (Fax)

Metro TeenAIDS, Teen AIDS Youth Coalition (founded in 1988), promotes, coordinates, supports, and conducts education, prevention, and referral programs to reduce the spread of HIV infection among youth and to serve the needs of those already infected. The Teen AIDS Information Center stocks brochures, posters, and videos, and gives youth a place to call and receive information about HIV and AIDS. The Youth Coalition has trained teen peer educators, who are HIV-negative, to speak to youth groups. TeenAIDS also sponsors the Annual TeenAIDS National Youth Conference, a national conference organized by teens to educate and empower high school students. Workshops for parents, educators, and youth service professionals give up-to-date information on HIV rates among adolescents, HIV transmission, and education and treatment. Youth Positive is a social and educational support group run by, and for, young people with HIV/AIDS. A resource directory provides referrals to HIV-antibody counseling and testing sites as well as to adolescent HIV-related services. Brochures are distributed.

Moonstone Group, Sexuality Services

935 Hanover St.
Yorktown Heights, NY 10598
(914) 245-3384
(914) 962-9841 (Fax)
E-mail: lwhbmh@prodigy.net

The Moonstone Group, Sexuality Services provides sex education programs for adults and teenagers with mental health deficits, mental retardation, and learning disabilities, as well as their families and caregivers. Conferences, training, and workplace education services are also offered to schools and professionals serving persons with developmental disabilities. Multidimentional, multisensory, interactive educational materials suited for persons with a range of developmental disabilities are available. Educational materials are disseminated to individuals or are available at the resource center. A video related to HIV prevention is offered.

National AIDS Fund (NAF)

1400 I St., NW, Suite 1220
Washington, DC 20005-2208
(202) 408-4848
(202) 408-1818 (Fax)

The National AIDS Fund (NAF) is a non-profit organization comprising many of the nation's top businesses, labor unions, and voluntary organizations which are committed to serving as leaders in responding to the impact of AIDS on the lives of working Americans. NAF publishes a broad range of guidelines, brochures, curricula, and manuals to assist both managers and employees, and provides industry specific, on-site problem solving, training, and education programs, with a special focus on developing organizational policies. Through its Workplace Resource Center (WRC), the Fund provides technical assistance for callers wanting to develop or improve personnel policies addressing HIV/AIDS. NAF answers questions from, and provides guidance to, employers, employees, and others about specific solutions for the challenge HIV/AIDS poses for the workplace. The Fund develops resources and provides guidance for fighting the spread of AIDS through effective workplace education policies and practices. Outreach and technical assistance are tailored to specific industries, geographic regions, companies, and trade associations.

National Asian Pacific American Families Against Substance Abuse (NAPAFASA)
1887 Maplegate St.
Monterey Park, CA 91755-6536
(213) 278-0031
(213) 278-9078 (Fax)

National Asian Pacific American Families Against Substance Abuse (NAPAFASA) is committed to eliminating alcohol and drug abuse among Asian and Pacific Islander families through public and private cooperation in support of the family's capacity to prevent the use of all forms of harmful drugs. The goals of NAPAFASA are to collect and disseminate information on the nature and extent of the problem of substance abuse among Asian and Pacific Islander communities in the U.S.; promote public education and national awareness among Asian and Pacific Islander groups in their own language regarding substance abuse prevention; establish an Asian and Pacific Islander curricula and related materials; establish a bilingual alcohol and drug abuse staff to translate publications; sponsor regional workshops; collaborate with government agencies to establish peer review groups to approve grants and contracts; develop alcohol and drug abuse literature; conduct training and technical assistance; support the development of model community programs; help develop educational materials on HIV/AIDS; and assist in the preparation of documentary films and public service announcements (PSAs) in various Asian and Pacific Islander languages. NAPAFASA sponsored an "HIV/AIDS Training Conference for Pacific Islanders" in Hawaii.

National Association on Drug Abuse Problems (NADAP)
355 Lexington Ave., 2nd Fl.
New York, NY 10017
(212) 986-1170
(212) 697-2939 (Fax)
Website: http://www.nadap.com

National Association on Drug Abuse Problems (NADAP) is a private, nonprofit organization dedicated to fighting drug and alcohol abuse. NADAP provides community and corporate education services, and employee assistance programs, as well as maintaining an information clearinghouse and referral bureau. NADAP's prevention services, including the Neighborhood Prevention Network (NPN), conduct anti-drug and anti-violence workshops for youth and support groups for parents. NADAP also provides vocational education and placement services for recovering drug and alcohol abusers who are in treatment.

National Coalition of Advocates for Students (NCAS)
Viviremos HIV Education Project
100 Boylston St., Suite 737
Boston, MA 02116
(617) 357-8507
(617) 357-9549 (Fax)
(800) 441-7192 (Resource information line)
E-mail: heartkey@aol.com

The National Coalition of Advocates for Students (NCAS), Viviremos HIV Education Project was established to ensure that children and youth with the greatest need would have access to quality health care and HIV education. Staff train health personnel and educators about how to educate farm worker youth and their parents about HIV. The Coalition has created a Spanish/English bilingual curriculum and set standards on effective HIV education programs.

National Organization on Adolescent Pregnancy, Parenting, and Prevention, Incorporated (NOAPP)
1319 F St., NW, Suite 400
Washington, DC 20004
(202) 783-5770
(888) 766-2777
(202) 783-5775 (Fax)
Website: http://www.noapp.erols.org
E-mail: noapp@noapp.org

657

The National Organization on Adolescent Pregnancy, Parenting, and Prevention, Incorporated (NOAPP) is a nonprofit organization that consists of a network of individuals and groups focused on adolescent pregnancy, care, and prevention issues, including AIDS. NOAPP offers technical assistance for program development, including the services of consultants; conducts training sessions for staff and volunteers; and maintains a resource center with data on programs and resources in each state. A national conference and regional training opportunities are held annually.

National Task Force on AIDS Prevention (NTFAP)
973 Market St., Suite 600
San Francisco, CA 94103
(415) 356-8100; (415) 356-8103 (Fax)

The National Task Force on AIDS Prevention (NTFAP) is a national minority organization advocating for, and assisting in, the development of HIV education and service programs by and for gay and bisexual men of color. NTFAP collaborates with local and national organizations to develop community-based programs that target disenfranchised populations. NTFAP provides technical assistance and training for African American, Asian and Pacific Islander, and multi-racial gay and bisexual men's organizations. The National Technical Assistance and Training program serves community groups composed of African American men who are gay or bisexual, an emerging network of Asian and Pacific Islander groups, AIDS service providers, and community-based organizations with programs targeting gay men of color. NTFAP serves as a consultant, providing assistance with needs assessment, capacity building and leadership skills, and partnership building on how to collaborate with other organizations. NTFAP produces safer sex materials, conducts research and evaluation activities, and sponsors national conferences. It also has produced Safer Sex Software, and Brothers, an award-winning interactive health video. The goal of the Each One Teach One (EOTO) Program is to establish a national network of HIV treatment education peer counselors among people of color.

Planned Parenthood Federation of America (PPFA)
810 7th Ave., New York, NY 10019
(212) 541-7800; (800) 829-7732 (National Office)
(800) 230-7526 (Connects to affiliate in caller's service area.)
(800) 669-0156 (Marketing Line); (212) 245-1845 (Fax)
Website: http://www.ppfa.org/ppfa

The Planned Parenthood Federation of America (PPFA) is a federation of family planning organizations that provides reproductive health care, family planning services, and sexuality education to persons worldwide. Contraception, abortion, sterilization, and infertility services are offered. PPFA also sponsors and advocates for biomedical, socioeconomic, and demographic research regarding reproductive health issues. PPFA produces educational materials, serves as a clearinghouse, and provides community education through affiliates. Most PPFA affiliates offer anonymous and/or confidential HIV-antibody testing and counseling to clients. All affiliates provide HIV-educational materials, safer sex counseling, and referral services.

Sexuality Information and Education Council of the U.S. (SIECUS)
130 W. 42nd St., Suite 350
New York, NY 10036-7802
(212) 819-9770; (212) 819-9776 (Fax)
Website: http://www.siecus.org

The Sexuality Information and Education Council of the U.S. (SIECUS) was founded to provide information and education on sexuality and related issues to health care professionals, educators, policy makers, students, and the general public. Under a federal grant from the Centers for Disease Control and Prevention (CDC), SIECUS initiated its National AIDS Education and Information Program. SIECUS also conducts workshops on issues related to sexuality and HIV/AIDS, provides information and technical assistance on sexuality, and runs train-the-trainer workshops. The SIECUS Mary S. Calderone library staff provide AIDS information to professionals and technical assistance and training to educators, health care professionals, and religious leaders. The AIDS collection comprises books, current journal articles, HIV/AIDS-related newsletters, and vertical files. SIECUS has a professional membership program, which includes a bimonthly journal, access to the library, and discounts on publications.

StandUP For Kids, National Office
1111 Osage St., Suite 205C
Denver, CO 80204
(303) 892-8328
(800) 365-4KID
(888) 453-1647 (Fax)
Website: http://www. standupforkids.org

StandUP For Kids, National Office, is an all-volunteer, non-profit organization that provides a range of support services to homeless adolescents and adolescents who are employed in the sex industry. It refers adolescents to a national network of volunteers who offer counseling, assistance with finding housing, and aid in returning to school. These volunteers also provide adolescents with help in getting medical attention. StandUP volunteers distribute a number of hygiene products to street youth, such as condoms and prenatal vitamins.

Teachers of English to Speakers of Other Languages (TESOL)
1600 Cameron St., Suite 300
Alexandria, VA 22314-2751
(703) 836-0774; (703) 836-7864 (Fax)
Website: http://www.tesol.edu

Teachers of English to Speakers of Other Languages (TESOL) is a membership organization whose mission is to strengthen the effective teaching and learning of English internationally. The AIDS and Health Education Committee provides information on HIV/AIDS for teachers, parents, and those learning English.

Wellness Councils of America (WELCOA)
7101 Newport Ave., Suite 311
Omaha, NE 68152-2175
(402) 572-3590; (402) 572-3594 (Fax)
http://www.welcoa.org

Wellness Councils of America (WELCOA) is a national nonprofit umbrella organization dedicated to promoting healthier lifestyles for all Americans, especially through health promotion activities at the worksite. WELCOA distributes health information via publications, videos, brochures, and a newsletter.

Women Organized to Respond to Life-Threatening Diseases (WORLD)
414 13th St.
Oakland, CA 94609
Box 11535
Oakland, CA 94612
(510) 658-6930; (510) 986-0341 (Fax)
Website: http://www.womenhiv.org

Women Organized to Respond to Life-Threatening Diseases (WORLD) works to provide support and information to women with HIV/AIDS and their friends, families, and loved ones; educate and inspire women with HIV/AIDS to advocate for themselves, one another, and their communities; and promote public awareness of women's HIV/AIDS issues and a compassionate response for all persons living with HIV/AIDS (PLWAs). WORLD offers retreats, maintains a speakers' bureau and an information hotline, provides information and referrals, and publishes a monthly newsletter. WORLD's AIDS Library contains newsletters, books, fact sheets, treatment updates, resource guides, videos, and tapes with special sections on women and children. WORLD hosts HIV University (HIVU), a free 10-week AIDS education class that deals with anatomy, gynecology, HIV symptoms, treatment options, clinical trials, and how to communicate with doctors.

YMCA of the USA
101 N. Wacker Dr.
Chicago, IL 60606
(312) 977-0031; (312) 977-9063 (Fax)
Website: http://www.ymca.net

The YMCA of the USA strives to educate and provide healthy alternatives to the misuse of alcohol and drugs across the nation. It provides counseling, training, and resources to local YMCA chapters, coordinates and encourages program development, and distributes selected materials to YMCA chapters. The National Advisory Committee meets annually to develop policy and guidelines for children with HIV/AIDS. Brochures regarding HIV/AIDS are also available, and referrals to housing and financial aid services are provided.

Services for the Incarcerated

American Civil Liberties Union (ACLU), National Prison Project (NPP)
(See listing under Policy and Legal Issues)

Critical Path AIDS Project
2062 Lombard St.
Philadelphia, PA 19146
(215) 545-2212
(215) 545-2212 (Fax)
Website: http://www.critpath.org

The Critical Path AIDS Project is a community-based project that provides information and referrals for crisis intervention and short term counseling through its AIDS treatment hotline. It also provides an Internet web page and an AIDS treatment newsletter. The project accepts collect calls from incarcerated persons living with HIV/AIDS (PLWAs).

National Commission on Correctional Health Care (NCCHC)
1300 Belmont Ave.
Chicago, IL 60657
(773) 880-1460
(773) 880-2424 (Fax)

The National Commission on Correctional Health Care (NCCHC) is a not-for-profit organization working to improve the quality of care in the nation's correctional facilities. NCCHC offers a wide range of services and programs designed to help correctional health care systems provide efficient, quality health care. It establishes standards for health care services in correctional facilities, operates a voluntary accreditation program for institutions that meet these standards, produces and disseminates resource publications, provides technical assistance, offers a quality review program, conducts educational trainings and conferences, and offers a certification program for correctional health professionals. NCCHC is supported by 36 national organizations representing the fields of health, law, and corrections. Each of these organizations has named a representative to the NCCHC Board of Directors. NCCHC provides educational services to incarcerated adolescents and adults, develops resource materials that address comprehensive health education within correctional environments, and provides a 3-day training session for educators, counselors, medical staff, and administrators of both adult and juvenile confinement facilities nationwide.

Osborne Association
AIDS in Prison Project
135 E. 15th St.
New York, NY 10003
(212) 673-6633; (212) 674-0800 — Collect calls accepted from inmates, Tues.–Thurs., 3-8pm
(212) 780-9878 (Fax)
Website: http://www.aidsnyc.org

The Osborne Association, AIDS in Prison Project, conducts research and recommends policy regarding HIV-positive inmates and people on parole. It established an AIDS/HIV clearinghouse and a bilingual hotline for inmates and former inmates. Staff and peer counselors provide inmates and former inmates, their advocates, family members, and friends with information on HIV prevention and treatment, TB prevention and treatment, discharge planning, inmate support groups, and medical parole.

Prison Fellowship Ministries, National Office
1856 Old Reston Ave.
Reston, VA 20190
P.O. Box 17500
Washington, DC 20041-0500
(703) 478-0100
(703) 478-0452 (Fax)
Website: http://www.pfm.org

The mission of the Prison Fellowship's Ministries, National Office, is to exhort, assist, and equip the church in its ministry to inmates, ex-inmates, victims, and their families and to advance Biblical standards of justice. Prison Fellowship, founded in 1976, is a nonprofit, volunteer organization. It provides Christian outreach through correctional seminars, bible studies, marriage seminars, life-planning seminars, a pen pal program, mentoring services, the Angel Tree project (to provide Christmas gifts for the children of inmates), and community service projects. A free bimonthly newspaper profiles athletes, celebrities, and political leaders who serve as positive role models. Special programs include Starting Line (entertainers visiting correctional facilities), Detroit Transition of Prisoners (TOP) (assists newly released inmates), and Neighbors Who Care (ministers to crime victims).

U.S. Department of Justice
Office of Justice Programs
National Criminal Justice Reference Service (NCJRS)
P.O. Box 6000
Rockville, MD 20849-6000
(800) 851-3420
(301) 519-5500 (Publication orders)
(301) 519-5212 (Fax)
Website: http://www.ncjrs.org

The National Criminal Justice Reference Service (NCJRS) provides a range of services and outreach activities to respond to the criminal justice information needs of professionals, practitioners, administrators, policymakers, and the general public. Information about HIV/AIDS in correctional facilities is available. The Reference Service links research findings with those who make policy at the state and local levels. NCJRS assists all Office of Justice Program agencies, including the National Institute of Justice (NIJ), the Office of Juvenile Justice and Delinquency Prevention, the Office for Victims of Crime (OVC), the Bureau of Justice Statistics (BJS), and the Bureau of Justice Assistance (BJA).

Support Services

Alcoholics Anonymous (AA), General Service Office
475 Riverside Dr.
New York, NY 10115
P.O. Box 459, Grand Central Station
New York, NY 10163
(212) 870-3400
(212) 870-3003 (Fax)
Website: http://www.alcoholics-anonymous.org

Alcoholics Anonymous (AA), General Service Office, is a fellowship of men and women who share their experiences in order to recover and help others recover from alcoholism. The General Services Office provides information about AA, including central office telephone numbers for each state and province in the U.S. and Canada.

At Risk Babies Crib Quilts (ABC)
569 First New Hampshire Turnpike, No. 3
Northwood, NH 03261
(603) 942-9211
(603) 942-9210 (Fax)

At Risk Babies Crib Quilts (ABC) provides baby quilts and booties for HIV-positive infants and children from birth to age 6 who have been affected by alcohol and other drugs, abandoned, or who are living in hospitals or foster care.

Gay Men's Health Crisis (GMHC)
(See listing under Policy and Legal Issues for additional information.)

Hemlock Society USA
(See listing under Policy and Legal Issues for additional information.)

NAMES Project Foundation
AIDS Memorial Quilt
310 Townsend St., Suite 310
San Francisco, CA 94107
(415) 882-5500; (415) 882-6200 (Fax)
Website: http://www.aidsquilt.org

The NAMES Project Foundation, AIDS Memorial Quilt, was founded in 1987 to memorialize all those who have died of AIDS-related illnesses and to illustrate the humanity behind the epidemic's statistics. The Memorial Quilt is comprised of thousands of individual fabric panels, each bearing the name of a single person lost to AIDS, sewn together to form one large quilt. The quilt now contains more than 30,000 panels made by individuals across the country and around the world. The NAMES Project displays portions of the Quilt more than 2,000 times a year to increase public awareness of the HIV/AIDS pandemic. The National Interfaith Quilt Display is an educational program using AIDS Memorial Quilt displays in religious settings. The Quilt is displayed to educate people about the epidemic, promote compassion, and send messages to prevent new infections. Places of worship are provided with a 12-foot section of the Quilt for up to one month. Educational materials, a videotape, a discussion guide, educational materials, and sermon outlines accompany the display. Technical assistance is also offered.

Narcotics Anonymous (NA), World Service Office (WSO)
19537 Nordhoff Place
Chatsworth, CA 91311
P.O. Box 9999
Van Nuys, CA 91409
(818) 773-9999; (818) 700-0700 (Fax)
Website: http://www.wsoinc.com

The Narcotics Anonymous (NA), World Service Office (WSO) is the international headquarters for the Fellowship of Narcotics Anonymous. NA is an international fellowship of men and women who come together to share their recovery. The only requirement for membership is the desire to stop using. Information about NA is available in several languages, on audiotape, and in Braille.

National Association on Drug Abuse Problems (NADAP)
355 Lexington Ave., 2nd Fl.
New York, NY 10017
(212) 986-1170
(212) 697-2939 (Fax)

National Association on Drug Abuse Problems (NADAP) is a private, nonprofit organization dedicated to fighting drug and alcohol abuse. NADAP provides community and corporate education services, and employee assistance programs, and maintains an information clearinghouse and referral bureau. NADAP's prevention services, including the Neighborhood Prevention Network (NPN), conduct anti-drug and anti-violence workshops for youth and support groups for parents. NADAP also provides vocational education and placement services for recovering drug and alcohol abusers who are in treatment.

National Council on the Aging (NCOA)
409 3rd St., SW
Washington, DC 20024
(202) 479-1200; (800) 424-9046
(202) 479-0735 (Fax)
Website: http://www.ncoa.org

The National Council on the Aging (NCOA) manages a national program called Family Friends, in which older volunteers help families with children who have special needs. Another NCOA initiative is the Family Friends HIVPositive Babies and Families project, which provides support and assistance to ill and disabled HIV-positive children and their families. Family Friends volunteers help by making sure that parents take their babies to the hospital for regular checkups and medication. They make certain that the parents also keep hospital or doctor appointments and take medication as prescribed. Family Friends volunteers help family members and future caregivers understand infectious diseases and necessary safe health practices and provide a role model for the family and the neighborhood through education.

National Family Caregivers Association (NFCA)
10605 Concord St., Suite 501
Kensington, MD 20895-2504
(301) 942-6430;
(301) 942-2302 (Fax)
Website: http://www.nfcacares.org

The National Family Caregivers Association (NFCA) is a nonprofit membership organization whose mission is to improve the overall quality of life for America's 18 million family caregivers. Membership is open to family caregivers, their friends, and the professionals and institutions supporting them. NFCA is the only national organization serving all family caregivers, regardless of their relationship to the person receiving care or the specifics of the medical situations they confront. Through its services to members in the areas of education and information, support and validation, public awareness and advocacy, NFCA strives to minimize the disparity between a caregiver's quality of life and that of mainstream Americans. Services include a newsletter, *Take Care!*; the Caregiver to Caregiver Support Network; Cards for Caregivers, a program of sending upbeat message cards to caregivers three times a year; a speakers' bureau; National Family Caregivers Week; and The Resourceful Caregiver, a guide to help caregivers take charge of their own lives.

National Hospice Organization (NHO)
1901 N. Moore St., Suite 901
Arlington, VA 22209
(703) 243-5900
(800) 658-8898 (Referrals line, Hospice helpline)
(703) 525-5762 (Fax)
Website: http://www.nho.org

The National Hospice Organization (NHO) is the nation's leading advocate for the terminally ill and a clearinghouse for locating hospice programs and information about hospice care. Its AIDS Resource Committee sponsored an AIDS Educational Summit to promote cooperative efforts between hospice and AIDS programs.

Omega Institute for Holistic Studies
260 Lake Drive
Rhinebeck, NY 12572
(914) 266-4444
(800) 944-1001 (Registration only)
(914) 266-4828 (Fax)
Website: http://omega-inst.org

The Omega Institute for Holistic Studies, established in 1977, is an holistic education center with experience in a variety of subject areas, from health and psychology to multicultural arts and spirituality. It organizes retreats to help women living with cancer develop a

667

better support system of friends, families, and caregivers, as well as retreats for AIDS caregivers in which support networks for persons living with HIV/AIDS (PLWAs) are established. The retreats focus on the role of families in helping PLWAs cope with social, medical, and emotional issues. The Institute also offers workshops in holistic health, psychological development, spiritual practice, the arts, family, and society. Training courses in stress therapy, yoga, dance therapy, and wellness are available.

Parents Families and Friends of Lesbians and Gays (PFLAG), National Office
(See listing under Policy and Legal Issues for additional information.)

Partnership for the Homeless
305 7th Ave.
New York, NY 10001-6008
(212) 645-3444
(800) 235-3444 (New York only)
(212) 477-4663 (Fax)
Website: http://www.partnershipforhomeless.org

The Partnership for the Homeless was founded in 1982 as a service-providing agency dealing exclusively with the issues of homelessness. The Partnership relies largely on volunteers, churches, and synagogues to help provide shelter, transitional and permanent housing, employment training, health, mental health, and other services. It locates housing for early-stage HIV-positive and symptomatic homeless men, women, and families who do not qualify for services elsewhere. It also locates other services including counseling and case management. Referrals to HIV-antibody testing, physicians, housing, and counseling are available.

Pediatric AIDS Foundation (PAF), Main Office
2950 31st Street, #125
Santa Monica, CA 90405
(310) 314-1459
(888) 499-HOPE
(310) 314-1469 (Fax)
Website: http://www. pedaids.org

The Pediatric AIDS Foundation (PAF)—founded by Elizabeth Glaser, Susan De Laurentis, and Susie Zeegen—funds pediatric AIDS research and provides financial assistance to hospitals that care for children with AIDS. PAF sponsors public education and school programs, especially those dealing with disclosure issues. It also distributes a video designed to help parents and educators discuss HIV with their children. PAF handles public education, fundraising, and media communications at its main office.

Theos International Foundation
322 Boulevard of the Allies, Suite 105
Pittsburgh, PA 15222
(412) 471-7779
(412) 471-7782 (Fax)

The Theos International Foundation provides support groups throughout the U.S. and Canada. These support groups help grieving people accept the death of a partner and adjust to the changed circumstances of their lives; help survivors re-establish personal identity and re-develop balanced social patterns; and help the general public appreciate and respond to the needs of those who mourn. It also provides conferences and workshops.

Visiting Nurse Associations of America (VNA-A)
11 Beacon St., Suite 910
Boston, MA 02108
(617) 523-4042
(617) 227-4843 (Fax)

The Visiting Nurse Associations of America (VNA-A) and the National Community AIDS Partnership (NCAP) are developing strategies to diagnose and treat the multi-leveled mental health complications arising from HIV infection for AIDS-diagnosed individuals receiving primary health care services in the home. Development of an effective model for the provision of integrated mental health services within the home setting will contribute to the quality and dignity of life for AIDS patients who rely on home-based primary care services.

Visual AIDS for the Arts, Incorporated
1170 Central Park West
New York, NY 10024
(212) 579-5440
(212) 579-5336 (Fax)

Visual AIDS for the Arts, Incorporated, is an organization of artists and art professionals that aims to heighten public awareness of the impact of the AIDS pandemic on cultural life and of the needs of persons living with HIV/AIDS (PLWAs), and to provide direct services to artists living with HIV/AIDS and their heirs. Visual AIDS originated and coordinates the Ribbon Project, Day Without Art (December 1), Night Without Light (December 1), Electric Blanket, and other awareness-oriented programs that utilize the talents of the arts community to advocate public action regarding AIDS-related issues. Visual AIDS operates the Archive Project, which offers direct services to artists with HIV/AIDS, including free photo documentation of their work, computer and hard copy archiving of this documentation, an artists' materials resource, special exhibition and publication opportunities, and referral services.

Technical Assistance

AIDS Housing of Washington (AHW)
(See listing under Housing for additional information.)

AIDS National Interfaith Network (ANIN)
1400 I St., NW, Suite 1220
Washington, DC 20005
(202) 842-0010
(202) 842-3323 (Fax)

The AIDS National Interfaith Network (ANIN) is a coalition of religious organizations founded in 1988 by people representing Jewish, Christian, Unitarian and other faith groups, as well as persons living with HIV/AIDS (PLWAs), their loved ones, and care providers. It assists AIDS ministries in developing local, regional, and national networks; disseminates culturally sensitive information; and offers technical assistance. As one of the national partners funded by the Centers for Disease Control and Prevention (CDC), ANIN coordinates the National AIDS Ministry Capacity Building for Prevention Projects. Through this project, ANIN will expand its assistance to build the capacity within national religious AIDS networks and will encourage individual AIDS ministries to participate in HIV prevention efforts.

American Association for Health Education (AAHE)
1900 Association Dr.
Reston, VA 20191
(703) 476-3437
(800) 213-7193
(703) 476-6638 (Fax)
Website: http://www.aahperd.org

The American Association for Health Education (AAHE) is a professional membership organization representing health educators and health promotion specialists from clinical, community health, and school settings. In cooperation with the Centers for Disease Control and Prevention (CDC), AAHE works through its HIV/AIDS Project to promote HIV prevention education and health education in schools via publications and collaborative training workshops. Health education programs target early childhood programs and youth in schools, college and university students, nonschool adults and the elderly, voluntary and community health agencies, preservice and inservice preparation for professionals, and research.

American Association for Marriage and Family Therapy
1133 15th St., NW, Suite 300
Washington, DC 20005
(202) 452-0109
(202) 223-2329 (Fax)
Website: http://www.aamft.org

The American Association for Marriage and Family Therapy is a national referral service available to consumers and family therapists dealing with AIDS and the family. It also provides conferences, educational materials, and a newsletter.

American Association for Respiratory Care (AARC)
11030 Ables Lane
Dallas, TX 75229
(972) 243-2272
(972) 484-2720 (Fax)
Website: http://www.aarc.org

The American Association for Respiratory Care (AARC) is a professional organization of respiratory therapists that encourages, develops, and provides educational programs for persons interested in respiratory therapy and diagnostics. It advances the science, technology, ethics, and art of respiratory care through institutes, meetings, lectures, and AIDS-related publications, including a video titled Pulmonary Manifestations of AIDS. AARC also facilitates cooperation and understanding among respiratory care personnel and the medical profession, allied health professions, hospitals, service companies, industry, governmental organizations, and others interested in respiratory care. It promotes pulmonary health and disease prevention to the general public.

American Federation of State, County, and Municipal Employees (AFSCME)
1625 L St., NW
Washington, DC 20036-5687
(202) 429-1000; (202) 429-1293 (Fax)
Website: http://www.afscme.org

The American Federation of State, County, and Municipal Employees (AFSCME) is a union representing public sector employees. Its AIDS programs consist of educating members about HIV/AIDS through workshops, printed materials, and train-the-trainer workshops for union leaders. The AFSCME AIDS Quilt provides a positive and creative means of expression for those whose lives have been affected by the epidemic. AFSCME's program also provides technical assistance to councils and locals. The workshops are tailored to specific audiences such as health care workers, correctional officers, and clerical staff. As one of the national partners funded by the Centers for Disease Control and Prevention (CDC), it operates the AFSCME AIDS Project: Education for Members, Staff, and Families About HIV/AIDS Risk Reduction.

American Foundation for the Blind (AFB), National Headquarters
11 Pennsylvania Plaza, Suite 300
New York, NY 10001
(212) 502-7600; (212) 502-7777 (Fax)
Website: http://www.afb.org

The American Foundation for the Blind (AFB), National Headquarters, is a national nonprofit organization that advocates, develops, and provides programs and services to enable persons who are blind or visually impaired to achieve equality of access and opportunity that will ensure freedom of choice in their lives. AFB is a national resource for people who are blind or visually impaired, the organizations that serve them, and the general public. Services include technical assistance, staff training, information, and referrals, books, pamphlets, periodicals, and audio cassettes, education through literature, social research, and legislative representation.

American Public Health Association (APHA)
1015 15th St., NW
Washington, DC 20005
(202) 789-5600; (202) 789-5661 (Fax)
Website: http://www.apha.org

The American Public Health Association (APHA), founded in 1872, is a professional organization of physicians, nurses, educators, social workers, health administrators, pharmacists, dentists, health planners, mental health professionals, and consumers. Its services include establishment of public health practices and procedures, research, education services, conferences, and publication of periodicals, books, and pamphlets. APHA committees include Equal Health Opportunity, Human Rights, International Health, Laboratory Standards and Practices, and Legal Practice. Databases, meetings, and policy analysis are available.

Asian and Pacific Islander American Health Forum (APIAHF)
Empowerment through Training and Technical Assistance (ETTA) Program
116 New Montgomery St., Suite 531
San Francisco, CA 94105
(415) 541-0866
(415) 512-3881 (Fax)

The Asian and Pacific Islander American Health Forum (APIAHF), Empowerment through Training and Technical Assistance (ETTA) Program, is a national advocacy organization that lobbies government agencies and collaborates with other organizations for improvement in the health status of Asian and Pacific Islander (API) Americans. The Empowerment Through Training and Technical Assistance Program provides technical assistance to API organizations in responding to HIV/AIDS and STDs. ETTA works with other API community organizations in the areas of program development, fundraising, administration, and improvement of available technologies.

Association of Black Psychologists (ABPsi)
National Technological AIDS Project
821 Kennedy St., NW
Washington, DC 20011
P.O. Box 55999
Washington, DC 20040-5999
(202) 722-0808
(202) 722-5941 (Fax)
Website: http://www.abpsi.org

The Association of Black Psychologists (ABPsi), was established in 1968 to promote and advance the profession of psychology, influence and affect social change, and develop programs whereby psychologists of African descent can assist in solving problems of Black communities and other ethnic groups. Its National Technological AIDS Project provides advocacy, training, and planning programs for Black professionals to meet the mental health needs of the Black community. The Association receives an ongoing training grant from the Centers for Disease Control and Prevention (CDC) to provide technical assistance and train members in HIV prevention. Technical assistance is provided for writing and proposal development, resource development, evaluation and quality control, needs assessment, and the production and distribution of printed materials. The train-the-trainer program provides information on workshops, networking, state and local health departments, AIDS service providers, and national and community-based organizations. The association publishes an AIDS newsletter for ABPsi members nationwide. The HIV/STD Project works in cooperation with the Agency for Health Care Policy and Research (AHCPR) to endorse the *Pneumocystis Carinii* Pneumonia (PCP) Prevention Awareness Campaign developed by the National Minority AIDS Council (NMAC).

Association of Nurses in AIDS Care (ANAC)
11250 Roger Bacon Dr., Suite 8
Reston, VA 20190-5202
(703) 925-0081; (800) 260-6780
(703) 435-4390 (Fax)
Website: http://www.anacnet.org/aids/

The Association of Nurses in AIDS Care (ANAC) was founded to foster the professional development of nurses involved in all aspects of AIDS and to promote the health, welfare, and rights of all persons living with HIV/AIDS (PLWAs). ANAC is striving to meet its goals by providing leadership to the nursing community, establishing standards of practice and education, promoting social awareness, creating an effective network, and serving as an advocate for HIV-infected persons. It also organizes conferences.

Association of Women's Health, Obstetric, and Neonatal Nurses (AWHONN)
2000 L St. NW, Suite 740
Washington, DC 20036
(800) 395-7373 (Facts On Demand)
(202) 737-0575 (Fax)
Website: http://www.awhonn.org

The Association of Women's Health, Obstetric, and Neonatal Nurses (AWHONN) is an independent, nonprofit association that promotes excellence in nursing practice to improve the health of women and newborns. AWHONN focuses on four aspects of nursing: education, research, practice, and policy. The organization produces guidelines on all aspects of women's health care.

Black Gay and Lesbian Leadership Forum
1436 U St. NW, Suite 200
Washington, DC 20009
(202) 483-6786
(202) 483-4970 (Fax)
Website: http://www.nblglf.org

The Black Gay and Lesbian Leadership Forum, established in 1988, provides opportunities for African American gay men and lesbians to exchange information and address urgent issues facing these communities. It educates and informs the African American community, as well as non-African American organizations, about unique contributions by black gays and lesbians to African American history. The primary function of the Forum has been to organize the Annual National Black Gay and Lesbian Conference and Institutes. The AIDS Prevention Team and the National Board of Governors are additional programs of the Forum. The AIDS Prevention Team articulates the voice of the HIV-positive African American community and provides HIV support groups, treatment updates, holistic counseling and treatments, and town meetings. The National Board of Governors of the Forum was founded to assist the Board of Directors and the Conference Steering Committee by providing input that reflects the broad diversity of issues relevant to the African American lesbian and gay communities.

CDC National AIDS Clearinghouse (CDC NAC)
P.O. Box 6003
Rockville, MD 20849-6003
(800) 458-5231
(800) 243-7012 (TTY)
(888) 282-7681 (Fax)
Website: http://www.cdcnac.org

The CDC National AIDS Clearinghouse (CDC NAC) is a national reference, referral, and publications distribution service for HIV and AIDS information. CDC NAC shares information and materials among professionals, including public health professionals, educators, social service workers, attorneys, employers, and human resource managers. CDC NAC maintains computerized information databases that are searched by reference specialists to refer requesters to appropriate organizations and help them locate needed materials, services, and funding information. The Clearinghouse also distributes a variety of government-approved AIDS and HIV-related publications. Resource centers in Rockville, MD, and Atlanta, GA, are available to visitors by appointment to search the Clearinghouse databases, review AIDS-related educational materials, and access CDC NAC'S many other services. Another important component of the Clearinghouse is the AIDS Clinical Trials Information Service (ACTIS), a central resource providing the latest information on federally and privately sponsored clinical trials currently being conducted to evaluate experimental drugs and other therapies for adults and children at all stages of HIV infection. ACTIS is a Public Health Service project provided collaboratively by the CDC, the Food and Drug Administration (FDA), the National Institute of Allergy and Infectious Diseases (NIAID), and the National Institutes of Health (NIH). The HIV/AIDS Treatment Information Service (ATIS) provides information about federally approved HIV/AIDS treatment guidelines to health care providers and persons living with HIV/AIDS (PLWAs). ATIS was developed through a coordinated Public Health Service effort by the Agency for Health Care Policy and Research (AHCPR), CDC, the Health Resources and Services Administration (HRSA), the Indian Health Service (IHS), the National Institutes of Health (NIH), and the Substance Abuse and Mental Health Services Administration (SAMHSA). The CDC Business and Labor Resource Service provides materials and technical assistance on workplace-based HIV and AIDS programs and information on national, state, and local resources. The Clearinghouse offers a variety of Internet services including a Web site, listserv of AIDS-related news, file transfer protocol, and gopher. Reference services are available by TTY for deaf and hearing impaired callers. Bilingual reference specialists can assist Spanish-speaking callers.

Dignity/USA, National AIDS Project
1500 Massachusetts Ave., NW, Suite 11
Washington, DC 20005
(202) 861-0017
(800) 877-8797
(202) 429-9808 (Fax)
Website: http://www.dignityusa.org

Dignity/USA, National AIDS Project, is a ministry for gay, lesbian, and bisexual Catholics. It has 85 local chapters nationwide to provide a unified voice and leadership and to be an instrument through which that voice can be heard by the church and society. The National AIDS Project offers social involvement, spiritual development, financial assistance, pastoral counseling, housing, educational services, recreational activities, and other practical support services for persons living with HIV/AIDS (PLWAs) and their caregivers. It also makes policy recommendations regarding feminist issues and HIV/AIDS.

Emory University, Rollins School of Public Health
Institute for Minority Health Research (IMHR)
1518 Clifton Rd., NE
Atlanta, GA 30322
(404) 727-9148
(404) 727-9170
(404) 727-1369 (Fax)
Website: http://www.sph.emory.edu/bshe/imhr

The Emory University, Rollins School of Public Health, Institute for Minority Health Research (IMHR), provides teaching, research, and services focused specifically on ethnic and racial minority populations in the United States. IMHR provides technical assistance to community-based organizations on program planning and evaluation.

Gay and Lesbian Medical Association (GLMA)
459 Fulton St., Suite 107
San Francisco, CA 94102
(415) 255-4547
(415) 255-4784 (Fax)
Website: http://www.glma.org

The Gay and Lesbian Medical Association (GLMA) was founded in 1981 to combat homophobia within the medical profession and in society at large, as well as to promote the best possible health care for lesbian, gay, and bisexual patients. GLMA provides a source of professional and personal support and affiliation for lesbian, gay, and bisexual physicians. Board meetings are open to all members. A newsletter is published quarterly. GLMA sponsors an annual lesbian physicians' retreat and a health care referral service for the lesbian and gay community. It provides speakers on lesbian and gay health issues. GLMA operates the Medical Expertise Retention Program (MERP),

677

which counsels health care professionals and physicians with AIDS or HIV-related problems. The Association maintains an AIDS Task Force; publishes position papers on important issues affecting the health of gay men, lesbians, and persons living with HIV/AIDS (PLWAs), and distributes health education materials. It also maintains a liaison with medical schools, training programs, and professional organizations regarding the needs of gay and lesbian patients. The Lesbian Health Fund provides grants for medical research on lesbian health issues, including educating health care workers about the health needs of lesbians and educating lesbians about risk reduction and early diagnosis of health problems.

The Grantsmanship Center (TGC)
1125 W. 6th St., 5th Fl.
Los Angeles, CA 90017
P.O. Box 17220
Los Angeles, CA 90017
(213) 482-9860
(213) 482-9863 (Fax)
Website: http://www.tgci.com

The Grantsmanship Center (TGC) is a training organization for the non-profit sector. The Center trains staff members of public and private agencies in grantsmanship, program management, and fundraising. Services target nonprofit and government human service agencies.

Howard University, College of Allied Health Sciences
National AIDS Minority Information and Education (NAMIE) Program
2139 Georgia Ave., NW, Suite 1C
Washington, DC 20001
(202) 865-3720
(202) 865-3799 (Fax)

Howard University, College of Allied Health Sciences, National AIDS Minority Information and Education (NAMIE) Program serves as a resource for communicating HIV/STD information to health care providers in the African American community and provides technical assistance to selected African American health care professional organizations and students for lowering the risk of HIV/STD transmission in their communities. It has a 5-year project designed to provide health professionals with expertise in discussing factual information about HIV disease, assessing high risk behaviors, promoting methods of preventing HIV transmission, counseling HIV infected persons, and providing AIDS education. The program utilizes leaders of the target groups in planning through an Executive Advisory Committee. The Program is funded through the Centers for Disease Control and Prevention (CDC) to develop, test, and implement a prototypic curriculum and training program at Howard University, with similar programs to be conducted in other geographic areas. Previously trained participants from the first cycle of the project will serve as facilitators and trainers at various collaborating sites.

Jackson State University
National Alumni AIDS Prevention Project (NAAPP)
(See listing under Prevention for additional information.)

Metro TeenAIDS, Teen AIDS Youth Coalition
(See listing under Prevention for additional information.)

National AIDS Fund (NAF)
(See listing under Prevention for additional information.)

National Alliance of State and Territorial AIDS Directors (NASTAD)
(See listing under Policy and Legal Issues for additional information.)

National Association of Community Health Centers (NACHC)
1330 New Hampshire Ave., NW
Washington, DC 20036
(202) 659-8008
(202) 659-8519 (Fax)
Website: http://www.aachc.com

The National Association of Community Health Centers (NACHC) is the trade association for the nation's community health centers, migrant health centers, and health care for the homeless projects. These clinics receive Federal Health Center funding to provide comprehensive primary care in medically underserved rural and urban communities nationwide. NACHC provides training to centers on funding and program development. It also educates health policymakers on the effectiveness of the Community Health Center model and works for increased attention to resources for meeting the health care needs of underserved communities.

National Association For Families and Addiction Research and Education (NAFARE)
122 S. Michigan Ave., Suite 1100
Chicago, IL 60603
(312) 541-1272
(312) 541-1271 (Fax)

The National Association for Families and Addiction Research and Education (NAFARE) provides a national network among professionals for the exchange of ideas regarding prevention of, and intervention with, families addiction, continuing professional education, research into the problems of families addiction, and the long-term outlook for infants and families. NAFARE translates current research on families addiction into public education programs and public health policy.

National Catholic AIDS Network (NCAN)
P.O. Box 422984
San Francisco, CA 94142-2984
(707) 874-3031
(707) 874-1433 (Fax)
Website: http://www.ncan.org

The National Catholic AIDS Network (NCAN) sponsors the National Catholic HIV/AIDS Ministry Conference and a national conference called HIV/AIDS: Its Impact on Clergy and the Religious. NCAN aims to foster effective communications, referrals, and training among Catholics affected by AIDS. It also assists religious congregations and dioceses in dealing with the impact of HIV/AIDS on their members.

National Clearinghouse for Alcohol and Drug Information (NCADI)
11426 Rockville Pike, Suite 200
Rockville, MD 20852-3007
P.O. Box 2345
Rockville, MD 20847-2345
(301) 468-2600; (800) 729-6686
(301) 468-6433 (Fax)

The National Clearinghouse for Alcohol and Drug Information (NCADI) is sponsored by the Center for Substance Abuse Prevention (CSAP) as the central point within the federal government for current print and audiovisual materials about alcohol and other drugs. NCADI's resources include databases on scientific findings; prevention programs and materials; field experts; federal grants; market research; tailored materials for parents, teachers, and youth; and information about organizations and groups concerned with alcohol and other drug problems. NCADI shares this information with the nation through free computerized literature searches, an audiovisual loan program, bulk distribution of federally developed materials, and exhibits at national conferences. PREVline is available to members of the professional community and the public on the Internet.

National Coalition of Hispanic Health and Human Services Organizations (COSSMHO)
Community HIV/AIDS Technical Assistance Network
1501 16th St., NW
Washington, DC 20036-1401
(202) 387-5000
(202) 797-4353 (Fax)

The National Coalition of Hispanic Health and Human Services Organizations (COSSMHO), Community HIV/AIDS Technical Assistance Network, is a coalition of community-based organizations (CBOS) and professionals working to improve the health and psychosocial well-being of Hispanics in the U.S. and Puerto Rico. COSSMHO's HIV and STD prevention efforts are carried out through its Community HIV and AIDS Technical Assistance Network (CHATAN). CHATAN provides technical assistance and advocacy at all levels of government by identifying, implementing, and evaluating culturally appropriate intervention strategies. It also trains professionals and lay persons serving Hispanic communities. In addition, CHATAN provides needs assessment and survey research, and develops educational and informational materials to help communities prevent the spread of HIV and STDs. Donations are provided to organizations serving Hispanic communities.

National Council of La Raza (NCLR)
(See listing under Policy and Legal Issues for additional information)

National Council of Negro Women (NCNW), National Office
633 Pennsylvania Ave., NW
Washington, DC 20004
(202) 737-0120
(202) 737-0476 (Fax)
Website: http://www.usbol.com./ncnw/

681

The National Council of Negro Women (NCNW), National Office, a coalition of more than 30 African American women's organizations, is dedicated to ensuring access to, and full participation of, African American women in the socio-economic political systems that impact the quality of life for all persons. To carry out this mission, NCNW works through and with affiliated organizations, individuals, and a diversity of agencies and organizations in both the public and private sectors. The NCNW's HIV/STD Training and Technical Assistance Project (TTAP) provides technical assistance and training to minority community-based organizations and collaborates with public health agencies in the effective delivery of HIV/STD prevention services targeting African American women and their families. TTAP Project goals are to identify and disseminate information on HIV/STD prevention strategies, build capacity of agencies providing HIV/STD prevention services to ensure cultural relevancy, provide planning, integration, and implementation training, establish a national network of culturally relevant HIV/STD programs, strengthen collaboration among community-based organizations and public health agencies, and establish NCNW as a national resource for HIV/STD training and technical assistance. NCNW also offers a speakers' bureau and research.

National Episcopal AIDS Coalition (NEAC)
1925 K St. NW
Washington, DC 20006
(202) 628-6628
(202) 872-1151 (Fax)
Website: http://www.neac.org

The National Episcopal AIDS Coalition (NEAC) works collaboratively for effective HIV/AIDS ministry on, and by, all levels of the Episcopal Church. This ministry includes educating all Episcopalians on HIV/AIDS issues and empowering them to act on that information; advocating for the physical, emotional, and spiritual health for persons living with HIV/AIDS (PLWAs); promoting pastoral care for PLWAs; and furthering the development of networks and communities of support for all those engaged in HIV/AIDS ministries in the Church. Among the activities promoted by NEAC is the National Day of Prayer, designated for all persons touched by the AIDS epidemic. It provides conferences and seminars, educational materials, and a database on AIDS ministries. It also participates in national and international Anglican Responses to HIV/AIDS.

National Family Planning and Reproductive Health Association (NFPRHA)

122 C St., Suite 380
Washington, DC 20001-2109
(202) 628-3535; (202) 737-2690 (Fax)
Website: http://www.nfprha.org

National Family Planning and Reproductive Health Association (NFPRHA) is a national membership organization representing family planning providers. NFPRHA's goal is to improve and expand the delivery of reproductive health care services throughout the U.S. Its members include state, county, and local health departments, hospitals, affiliates of the Planned Parenthood Federation of America, and independent clinics, physicians, nurses, and consumers. NFPRHA monitors legislative developments relating to AIDS and other reproductive health matters.

National Hemophilia Foundation (NHF)

Hemophilia and AIDS Network for the Dissemination of Information (HANDI)
(See listing under Policy and Legal Issues for additional information.)

National Latino/a Lesbian and Gay Organization (LLEGO), Incorporated

1612 K St., NW, Suite 500
Washington, DC 20006
(202) 466-8240; (202) 466-8530 (Fax)
Website: http://www.llego.org

The National Latino/a Lesbian and Gay Organization (LLEGO), Incorporated, founded in 1987, is a nonprofit nationwide network of lesbian and gay Latino/as. LLEGO maintains a database and directory of resources for gay Latinos and lesbian Latinas and holds regional conferences yearly. It also operates the Technical Assistance and Training for AIDS (TATA) project for Latino/a lesbian and gay community-based organizations (CBOs), mainstream Latino/a organizations, and non-Latino/a AIDS service organizations. LLEGO provides seed funding for lesbian and gay organizations and works to promote civil rights issues.

National Lesbian and Gay Health Association (NLGHA)

(See listing under Policy and Legal Issues for additional information.)

National Mental Health Association (NMHA)
1021 Prince St.
Alexandria, VA 22314-2971
(703) 684-7722
(800) 433-5955 (TTY)
(703) 684-5968 (Fax)
Website: http://www.nmha.org

The National Mental Health Association (NMHA) is a nonprofit organization that publishes information on multiple mental health issues, including AIDS. Referrals to HIV-antibody testing, physicians, financial aid, and housing services are available. A newsletter and brochures are also distributed.

National Minority AIDS Council (NMAC)
(See listing under Policy and Legal Issues for additional information.)

National Native American AIDS Prevention Center (NNAAPC)
134 Linden St.
Oakland, CA 94607
(510) 444-2051; (800) 283-2437
(800) 283-6880 (24-hour fax on demand)
(510) 444-1593 (Fax)
Website: http://www.nnaapc.org

The National Native American AIDS Prevention Center (NNAAPC) is an organization directed and managed by and for Native Americans, Alaskan Natives, and Hawaiian Natives. It provides training and technical assistance to local Native communities to encourage them to begin HIV prevention activities. The Center also operates a clearinghouse for Native-specific AIDS and STDs information and publishes a quarterly newsletter. NNAAPC also operates two community-based demonstration programs (Tulsa, OK and Oklahoma City, OK) to provide case management and client advocacy to Native Americans with HIV. As one of the national partners funded by the Centers for Disease Control and Prevention (CDC), NNAAPC coordinates the National Native American AIDS Prevention Media Services campaign. The campaign provides HIV/AIDS resources to native media outlets, offers HIV information via fax-on-demand and electronic bulletin boards, and provides technical assistance on the development of Native American–focused HIV materials.

National Network for Youth, Inc.
Safe Choices Project
1319 F St., NW, Suite 401
Washington, DC 20004
(202) 783-7949
(800) 878-2437 (Safe Choices Technical Assistance)
(202) 783-7955 (Fax)

The National Network for Youth, Inc., Safe Choices Project provides innovative HIV prevention training, technical assistance, and telephone consultation to professionals working with youth in high-risk situations. It also distributes the Safe Choices Guide, a skills-based HIV/STD prevention manual for youth workers.

National Organization of Black County Officials (NOBCO)
National Minority HIV/AIDS Project
440 1st St., NW, Suite 410
Washington, DC 20001
(202) 347-6953; (202) 393-6596 (Fax)
Website: http://www.nobco.org

The National Organization of Black County Officials (NOBCO) is the service arm of the National Association of Black County Officials (NABCO) and provides a mechanism for effective minority representation and participation within the National Association of Counties (NACo). It offers technical assistance, conferences, information exchange, and program planning to Black elected and appointed county officials. It coordinates and facilitates county-related activities for its members and serves as a clearinghouse for the exchange of technical information. Under a Cooperative Agreement with the Centers for Disease Control and Prevention (CDC), NOBCO works to increase the level of knowledge and skill among staff of community-based organizations, health and human services agencies, and national programs targeting ethnic minority youth to better enable them to plan and implement state-of-the-art approaches to HIV/AIDS prevention education. Under a supplemental cooperative agreement, NOBCO provides technical assistance to state, territorial, and local health departments who are developing HIV prevention community planning boards.

National Organization on Adolescent Pregnancy Parenting and Prevention Incorporated (NOAPP)
(See listing under Prevention for additional information.)

National Task Force on AIDS Prevention (NTFAP)
(See listing under Prevention for additional information.)

National Women's Health Resource Center (NWHRC)
120 Albany St., Suite 820
New Brunswick, NJ 08901
(732) 828-8575
(877) 986-9472 (toll free)
(732) 249-4671 (Fax)
Website: http://www.healthywomen.org

The National Women's Health Resource Center (NWHRC), incorporated in 1988, is a non-profit membership organization that serves as the national clearinghouse and information resource for women's health information, providing information to enable women and their care providers to make informed health decisions. NWHRC uses its Information Database to provide current information on women's health issues in response to written inquiries from throughout the country. It publishes a comprehensive women's health newsletter, collaborates with national corporations to develop women's health campaigns, disseminates information to women, and provides educational materials and information to companies via Worksite Wellness Programs. Using the Center's National Referral Database, the NWHRC refers callers to women's health care providers, including HIV/AIDS service organizations, in all regions of the U.S.

Polaris Research and Development
Center for AIDS Prevention and Education
390 4th St.
San Francisco, CA 94107
(415) 777-3229
(800) 871-6688
(415) 512-0212 (Fax)
Website: http://www.polarisinc.com

Polaris Research and Development, Center for AIDS Prevention and Education is a minority research and development firm whose work includes AIDS awareness surveys in the African American community, as well as surveys of juvenile male prostitution. Other populations studied include the developmentally disabled and those with mental health problems. It has developed risk-reduction and media campaign materials for underserved populations, including injection drug users and migrant workers. The training programs include a cross-cultural training program, AIDS training of trainers, a Basic AIDS Training, and focus group facilitator training. Insights for Psychologists About HIV Disease and Ethnic Minority Clients provides a means for health care professionals to explore their own attitudes, values, and judgments, and understanding of their clients and their ability to work successfully with persons living with HIV/AIDS (PLWAs). The AIDS Risk Assessment Program teaches counselors how to identify men and women who are at high risk of becoming infected with HIV.

Public Health Foundation (PHF)
(See listing under Policy and Legal Issues for additional information.)

United Church Board for Homeland Ministries
HIV/AIDS Ministry Program
700 Prospect Ave.
Cleveland, OH 44115-1100
(216) 736-3270
(216) 736-3263 (Fax)

The United Church Board for Homeland Ministries, HIV/AIDS Ministry Program, coordinates HIV/AIDS activities within the United Church of Christ (UCC). The Program provides information resources to UCC churches and UCC-related institutions about HIV/AIDS. UCC also provides referrals and maintains a relationship with the United Church AIDS/HIV network. UCC produces Affirming Persons-Saving Lives, a comprehensive curriculum for HIV/AIDS awareness and prevention education, designed for Christian education settings.

U.S. Conference of Mayors Health Programs (USCM)
(See listing under Policy and Legal Issues for additional information.)

U.S. Department of Health and Human Services
National Aging Information Center (NAIC)
330 Independence Ave., SW, Rm. 4656
Washington, DC 20201
(202) 619-7501
(202) 401-7620 (Fax)
Website: http://www.ageinfo.org

The U.S. Department of Health and Human Services, Administration on Aging, National Aging Information Center (NAIC) compiles, houses, and disseminates information on key aspects of aging. This information includes statistics on services and activities supported by the Older Americans Act; demographic data; information on the health, economic, and social conditions of older people; and services. NAIC provides bibliographic searches for HIV/AIDS related material. Other services include responding to written and telephone requests for information and distributing materials. An electronic bulletin board and public reading room are also available.

U.S. Department of Labor

Occupational Safety and Health Administration (OSHA)
200 Constitution Ave., NW
Washington, DC 20210
(202) 219-8151
(202) 219-5986 (Fax)
Website: http://www.osha.gov

The Occupational Safety and Health Administration (OSHA) was created within the U.S. Department of Labor as a regulatory agency to encourage employers and employees to reduce workplace hazards and implement new or improved safety and health programs. OSHA provides for research to develop innovative ways of dealing with occupational safety and health problems; establishes responsibilities and rights for safety and health conditions; maintains a reporting and record keeping system to monitor job-related injuries and illnesses; establishes training programs to increase the number and competence of occupational safety and health personnel; develops mandatory job safety and health standards and enforce them effectively; and provides for the development, analysis, evaluation, and approval of state occupational safety and health programs. Coverage extends to all employers and employees in the U.S., Puerto Rico, and all other territories under federal government jurisdiction and is provided either directly by federal OSHA or through an OSHA-approved state program. State programs are required to provide standards and enforcement programs as well as voluntary compliance activities which are at least as effective as the federal programs. OSHA's area offices are full-service centers offering a variety of informational services, such as availability for speaking engagements, publications, audiovisual aids on workplace hazards, and technical advice. OSHA also provides a limited number of grants to nonprofit organizations to conduct workplace training and education in subjects where there are unmet safety and health education needs. OSHA's primary focus on AIDS is to prevent occupational exposure to bloodborne pathogens, thus reducing the risk of contracting Hepatitis B and AIDS on the job.

Treatment

AIDS Clinical Trials Information Service (ACTIS)
P.O. Box 6421
Rockville, MD 20849-6421
(800) 874-2572
(800) 243-7012
(301) 519-0459 (international)
(301) 519-6616 (Fax)
Website: http://www.actis.org

The AIDS Clinical Trials Information Service (ACTIS) is a Public Health Service (PHS) project provided collaboratively by the Centers for Disease Control and Prevention (CDC), the Food and Drug Administration (FDA), the National Institute of Allergy and Infectious Diseases (NIAID), and the National Library of Medicine (NLM), and offered through the CDC National AIDS Clearinghouse (CDC NAC). This service is a central resource providing current information on federally and privately sponsored clinical trials for HIV-infected individuals and on the drugs being investigated in these trials. Callers to the service are linked with experienced health specialists who access online databases offering up-to-date information on more than 500 studies and more than 200 drugs. Studies are presently in progress for adults and children at all stages of HIV infection, including those who are HIVinfected but have no symptoms. Callers are provided with specific information on various study requirements, including eligibility, exclusion criteria, duration, location, and the names and telephone numbers of contacts at each study site. Callers may also obtain a printout of a custom search of the databases. Reference specialists are available to answer questions from HIV-positive individuals and their families, as well as health professionals.

AIDS Medicine and Miracles (AMM)
P.O. Box 20650
Boulder, CO 80308-3650
(303) 447-8777
(800) 875-8770
(303) 447-3902 (Fax)
Website: http://www.ares.csd.net/~amm/

Founded in 1987, AIDS, Medicine and Miracles (AMM) holds healing conferences that educate, nurture, and empower persons living with HIV/AIDS (PLWAs), and their caregivers and loved ones. Three annual national conferences and two or three 1-day institutes at other national AIDS conferences explore medical and complementary therapies and psychosocial and spiritual issues in a supportive setting.

AIDS Treatment Data Network
611 Broadway, Suite 613
New York, NY 10012-2809
(212) 260-8868
(800) 734-7104
(212) 260-8869 (Fax)
Website: http://www.aidsnyc.org/network

The AIDS Treatment Data Network is a nonprofit organization that offers a computerized registry of clinical trials of promising AIDS drugs open in New York, Connecticut, Pennsylvania, and New Jersey. Other services include case management, support, and referrals. Services are targeted towards Hispanics and also to people who have low literacy skills.

American Association of Naturopathic Physicians (AANP)
(See listing under Policy and Legal Issues for additional information.)

Consumer Health Information Research Institute (CHIRI)
300 Pink Hill Rd.
Independence, MO 64057
(816) 228-4595
(816) 228-4995 (Fax)

The Consumer Health Information Research Institute (CHIRI) provides information on AIDS fraud, AIDS misinformation, and AIDS propaganda relating to products, literature, procedures, devices, and treatments.

Critical Path AIDS Project
(See listing under Support Services for additional information.)

Gay Men's Health Crisis (GMHC)
(See listing under Policy and Legal Issues for additional information.)

HIV/AIDS Treatment Information Service (ATIS)
P.O. Box 6303
Rockville, MD 20849-6303
(800) 448-0440; (301) 519-6616 (Fax)
Website: http://www.hivatis.org

The HIV/AIDS Treatment Information Service (ATIS) is a toll-free reference service that provides federally approved treatment guidelines and timely, accurate information to assist health care and service providers in dealing with patients with HIV/AIDS. It is also a free reference service for persons living with HIV/AIDS (PLWAs), their families, and friends. Staff answer questions using databases including those of the National Library of Medicine. Copies of federally approved HIV/AIDS treatment guidelines are available, and bilingual reference specialists can handle inquiries in Spanish and English. The service is offered through the CDC National AIDS Clearinghouse (NAC) and sponsored by the Agency for Health Care Policy and Research (AHCPR), the Centers for Disease Control and Prevention (CDC), the Health Resources and Services Administration (HRSA), the Indian Health Service (IHS), the Office of HIV/AIDS Policy (OHAP), the National Institutes of Health (NIH), and the Substance Abuse and Mental Health Services Administration (SAMHSA).

International Association of Physicians in AIDS Care (IAPAC)
(See listing under Policy and Legal Issues for additional information.)

National Association For Families and Addiction Research and Education (NAFARE)
(See listing under Technical Assistance for additional information.)

National Institutes of Health (NIH)
Office of Research on Women's Health (ORWH)
(See listing under Policy and Legal Issues for additional information.)

National Mental Health Association (NMHA)
1021 Prince St.
Alexandria, VA 22314-2971
(703) 684-7722; (800) 969-6642
(800) 433-5955 (TTY)
(703) 684-5968 (Fax)
Website: http://www.nmha.org

The National Mental Health Association (NMHA) is a nonprofit organization that publishes information on multiple mental health issues, including AIDS. Referrals to HIV-antibody testing, physicians, financial aid, and housing services are available. A newsletter and brochures are also distributed.

National Minority AIDS Council (NMAC)
(See listing under Policy and Legal Issues for additional information.)

Pediatric AIDS Foundation (PAF), Research Division
2950 31st Street, #125
Santa Monica, CA 90405
(310) 395-9051; (310) 395-5149 (Fax)

The Pediatric AIDS Foundation (PAF), Research Division, prioritizes, defines, funds, and conducts research that impacts the diagnosis, treatment, and prevention of HIV/AIDS. Research projects include topics such as the transmission of HIV from mothers to their unborn children, HIV/AIDS gene therapy, long-term survivors, AZT resistance, and new technologies.

Positive Images and Wellness (PIW), Incorporated
National Center for Wellness and Health Promotion
13100 New Hampshire Ave.
Silver Spring, MD 20904
(301) 236-4614; (301) 236-4609 (Fax)
Website: http://www.erols.com

Positive Images and Wellness Incorporated (PIW), National Center for Wellness and Health Promotions, was founded by an occupational therapist committed to holistic health, especially in the areas of HIV/AIDS rehabilitation and education. Classes are offered in holistic health and health professionals are offered continuing education. The organization sponsors two annual conferences: the Integrative Medicine and Wellness Conference and the Children Health and Well-Being Conference.

Project Inform, HIV Treatment Hotline
205 13th Street, #2001
San Francisco, CA 94103
(800) 822-7422
(415) 558-8669; (415) 558-0684 (Fax)
Website: http://www.projinf.org/

Project Inform, a nonprofit, volunteer organization, was founded in 1985 to collect, review, and distribute information on experimental drug treatments for HIV/AIDS. The HIV Treatment Hotline gives information on treatment options and distributes printed materials. Fact sheets are prepared on treatments that meet Project Inform's criteria of established safety, reasonable expectation of efficacy, and general availability. The information provided summarizes current research findings, reports by users, known side effects, overall risks and benefits, and correct use of treatments. Project Inform is collaborating with other organizations in a nationwide effort to reinvigorate AIDS research and to fight for effective AIDS treatments. Services are also available online.

University of Miami, School of Medicine
Touch Research Institute (TRI)
Dept. 820
1601 NW 12th Ave.
P.O. Box 016250
Miami, FL 33101
(305) 243-6781
(305) 243-6488 (Fax)
Website: http://gehon.ir.miami.edu/ped

The University of Miami, School of Medicine, Touch Research Institute (TRI), is the first center in the world for basic and applied research on the sense of touch. TRI works to obtain further knowledge in health, development, and the treatment of disease through the use of massage and touch therapies. Research projects include enhancing the immune function in AIDS patients, cancer patients, and premature infants. The behavioral and immune functioning of HIV-exposed infants is also investigated. TRI also provides training programs, a newsletter, and other educational materials.

U.S. Department of Health and Human Services, Public Health Service
National Institutes of Health, National Institute of Allergy and Infectious Diseases (NIAID)
31 Center Dr., MSC 2520
Bethesda, MD 20892-2520
(301) 496-5717
(301) 402-0120 (Fax)
Website: http://www.nih.niaid.gov

The National Institute of Allergy and Infectious Diseases (NIAID) conducts and supports biomedical research on allergic, immunologic, and infectious diseases including HIV infection and AIDS. Through its outreach program, the Institute provides information on research results to health professionals. NIAID provides written materials describing its research on HIV/AIDS and lay language publications related to HIV/AIDS.

U.S. Department of Health and Human Services, Public Health Service

National Institutes of Health, National Cancer Institute (NCI), Cancer Information Service (CIS)
31 Center Dr., MSC2580 Bldg. 31, Rm. 10A07
Bethesda, MD 20892-2580
(301) 496-5583 (Ext. 241)
(800) 422-6237 (Information line)
(301) 402-2594 (Fax)
Website: http://www.nci.nih.gov/

The National Cancer Institute (NCI), Cancer Information Service (CIS), is a toll-free service where trained professionals answer questions about the causes, symptoms, and treatment of cancer. Accurate, confidential, personalized information on cancer is provided to patients and their families, health professionals, and the general public. Referrals to cancer specialists and investigational treatment studies and also provided. Free publications are available.

Chapter 63

Mental Health Services for People with HIV/AIDS

Introduction

A diagnosis of HIV/AIDS can be emotionally devastating. Yet, many people with HIV/AIDS do not have the support of family and friends to help them cope with the isolation or stigma associated with HIV. People with HIV, the virus that causes AIDS, can experience adjustment disorders, depression, or mood disorders as a complication of the disease. Research also shows that the virus may infect the brain, impairing the central nervous system and causing neuropsychiatric problems such as AIDS Dementia. Any one of these conditions can compromise one's mental and physical health, as well as one's quality of life.

To address these compelling and complex needs, the federal Center for Mental Health Services (CMHS) launched HIV/AIDS Mental Health Services Demonstration Program in 1994. This effort supports 11 service demonstration projects and one coordinating center.

The 11 projects provide a range of high quality, culturally appropriate mental health services including diagnostic services, treatment, group therapy, buddy programs, and family therapy. All services welcome the participation of family members, partners, and significant others. Many projects also provide case management, outreach, and home-based mental health services. They also utilize local advisory

Department of Health and Human Services (DHHS) Publication No. (SMA) 96-3121, Substance Abuse and Mental Health Services Administration, 1996; contact information verified in 1998.

boards comprised of representatives of community-based service organizations and consumers. [Contact information is provided below for the sites that could be located in 1998.]

All sites are being evaluated to determine which are most effective on delivering mental health services to people affected by and living with HIV/AIDS who need them. The most effective interventions can be replicated in other communities. We are also learning the types of people who are served by the Program, what services they receive and the impact of those services on the quality of life.

CMHS is a component of the Substance Abuse and Mental Health Services Administration (SAMHSA) in the U.S. Department of Health and Human Services. The HIV/AIDS Mental Health Services Demonstration Program is a joint effort among SAMHSA, the Health Resources and Services Administration and the National Institutes of Health.

Grantees

California

SPECTRUM Mental Health

- Linkage of HIV services in South Central Los Angeles
- "One-stop" mental health and medical services
- English and Spanish counseling, evaluation and treatment

Eric Bing, MD, MPH
SPECTRUM Mental Health
Drew University of Medicine and Science
774 E. 118th Street, MP 19B, Bldg. K
Los Angeles, CA 90059
Tel:(213) 563-4939
Fax:(213) 563-9333
E-mail:EGBDrew@aol.com

The Walden House Planetree Assessment and Treatment Services

- Assessment and mental health services for people with addictions (including the incarcerated)
- Provides detoxification and long/short term residential and outpatient drug treatment
- Psychiatric training for paraprofessionals

Brian Greenberg, PhD
The Walden House Planetree Assessment
and Treatment Services
520 Townsend Street
San Francisco, CA 94103
Tel:(415) 554-1100, ext. 103
Fax:(415) 554-1122
E-mail:editor@waldenhouse.org

Georgia

CAMS Project

- Linkages among HIV-related mental health service agencies
- Network evaluates consumer needs and services delivery
- Comprehensive, multidisciplinary mental health services

J. Stephen McDaniel, MD
CAMS Project
Emory University, Center for AIDS/HIV Mental Health Services
Grady Health System Infectious Disease Program
341 Ponce de Leon Avenue
Atlanta, GA 30308
Tel:(404) 616-6310
Fax: (404) 616-9700

Illionis

CHHAPS Project

- Integrated mental health and primary care services
- Collaboration among county and city health agencies
- Ongoing clinical and HIV specific training

Tomas Soto, PhD
CHHAPS Project
Chicago HIV Health and Psychological Support Project
CCH HIV Primary Care Center
1900 W. Polk, Room 1256
Chicago, IL 60612
Tel: (312) 633-7328
Fax: (312) 633-3002

Nebraska

Harambee Mental Health Project

- Support groups for African Americans
- Extensive case management and support
- Home-based mental health services
- Integrated with HIV prevention strategies

Suzanne Myers, MSW
Harambee Mental Health Project, Charles Drew Health Center, Inc.
Mental Health Services
2915 Grant Street
Omaha, NE 68111
Tel: (402) 453-3913; Fax: (402) 453-1970
E-mail: 103064.2776@compuserve.com

New Jersey

Kinship Connection Project

- Help families plan for care of children upon death of the parent [permanency planning]
- Individual and family services provided in home
- Individual and family services for potential guardian
- Bi-lingual services [Spanish]

Charlene Mason-Reese, MSW
Kinship Connection Project
Elizabeth General Medical Center, Monastery
655 East Jersey Street
Elizabeth, NJ 07201
Tel: (908) 965-7123; Fax: (908) 965-7127

New York

The Special Needs Clinic

- Integrated liaison model identifies and engages HIV-affected families in adult and pediatric AIDS medical care settings
- Provides comprehensive family-based mental health services to both children and adults in one clinical site
- Continuity of treatment for children following parental health

Jennifer Havens, MD
The Special Needs Clinic
Presbyterian Babies Hospital
619 North, 622 W. 168th Street, VC4-E
New York, NY 10032
Tel: (212) 305-9909; Fax: (212) 305-7400
E-mail: JHAVENS@INTERPORT.NET

Virginia

Alexandria Mental Health HIV / AIDS Project

- Outreach to minority and hard-to-engage populations
- Coordinated interagency case management
- Caregiver support
- Prevention education

Andrea Ronhovde, LCSW
Alexandria Mental Health HIV/AIDS Project/AMHAP
Alexandria Community Services Board
Division of Mental Health Services
720 N. Saint Asaph Street
Alexandria, VA 22314
Tel: (703) 838-6400; Fax: (703) 838-5062
Email: HPCY76A@Prodigy.com

Mini Mental Health Center

- Focuses on women and those with substance abuse or AIDS dementia
- Mental health, substance abuse. and neuropsychological assessment
- Psychoeducational groups promote "Living with HIV/AIDS" and "Risk Reduction"

Deborah Haller, PhD
Mini Mental Health Center (MMHC)
Medical College of Virginia, Department of Psychiatry
P.O. Box 980109
Richmond, VA 23298
Tel: (804) 828-9925; Fax: (804) 828-9906
E-mail: DHALLER@HSC.VCU.EDU

Coordinating Center

Research Triangle Institute

- Primary responsibility for the design and conduct of the multisite evaluation in collaboration with 11 service projects
- Collects and maintains data from service projects
- Prepares annual progress reports and final evaluation reports

William E. Schlenger, PhD
Research Triangle Institute (RTI)
P.O. Box 12194
Research Triangle Park, NC 27709-2194
Tel: (919) 541-6372
Fax: (919) 541-5945
E-mail: FP$BS@RTI.ORG

CHMS Program Director

Elaine Dennis, MSp
HIV/AIDS Mental Health Services Demonstration Program
Center for Mental Health Services
5600 Fishers Lane, Room 15-81
Rockville, MD 20857
Tel: (301) 443-7817
Fax: (301) 443-0737
E-mail: EDENNIS@SAMHSA.GOV

Consumer Representative

Mickey W. Smith, BASW
1315 T Street, NW, #1
Washington, DC 20009
Tel: (202) 462-7756
Fax: (202) 745-3733
E-mail: DCMICKEY@aol.com

Chapter 64

State HIV/AIDS Hotlines and Prevention Program Coordinators

HIV/AIDS Hotlines by State

Alabama

Alabama AIDS Hotline
201 Monroe St.
Montgomery, AL 36104
(334) 206-5364 (Administrative)
(800) 228-0469 (Alabama only)
(334) 206-2092 (Fax)

Alaska

Alaskan AIDS Hotline
1057 W. Fireweed Ln., Suite 102
Anchorage, AK 99503-1736
(907) 263-2050 (Administrative)
(907) 276-4880 (Nationwide)
(800) 478-2437 (Alaska only)
(907) 263-2051 (Fax)

California

So. CA HIV/AIDS Hotline
1313 N. Vine St.
Los Angeles, CA 90028-8107
(213) 993-1600 (Administrative)
(213) 876-2437 (So. CA only)
(800) 553-2437 (TTY, So. CA)
(800) 922-2437 (So. CA only)
(213) 993-1598 (Fax)

San Francisco AIDS Foundation
Northern California Trilingual
AIDS Hotline
10 United Nations Plz.
San Francisco, CA 94102-4910
P.O. Box 426182
San Francisco, CA 94142-6182
(415) 487-3000 (Administrative)
(415) 863-2437 (Nationwide)
(800) 367-2437 (No. CA only)
(800) 367-2437 (Spanish, Northern California only)
(415) 487-8089 (Fax)

Excerpted from *National Organizations Providing HIV/AIDS Services*, CDC National AIDS Clearinghouse, September 1997; verified and updated in October 1998.

Colorado

Colorado Department of Health
AIDS Education and Training
Program
Colorado AIDS Hotline
4300 Cherry Creek Dr., S., A3
Denver, CO 80222-1530
(303) 692-2720 (Administrative)
(303) 782-5186 (Nationwide)
(800) 252-2437 (Colorado only)
(303) 782-0904 (Fax)

Connecticut

Connecticut Department of Public Health and AIDS Division
401 Capitol Ave.
Hartford, CT 06104
(860) 509-7801 (Administrative)
(800) 342-AIDS (Nationwide)
(800) 322-3222 (Publications)
(860) 509-7854 (Fax)

Delaware

Delaware AIDS Hotline
100 W 10th, Suite 315,
Suite 820
Wilmington, DE 19801
(302) 652-6776 (Administrative)
(800) 422-0429 (Delaware only)
(302) 652-5150 (Fax)

District of Columbia

District of Columbia AIDS
Information Line
1407 S. St., NW
Washington, D.C. 20009-3819
(202) 939-7822
(Administrative)
(202) 332-2437 (Nationwide)
(202) 939-7814 (TTY)
(202) 797-3504 (Fax)

Florida

Florida HIV/AIDS Hotline
P.O. Box 10950
Tallahassee, FL 32302
(850) 681-9131 (Administrative)
(800) 352-AIDS (Florida only)
(904) (888)503-7118 (TTY)
(800) 243-7101 (Haitian Creole,
Florida only)
(800) 545-SIDA (Spanish, Florida
only)
(850) 561-3443 (Fax)

Georgia

Georgia AIDS Information Line
1438 W. Peachtree St., Suite 100
Atlanta, GA 30309-2955
(404) 876-9944 (Administrative)
(404) 876-9944 (Nationwide)
(404) 885-6794 (TTY)
(800) 551-2728 (Georgia only)
(404) 885-6799 (Fax)

Hawaii

Hawaii STD/AIDS Hotline
277 Ohua Ave.
Honolulu, HI 96815-3643
(808) 922-4787 (Administrative)
(808) 922-1313 (Nationwide)
(800) 321-1555 (Hawaii only)
(808) 922-4794 (Fax)

Idaho

Idaho AIDS Foundation Hotline
1602 W. Franklin St.
Boise, ID 83702
P.O. Box 421
Boise, ID 83701-0421
(208) 345-2277 (Administrative)
(800) 677-2437 (Idaho only)
(208) 336-0303 (Fax)

State HIV/AIDS Hotlines and Prevention Program Coordinators

Illinois

Illinois AIDS Hotline
Test Positive Aware Network
1258 W. Belmont St.
Chicago, IL 60657
(773) 404-8726 (Administrative)
(800) 782-0423 (TTY, Illinois only)
(800) 243-2437 (Illinois only)
(773) 404-1040 (Fax)
 (800) 342-2437(National)

Indiana

Indiana HIV/STD Hotline
3951 N. Meridian St.
Suite 101
Indianapolis, IN 46208
P.O. Box 1964
Indianapolis, IN 46202-1964
(317) 920-1200 (Administrative)
(800) 848-2437 (Indiana only)
(800) 972-5123 (TTY, Indiana only)
(317) 926-7823 (Fax)
(800) 848-AIDS (National)

Iowa

Iowa Statewide AIDS Hotline
2116 Grand Ave.
Des Moines, IA 50312-5368
(515) 244-6700 (Administrative)
(800) 445-2437 (Iowa only)

Kentucky

Kentucky AIDS Hotline
152 W. Zandal
Lexington, KY 40503
(606) 278-7494 (Administrative)
(606) 278-9667 (Fax)

Louisiana

Louisiana AIDS Hotline
NO AIDS Task Force
1407 Decatur St.
New Orleans, LA 70116
(504) 945-4000 (Administrative)
(504) 944-2437 (Nationwide)
(800) 99A-IDS9 (Nationwide)
(504) 945-4048 (Fax)

Maine

Maine AIDS Hotline
W. 615 Congress St.
Portland, ME 04101-4031
P.O. Box 5305
Portland, ME 04101
(207) 774-6877 (Administrative)
(800) 851-2437 (Maine only)
(207) 879-0761 (Fax)

Maryland

Maryland AIDS Hotline
11141 Georgia Avenue
Suite 312
Wheaton, MD 20902-4658
(410) 333-2437
(800) 584-8183 (Testing)
(900) 680-4HIV (Counseling)
(800) 590-2437 (National)

Massachusetts

Massachusetts AIDS Hotline/
AIDS Action Hotline
AIDS Action Committee
131 Clarendon St., 5th Fl.
Boston, MA 02116-5131
(617) 437-6200 (Administrative)
(888) 436-6200 (Nationwide)
(617) 437-1394 (TTY)
(617) 437-6445 (Fax)

Michigan

AIDS Partnership Michigan
2751 E. Jefferson, Suite 301
Ferndale, MI 48207
(313) 446-9800 (Administrative)
(800) 750-TEEN (TeenLink
Hotline)
(800) 332-0849 (TTY)
(800) 872-2437 (Michigan only)
(800) 515-3434 (Client Services)
(313) 446-9839 (Fax)
(800) 522-0399 (Health Care
Workers Hotline)

Minnesota

Minnesota AIDS Project
Minnesota AIDS Line
1400 Park Ave. S.
Minneapolis, MN 55404-1550
(612) 373-2437 (Administrative)
(888) 820-2437 (Minnesota
only)
(612) 341-3804 (Fax)

Mississippi

CONTACT the Crisis Line
CONTACT AIDS Hotline
P.O. Box 5192
Jackson, MS 39296-5192
(601) 713-4099 (Administrative)
(601) 713-4098 (Fax)

Missouri

Missouri AIDS Information Line
3030 Walnut St.
Kansas City, MO 64108
(816) 561-8784 (Administrative)
(800) 533-2437 (Nationwide)
(816) 561-9518 (TTY)
(816) 531-7199 (Fax)

Montana

Montana Department of Health
and Human Services
STD/HIV Prevention Program
1400 Broadway, Cogswell Bldg.
Rm C305
Helena, MT 59620
(406) 444-3565 (Administrative)
(800) 233-6668 (Montana only)
(406) 444-2920 (Fax)
(800)675-2437 (E. Montana)
(800)663-9002 (W. Montana)

Nebraska

Nebraska AIDS Project
Nebraska AIDS Hotline
3610 Dodge Street
Suite 11 O-W
Omaha, NE 68131
(402) 342-6367 (Administrative)
(800) 782-2437 (Nationwide)
(402) 342-9073 (Fax)

Nevada

Nevada AIDS Hotline
505 E. King Street
Room 304
Carson City, NV 89701-4761
(702) 687-4804 (Administrative)
(800) 842-2437 (Nationwide)
(702) 687-4988 (Fax)

New Hampshire

STD/HIV Program
6 Hazen Dr.
Concord, NH 03301-6501
(603) 271-4502 (Administrative)
(800) 752-2437 (New Hampshire
only)
(800) 735-2964 (TTY)
(603) 271-4934 (Fax)

New Jersey

New Jersey AIDS Hotline
201 Lyons Ave.
Newark, NJ 07112-2027
(973) 926-7443 (Administrative)
(800) 624-2377 (New Jersey only)
(973) 926-8008 (TTY)
(973) 926-0013 (Fax)

New Mexico

New Mexico AIDS Hotline
525 Camino De Los Marquez, Suite 1
Santa Fe, NM 87501
(505) 476-8475 (Administrative)
(800) 545-2437 (New Mexico only)
(505) 476-8527 (Fax)

New York

New York State AIDS/HIV Hotlines
Elm & Carlton Sts.
Buffalo, NY 14263-0001
(716) 845-3170 (Administrative)
(800) 872-2777 (New York only)
(800) 541-2437 (New York only)
(716) 845-8178 (Fax)

Ohio

Ohio AIDS Hotline
Columbus AIDS Task Force
1500 W. Third Avenue
Suite 329
Columbus, OH 43212-2856
(614) 488-2437 (Administrative)
(800) 332-3889 (TTY, Ohio only)
(800) 332-2437 (Ohio only)
(614) 487-5962 (Fax)

Oklahoma

OK AIDS Hotline, Dept. of Health
HIV/STD Service
1000 NE 10th St. Mail Drop 0308
Oklahoma City, OK 73117-1299
(405) 271-4636 (Administrative)
(800) 535-AIDS (TTY)
(800) 535-AIDS (Oklahoma only)
(405) 271-5149 (Fax)

Oregon

Cascade AIDS Project
620 SW 5th Ave., Suite 300
Portland, OR 97204-1418
(503) 223-5907 (Administrative)
(503) 223-2437 (Nationwide)
(503) 223-2437 (TTY)
(800) 777-2437 (Area codes 503, 206, and 208 only)
(503) 223-7087 (Fax)

Pennsylvania

Pennsylvania Dept.of Health
Bureau of HIV/AIDS
Forester & Commonwealth, #912
Harrisburg, PA 17120
P.O. Box 90
Harrisburg, PA 17108
(215) 783-0479 (Administrative)
(800) 662-6080 (PA only)
(215) 772-4309 (Fax)
(215) 545-2212 (Critical Path)

Rhode Island

RI Project AIDS Hotline
232 W. Exchange St.
Providence, RI 02903
P.O. Box 1024
Providence, RI 02903-1024
(401) 831-5522 (Administrative)
(800) 726-3010 (Nationwide)
(401) 454-0299 (Fax)

South Carolina

SC HIV/AIDS Hotline
South Carolina Dept. of Health
and Environmental Control
HIV/AIDS Division
1751 Calhoun St.
Columbia, SC 29211
P.O. Box 101106
Columbia, SC 29211-0106
(803) 737-4110 (Administrative)
(800) 322-2437 (S.C. only)
(803) 737-3979 (Fax)

Tennessee

Tennessee AIDS Hotline
Tennessee HIV/AIDS Program
426 5th Ave., N., 4th Fl.
Nashville, TN 37247-4911
(615) 741-7500 (Administrative)
(800) 525-2437 (Tennessee only)
(615) 741-3857 (Fax)

Texas

Texas HIV and STD Infoline
Texas Department of Health
Bureau of HIV/STD Prevention
1100 W. 49th St.
Austin, TX 78756-3101
(512) 490-2500 (Administrative)
(800) 299-2437 (Texas only)
(800) 252-8012 (TTY)
(512) 490-2538 (Fax)

Utah

AIDS Information Hotline
Utah AIDS Foundation
1408 S., 1100 E.
Salt Lake City, UT 84105-2435
(801) 487-2323 (Administrative)
(801) 487-2100 (Nationwide)
(800) 366-2437 (Utah only)
(801) 486-3978 (Fax)

Vermont

Vermont AIDS Hotline
Vermont Department of Health
108 Cherry St.
Burlington, VT 05402
P.O. Box 70
Burlington, VT 05402-0070
(802) 863-7245 (Administrative)
(800) 882-2437 (Vermont only)
(800) 319-3141 (TTY, VT only)
(802) 863-7314 (Fax)

Virgin Islands

Virgin Islands AIDS Hotline
6&7 Estate Diamond & Ruby
Christiansted, VI 00820
(809) 778-6105 (Administrative)
(809) 773-2437 (Nationwide)

Virginia

Virginia Department of Health
Virginia STD/AIDS Hotline
P.O. Box 2448, Rm. 112
Richmond, VA 23218-2448
(804) 487-2323 (Administrative)
(800) 533-4148 (TTY, VA only)
(800) 533-4148 (Virginia only)
(800) 322-7432 (Spanish, Virginia only)
(804) 225-3517 (Fax)

Washington

Washington HIV/AIDS Hotline
Airdustrial Park Bldg. 9
MS 47840
Olympia, WA 98504-7840
P.O. Box 47840
Olympia, WA 98504-7840
(360) 586-3887 (Administrative)
(800) 272-2437 (WA only)
(360) 586-5525 (Fax)

West Virginia

West Virginia AIDS Hotline
West Virginia Office of Health
and Human Resources
AIDS Program
1422 Washington St., E.
Charleston, WV 25301-1978
(304) 558-2950 (Administrative)
(800) 642-8244 (WV only)
(304) 558-6335 (Fax)

Wyoming

Wyoming AIDS Hotline
Hathaway Bldg., 4th Fl.
2300 Capitol Ave.
Cheyenne, WY 82002-0710
(307) 777-5800 (Administrative)
(800) 327-3577 (Nationwide)
(307) 777-5402 (Fax)

State HIV/AIDS Prevention Program Coordinator Offices

Alabama

Alabama Department of Public
Health
Division of HIV/AIDS Prevention
Sexually Transmitted Disease
Branch
RSA Tower, Suite 1410
Montgomery, AL 36130-3017
P.O. Box 30317
Montgomery, AL 36130-3017
(334) 206-5364

Alaska

Alaska Department of Health
and Social Services
Division of Public Health Section of Epidemiology
AIDS/STD Program
3601 C St., Suite 540
Anchorage, AK 99503-0249
P.O. Box 240249
Anchorage, AK 99524-0249
(907) 269-8000
(907) 465-2898 (Fax)

American Samoa

American Samoa Department of
Health Services
LBJ Tropical Medical Center
Pago Pago, AS 96799
(684)699-1529

Arizona

Arizona Department of Health
Services
Division of Disease Prevention
Office of HIV/AIDS Services
3815 N. Black Canyon Fwy.
Phoenix, AZ 85015-5351
(602) 230-5819
(602) 230-5973 (Fax)

Arkansas

Arkansas Department of Health
Sexually Transmitted Diseases
Div. AIDS Prevention Program
4815 W. Markham, Slot 33
Little Rock, AR 72205-3867
(501) 661-2408

California

Los Angeles County Dept. of
Health Services
AIDS Programs
600 S. Commonwealth Ave., 6th Fl.
Los Angeles, CA 90005
(213) 351-8000
(213) 738-0825 (Fax)

CA Dept. of Health Services
Office of AIDS
830 S St.
Sacramento, CA 95814
P.O. Box 942732
Sacramento, CA 94234-7320
(916) 323-4314

S. F. Dept. of Public Health
AIDS Surveillance Office
25 Van Ness Ave., Suite 500
San Francisco, CA 94102
(415) 554-9050
(415) 431-0353 (Fax)

Colorado

Colorado Department of Health
Disease Control and Environmental Epidemiology
4300 Cherry Creek Dr. S, Ste. A3
Denver, CO 80220-1530
(303) 692-2700
(303) 782-0904 (Fax)

Connecticut

Conn. Dept. of Public Health
AIDS Division
410 Capital Ave., MS 11, APV
Hartford, CT 06134-0308
P.O. Box 340308
Hartford, CT 06134-0308
(860) 509-7801

Delaware

Deleware Department of Health
and Social Services
Division of Public Health
Health Monitoring and Program
Consultation
Federal & Water St.
Dover, DE 19903
P.O. Box 637
Dover, DE 19903
(302) 739-3033
(302) 739-6617 (Fax)

District of Columbia (Washington DC)

District of Columbia Commission of Public Health
Department of Human Ser-
vices for HIV/AIDS
Division of HIV Prevention
717 14th St., NW
Suite 600
Washington, D.C. 20005
(202) 727-2500
(202) 727-0577 (TTY)
(202) 727-8471 (Fax)

Florida

Florida Department of Health
and Rehabilitative Services
Bureau of Disease Intervention
Program Planning and Man-
agement
1309 Winewood Blvd.
Bldg. 6
Rm 4r
Tallahassee, FL 32399-0700
(850) 922-6675
(850) 922-4202 (Fax)

Georgia

GA Dept. of Human Resources
Division of Public Health
Communicable Disease Branch
AIDS Section
2 Peachtree St., NW., Suite 400
Atlanta, GA 30303-3186
(404) 657-3110
(404) 876-9944 (TTY)
(404) 657-3133 (Fax)

Hawaii

Hawaii Department of Health
Communicable Disease Division
STD/AIDS Prevention Branch
3627 Kilauea Ave., Suite 306
Honolulu, Hi 96816
(808) 733-9010
(808) 733-9015 (Fax)

Hawaii Department of Health
Communicable Disease Division
STD/AIDS Prevention Branch
Hawaii Seropositivity and Medical Management Program
3627 Kilauea Ave., Suite 306
Honolulu, HI 96816
(808) 732-0026
(808) 735-8529 (Fax)

Idaho

ID Dept. of Health and Welfare
Div. of Health, Br. of Clinical
and Preventive Service
STD/AIDS Program
450 W. State St., 4th Fl.
Boise, ID 83720-0034
P.O. Box 83720
Boise, ID 83720-0036
(208) 334-5937
(208) 332-7346 (Fax)

Illinois

Chicago Department of Health
Division of HIV/AIDS
Office of Public Policy and Programs
333 S. State Street
2nd Fl., Rm. 200
Chicago, IL 60604-3972
(312) 747-2437
(312) 744-4284 (TTY)
(312) 747-9663 (Fax)

Illinois Department of Public Health
Division of Infectious Diseases
AIDS Activity Section
525 W. Jefferson Street
1st Floor
Springfield, IL 62761
(217) 524-5983
(217) 524-6090 (Fax)

Illinois Department of Public Health
Division of Infectious Diseases
HIV/AIDS Section
160 N. Lasalle St., 7th Fl. S.
Chicago, IL 60601
(312) 814-4846
(312) 814-4844 (Fax)

Indiana

Indiana Department of Health
Division of HIV/STD
AIDS Program
2 N. Meridian St.
Indianapolis, IN 46202
P.O. Box 1964
Indianapolis, IN 46402-1964
(317) 233-7867
(317) 233-7663 (Fax)

Iowa

Iowa Department of Public
Health
Division of Health Protection
AIDS Prevention Program
321 E. 12th St.
Des Moines, IA 50319-0075
(515) 242-5838

Kansas

Kansas Department of Health
and Environment
Bureau of Disease Prevention
and Health Promotion
AIDS Section
109 SW 9th Street
Suite 605
Topeka, KS 66612-1271
(785) 296-6173
(785) 296-4197 (Fax)

Kentucky

Kentucky Department for
Health Service
Communicable Disease Branch
Epidemiology Division
HIV/AIDS Program
275 E. Main Street
2nd Fl.
Frankfort, KY 40621
(502) 564-6539
(502) 564-9865 (Fax)

Louisiana

Office of Public Health
Louisiana AIDS Prevention and
Surveillance Program
325 Loyola Ave., Rm. 618
New Orleans, LA 70112
(504) 568-7525
(508) 568-5507 (Fax)

Maryland

Maryland Department of Health
and Mental Hygiene
AIDS Administration Center for
AIDS Education
500 N. Calvert St., 5th Fl.
Baltimore, MD 21202
(410) 767-5019
(410) 333-4800 (TTY)
(410) 333-6333 (Fax)

Maine

ME Dept. of Human Services
Disease Control Division
HIV/STD Program
157 Capitol St.
Augusta, ME 04330
State House Station #11
Augusta, ME 04333
(207) 287-3747
(207) 287-6865 (Fax)

Massachusetts

MA Dept. of Public Health
HIV/AIDS Bureau
250 Washington St., 3rd Fl.
Boston, MA 02108-4619
(617) 624-5300
(617) 624-5399 (Fax)

Michigan

MI Dept. of Public Health
HIV/AIDS Prevention and Intervention Section
3423 Martin Luther King Blvd.
Lansing, MI 48906
P.O. Box 30195
Lansing, MI 48909
(517) 335-8371
(517) 335-9611 (Fax)

Minnesota

MN Dept. of Health
Div. of Disease Prev. and Ctrl.
AIDS/STD Prev. Services Section
717 Delaware St., SE
Minneapolis, MN 55440-9441
P.O. Box 9441
Minneapolis, MN 55440
(612) 676-5698
(612) 676-5739 (Fax)

Mississippi

MS State Dept. of Health
Division STD/HIV, Prev. Prog.
2423 N. State St.
Jackson, MS 39215
P.O. Box 1700
Jackson, MS 39215-1700
(601) 960-7723
(601) 960-7909 (Fax)

Missouri

Missouri Department of Health
Dept.of Epidemiology and Env.
Health, Br. of STD/HIV Prev.
930 Wildwood Dr.
Jefferson City, MO 65109
P.O. Box 570
Jefferson City, MO 65102-0570
(573) 526-7303
(573) 751-6417 (Fax)

Montana

MT Dept. of Public and Human
Services, AIDS/STD Program
1400 Broadway, Rm. C-305
Helena, MT 59620-9521
P.O. Box 202951
Helena, MT 59620-2951
(406) 444-3565
(406) 444-6842 (Fax)

Nebraska

NE Dept. of Health, Div. of Disease Control, HIV/AIDS Program
301 Centennial Mail S.
Lincoln, NE 68508
P.O. Box 95007
Lincoln, NE 68509-5007
(402) 471-2937
(800) 782-AIDS (TTY)
(402) 471-6426 (Fax)

New Hampshire

New Hampshire Department of
Health and Human Services
Div. of Public Health Services
STD/HIV Program
6 Hazen Dr.
Concord, NH 03301
(603) 271-4576
(603) 271-4934 (Fax)

New Jersey

New Jersey Dept. of Health
Office of the Asst. Commissioner
Div. of AIDS Prevention and Ctrl.
50 E. State St., PO Box 363
Trenton, NJ 08625-0363
(609) 984-5874
(609) 292-4244 (Fax)

New Mexico

New Mexico Health Department
Public Health Division
HIV/AIDS/STD Prevention and
Services Bureau
525 Camino de los Marquez, Ste. 1
Santa Fe, NM 87501
P.O. Drawer 26110
Santa Fe, NM 87501
(505) 476-8456
(505) 476-8527 (Fax)

New York

New York Department of Health
Office of Public Health
AIDS Institute
Corning Tower, Rm. 342
Empire State Plz.
Albany, NY 12237-0684
(518) 473-4229
(518) 473-7286 (Fax)

Nevada

NV Dept. of Human Resources
Sexually Transmitted Disease/
HIV Office, Br. of Disease Control and Intervention Services
505 E. King St., Rm. 304
Carson City, NV 89710
(702) 687-4800
(702) 687-4988 (Fax)

North Carolina

NC Dept. of Env. Health and
Natural Resources, Communicable Disease Control Section
HIV/STD Control Branch
225 N. McDowell St.
Raleigh, NC 27611-7687
P.O. Box 29601
Raleigh, NC 27611-7687
(919) 733-7301
(919) 733-1020 (Fax)

North Dakota

ND Dept. of Health and Consolidated Laboratories
Division of Disease Control
AIDS Program
600 E. Boulevard Ave., Dept. 301
Bismarck, ND 58505-0200
(701) 328-2378
(701) 328-1412 (Fax)

Ohio

Ohio Department of Health
Division of Preventive Medicine
AIDS Unit
35 E. Chestnut St.
Columbus, OH 43266-0588
P.O. Box 118
Columbus, OH 43266-0118
(614) 644-1838
(614) 728-0876 (Fax)

Oklahoma

Oklahoma Department of Health
HIV/STD Services
1000 NE 10th St.
Oklahoma City, OK 73117-1299
(405) 271-4636
(405) 271-5149 (Fax)

Oregon

Oregon Health Division
HIV Program
800 N.E. Oregon St., Room 745
Portland, OR 97232-2109
P.O. Box 14450
Portland, OR 97214
(503) 731-4029
(541) 732-4031 (TTY)
(503) 731-4608 (Fax)

Pennsylvania

PA Dept. of Health, Br. of Communicable Diseases
Forester & Commonwealth Ave., Rm. 912
Harrisburg, PA 17120
P.O. Box 90
Harrisburg, PA 17108
(717) 783-0479
(717) 772-4309 (Fax)

Philadelphia Department of Public Health
AIDS Activities Coordinating Office
500 S. Broad St.
Philadelphia, PA 19146
(215) 875-6570
(215) 685-6714 (Fax)

Puerto Rico

Puerto Rico Dept. of Health
AIDS Affairs and Communicable Diseases Program
P.O. Box 70184
San Juan, PR 00936-8184
(787) 274-5591
(787) 274-5592 (Fax)

Rhode Island

Rhode Island Dept. of Health
Division of Disease Control
Office of AIDS/STD
3 Capitol Hill, Rm. 106
Providence, RI 02908-5097
(401) 222-2320
(401) 222-2506 (TTY)
(401) 272-3771 (Fax)

South Carolina

South Carolina Dept. of Health and Environmental Control
Bureau of Preventive Health Services
HIV/AIDS Division
AIDS Prevention Program
2600 Bull St.
Columbia, SC 29201
Box 101106
Columbia, SC 29211
(803) 898-0749
(803) 898-0573 (Fax)

South Dakota

South Dakota Dept. of Health
Office of Disease Prevention
AIDS Prevention Project
615 E. 4th St.
Pierre, SD 57501-1700
(605) 773-4470
(605) 773-5509 (Fax)

Tennessee

Tennessee Dept. of Health
Communicable and Environmental Disease Services
STD/HIV Surveillance
425 5th Ave. N., Cordell Hull, 4th Fl.
Nashville, TN 37247-4911
(615) 741-7500
(615) 741-3857 (Fax)

Texas

Texas Department of Health
Br. of HIV and STD Prevention
HIV/STD Health Resources Div.
Epidemiology
1100 W. 49th St.
Austin, TX 78756-3199
(512) 490-2535
(512) 490-2538 (Fax)

Utah

Utah Department of Health
Div. of Community Health Services
Bureau of HIV/AIDS Tuberculosis Control and Refugee Help
288 N., 1460 W
Cannon Health Bldg.
Salt Lake City, UT 84114-2867
P.O. Box 142867
Salt Lake City, UT 84114-2867
(801) 538-6096
(801) 538-9913 (Fax)

Vermont

Vermont Department of Health
Division of Epidemiology
AIDS Program
108 Cherry St.
Burlington, VT 05401
P.O. Box 70
Burlington, VT 05402
(802) 863-7200
(802) 863-7314 (Fax)

Virgin Islands

Virgin Islands Dept. of Health
Community Health Services
AIDS Prevention Program
c/o 48 Sugar Estates
St. Thomas, VI 00802
(340) 774-0177
(340) 777-4001 (Fax)

Virginia

Virginia Dept. of Health
Division of Communicable Disease Control
Division of STD/AIDS
1500 E. Main St., Rm. 112
Richmond, VA 23219
Main St. Stn. P.O. Box 2448
Richmond, VA 23218
(804) 786-6267
(800) 828-1120 (TTY)
(804) 225-3517 (Fax)

Washington

Washington Dept. of Health
HIV/AIDS Client Services
Airdustrial Pk., Bldg. 9
Olympia, WA 98504
P.O. Box 47840
Olympia, WA 98504-7840
(360) 236-3427

West Virginia

West Virginia Department of
Health and Human Resources
Bureau of Public Health
Division of Surveillance and
Disease Control
1422 Washington St., E.
Charleston, WV 25301
(304) 558-5358
(304) 558-6335 (Fax)

Wisconsin

Wisconsin Department of
Health and Social Services
Division of Health
Bureau of Public Health
AIDS/HIV Program
1414 E. Washington Ave., Room 241
Madison, WI 53703-3044
(608) 267-5287
(608) 266-2906 (Fax)

Wyoming

Wyoming Department of Health
Preventive Medicine Services
AIDS Prevention Program
2300 Capitol Ave., Rm. 488
Cheyenne, WY 82002-0710
(307) 777-5800
(307) 777-5402 (Fax)

Index

Index

Page numbers followed by 'n' indicate a footnote. Page numbers in *italics* indicate a table or illustration.

Numeric

3TC (lamivudine)
  defined 585
  FDA approval 7, 22, *229*
  HIV treatment *201–2*, 240–53, 445
    children 50
1592U89, HIV treatment 50

A

AA *see* Alcoholics Anonymous (AA)
AAC *see* AIDS Action Council (AAC)
AAHE *see* Health Education, American Association for (AAHE)
AANP *see* Naturopathic Physicians, American Association of
AARC *see* Respiratory Care, American Association for (AARC)
AARP *see* Retired Persons, American Association of (AARP)

ABA *see* American Bar Association (ABA)
ABC *see* At Risk Babies Crib Quilts (ABC)
ABPsi *see* Black Psychologists, American Association of (ABPsi)
ACA *see* Counseling Association, American (ACA)
accelerated benefits *see* viatical settlements
ACLU *see* American Civil Liberties Union (ACLU)
acquired immune deficiency syndrome *see* AIDS (acquired immune deficiency syndrome)
ACTIS *see* AIDS Clinical Trials Information Service (ACTIS)
ACT-UP *see* AIDS Coalition To Unleash Power (ACT-UP)
acupuncture, defined 504
acyclovir, described 504
ADCC *see* antibody-dependent cell-mediated cytotocicity (ADCC)
adenoids, HIV infection 24
  see also lymphoid organs
adenopathy, defined 504
adjuvant, defined 504
adjuvant therapy 482
administration route, defined 504–5

717

body fluids
    defined 514
    HIV transmission 14–15, 68, 146, 260
    barriers, described 146, 264
    see also blood; mucous membranes;
        semen; sweat; tears; urin; vagi-
        nal secretions
bone marrow, defined 514
bone marrow suppression, defined
    515
booster, defined 515
Boys and Girls Club of America
    (B&GCA) 650
branched DNA assay (bDNA) 182,
    199, 515
breastfeeding
    cytomegalovirus 327
    HIV transmission 4, 41, 47, 260, 427
Breithard, William 346
BRM *see* biological response modifi-
    ers (BRM)
Business and Labor Resource Service
    (BLRS; CDC) 622

C

cachexia (emaciation)
    defined 515
    treatment 174
California
    AIDS/HIV hotline 701
    AIDS/HIV prevention offices 708
    AIDS/HIV statistics *84, 90, 112*
    prison inmates *138*
    HIV-2 reported cases 34
    HIV/AIDS mental health services
        696–97
California, University of (San Fran-
    cisco)
    Institute for Health Policy Studies
        645–46
canarypox 482–83, 508
    defined 515–16
Cancer Care 350
Cancer Institute, National (NCI)
    described 560
    Kaposi's sarcoma 343
    PDQ database, described 343–44

cancers
    AIDS-related
        defined 506–7
        Kaposi's sarcoma 5, 8, 174
        lymphomas 5
        treatment 8
    cervical
        defined 519
        Social Security benefits 357
        HIV infection 17–18
        immune system 3
        treatment 7
Candida albicans
    defined 516
    treatment 305–6
candidiasis
    children 50
    Social Security benefits 357
    see also yeast infections
carcinogen, defined 516
caregivers
    HIV prevention 13
    home care 257–79
    resource information 278–79, 666–
        67
    self-protection 268–72
Caribbean, HIV/AIDS epidemic 157–58
Catania, Joseph 67
Catholic AIDS Network, National
    (NCAN) 680
CAT scan, defined 526
causes of death
    AIDS-related *74,* 91, 373, 400
        men 133
        prison inmates 139, 142
    HIV infection 101, 149
        children 46
    opportunistic infections 5
        children 50
    tuberculosis 318
CCR5 (chemokine receptor 5)
    described 25
    HIV protection 475–76
CD4+T cells
    AIDS definition 5
    described 17–18, 516–17
    HIV infection 22, 26–30, 184, 213–14
    quantities 5–6, 17–18, 24–26,
        188–89, 478

children, continued
  HIV/AIDS-associated deaths
    statistics 18
  HIV/AIDS epidemic 150–52
  HIV infection
    pneumonia treatment 8
    statistics 77, *84–90*
  HIV treatment 241
  Mycobacterium avium complex 326
  opportunistic infections
    AIDS-related 5, 50–51
  Social Security benefits 354, 359
Children's Defense Fund (CDF) 632
CHIRI *see* Consumer Health Information Research Institute (CHIRI)
chlamydia
  defined 520
  HIV transmission 4, 40
CHO cell, defined 520
CHOICE *see* Concern for Health Options, Information, Care, and Education (CHOICE)
chronic idiopathic demyelinating polyneuropathy (CIPD), defined 520
CIPD *see* chronic idiopathic demyelinating polyneuropathy (CIPD)
circumoral paresthesia, defined 520
clade, defined 520–21, 582
clinical, defined 521
clinical practice guidelines, defined 521
clinical trials
  AIDS therapies 491–99, 505
  community-based, defined 522
  defined 521
  fluconazole 305
  HIV medications 472–74
  HIV vaccines 486–89
  HIV wasting syndrome 281, 283
  Internet information 607–8
  intravenous immunoglobulin (IVIG) 51
  Kaposi's sarcoma 342
  pediatric AIDS 45, 47–48
  pediatric HIV disease 50
  phases, described 569–70
  protease inhibitors 50
  see also AIDS Clinical Trials Information Service
clone, defined 521

clotimazole (Lotrimin; Mycelex), thrush treatment 302
cluster designation 4 *see* CD4+T cells
CMHS *see* Mental Health Services, Center for (CMHS)
CMV *see* cytomegalovirus (CMV)
coagulation disorder, AIDS/HIV statistics *85, 87–89*, 110
  see also hemophilia
coccidioidomycosis, defined 521
codon, defined 522
cofactors, defined 522, 526
cognitive impairment, defined 522
cohort, defined 522
Colorado
  AIDS/HIV hotline 702
  AIDS/HIV prevention office 708
  AIDS/HIV statistics *84, 90, 112*
  prison inmates *138*
  HIV-2 reported cases 34
combination therapy
  defined 522
  HIV treatment 7, *201*, 451–53
  toxoplasmosis treatment 310
Combivir, FDA approval *229*
community-based organizations
  defined 523
  HIV/AIDS education 59, 103
Community Health Centers, National Association of (NACHC) 636–37, 679
community planning, defined 523
compassionate use, defined 523
complement, defined 523
complementary therapy, defined 523
computed tomography, defined 526
Concern for Health Options, Information, Care, and Education (CHOICE) 650–51
concomitant medications, defined 523
concorde study, defined 524
condoms
  distribution 415
  education programs 58
  female 171, 392
  HIV prevention 8, 15–16, 170–71, 389–93
  older adults 67
  women 124–25, 171
  young persons 104

G

Guidelines for the Prevention of Opportunistic Infections (CDC) 313, 319, 329
Guidelines for the Use of Antiretroviral Agents in HIV-Infected Adults and Adolescents (DHHS) 37
"Guide to Selected HIV/AIDS-Related Internet Resources" (CDC) 583n

H

HAART see antiretroviral therapies, highly active (HAART)
half-life, defined 538
Hammett, Theodore 143
hand washing
cryptosporidiosis prevention 294–95
HIV prevention 13
toxoplasmosis prevention 309–10
Harlow, Caroline Wolf 143
Harvard AIDS Institute 633
Hawaii
AIDS/HIV hotline 702
AIDS/HIV prevention offices 709
AIDS/HIV statistics 84, 90, 112
prison inmates 138
HDI see Hispanic Designers Incorporated (HDI)
Health and Human Services, Department of (DHHS) 695n
contact information 623–24, 687–88
described 528
HIV infection treatments 37, 423n
antiretroviral therapies 185–86, 188–89
protease inhibitors 237
Health Care Policy and Research, Agency for (AHCPR)
cancer pain management 345
see also Public Health Service
health care workers
HIV infection 145–48
needle sticks 4, 11, 442–44
post-exposure treatment 386, 441–49
sexual identity issues 125
home caregivers 258–59

health care workers, continued
tuberculosis 319–20
Health Education, American Association for (AAHE) 670–71
Health Resources and Services Administration (HRSA)
described 538
HIV/AIDS research 65
program development grants 62
Healthy People 2000, HIV infection 374
hematotoxic, defined 539
hematrocrit, defined 538
Hemlock Society USA 634
hemoglobin, defined 539
hemolysis, defined 539
hemophilia
AIDS/HIV statistics 85, 87–89
men 129–31
defined 539
HIV infection
women 118–20
see also coagulation disorder
Hemophilia Foundation, National (NHF) 640
Henry J. Kaiser Foundation, HIV treatment panel 185, 188–89
hepatic, defined 539
hepatitis
defined 539
prevention 195, 442
hepatomegaly, defined 539
herpes
defined 539
HIV transmission 4, 40
herpes simplex
defined 539–40
HIV infection 269
Social Security benefits 357
herpes varicella zoster virus (VZV), defined 540, 589
Hester, Tom 143
HGH see human growth hormone (HGH)
Hispanic Designers Incorporated (HDI) 652–53
Hispanic Health and Human Services Organizations, National Coalition of (COSSMHO) 681

730

immune system, continued
defined 544–45
HIV infection 3, 17–18, 22, 24, 30–31, 467–68, 481
protection 477–78
research 64
immune thrombocytopenia purpura (ITP), defined 545
immunity, defined 545
immunizations, defined 545
see also vaccines
immunocompetent, defined 545
immunocompromised, defined 545
immunodeficiency, defined 545
immunogen, defined 545
immunogenicity, defined 545
immunogenicity, described 478
immunoglobulin, defined 545
immunomodulator, defined 545
immunostimulant, defined 546
immunosuppression, defined 546
immunotherapy, defined 546, 567
immunotoxin, defined 546
incidence, defined 546
inclusion criteria (clinical trials), defined 533, 546
incubation period, defined 546
Indiana
AIDS/HIV hotline 703
AIDS/HIV prevention office 709
AIDS/HIV statistics *84, 90, 112*
prison inmates *138*
Indian Health Service (IHS), described 546
indinavir (Crixivan)
defined 546
FDA approval 7, 23, *229*
HIV treatment *201, 204–6, 208, 210, 218, 225,* 239–53, 445
infants
HIV diagnosis 45
HIV infection tests 6
HIV transmission 11, 41
HIV treatment 424
tuberculosis 321
infections
bacterial
pediatric HIV disease 50
defined 546–47

infections, continued
ear 5
eye 5, 8, 526, 534
fungal 8
HIV provirus 22
immune system
HIV infection 3, 18
subclinical, defined 581
yeast 8
see also opportunistic infections; viruses
infectious, defined 547
infectious diseases, breastfeeding 47
Infectious Diseases Society of America 190, 313, 319
informed consent, defined 547
infusion, defined 547
injection drug users
AIDS/HIV statistics 18, *85, 88–89,* 373–76
men *129–31*
HIV-2 transmission 37
HIV infection 406–7
women *118–20*
HIV prevention 386
HIV transmission 4, 11, 101, 380
prison inmates 135, *141*
Inmates in State Correctional Facilities, Survey of 136–37
inoculation, defined 547
see also immunizations; vaccines
insects
HIV transmission 43, 68
insects, HIV transmission 14–15
institutional review board (clinical trials), defined 547–48
Insurance Commissioners, National Association of 369
integrase
defined 548
described 20, 22, 468
integration, defined 548
intent to treat, defined 548
interferon alfa-2a (Roferon-A), FDA approval 174
interferon alfa-2b (Intron-A), FDA approval 174
interferons
defined 507, 548

sexual activity, continued
  HIV infection 3, 8, 15
    adolescents 54
    anal sex 8, 15, 41
    oral sex 8, 15, 41
    women 125
  HIV transmission 4, 11, 23, 39–43,
    68
sexual behavior
  heterosexual
    AIDS/HIV epidemic 101–4
    HIV infection statistics 18, *85–90,*
      94, 117–20, 380, 405
  homosexual
    AIDS/HIV statistics *84–90, 94–97,*
      123–34
    see also bisexuals; gay people; ho-
      mophobia; lesbians
sexual development, emotional issues
  55–56
  see also adolescents
Sexuality Information and Education
  Council of the U.S. (SIECUS) 659
sexually transmitted diseases (STD)
  adolescents 54, 101–3
    education 57–58
  defined 579
  HIV prevention 8, 387–88, 389,
    395–98
  Hispanics 107–8
  HIV transmission 4, 40
  Internet information 606
  prevention 16
    condoms 171
SFAF *see* San Francisco AIDS Foundation (SFAF)
SGOT *see* serum glutamic oxaloacetic
  transaminase (SGOT)
SGPT *see* serum glutamic pyruvate
  transaminase (SGPT)
Sherman, Betty 143
shingles *see* herpes varicella zoster
  virus (VZV)
side effects, described 580
SIECUS *see* Sexuality Information
  and Education Council of the U.S.
  (SIECUS)
simian immunodeficiency virus (SIV)
  19, 458, 483, 580

SIV *see* simian immunodeficiency virus (SIV)
skin patches, pain management 348–
  51
slow viruses *see* lentiviruses
Social Health Association, American
  648–49
Social Security Administration (SSA)
  69–70
Social Security benefits, HIV infection 353–63
Social Security Disability Insurance
  (SSDI), described 354
social services, HIV-positive adolescents 62
somatropin (Serostim), HIV wasting
  syndrome 282
South Carolina
  AIDS/HIV hotline 706
  AIDS/HIV prevention office 713
  AIDS/HIV statistics *84, 90, 112*
  prison inmates *138*
South Dakota
  AIDS/HIV prevention office 713
  AIDS/HIV statistics *84, 90, 112*
spenomegaly, defined 580
spermicides, HIV infection 8, 393
spinal tap *see* lumbar puncture
spleen
  defined 580
  HIV infection 24
  see also lymphoid organs
Sporanox Oral Solution
  (itraconazole), thrush treatment
  303
sputum analysis, defined 580
SSA *see* Social Security Administra-
  tion (SSA)
SSDI *see* Social Security Disability
  Insurance (SSDI)
SSI *see* Supplemental Security Income (SSI)
Stall, Ron 67
standards of care, defined 580
StandUP For Kids 659–60
staphylococcus, defined 580
State, County, and Municipal Employees, American Federation of
  (AFSCME) 672

Contagious & Non-Contagious Infectious Diseases Sourcebook

Basic Information about Contagious Diseases like Measles, Polio, Hepatitis B, and Infectious Mononucleosis, and Non-Contagious Infectious Diseases like Tetanus and Toxic Shock Syndrome, and Diseases Occurring as Secondary Infections Such as Shingles and Reye Syndrome, Along with Vaccination, Prevention, and Treatment Information, and a Section Describing Emerging Infectious Disease Threats

Edited by Karen Bellenir and Peter D. Dresser. 566 pages. 1996. 0-7808-0075-3. $78.

■

Death & Dying Sourcebook

Basic Information for the Layperson about End-of-Life Care and Related Ethical and Legal Issues, Including Chief Causes of Death, Autopsies, Pain Management for the Terminally Ill, Life Support Systems, Coma, Euthanasia, Assisted Suicide, Hospice Programs, Living Wills, Near-Death Experiences, Counseling, Mourning, Organ Donation, Cryogenics and Physician Training and Liability, Along with Statistical Data, a Glossary, and Listings of Sources for Additional Help and Information

Edited by Annemarie Muth. 600 pages. 1999. 0-7808-0230-6. $78.

■

Diabetes Sourcebook, 1st Edition

Basic Information about Insulin-Dependent and Noninsulin-Dependent Diabetes Mellitus, Gestational Diabetes, and Diabetic Complications, Symptoms, Treatment, and Research Results, Including Statistics on Prevalence, Morbidity, and Mortality, Along with Source Listings for Further Help and Information

Edited by Karen Bellenir and Peter D. Dresser. 827 pages. 1994. 1-55888-751-2. $78.

"...very informative and understandable for the layperson without being simplistic. It provides a comprehensive overview for laypersons who want a general understanding of the disease or who want to focus on various aspects of the disease." — Bulletin of the MLA, Jan '96

■

Diabetes Sourcebook, 2nd Edition

Basic Consumer Health Information about Type 1 Diabetes (Insulin-Dependent or Juvenile-Onset Diabetes), Type 2 (Noninsulin-Dependent or Adult-Onset Diabetes), Gestational Diabetes, and Related Disorders, Including Diabetes Prevalence Data, Management Issues, the Role of Diet and Exercise in Controlling Diabetes, Insulin and Other Diabetes Medicines, and Complications of Diabetes Such as Eye Diseases, Periodontal Disease, Amputation, and End-Stage Renal Disease; Along with Reports on Current Research Initiatives, a Glossary, and Resource Listings for Further Help and Information

Edited by Karen Bellenir. 725 pages. 1998. 0-7808-0224-1. $78.

■

Diet & Nutrition Sourcebook, 1st Edition

Basic Information about Nutrition, Including the Dietary Guidelines for Americans, the Food Guide Pyramid, and Their Applications in Daily Diet, Nutritional Advice for Specific Age Groups, Current Nutritional Issues and Controversies, the New Food Label and How to Use It to Promote Healthy Eating, and Recent Developments in Nutritional Research

Edited by Dan R. Harris. 662 pages. 1996. 0-7808-0084-2. $78.

"Useful reference as a food and nutrition sourcebook for the general consumer."
— Booklist Health Sciences Supplement, Oct '97

"Recommended for public libraries and medical libraries that receive general information requests on nutrition. It is readable and will appeal to those interested in learning more about healthy dietary practices."
— Medical Reference Services Quarterly, Fall '97

"With dozens of questionable diet books on the market, it is so refreshing to find a reliable and factual reference book. Recommended to aspiring professionals, librarians, and others seeking and giving reliable dietary advice. An excellent compilation." — Choice, Feb '97

■

Diet & Nutrition Sourcebook, 2nd Edition

Basic Consumer Health Information about Dietary Guidelines, Recommended Daily Intake Values, Vitamins, Minerals, Fiber, Fat, Weight Control, Dietary Supplements, and Food Additives; Along with Special Sections on Nutrition Needs throughout Life and Nutrition for People with Such Specific Medical Concerns as Allergies, High Blood Cholesterol, Hypertension, Diabetes, Celiac Disease, Seizure Disorders, Phenylketonuria (PKU), Cancer, and Eating Disorders, and Including Reports on Current Nutrition Research and Source Listings for Additional Help and Information

Edited by Karen Bellenir. 600 pages. 1999. 0-7808-0228-4. $78.

■

Domestic Violence Sourcebook

Basic Information about the Physical, Emotional and Sexual Abuse of Partners, Children, and Elders, Including Information about Hotlines, Safe Houses, Safety Plans, Resources for Support and Assistance, Community Initiatives, and Reports on Current Directions in Research and Treatment; Along with a Glossary, Sources for Further Reading, and Listings of Governmental and Non-Governmental Organizations

Edited by Helene Henderson. 600 pages. 1999. 0-7808-0235-7. $78.

■

Ear, Nose & Throat Disorders Sourcebook

Basic Information about Disorders of the Ears, Nose, Sinus Cavities, Pharynx, and Larynx, Including Ear Infections, Tinnitus, Vestibular Disorders, Allergic and Non-Allergic Rhinitis, Sore Throats, Tonsillitis, and Cancers That Affect the Ears, Nose, Sinuses, and Throat, Along with Reports on Current Research Initiatives, a Glossary of Related Medical Terms, and a Directory of Sources for Further Help and Information

Edited by Karen Bellenir and Linda M. Shin. 592 pages. 1998. 0-7808-0206-3. $78.

Endocrine & Metabolic Disorders Sourcebook

Basic Information for the Layperson about Pancreatic and Insulin-Related Disorders Such as Pancreatitis, Diabetes, and Hypoglycemia; Adrenal Gland Disorders Such as Cushing's Syndrome, Addison's Disease, and Congenital Adrenal Hyperplasia; Pituitary Gland Disorders Such as Growth Hormone Deficiency, Acromegaly, and Pituitary Tumors; Thyroid Disorders Such as Hypothyroidism, Graves' Disease, Hashimoto's Disease, and Goiter; Hyperparathyroidism; and Other Diseases and Syndromes of Hormone Imbalance or Metabolic Dysfunction, Along with Reports on Current Research Initiatives

Edited by Linda M. Shin. 632 pages. 1998. 0-7808-0207-1. $78.

Environmentally Induced Disorders Sourcebook

Basic Information about Diseases and Syndromes Linked to Exposure to Pollutants and Other Substances in Outdoor and Indoor Environments Such as Lead, Asbestos, Formaldehyde, Mercury, Emissions, Noise, and More

Edited by Allan R. Cook. 620 pages. 1997. 0-7808-0083-4. $78.

". . . a good survey of numerous environmentally induced physical disorders . . . a useful addition to anyone's library."
— Doody's Health Science Book Reviews, Jan '98

". . . provide[s] introductory information from the best authorities around. Since this volume covers topics that potentially affect everyone, it will surely be one of the most frequently consulted volumes in the Health Reference Series." — Rettig on Reference, Nov '97

"Recommended reference source."
— Booklist, Oct '97

Ethical Issues in Medicine Sourcebook

Basic Information about Controversial Treatment Issues, Genetic Research, Reproductive Technologies, and End-of-Life Decisions, Including Topics Such as Cloning, Abortion, Fertility Management, Organ Transplantation, Health Care Rationing, Advance Directives, Living Wills, Physician-Assisted Suicide, Euthanasia, and More; Along with a Glossary and Resources for Additional Information

Edited by Helene Henderson. 600 pages. 1999. 0-7808-0237-3. $78.

Fitness & Exercise Sourcebook

Basic Information on Fitness and Exercise, Including Fitness Activities for Specific Age Groups, Exercise for People with Specific Medical Conditions, How to Begin a Fitness Program in Running, Walking, Swimming, Cycling, and Other Athletic Activities, and Recent Research in Fitness and Exercise

Edited by Dan R. Harris. 663 pages. 1996. 0-7808-0186-5. $78.

"A good resource for general readers."
— Choice, Nov '97

"The perennial popularity of the topic . . . make this an appealing selection for public libraries."
— Rettig on Reference, Jun/Jul '97

Food & Animal Borne Diseases Sourcebook

Basic Information about Diseases That Can Be Spread to Humans through the Ingestion of Contaminated Food or Water or by Contact with Infected Animals and Insects, Such as Botulism, E. Coli, Hepatitis A, Trichinosis, Lyme Disease, and Rabies, Along with Information Regarding Prevention and Treatment Methods, and a Special Section for International Travelers Describing Diseases Such as Cholera, Malaria, Travelers' Diarrhea, and Yellow Fever, and Offering Recommendations for Avoiding Illness

Edited by Karen Bellenir and Peter D. Dresser. 535 pages. 1995. 0-7808-0033-8. $78.

"Targeting general readers and providing them with a single, comprehensive source of information on selected topics, this book continues, with the excellent caliber of its predecessors, to catalog topical information on health matters of general interest. Readable and thorough, this valuable resource is highly recommended for all libraries."
— Academic Library Book Review, Summer '96

"A comprehensive collection of authoritative information." — Emergency Medical Services, Oct '95

Continues next page

Gastrointestinal Diseases & Disorders Sourcebook

Basic Information about Gastroesophageal Reflux Disease (Heartburn), Ulcers, Diverticulosis, Irritable Bowel Syndrome, Crohn's Disease, Ulcerative Colitis, Diarrhea, Constipation, Lactose Intolerance, Hemorrhoids, Hepatitis, Cirrhosis, and Other Digestive Problems, Featuring Statistics, Descriptions of Symptoms, and Current Treatment Methods of Interest for Persons Living with Upper and Lower Gastrointestinal Maladies

Edited by Linda M. Ross. 413 pages. 1996. 0-7808-0078-8. $78.

". . . very readable form. The successful editorial work that brought this material together into a useful and understandable reference makes accessible to all readers information that can help them more effectively understand and obtain help for digestive tract problems." — *Choice, Feb '97*

Genetic Disorders Sourcebook

Basic Information about Heritable Diseases and Disorders Such as Down Syndrome, PKU, Hemophilia, Von Willebrand Disease, Gaucher Disease, Tay-Sachs Disease, and Sickle-Cell Disease, Along with Information about Genetic Screening, Gene Therapy, Home Care, and Including Source Listings for Further Help and Information on More Than 300 Disorders

Edited by Karen Bellenir. 642 pages. 1996. 0-7808-0034-6. $78.

"Provides essential medical information to both the general public and those diagnosed with a serious or fatal genetic disease or disorder." — *Choice, Jan '97*

"Geared toward the lay public. It would be well placed in all public libraries and in those hospital and medical libraries in which access to genetic references is limited." — *Doody's Health Sciences Book Review, Oct '96*

Head Trauma Sourcebook

Basic Information for the Layperson about Open-Head and Closed-Head Injuries, Treatment Advances, Recovery, and Rehabilitation, Along with Reports on Current Research Initiatives

Edited by Karen Bellenir. 414 pages. 1997. 0-7808-0208-X. $78.

Health Insurance Sourcebook

Basic Information about Managed Care Organizations, Traditional Fee-for-Service Insurance, Insurance Portability and Pre-Existing Conditions Clauses, Medicare, Medicaid, Social Security, and Military Health Care, Along with Information about Insurance Fraud

Edited by Wendy Wilcox. 530 pages. 1997. 0-7808-0222-5. $78.

"The layout of the book is particularly helpful as it provides easy access to reference material. A most useful addition to the vast amount of information about health insurance. The use of data from U.S. government agencies is most commendable. Useful in a library or learning center for healthcare professional students." — *Doody's Health Sciences Book Reviews, Nov '97*

Healthy Aging Sourcebook

Basic Consumer Health Information about Maintaining Health through the Aging Process, Including Advice on Nutrition, Exercise, and Sleep, Along with Help in Making Decisions about Midlife Issues and Retirement, Practical and Informed Choices in Health Consumerism, and Data Concerning the Theories of Aging, Aging Now, and Aging in the Future, Including a Glossary and Practical Resource Directory

Edited by Jenifer Swanson. 500 pages. 1999. 0-7808-0390-6. $78.

Immune System Disorders Sourcebook

Basic Information about Lupus, Multiple Sclerosis, Guillain-Barré Syndrome, Chronic Granulomatous Disease, and More, Along with Statistical and Demographic Data and Reports on Current Research Initiatives

Edited by Allan R. Cook. 608 pages. 1997. 0-7808-0209-8. $78.

Kidney & Urinary Tract Diseases & Disorders Sourcebook

Basic Information about Kidney Stones, Urinary Incontinence, Bladder Disease, End Stage Renal Disease, Dialysis, and More, Along with Statistical and Demographic Data and Reports on Current Research Initiatives

Edited by Linda M. Ross. 602 pages. 1997. 0-7808-0079-6. $78.

Learning Disabilities Sourcebook

Basic Information about Disorders Such as Dyslexia, Visual and Auditory Processing Deficits, Attention Deficit/Hyperactivity Disorder, and Autism, Along with Statistical and Demographic Data, Reports on Current Research Initiatives, an Explanation of the Assessment Process, and a Special Section for Adults with Learning Disabilities

Edited by Linda M. Shin. 579 pages. 1998. 0-7808-0210-1. $78.

Medical Tests Sourcebook

Basic Consumer Health Information about Medical Tests, Including Periodic Health Exams, General Screening Tests, X-ray and Radiology Tests, Electrical Tests, Tests of Body Fluids and Tissues, Scope Tests, Lung Tests, Gene Tests, Pregnancy Tests, Newborn Screening Tests, Sexually Transmitted Disease Tests, and Computer Aided Diagnoses; Along with a Section on Paying for Medical Tests, a Glossary, and Resource Listings

Edited by Joyce B. Shannon. 600 pages. 1999. 0-7808-0243-8. $78.

Men's Health Concerns Sourcebook

Basic Information about Health Issues That Affect Men, Featuring Facts about the Top Causes of Death in Men, Including Heart Disease, Stroke, Cancers, Prostate Disorders, Chronic Obstructive Pulmonary Disease, Pneumonia and Influenza, Human Immunodeficiency Virus and Acquired Immune Deficiency Syndrome, Diabetes Mellitus, Stress, Suicide, Accidents and Homicides; and Facts about Common Concerns for Men, Including Impotence, Contraception, Circumcision, Sleep Disorders, Snoring, Hair Loss, Diet, Nutrition, Exercise, Kidney and Urological Disorders, and Backaches

Edited by Allan R. Cook. 760 pages. 1998. 0-7808-0212-8. $78.

Mental Health Disorders Sourcebook

Basic Information about Schizophrenia, Depression, Bipolar Disorder, Panic Disorder, Obsessive-Compulsive Disorder, Phobias and Other Anxiety Disorders, Paranoia and Other Personality Disorders, Eating Disorders, and Sleep Disorders, Along with Information about Treatment and Therapies

Edited by Karen Bellenir. 548 pages. 1995. 0-7808-0040-0. $78.

"This is an excellent new book . . . written in easy-to-understand language."
— *Booklist Health Science Supplement, Oct '97*

". . . useful for public and academic libraries and consumer health collections."
— *Medical Reference Services Quarterly, Spring '97*

"The great strengths of the book are its readability and its inclusion of places to find more information. Especially recommended." — *RQ, Winter '96*

". . . a good resource for a consumer health library."
— *Bulletin of the MLA, Oct '96*

"The information is data-based and couched in brief, concise language that avoids jargon. . . . a useful reference source." — *Readings, Sept '96*

"The text is well organized and adequately written for its target audience." — *Choice, Jun '96*

". . . provides information on a wide range of mental disorders, presented in nontechnical language."
— *Exceptional Child Education Resources, Spring '96*

"Recommended for public and academic libraries."
— *Reference Book Review, '96*

Ophthalmic Disorders Sourcebook

Basic Information about Glaucoma, Cataracts, Macular Degeneration, Strabismus, Refractive Disorders, and More, Along with Statistical and Demographic Data and Reports on Current Research Initiatives

Edited by Linda M. Ross. 631 pages. 1996. 0-7808-0081-8. $78.

Oral Health Sourcebook

Basic Information about Diseases and Conditions Affecting Oral Health, Including Cavities, Gum Disease, Dry Mouth, Oral Cancers, Fever Blisters, Canker Sores, Oral Thrush, Bad Breath, Temporomandibular Disorders, and other Craniofacial Syndromes, Along with Statistical Data on the Oral Health of Americans, Oral Hygiene, Emergency First Aid, Information on Treatment Procedures and Methods of Replacing Lost Teeth

Edited by Allan R. Cook. 558 pages. 1997. 0-7808-0082-6. $78.

"Recommended reference source." — *Booklist, Dec '97*

Pain Sourcebook

Basic Information about Specific Forms of Acute and Chronic Pain, Including Headaches, Back Pain, Muscular Pain, Neuralgia, Surgical Pain, and Cancer Pain, Along with Pain Relief Options Such as Analgesics, Narcotics, Nerve Blocks, Transcutaneous Nerve Stimulation, and Alternative Forms of Pain Control, Including Biofeedback, Imaging, Behavior Modification, and Relaxation Techniques

Edited by Allan R. Cook. 667 pages. 1997. 0-7808-0213-6. $78.

"The information is basic in terms of scholarship and is appropriate for general readers. Written in journalistic style . . . intended for non-professionals. Quite thorough in its coverage of different pain conditions and summarizes the latest clinical information regarding pain treatment." — *Choice, Jun '98*

"Recommended reference source."
— *Booklist, Mar '98*

Continues next page

Physical & Mental Issues in Aging Sourcebook

Basic Consumer Health Information on Physical and Mental Disorders Associated with the Aging Process, Including Concerns about Cardiovascular Disease, Pulmonary Disease, Oral Health, Digestive Disorders, Musculoskeletal and Skin Disorders, Metabolic Changes, Sexual and Reproductive Issues, and Changes in Vision, Hearing, and Other Senses; Along with Data about Longevity and Causes of Death, Information on Acute and Chronic Pain, Descriptions of Mental Concerns, a Glossary of Terms, and Resource Listings for Additional Help

Edited by Heather E. Aldred. 625 pages. 1999. 0-7808-0233-0. $78.

Pregnancy & Birth Sourcebook

Basic Information about Planning for Pregnancy, Maternal Health, Fetal Growth and Development, Labor and Delivery, Postpartum and Perinatal Care, Pregnancy in Mothers with Special Concerns, and Disorders of Pregnancy, Including Genetic Counseling, Nutrition and Exercise, Obstetrical Tests, Pregnancy Discomfort, Multiple Births, Cesarean Sections, Medical Testing of Newborns, Breastfeeding, Gestational Diabetes, and Ectopic Pregnancy

Edited by Heather E. Aldred. 737 pages. 1997. 0-7808-0216-0. $78.

". . . for the layperson. A well-organized handbook. Recommended for college libraries . . . general readers."
— *Choice, Apr '98*

"Recommended reference source."
— *Booklist, Mar '98*

"This resource is recommended for public libraries to have on hand."
— *American Reference Books Annual, '98*

Public Health Sourcebook

Basic Information about Government Health Agencies, Including National Health Statistics and Trends, Healthy People 2000 Program Goals and Objectives, the Centers for Disease Control and Prevention, the Food and Drug Administration, and the National Institutes of Health, Along with Full Contact Information for Each Agency

Edited by Wendy Wilcox. 698 pages. 1998. 0-7808-0220-9. $78.

Rehabilitation Sourcebook

Basic Information for the Layperson about Physical Medicine (Physiatry) and Rehabilitative Therapies, Including Physical, Occupational, Recreational, Speech, and Vocational Therapy; Along with Descriptions of Devices and Equipment Such as Orthotics, Gait Aids, Prostheses, and Adaptive Systems Used during Rehabilitation and for Activities of Daily Living, and Featuring a Glossary and Source Listings for Further Help and Information

Edited by Theresa K. Murray. 600 pages. 1999. 0-7808-0236-5. $78.

Respiratory Diseases & Disorders Sourcebook

Basic Information about Respiratory Diseases and Disorders, Including Asthma, Cystic Fibrosis, Pneumonia, the Common Cold, Influenza, and Others, Featuring Facts about the Respiratory System, Statistical and Demographic Data, Treatments, Self-Help Management Suggestions, and Current Research Initiatives

Edited by Allan R. Cook and Peter D. Dresser. 771 pages. 1995. 0-7808-0037-0. $78.

"Designed for the layperson and for patients and their families coping with respiratory illness. . . . an extensive array of information on diagnosis, treatment, management, and prevention of respiratory illnesses for the general reader."
— *Choice, Jun '96*

"A highly recommended text for all collections. It is a comforting reminder of the power of knowledge that good books carry between their covers."
— *Academic Library Book Review, Spring '96*

"This sourcebook offers a comprehensive collection of authoritative information presented in a nontechnical, humanitarian style for patients, families, and caregivers."
— *Association of Operating Room Nurses, Sept/Oct '95*

Sexually Transmitted Diseases Sourcebook

Basic Information about Herpes, Chlamydia, Gonorrhea, Hepatitis, Nongonoccocal Urethritis, Pelvic Inflammatory Disease, Syphilis, AIDS, and More, Along with Current Data on Treatments and Preventions

Edited by Linda M. Ross. 550 pages. 1997. 0-7808-0217-9. $78.